STANDARDS AND PRACTICE OF HOMECARE THERAPEUTICS

Second Edition

STANDARDS AND PRACTICE OF HOMECARE THERAPEUTICS

Second Edition

Edited by

Michael M. Rothkopf, M.D., F.A.C.P., F.A.C.N.

Assistant Clinical Professor of Medicine

Columbia University College of Physicians and Surgeons

New York, New York

Metabolic Associates, P.A.

Florham Park, New Jersey

formerly

National Medical Director

Clinical Homecare, Ltd.

Fairfield, New Jersey

Senior Vice President of Medical Affairs

Curaflex Health Services, Inc.

Ontario, California

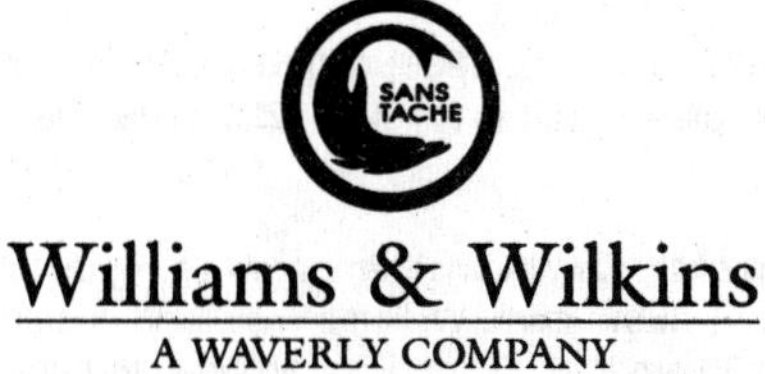

Williams & Wilkins

A WAVERLY COMPANY

BALTIMORE • PHILADELPHIA • LONDON • PARIS • BANGKOK
BUENOS AIRES • HONG KONG • MUNICH • SYDNEY • TOKYO • WROCLAW

Editor: Jonathan W. Pine, Jr.
Managing Editor: Leah Ann Kiehne Hayes
Production Coordinator: Raymond E. Reter
Copy Editor: Thomas Lehr
Designer: Silverchair Science + Communications, Inc.
Illustration Planner: Lorraine Wrzosek
Typesetter: Peirce Graphic Services, Inc.
Printer & Binder: Vicks Lithograph & Printing Corp.

351 West Camden Street
Baltimore, Maryland 21201-2436 USA

Rose Tree Corporate Center
1400 North Providence Road
Building II, Suite 5025
Media, Pennsylvania 19063-2043 USA

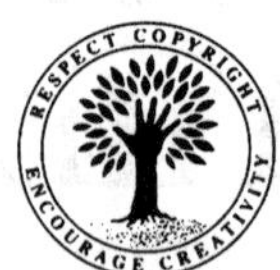

Accurate indications, adverse reactions, and dosage schedules for drugs are provided in this book, but it is possible that they may change. The reader is urged to review the package information data of the manufacturers of the medications mentioned.

Printed in the United States of America

First Edition, 1992, published as *Intensive Homecare*

Library of Congress Cataloging-in-Publication Data

Standards and practice of homecare therapeutics / [edited by] Michael
    M. Rothkopf.—2nd ed.
        p.   cm.
    Rev. ed. of: Intensive homecare. c1992.
    Includes bibliographical references and index.
    ISBN 0-683-07375-3
    1. Home care services.   2. Critical care medicine.   I. Rothkopf, Michael M.
II. Intensive homecare.
        [DNLM: 1. Home Care Services. WY 115 S7848 1997]
    RA645.3.I58 1997
    362.1′4—dc20
    DNLM/DLC
    for Library of Congress   96-20733
                                                                              CIP

The Publishers have made every effort to trace the copyright holders for borrowed material. If they have inadvertently overlooked any, they will be pleased to make the necessary arrangements at the first opportunity.

To purchase additional copies of this book, call our customer service department at **(800) 638-0672** or fax orders to **(800) 447-8438.** For other book services, including chapter reprints and large quantity sales, ask for the Special Sales department.

Canadian customers should call **(800) 268-4178,** or fax **(905) 470-6780.** For all other calls originating outside of the United States, please call **(410) 528-4223** or fax us at **(410) 528-8550.**

Visit Williams & Wilkins on the Internet:http://www.wwilkins.com or contact our customer service department at **custserv@wwilkins.com.** Williams & Wilkins customer service representatives are available from 8:30 am to 6:00 pm, EST, Monday through Friday, for telephone access.

                                                                    96 97 98 99 00
                                                                    1 2 3 4 5 6 7 8 9 10

This book is dedicated to:
The patient-pioneers, whose courage and independence
permitted the evolution of intensive homecare.
The homecare nurses, pharmacists, and other professionals whose
careful caring make intensive homecare a practical reality.
My family, whose loving support is the cornerstone of my success.

FOREWORD

Change continues to occur in a dramatic and significant manner in virtually all aspects of the practice of medicine in this country and throughout the world. Indeed, developments in the economic, social, political, legal, technological, fundamental, and practical application areas of endeavor are approaching a 5-year doubling rate. Accordingly, it is imperative that all physicians, surgeons, and other members of the healthcare profession maintain a concerted effort to remain abreast of the great wealth of ideas, knowledge, experience, techniques, modalities, and philosophies that are being generated and promulgated to increase the effectiveness and efficiency of therapeutic and prophylactic healthcare. This volume is an outstanding compendium of chapters summarizing the experience and wisdom of a group of practitioners in the relatively new specialized arena of homecare therapeutics. It is clearly the most comprehensive reference source of information in this most exciting, important, and rapidly developing field of healthcare.

Historically, care in the home was the only form of medicine practiced in colonial America prior to the founding of Pennsylvania Hospital in Philadelphia in 1751 by Benjamin Franklin and Dr. Thomas Bond. Patients who could afford healthcare services received them primarily in their own homes or in their personal physicians' offices.

The early hospitals were established to provide medical care to indigent or indentured patients who had no homes of their own or no family or servants to help care for them at home. Eventually, as the complexity and sophistication of diagnostic and therapeutic techniques advanced, hospitals underwent an evolution to become the centers for administering all but relatively basic and hygienic care to patients. As the metamorphosis of hospitals unfolded, nursing care continued to be available for some patients at home through a system of professional nursing associations and private contracts, and doctors continued to make house calls. By the middle of the 20th century following World War II, the geometric advances of knowledge and technology in medicine virtually mandated that all but the simplest medical and surgical procedures and treatments be undertaken in hospitals. At the time, homecare was limited essentially to patients requiring convalescent, rehabilitative, educational, or custodial care.

As has occurred repeatedly in the past, the pendulum is now swinging back in the other direction, and major changes in the manner in which medicine is being practiced and in which healthcare is being provided are well under way.

Nearly three decades ago, total parenteral nutrition—or intravenous hyperalimentation, as it is also known—was successfully inaugurated and applied as a useful therapeutic technique in the management of critically ill, malnourished, hospitalized patients. Since then, this feeding technique has not only been instrumental in saving countless lives, improving physiologic function, and increasing quality of life, but it has also clearly demonstrated the relevance of adequate nutritional support to the achievement of optimal clinical results in critically ill and complex medical and surgical patients who previously were not thought to be salvageable. Subsequently, these results have led to a monumental increase in the use of enteral feedings in patients whose oral intake has been inadequate to support normal nutritional and metabolic status. Within a short period of time, the need for ambulatory and home parenteral and enteral feeding techniques to maintain patients with no other indications for hospital confinement pioneered the development of commercial home healthcare agencies and the homecare industry. Subsequently, once it had been demonstrated that a technique as complex and technically demanding as total parenteral nutrition could be carried out safely and efficaciously at home, it became apparent that many other procedures and therapies that had previously been thought to require hospital admission could now be accomplished as well or better at home. A rampant growth and natural maturation of the medical technologies, principles, and practices in this developing field followed. Furthermore, innovative developments and applications continue; these promising developments are apparently unlimited, as manifested by this volume, which serves to facilitate and complement the practice of intensive homecare and home therapeutics.

The editor, Michael M. Rothkopf, M.D., has assembled an outstanding group of experts who have authored a comprehensive list of topics dealing with home management of patients requiring a wide range of specialized intensive care services. The 30 chapters are well organized and are presented in two sections dealing first with fundamentals and basic principles, followed by presentation of specific conditions and therapeutic situations in a homecare setting. Many of the chapters that appeared in the first edition have been extensively rewritten and updated. To complement these chapters, the new edition has been greatly expanded to include additional chapters dealing with the economic impact of homecare, homecare for the pediatric patient, homecare of the transplant patient, and home emergency care. Each of these chapters is quite unique, and the authors present and discuss their subject matter in an elegant style and understandable manner.

We are in the midst of a revolution in the means and methods by which health care services will be provided, not only for patients with routine problems, but also for patients requiring more intricate and intensive aspects of care in institutions and at home. For those in the medical profession who wish to exert the leadership for—or to remain abreast of—the rapidly evolving area of home therapeutics, the subject matter presented herein is required reading and is excellent reference material. The authors, editor, and publisher merit congratulations for their insight, initiative, generosity, and effectiveness in producing this compilation of critically important information and experience for our consideration, consumption, and application to the benefit of our patients.

Stanley J. Dudrick, M.D.
Clinical Professor of Surgery
Yale University School of Medicine
New Haven, Connecticut
Program Director and Associate Chairman
Department of Surgery
St. Mary's Hospital
Waterbury, Connecticut

PREFACE

We are practicing medicine in a transitional age. There is little doubt that hospital care as we know it will someday be available only for the most unstable of patients who require continuous attention from a team of physicians. Practically all other medical care will take place in an outpatient center or at home. The "hospital era" will give way to the "homecare era."

When I prepared the first edition of this book 5 years ago, homecare was a very young field. There was much enthusiasm for homecare in theory, but support was tentative, contingent upon the results of clinical experience. Basic questions regarding the safety and efficacy of medical care at home, and of the dramatic shift to patient responsibility, were still unanswered.

The first edition, *Intensive Homecare,* was itself a pioneering effort. It was among the first books to compile reviews on the emerging field of homecare therapeutics. I could see the need for this book from my vantage point as medical director of a national homecare organization. But it was difficult to produce a textbook for an area still in a rapid growth phase. The first edition was like a snapshot of a fast-moving train. You get a glimpse of the object, and its speed, but not a comprehensive understanding. After a brief interval, I realized that an updated version would be necessary.

In the years since the first edition's publication, the practicality of homecare has been established. The basic questions are being addressed and initial resistance has diminished. Homecare therapeutics has proved to be safe and effective.

While its initial impetus may have been economic, homecare has been shown to have several other important advantages over hospital care. It separates the patient from the multiply resistant hospital microorganisms, reducing the risk of nosocomial infection. It calms the patient emotionally and may thereby improve immunity and the tolerance of toxic treatments such as chemotherapy. It allows adults the option of returning to work and children the option of returning to school sooner, and more productively. It improves quality of life, especially for terminally ill patients.

The growth of homecare programs has given new and expanded responsibilities for each of the professional disciplines it employs. Thus, there have emerged homecare nurses, homecare pharmacists, homecare dietitians, physical therapists, etc. Each has received specialized training and guidelines for the application of homecare in their respective fields. Each has a documented set of standards on which to rely that define their role in the care of the patient at home.

However, the glaring exception to this phenomenon is the physician! The physician is offered no special training, education, or even established guidelines to follow for homecare. We have received no formal training in its use, during either medical school or residency. Although physicians remain ultimately responsible for a patient on homecare, they do not realize the scope of their responsibilities in referring or managing the patient at home.

Even experienced, hospital-based physicians find themselves at a loss when it comes to homecare. I commonly overhear seasoned, well-respected physicians relating discomfort in managing therapeutics at home. Physicians are simply out of their element in homecare.

It is not that physicians are unwilling to learn, but that limited resources are available to instruct the physician about homecare. The literature is scant. There are few large-scale comprehensive studies. Most physicians have been left to struggle through self-training in homecare based on their clinical judgment.

In addition to training, there are two other obstacles that interfere with physicians' participation in homecare: time and reimbursement. Physicians will have difficulty budgeting the amount of time required for homecare while already under the strains imposed by such programs as managed care plans. On the other hand, there is little financial incentive to make time for these activities because physician reimbursement for homecare services is poor—generally lower than for nurses or physical therapists.

Thus, while homecare is quickly moving to replace hospital care, the physician's involvement has been limited. In a real sense, an appropriate physician component has been left out of the homecare equation.

Physicians should be the leaders of the homecare movement. They should control patient care and the actions of the homecare team. Yet they cannot do so without first knowing what the team consists of and what its function is. They need guidelines on which to judge the appropriateness of the care rendered at home. Importantly, they need standards on which to judge the quality of an organization to which they refer their patients.

The purpose of this book is to provide comprehensive, physician-oriented instruction about homecare. In the absence of a curriculum on homecare, this book can provide a framework on which to base an emerging practice area.

Doctors need to know what homecare is and what it is not; which homecare services are appropriate and which patients are most likely to benefit. Conversely, they need to know what therapies and patients should be excluded. Physicians must also understand the practical aspects of homecare, such as the devices used and the structure of the organization supplying services to their patient. They must more fully understand what the physician's role is in the setting and what liabilities accrue.

Until now, physicians have had little to draw upon in assisting them with developing homecare practices. This book attempts to correct that deficiency. Every chapter has been designed with the intention of informing the physician-reader on how to practice medicine in a hospital without walls.

The authors were selected not only because they had theoretical knowledge but because they had special insight and experience in homecare therapeutics. This book has been written by the real "doers" in the field. This was necessary, because it is impossible to do a "review of the literature" when no significant literature exists. But it was also critical because the purpose of this book was to provide practical information that physicians could immediately apply.

I am indebted to Leah Hayes, Tom Lehr, and the staff at Williams & Wilkins for their hard work and dedication. My wife, Gail, also deserves extra recognition, as she was the de facto coeditor. Many others helped with the second edition, but especially Ruth Elliot, who coordinated the early phase, and Nora Cardone, who worked on the finishing touches.

I hope this book will prepare physicians for the practice of homecare therapeutics. Homecare has many strengths and advantages over hospital care. Active physical involvement will enhance it further.

CONTRIBUTORS

Jeffrey Askanazi, M.D.

Chief Executive Officer
Pain Centers Incorporated
Greenville, Michigan

John R. Bach, M.D., F.A.A.P.M.R., F.C.C.P.

Associate Professor and Vice Chairman
Department of Physical Medicine and
  Rehabilitation
Co-Director, Jerry Lewis Muscular
  Dystrophy Association Clinic
University of Medicine and Dentistry of
  New Jersey
New Jersey Medical School
University Hospital
Newark, New Jersey
Director, Center for Ventilatory
  Management Alternatives
Kessler Institute for Rehabilitation and
  University Hospital
West Orange, New Jersey

Monica Bais, M.D.

Resident in Medicine
St. Barnabas Medical Center
Livingston, New Jersey

Warren Balinsky, Ph.D.

Associate Professor of Health Services
  Management and Policy
New School for Social Research
Graduate School of Management and Urban
  Policy
New York, New York

C. Gresham Bayne, M.D.

Associate Clinical Professor of Medicine
University of California, San Diego, School
  of Medicine
President, Call Doctor Medical
  Group, Inc.
Director, American Academy of Home Care
  Physicians
San Diego, California

Leonard Bielory, M.D.

Director, Division of Allergy and
  Immunology
University of Medicine and Dentistry of
  New Jersey
New Jersey Medical School
Newark, New Jersey

Christopher R. Blagg, M.D., F.R.C.P.

Professor of Medicine
Division of Nephrology
University of Washington School of
   Medicine
Executive Director, Northwest Kidney
   Centers
Seattle, Washington

Ghias U. Butt, M.D., M.R.C.P.

Fellow in Nephrology
Georgetown University School of Medicine
Georgetown University Medical Center
Washington, D.C.

Niculae Ciobanu, M.D., F.A.C.P.

Associate Professor of Clinical Medicine
Albert Einstein College of Medicine of
   Yeshiva University
Director, Stem Cell Transplant Program
St. Vincent's Hospital and Medical Center
   of New York
Chief Executive Officer and Medical
   Director
Stem Cell Sciences, Inc.
New York, New York

Gigi R. Diamond, M.D.

Clinical Assistant Professor of Medicine
University of Medicine and Dentistry of
   New Jersey
New Jersey Medical School
Newark, New Jersey

Ruth A. Elliot

Metabolic Associates, P.A.
Florham Park, New Jersey

Kevin J. Ferrick, M.D.

Assistant Professor of Medicine
Division of Cardiology
Albert Einstein College of Medicine of
   Yeshiva University
Montefiore Medical Center
Bronx, New York

Fran L. Freeman, M.S.

Director, Division of Administration
Department of Pediatrics
Albert Einstein College of Medicine of
   Yeshiva University
Montefiore Medical Center
Bronx, New York

Allen I. Goldberg, M.D., M.M., F.A.A.P., F.C.C.P., F.A.C.P.E.

Professor of Pediatrics
Stritch School of Medicine
Loyola University Chicago
President, American Academy of Home
   Care Physicians
Treasurer, American College of Chest
   Physicians
Chicago, Illinois

Mark H. Goldberger, M.D.

Assistant Professor of Medicine
Albert Einstein College of Medicine of
   Yeshiva University
Director, Division of Cardiology
North Central Bronx Hospital
Montefiore Medical Center
Bronx, New York

Hervé Gouraige, Esq., J.D.

Of Counsel
Department of Litigation
Latham & Watkins
Newark, New Jersey

Lisa P. Haverstick, R.D., C.N.S.D.

Research Dietitian
Metabolic Associates, P.A.
Florham Park, New Jersey

Monroe S. Karetzky, M.D.

Associate Professor of Medicine
University of Medicine and Dentistry of
   New Jersey
New Jersey Medical School
Director, Sleep Disorders Center
Director, Division of Pulmonary and Critical
   Care
Assistant Director of Medicine
Beth Israel Medical Center
Newark, New Jersey

Stuart D. Katz, M.D.

Assistant Professor of Medicine
Division of Circulatory Physiology
Columbia University College of Physicians
 and Surgeons
Director, Clinical Service
The Heart Failure Center
Columbia Presbyterian Medical Center
New York, New York

Richard Lander, M.D., F.A.A.P.

Clinical Assistant Professor of Pediatrics
University of Medicine and Dentistry of
 New Jersey
New Jersey Medical School
Newark, New Jersey

Christine Lawrence, R.N., C.S., M.S., A.N.P

Adult Nurse Practitioner
Division of Circulatory Physiology
Columbia-Presbyterian Medical Center
New York, New York

Rosanna Leveriza, M.D.

Resident in Medicine
St. Barnabas Medical Center
Livingston, New Jersey

Grace Cumming Long, Ph.D.

Research Assistant in Medicine
Division of Allergy and Immunology
University of Medicine and Dentistry of
 New Jersey
New Jersey Medical School
Newark, New Jersey

William D. Marino, M.D.

Associate Professor of Clinical Medicine
New York Medical College
Valhalla, New York
Department of Medicine
Our Lady of Mercy Medical Center
Bronx, New York

Nuala Ronan, R.N., C.C.R.N.

Nurse Coordinator
Heart Failure Unit
Columbia Presbyterian Medical Center
New York, New York

Gail S. Rothkopf, Ph.D.

Research and Editorial Assistant
Metabolic Associates, P.A.
Florham Park, New Jersey

Michael M. Rothkopf, M.D., F.A.C.P., F.A.C.N.

Assistant Clinical Professor of Medicine
Columbia University College of Physicians
 and Surgeons
New York, New York
Metabolic Associates, P.A.
Florham Park, New Jersey

Leonard H. Sigal, M.D., F.A.C.P., F.A.C.R.

Associate Professor of Medicine, Pediatrics,
 and Molecular Genetics and Microbiology
Chief, Division of Rheumatology
University of Medicine and Dentistry of
 New Jersey
Robert Wood Johnson Medical School
New Brunswick, New Jersey

Bjørn Skeie, M.D., Ph.D.

Director, Intensive Care Unit
Department of Anesthesiology
Rikshospitalet
Oslo, Norway

Kimberly N. Stewart, R.N., B.S.N.

Department of Pediatric Hematology
Children's Hospital of The King's
 Daughters
Norfolk, Virginia
Nurse Coordinator
Hemophilia Comprehensive Care Program
Tidewater, Virginia

Michael H. Torosian, M.D.

Associate Professor of Surgery
Division of Surgical Oncology
University of Pennsylvania School of
   Medicine
Hospital of the University of Pennsylvania
Philadelphia, Pennsylvania

Eric J. Werner, M.D.

Associate Professor of Pediatrics
Eastern Virginia Medical School
Division of Pediatric Hematology
Children's Hospital of the King's Daughters
Norfolk, Virginia

James F. Winchester, M.D., F.R.C.P.

Professor of Medicine
Division of Nephrology
Georgetown University School of Medicine
Georgetown University Medical Center
Washington, D.C.

CONTENTS

Section I — Fundamentals and Basic Principles

I

FUNDAMENTALS AND BASIC PRINCIPLES

1

OVERVIEW OF HOMECARE THERAPEUTICS:

Concept and Scope of Intensive Homecare

Michael M. Rothkopf

CHAPTER AT A GLANCE: Homecare therapeutics has evolved in a path that parallels the development of the hospital system a century ago. Economic issues, patient awareness, and hospital-acquired illness have provided growing pressures for early discharge. Established programs for "intensive homecare" have provided a new standard of care for chronically ill patients.

Introduction

Why homecare? The obvious answer to this central question is that homecare therapeutics offers quality and effectiveness at a lower cost than hospital care. However, homecare offers benefits that exceed financial concerns. These include improved quality of life for the patient and family members, continued participation in social and workplace activities, occupational therapy, and even improved quality of care. When these aspects are combined with the derived economic efficiencies, homecare therapeutics emerges as a powerful force among today's developing trends.

Home healthcare has been described as a "hospital without walls," and it is capable of providing many of the services traditionally considered hospital-level care. In the push for efficiency, many hospitals are allowing only the sickest patients to enter or remain within their facility. The increased level of acuity within the hospital has been made possible through the extensive use of outpatient services, which provide a therapeutic delivery method for more stable patients.

However, in the rush to develop alternative care methods and discharge the patient early, has the physician been left behind? While many years have been spent in training for hospital care and office procedures, little established training is available for the physician with patients in homecare. How does one practice medicine in a hospital without walls?

If the homecare setting is to replace much of the hospitalization we are accustomed to, what changes in responsibilities do physicians face in this new arena? Physicians can expect scrutiny of their treatment of homecare patients, their supervision of homecare nurses, and their choice of homecare companies. Thus, there are new issues of liability beyond those of malpractice.

Homecare is not merely the replacement of hospital care at home. It is an entirely different system of care. Each participant's role has been modified to meet the venue. The nurse, pharmacist, physical therapist, and certainly the patient have evolved new approaches to meet the demands of homecare. What about the physician?

To face the challenges of this new healthcare movement, physicians can apply standards that parallel those they have followed in the past. However, there are new concerns that will have to be addressed. The physician should be prepared to judge the effectiveness of therapy and the appropriateness of care rendered by the homecare team. Practice patterns may need to be adjusted to accommodate the patient receiving homecare. The physician will be expected to extend himself administratively, professionally, and personally.

Evolution of Modern Homecare Therapeutics

As is the case with other advancements in healthcare, homecare therapeutics has developed because of new technology and societal trends. New approaches in medicine often go through a rite of passage that includes initial enthusiasm, rebound skepticism, and then general acceptance. As of this writing, we believe homecare is entering the third phase.

Before the 20th century, medicine was an art practiced predominantly at a patient's home. The housecall was a central focus of a doctor's work day. Patients who were ill could not travel to an office. The expected norm was that the doctor would visit the patient. The reasons for this are partly related to the difficulties surrounding patient travel before the emergence of the automobile and an organized ambulance system. But also, medicine was simple, and much of what could be done did not require sophisticated equipment. The doctor carried his tools and medications with him. For example, Laënnec invented the stethoscope about 1810, and von

Helmholtz devised the ophthalmoscope around 1850. These implements, and most other devices, were intended for use at the patient's home. Even surgeries were performed there. Acute care could be given anywhere the doctor had access to the patient. This included the home, office, or practically anywhere else. The hospital was probably a less convenient place than most.

The hospital's role in earlier times was limited to providing custodial long-term care to the infirm and invalid, many of whom were destitute. They were far from today's centers of medical excellence and scientific learning. Anyone with means sought to avoid them.

Since modern nursing did not exist yet, the patient's family served as the caregivers. They administered medicines and treatments according to the doctor's instructions and provided comfort and solace to the patient using home remedies.

19th-Century Advances

Significant changes of the industrial revolution and the era of enlightenment slowly carried into medical practice. Ongoing medical studies in the 19th century brought advances that revolutionized medical care in the 20th century. The application of sulfuric ether in minor surgery by Long in 1842 was among the most significant steps. This led to techniques that involved longer and more complex operations. Such figures as Billroth, Sims, Halstead, and Horsley devised new surgical approaches to diseases of the neck, chest, abdomen, and central nervous system.

Florence Nightingale's (1820–1910) innovating efforts led to a professional status for nurses. Her selflessness during the care of British wounded of the Crimean War (1854–1855) led to the establishment of educational institutions that graduated women with nursing degrees. In a parallel development, Jean Henri Dunant, a Swiss banker, founded the Red Cross in 1859 after observing the appalling care rendered to men after battle. This established the idea of transporting the sick and injured to centralized places for treatment.

The concept of asepsis and the germ theory was accepted only after much dissent. Holmes, Semmelweis, and Lister each described its importance. However, many surgeons remained skeptical about sterilization. It was not until the early 20th century that these concepts were universally accepted.

Pasteur, building on the foundation laid by Jenner and Koch, produced a monumental amount of work in the latter part of the 19th century. This led finally to the broad acceptance of the bacterial basis of infection, antisepsis, and inoculation of attenuated organisms (1). After some rebound skepticism, these advances gradually became an important part of a new standard of care.

In 1895, Röntgen discovered x-rays (2), which led quickly to the medical application of radiography. A few years later, Einthoven described a practical system of galvanometry that led to the modern electrocardiogram.

The Hospital Era

As medicine slowly adapted to the emerging science, physicians added the new methods to their practices. Most of these methods could not be applied in the patient's home, however. They required equipment and qualified personnel. A new kind of hospital evolved and expanded with physician leadership. Some of these facilities were actually begun within the physicians' homes or as entrepreneurial ventures by the physicians. Eventually they became mammoth institutions, many of which are now passing their 100-year milestones.

Another medical development of the late 19th century was the "teaching hospital," exemplified by The Johns Hopkins Hospital. Hopkins combined a medical treatment center with a school of medicine (3). Other schools soon emulated this concept.

The new teaching hospitals were not custodial care institutions but centers for medical research, treatment, and modern therapy. Here medical science evolved rapidly and the practice of medicine became progressively complex. The mushrooming of medical knowledge provided tremendous insight into diseases and treatments. Physicians became more scientific as each new method extended the boundaries of possibilities. Treatments considered impossible decades earlier—such as open-heart surgery, renal dialysis, and mechanical respiratory support—developed and became commonplace.

As new information and apparatus entered daily practice, physicians became uncomfortable in the home setting. More and more treatments were taking place within the hospital. In the course of progress, the long heritage of the housecall was all but abandoned.

From the patient's perspective, the dissociation between healing and home brought mixed reactions. Physicians were criticized for not making housecalls but were glorified for the use of modalities that saved patients previously considered terminal. Hospitals were viewed as sanctuaries where miraculous cures were possible, but their cold, sterile environment made patients apprehensive.

Despite its sophistication, the hospital was not without its drawbacks. It became clear that hospitalization itself posed significant risk to the patient (Fig. 1.1). It produced emotional stress, which could alter the response to therapy and effect recovery (4). It exposed the patients to highly resistant bacteria that could produce fatal infections. Nutritional status often declined significantly during hospitalization, impairing healing (5). These observations led to the recognition of a new group of diseases, termed "hospital-acquired."

Medical Consumerism

After World War II, general society became more technologically literate. Americans were introduced to more appliances, machines, and electronics for the home. Devices such as videotape recorders and home computers gained broad use despite the fact that the average person had practically no notion of the functional principles. Consumers with a minimum of education could be taught, in a step-by-step process, to operate these units and make them useful in the home. We have termed such developments "simplified sophistication" to recognize the combination of complex equipment and computerization, in

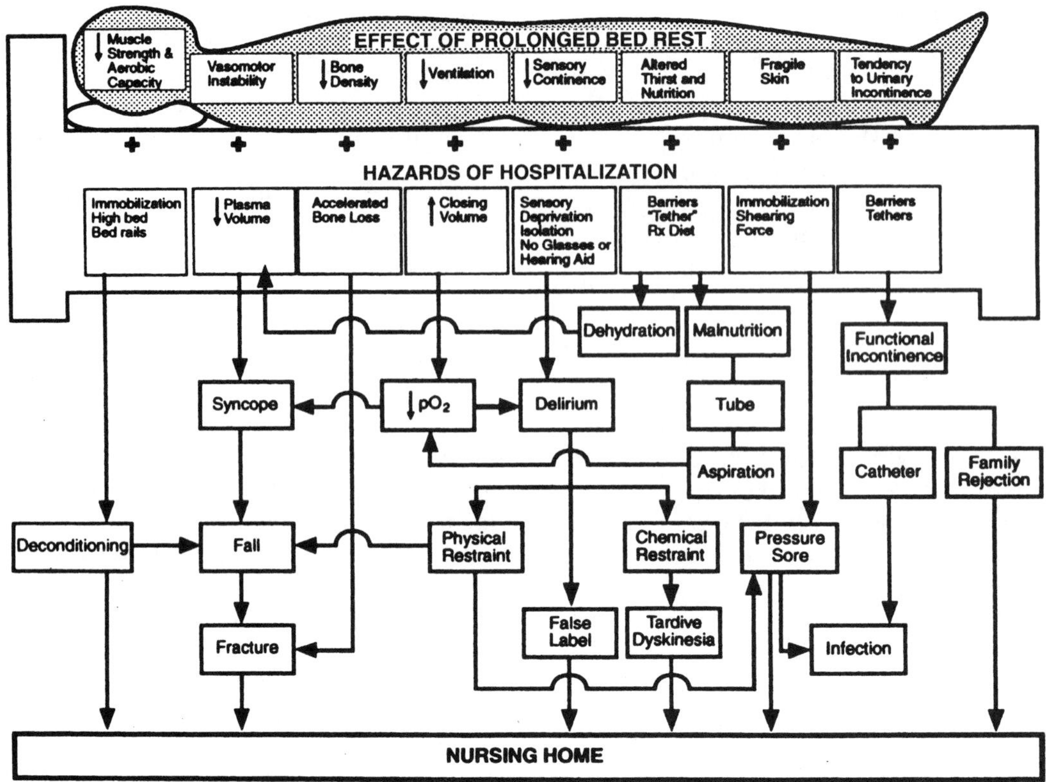

Figure 1.1.   Hazards of hospitalization. (Modified from Creditor, MC. Hazards of hospitalization of the elderly. Ann Intern Med 1993;118:219–223.)

which a single button activates a variety of functions. This concept has carried over to the use of medical devices at home.

An informal education in healthcare was already occurring. News media included coverage of health and medicine into their formats. Press releases from researchers and medical journals began to appear regularly in the lay press. Devices traditionally reserved for use by doctors such as pulse meters, otoscopes, and sphygmomanometers began to appear in formats for use in patients' homes. Performance of blood glucose measurement, pregnancy testing, and even cholesterol measurement became common using commercial kits sold over the counter at the local pharmacy.

Socially, postwar America was a culture in constant flux. Among the many changes in the social fabric was the development of consumerism, health foods, and alternative medicines. These movements encouraged people to assert themselves and take health matters into their own hands. When individuals with this perspective became ill, they did not accept the status quo, but sought methods to "take charge."

Knowledgeable medical consumers emerged who wanted a more active role in their care process. As a sign of their independence, patient support groups were formed for many chronic illnesses. These groups focused on the patients' needs rather than the medical aspects of the disease. This group of activist/patients played a definite role in the emergence of modern homecare therapeutics.

Economic Factors

Economic and utilization concerns have provided an incentive to reduce hospital admissions and lengths of stay. In the United States, healthcare expenditure showed consistent growth in excess of other sectors in the economy from the mid-1970s until 1994 (6). For example, the 1987 U.S. healthcare expenditure was $500 billion (11.1% of GNP). By 1993 it had risen to $900 billion (14%).

Beginning in the early 1980s, professional review organizations (PROs) and in-hospital utilization review (UR) groups monitored the use of patient services and provided pressure to reduce the time and expense of hospitalizations. Health maintenance organizations (HMOs) focused on providing preventive measures that would lessen the use of hospital care. Patients participating in HMOs were limited to seeing participating physicians who had agreed to abide by HMO guidelines. Physicians were strongly encouraged to minimize hospital use. Some took up this challenge by spearheading the efforts to develop homecare organizations. As with the hospital-era emergence 100 years earlier, some physicians added homecare services to their practices or developed new companies through entrepreneurship.

The economic advantages of intensive homecare are overwhelming. The National League of Nursing estimated in 1988 that patients requiring nursing care following surgery accrue hospital costs ranging from $300 to $500 per day compared to $25 to $75 per day for the same care at home. In the more intensive area, a baby requiring ventilatory and nutritional support had hospital costs of $60,900 per month compared to equivalent care at home for $20,200 per month.

A 1989 study on the cost of treating AIDS patients showed that the average hospital cost was $750 per day compared to $200 per day for comparable care at home (7). Furthermore, based on existing reimbursement standards, the average hospital lost money treating AIDS patients, whereas the homecare company profited. A more in-depth analysis of the economic impact of homecare is found in Chapter 9.

Quality-of-Life Issues

The trend toward more homecare occurs at a time of increasing awareness regarding a patient's quality of life. These issues include the patient's perception of his illness and the comfort of the therapy. The patient's functional activity level, perception, appetite, and social interactions are carefully considered in this light.

The complexity of the hospital system reduces the patient's individuality and freedom. Personal needs are often considered secondary to the ongoing process of hospital regimens. The patient comes to feel lost within the bureaucracy.

Hospital-based care practice focuses almost entirely on the length of survival for each illness. Quality-of-life studies ask the question of the value of the time extended. Using this type of analysis, some standard medical approaches are clearly deficient (8). Specific methods for assessing quality of life have been developed for cancer (9), joint disease (10), heart disease (11), and chronic lung disease (12). Once validated, these methods are expected to give insight to the usefulness of treatment regimens from the patient's perspective. Since many treatments currently employed are considered palliative rather than curative, it is important to objectively determine whether or not they truly offer comfort.

For example, when healthy volunteers were asked to choose hypothetical options for the treatment of laryngeal carcinoma, 20% chose radiation rather than surgery despite having been informed of the substantially reduced 3-year survival (13). These individuals apparently valued voice preservation over longevity.

In a study of the patient perception of chemotherapy side effects, 54% of the most severe symptoms were nonphysical (14). Although the patients did complain of vomiting, alopecia, and weight loss, they were more disturbed by the process of treatment, feeling tired, constantly sleeping, and the manner in which the treatment affected their family and their ability to perform usual activities. These emotional concerns often outweighed the physical side effects of treatments.

A key element in improving the quality-of-life aspects of illness is related to the patient's ability to return to his normal home environment (15). Therefore, this area of investigation has provided significant support for the concept of homecare. Based on quality-of-life studies, it is clear that homecare should be viewed as more than an alternative to standard hospital therapy.

Homecare can also be effectively utilized as preventive therapy, which focuses on maintaining quality of life. Two recent studies of elderly patients demonstrated that delaying disability and reducing hospital use were benefits of homecare (16, 17).

Quality-of-Care Issues

The complexity of interactions required to practice modern medicine within the hospital may result in an increased probability of unfortunate errors. Policy and procedures manuals are an attempt to maintain consistency. However, the practical aspects of care are rarely reflected in these tomes.

Medical treatment errors are often the result of inadequate communication between caregivers. The error frequency is increased by the number of professionals involved in the patient's care. The chart can include notes by different physicians, nurses, respiratory therapists, physical therapists, dietitians, and social workers. All of them write brief summaries of the patient's progress in the chart but do not always communicate directly with one another.

The medical record itself was not well designed for such an overwhelming amount of activity (18). Hospital charts must fit on racks and are often "thinned" by ward secretaries, resulting in loss of information. Synthesis of the data contained in the chart does not occur until the discharge summary is prepared. The development of computerized patient records may alleviate some of these problems, but it has been slow to develop.

Communication errors among the treatment team of physicians, nurses, and other professionals eventually filter down to the patient and produce consternation. In studies in which patients were asked to participate in their own medical record keeping, increased patient satisfaction as well as improved administration resulted (19). Astute patients have learned to respond to these situations by becoming educated "healthcare consumers" (20).

In response to these concerns, an area of nursing research has developed methods to evaluate the patient's ability to provide his or her own care. These concepts focus on a variety of factors that have an impact on the delivery of healthcare to the individual.

Although the self-care concept was initially considered for use with hospital patients, it can easily be adapted to homecare. In fact, a patient who is making full use of such a system might be inclined to ask himself why he needs to be in the hospital at all.

Homecare-Specific Therapy

Since the inception of homecare, several diseases and treatments have become recognized as being well suited for home therapy. These treatments have proved the value of homecare, often producing results superior to those observed in the hospital. They illustrate some of the significant medical advantages of the home environment, not the least of which is its microbiologic simplicity with regard to resistant bacteria. Gradually, home therapies have been developed for other medical conditions that were also well suited to the home setting. For example, total parenteral nutrition (TPN), peritoneal dialysis, and ventilatory support were pioneering therapies that established the efficacy of ongoing hospital-level care at home. As the pressure for early hospital discharge continued, treatments such as intravenous administration of antibiotics or pain management were also seen as being appropriate for homecare. Today, a wide variety of treatments are given at home, but most focus on a finite group of diagnoses or treatments that have been shown to be particularly amenable to homecare therapy. This list of conditions, which we term "homecare-specific," includes diseases and treatments for which the current standard of practice involves homecare therapeutics.

The physician encountering such conditions should consider a role for homecare early in the treatment. Extra effort to prepare the patient for homecare is worthwhile in these circumstances. The issue of homecare should be discussed with the patient and family soon after diagnosis and treatment begin. Appropriate personnel and vendors should be notified as soon as possible to make appropriate preparations.

The following is a partial list of homecare-specific conditions. Obviously, the list is evolving and is expected to lengthen over time. This is because safety and efficacy continue to be documented with growing experience in homecare.

- *Nutritional support:* Long-term TPN; long-term enteral feeding; short-term TPN (1–4 weeks)
- *Infectious diseases:* AIDS; endocarditis; osteomyelitis; Lyme disease.
- *Nephrology:* Peritoneal dialysis; hemodialysis; intradialytic parenteral nutrition (IDPN).
- *Respiratory care:* Oxygen supplementation; chronic mechanical ventilation; ventilatory assist devices.
- *Cardiology:* Inotrope infusions; arrhythmia detection; defibrillation.
- *Obstetrics:* Intrauterine monitoring; tocolytic therapy; hyperemesis gravidarum.

Standard of Care

All of the conditions listed above have at least one thing in common: the anticipated role of homecare therapy. In most of them, hospital care is provided only at short intervals—either to prepare the patient for homecare or to treat its complications. Thus, the standard of practice for these conditions involves homecare to such an extent that hospitalization for them is viewed as unusual. For example, few physicians today would consider hospitalizing a patient for Lyme disease unless the condition was advanced and involved the heart and central nervous system. Most patients are diagnosed in an outpatient setting and started on oral antibiotics. If IV antibiotics are needed, they are started at home. One can predict that admitting such a patient to the hospital would result in the physician receiv-

ing a spate of calls from utilization reviewers and case managers.

The other conditions listed above are similarly so entwined with homecare that it is inconceivable today to treat them without some consideration of outpatient therapy.

How did the standard of practice for these conditions shift from hospital to homecare? Who determines this standard? How is it enforced? Although these may seem amorphous concepts, they have great relevance for homecare. The physician will be the sole decision maker in the homecare setting without the assistance of safeguards that exist within a hospital. Therefore, his liability exposure has increased and he should rightly seek to conform to the standards of practice.

Physicians, administrators, insurers, and even malpractice attorneys know that standards of practice are local issues set within the community. They involve the concept of what is accepted medical care on a larger scale but also take into account the type and number of consultants available and the level of aggressiveness expected in patient care. This may vary from hospital to hospital and even within groups of physicians at a single hospital.

Physicians should feel secure that they are participating within an acceptable standard of their community; if in doubt, they should discuss the matter with their colleagues. Homecare companies and the Joint Commission on Accreditation of Healthcare Organizations (JCAHO) apply standards of practice, although these are generally not directed at the physician. However, many homecare companies appoint medical advisory boards, which may be of service to physicians in judging appropriate therapy.

A key issue in supervising homecare is that the physician should be satisfied that a local standard of care will be met. This should be one that meets both established guidelines (i.e., JCAHO) and the physician's personal standards.

The physician should be satisfied that his patient is receiving the best quality of care available for the individual circumstances and locale. As noted above, this is based on a local standard, but physicians should be mindful of national trends and their own ability to set a higher standard by adapting a treatment. For example, information presented in a journal or conference can be taken into practical use within the community, thereby setting a new standard.

Standards of care are almost never written or even talked about. It may be little more than a passing comment in the hallway or doctor's lounge such as: "this is how we do things here." Personal experience obtained during the physician's training (medical school, residency, etc.) is also important in setting standards. Still, for homecare to become an accepted standard of practice for the conditions listed above required more than personal experience or local influence. Each hospital, for example, has only a small number of appropriate candidates for these homecare-specific therapies. Therefore, the process of standardizing these practice parameters must have involved communication over a larger geographic area.

The initial impetus may have been provided by efforts of the insurance carriers focusing on cost savings and by the profit motives of the homecare suppliers. The role of the patient as healthcare consumer must also be recognized in this regard. This appears to be another example of the evolution of homecare in parallel to the hospital system. As hospitals made use of homecare to accommodate early discharges, standards of practice carried over from hospital to home. The JCAHO's accreditation process also assisted in this effort because hospital accreditation includes documentation of adequate standards for affiliated organizations. Eventually, the JCAHO extended its process directly over homecare organizations.

Any condition deemed appropriate for homecare can be judged in comparison to the homecare-specific conditions listed above. From these, the general principles create a criterion that a physician may use in determining an appropriate standard of care. For example, if the patient requirements or drug administration methods are similar to those of homecare-specific conditions, the condition is probably appropriate for homecare.

As a general rule, homecare therapeutics can be considered an appropriate standard of care whenever (*a*) the condition being treated is of a long-term nature that would require prolonged complex care, and (*b*) the clinical status is sufficiently stable that it requires a minimum of monitoring activity to treat it safely.

The Homecare Era

As the trends mentioned above progressed, almost independently a national consciousness developed that resulted in the development of a new form of homecare. The factors involved included:

- Advances in medical techniques
- Application of "simplified sophistication" to medical equipment
- Increase in technological awareness among the general population
- Dissemination of medical knowledge to the public
- Increase in assertiveness and self-reliance among patients
- Increase in the risk of hospital care
- Increase in the cost of hospital care

These trends focused on the care of patients with chronic illness (Fig. 1.2), allowing the emergence of a new concept that both offered opportunities and resolved many problems. This concept made use of homecare in an advanced way that differentiated it from such programs as visiting nurse services or home health aids. The new homecare concept involved not only durable medical equipment (DME) but also hospital-level therapies such as ventilators and intravenous

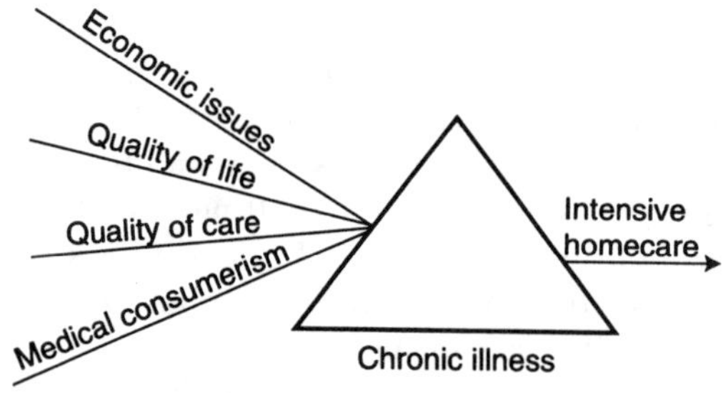

Figure 1.2.   "Intensive homecare" prism.

medications. It became known as high-tech or aggressive homecare.

In 1992, we coined the term "intensive homecare" to delineate the grouping of homecare therapeutics from supplier "lower-tech" methods. These therapies rely on the expectation that the patient himself—with the proper training, support services, and back-up professional staff—can administer advanced medical care in the home environment.

Infusion Services

Home infusion therapy is among the most commonly used aspects of intensive homecare. Parenteral nutrition, antibiotics, cancer chemotherapeutic agents, narcotics, cardiac medications, and even anticoagulants have been safely administered in the home. In some states, administration of blood products under the auspices of homecare is also permitted.

Homecare infusions initially used simple venous catheters similar to those used in hospitals. However, these were impractical, as they required a nurse or physician to perform re-insertion on a frequent basis. The availability of safe, reliable, long-term vascular access such as the Hickman/Broviac catheter was a major development in the technical ability to provide home infusions. Such catheters could remain in place for months or years, requiring only basic care methods rather than expert medical or nursing attention.

Catheters that exit the skin so that the infusion site can be entered directly are generally preferred for patients who require daily infusions such as TPN. Totally implanted devices (Port-A-Cath, etc.) that must be entered through a needle puncture of the skin are mostly used for patients who require intermittent infusions, such as chemotherapy.

Home infusion solutions are generally prepared by the homecare pharmacy using sterile conditions under a laminar flow hood. Early patients performed some of the solution mixing in a process referred to as "self-mix." This method was preferred by some homecare pharmacists because of concerns about the stability of particular intravenous components over time. Recent data have shown that intravenous vitamins, dextrose,

amino acids, lipids, and many of the antibiotics are stable for several days after mixing, provided they are kept in refrigerated storage (21). Thus, current practice employs the widespread use of solutions mixed by a pharmacist and delivered, user-ready, to the patient's home.

The patient's home must also be outfitted with the necessary supplies and equipment to perform the infusion. These include intravenous tubing, infusion pump, dressing kits, heparin flushes, alcohol swabs, etc.

Ventilatory Support

Home artificial ventilation has been in use since the polio epidemic of the 1950s. Advances in equipment and techniques have expanded the applications to include many patients with end-stage pulmonary disease.

Patients receiving home ventilation range from those who are completely dependent on mechanical ventilators to those who require assistance only part of the day. For the former group, the home becomes an approximation of a fully staffed respiratory unit with nurses, respiratory therapists, and family members participating in patient care. Activities such as chest physiotherapy, tracheal suctioning, and administration of nebulized medications generally require the assistance of someone other than the patient. However, occasionally patients may even perform these activities for themselves.

For this level of home ventilation, a review for adequate environmental conditions may be necessary. For example, some ventilators require special electrical current and backup. Facilities must be in place to provide for continued therapy in the event of a power failure. When high-concentration oxygen is used at home, proper storage facilities are required as well as fire safety precautions.

For patients receiving intermittent ventilatory support at home, such as a nighttime rest with assisted ventilation, less additional staff and equipment are required. Many of these patients depend only on their spouse or other family member to help them prepare for the therapy.

Noninvasive methods of ventilatory support, such as the Carass ventilator, have been adapted for home use. Several newer devices for providing negative-pressure ventilatory assistance have also been developed and are undergoing refinement.

Home Dialysis

Approximately 20,000 patients each year undergo some form of dialysis procedures at home. The majority of these are patients receiving continuous ambulatory peritoneal dialysis (CAPD). CAPD is a simple procedure in which a dialysate fluid is infused into the peritoneal cavity, allowed to remain for a given length of time, and then simply drained out and replaced by a fresh solution. The entire procedure is performed using gravity drips. Generally, the solutions are changed only four times per day, allowing for continuous, gradual dialysis without significant interruption of lifestyle.

However, a growing percentage of patients are opting for machine-delivered home dialysis methods. These include several peritoneal methods as well as hemodialysis. Such methods as intermittent peritoneal dialysis (IPD), continuous-cycling peritoneal dialysis (CCPD), nocturnal peritoneal dialysis (NPD), and tidal peritoneal dialysis (TPD) have been shown to be of value in selected patients.

Hemodialysis may also be performed at home. Home hemodialysis (HHD) has been utilized since the early days of dialysis and actually predates many other methods. Although its use has leveled off because of financial constraints, HHD deserves reexamination as an alternative for motivated patients.

Although technically similar to in-center hemodialysis, HHD offers quality-of-life benefits that should not be overlooked.

Pain Management

The premier tenet of medicine is to alleviate suffering and obviate pain. The development of a specialty area in this field has brought with it new concepts that allow patients to receive hospital-level pain control without confinement.

Morphine and its semisynthetic derivatives have been administered by continuous drip with excellent results at home. The dosage may be adjusted to produce pain control without clouding mental status. Such systems can utilize intravenous, subcutaneous, or epidural routes. They generally employ small infusion pumps, which carry on-board computer units that can be programmed to continuously deliver the correct dosage. Additional bolus doses can also be programmed into the units with predefined restrictions per the physician's order. For example, the physician may order a morphine drip to run subcutaneously over 24 hours to control intractable pain. If the patient experiences a sudden increase in symptoms that require more control, an additional bolus dose can be administered under the patient's control. However, this bolus dosage is preprogrammed to allow only a limited number of additional doses per hour. This should ensure that the patient receives pain relief without sacrificing safety.

Summary

The concept of intensive homecare will eventually bring the medical revolution of the 20th century full circle and return many aspects of patient care to the home setting. The patient or his family members can be trained to perform many of the activities traditionally done by hospital personnel.

Combining life-sustaining therapy and homecare into a single entity has created a new field of medicine with special advantages for the patient and new challenges for the physician. Ongoing studies in the field will undoubtedly result in further developments in techniques and equipment.

References

1. Lyons AS, Petrucelli RJ. Medicine, An Illustrated History. New York: Harry N. Abrams, 1978.
2. Glasser, O. Dr. W. C. Röntgen. Springfield, IL: Charles C Thomas, 1945, and William Conrad Röntgen, 1934.
3. Relman AS. The Johns Hopkins Centennial. N Engl J Med 1989;320:1411–1412.
4. Coccaro EF, Prudic J, Rothpearl A, Nurnberg HG. Effect of hospital admission of DST results. Am J Psychiatry 1984;141:982–985.

5. Bistrian BR, Blackburn GL, Vitale J, et al. Prevalence of malnutrition in general medical patients. JAMA 1976; 235:1567–1570.
6. Data from the Office of National Cost Estimates. Washington, DC: Health Care Financing Administration, Office of the Actuary, October 1988.
7. Andrulis DP, Beers-Weslowski V, Gage LS. The 1987 U.S. hospital AIDS survey. JAMA 1989;262:784–794.
8. Sage WM, Rosenthal MH, Silverman JF. Is intensive care worth it? An assessment of input and outcome for the critically ill. Crit Care Med 1986;14:777–794.
9. Spitzer WO, Dobson AJ, Hall J, et al. Measuring the quality of life of cancer patients. J Chronic Dis 1981; 34:585–597.
10. Fries JF, Spitz PW, Young DY. The dimensions of health outcomes: the health assessment questionnaire, disability and pain scales. J. Rheumatol 1982;5: 789–793.
11. Goldman L, Hashimoto D, Cook EF. Comparative reproducibility and validity of systems for assessing cardiovascular functional class: advantages of a new specific activity scale. Circulation 1981;64:1227–1234.
12. Mahler DA, Weinberg DH, Wells CK, et al. Measurement of dyspnea: description of two new indices, interobserver agreement and physiological correlations. Am Rev Respir Dis 1982;24 (Suppl 1):138.
13. McNeil BJ, Weichselbaum R, Parker SG. Speech and survival: trade-offs between quality and quantity of life in laryngeal cancer. N Engl J Med 1981;305:982–987.
14. Coates A, Abraham S, Kaye SB, et al. On the receiving end—patient perception of the side-effects of cancer chemotherapy. Eur J Clin Oncol 1983;19:204–208.
15. Presant CA. Quality of life in cancer patients—who measures what? Am J Clin Oncol 1984;7:571–573.
16. Stuck, AE, Aronow, HU, Steiner, A, et al. A trial of annual in-home comprehensive geriatric assessments for elderly people living in the community. N Engl J Med 1995;333:1184–1189.
17. Rich, MW, Beckham, V, Witenberg, C, et al. A multidisciplinary intervention to prevent the readmission of elderly patients with congestive heart failure. N Engl J Med 1995;333:1190–1195.
18. Weed LL. Medical records, medical education and patient care: the problem oriented record as a basic tool. Cleveland, OH: The Press of Case Western Reserve University, 1971, 25:98–108.
19. Lovell A, Zander LI, James CE, et al. The St. Thomas's Hospital maternity case notes study: a randomised controlled trial to assess the effects of giving expectant mothers their own maternity case notes. Paediatr Perinatol Epidemiol 1987;1:57–66.
20. Oley Foundation Report. Lifeline Letters. Albany, NY: The Oley Foundation for Home Parenteral and Enteral Nutrition.
21. Barat AC, Harrie K, Jacob M, et al. Effect of amino acid solutions on total nutrient admixture stability. J Parenter Enteral Nutr 1987;11:384–388.

2

THE PHYSICIAN'S ROLE IN HOMECARE:

Doctoring in a Hospital Without Walls

Michael M. Rothkopf

CHAPTER AT A GLANCE: Homecare therapeutics developed during a period in which physicians had all but abandoned the housecall in favor of hospital care. This has resulted in a serious lack of physician leadership in homecare, which must be reversed. The physician referring a patient for homecare services faces new responsibilities and exposure. The doctor-patient relationship and the psychosocial needs of the patient receiving homecare will need adaptation. Physicians with heavy homecare responsibilities may need to modify their practices to accommodate these complex issues.

Introduction

Although the physician plays a pivotal role in the homecare process, few doctors referring a patient for home health services realize the scope of their responsibilities for this type of therapy (Table 2.1).

Unlike more traditional approaches, in which established systems apply checks and balances, the physician is often not only the key decision maker in a homecare case, but the *only* decision maker. In some ways, this is a liberating concept for the physician. Hospital bureaucracies, quality assurance monitors, peer review organizations, and case managers have all eroded the autonomy of the individual physician in recent years. The homecare setting, in a very real sense, restores that autonomy and the simple bilaterality of the doctor-patient relationship.

However, with this added freedom comes many new responsibilities for which the physician must be prepared. These exist at virtually every level of the homecare process. From the point at which homecare is first explained to the patient until he or she is discharged from service, additional information and decisions are needed. Unfortunately, most physicians are unprepared to deal with the complex issues associated with this role.

The physician generally knows little about the process of preparing the patient for homecare and even less about criteria on which to judge homecare quality. However, while these activities are not familiar to the physician, he will often be expected to sign his approval for them, authorizing payment for Medicare or other agencies.

The Need for Physician Leadership in Homecare

The physician must view himself as the director of various homecare services for the patient. Although it is true that discharge planners

Table 2.1. Physician Responsibilities in Structuring Therapeutics for Homecare

1. Configure medication/therapy to comply with the homecare setting.
2. Develop a therapeutic plan.
3. Confirm adequacy of training of the patient/family.
4. Select the homecare vendor(s).
5. Select the homecare nursing service.
6. Monitor therapy for efficacy.
7. Monitor therapy for complications.
8. Supervise other professionals: RN, RP, RD.
9. Complete therapy and discharge patient from service.

generally take on the tedious aspects of coordinating homecare, it is important that the physician remain actively involved in it.

The doctor should retain the right to decide who will be involved in the care of his patients. Just as he has the right and responsibility to call consultants in the hospital, the physician must control the case at home. He should resist relegating these duties to other members of the team. Although this is tempting because of the effort involved, it is a slippery slope that may lessen the physician's authority. An alternative for physicians with a heavy homecare load is to assign a member of their office staff as a homecare coordinator.

Physicians remain legally responsible for the quality and continuity of care, complications of therapy, and the outcome of events in homecare. There are even statutes in some states that provide for legal liability of inadequate supervision for ancillary staff. For example, a New Jersey anesthesiologist was effectively prosecuted for failing to supervise and train a nurse anesthetist working in an outpatient surgi-center. Although the anesthesiologist was not required either by law or by the policies and procedures of the center to be present during the nurse anesthetist's activities, the State Board of Medical Examiners held that he was directly responsible for her training and for adherence to quality standards. On that basis, the physician's license to practice medicine in the state of New Jersey was suspended. Therefore, although the physician was not liable for malpractice, there were additional liabilities related to his role as a supervisor of a professional team (1).

This case has particular relevance to the homecare physician. The physician is *the pivotal decision maker,* responsible for the delivery of services and the maintenance of standards and quality. If he feels members of the team are not performing to appropriate levels, he must intervene. Furthermore, all members of the team should understand the physician's authority and the requirement to follow his instructions.

The AMA recently observed that the expansion of home health services has occurred in an era when most physicians have decreased their involvement (2). As outlined in Chapter 1, physicians have focused on developments in hospital therapies and have all but abandoned the housecall. The combination of these trends has produced a serious lack of medical leadership in homecare.

Based on a report prepared jointly by the Council on Medical Education and the Council of Scientific Affairs, the AMA calls for intensified involvement by physicians in home health care. They recommended steps be undertaken to increase physician training and familiarity with homecare, and that physicians be encouraged to take the lead in such important issues as quality standards, public policy, utilization, and reimbursement for homecare services. Similar statements have been made by other organizations, including the American College of Physicians (3) and the American Academy of Home Care Physicians (4).

The larger view takes the perspective of homecare as being parallel to the hospital system, which it is gradually replacing. At best, physicians should participate in committees and other administrative duties within homecare organizations just as they do in the hospital. At the very least, physicians should be reminded that they must not relinquish their authority in the direct control of their patients' care at home.

Role of the Referring Physician

Hospital-level services, such as intravenous therapy and mechanical ventilation, are performed using a team of health professionals. Nurses, pharmacists, respiratory therapists, and a variety of paraprofessional assistants all contribute to the delivery of these services. Few or none of these individuals will be present in the patient's home after discharge from the hospital. Therein lies the most significant difference in the care setting and its most important challenges: if the patient is expected to provide most services for himself, or possibly with the help of a family member, how can he replace the many staff members and their expertise?

The physician must play an active role in the homecare process. His first duty is to carefully review the patient's status to determine the appropriateness for homecare. A number of questions should be answered as a preparatory sequence:

1. Are there any obvious exclusions to homecare for this patient? For example, is the therapy too complex or does it require specialized monitoring? Is the patient too unstable to be safely cared for at home? Is the home environment adequate? Are there family members available to assist with patient care?
2. Is the patient an appropriate homecare candidate? For example, can he or she learn the necessary procedures? Does the patient have any visual or physical impairment that limits dexterity? Does the patient possess sufficient reading and comprehension skills?
3. Is the treatment appropriate for homecare; i.e., does it conform to a community standard of practice? Does it require extensive preparation? Does it require special equipment, training, or monitoring? Can it be modified to allow the patient intervals of normal living away from the therapy with the least amount of interference? Will it require special methods for waste disposal?
4. Are there quality homecare vendors available to supply the prescribed therapy or services? Do they have the respect of other physicians in the community? Do they have JCAHO approval?
5. Are there experienced homecare nurses available to carry out the therapeutic plan and monitor the patient? Are they willing to follow the physician's orders and inform him of deviations in the patient's condition?

Obviously, not every hospital treatment can be considered appropriate for homecare. For example, few people would recommend a high dose of dopamine or Levophed drip in a homecare setting. Although the drugs could be delivered, their appropriate monitoring would require full-time staffing and costly equipment.

Patient Selection (See Also Chapter 3)

A concept of the appropriateness of treatment for homecare must emerge for each physician and involves previous experience and published results. An additional subjective factor involves patient tolerance and acceptance. Some patients are very capable, very motivated, and very anti-hospital. Such patients are excellent homecare candidates and can often push the limit of what is acceptable therapy at home.

For example, we have treated AIDS patients at home receiving a combination of TPN, ganciclovir, and aerosolized pentamidine. Each of these patients kept detailed log books that included vital signs, symptoms, fluid intake and output, and even lab flow sheets. For this type of patient, it is a reasonable decision to make extensive use of homecare therapeutics. One can expect that quality of care will be maintained and that the clinical outcome will equal or surpass hospital care.

On the other hand, some patients are clearly overwhelmed by the concept and process of self-care. Such individuals require significant assistance from staff, including visiting nurses and home health aids. They often call out for help during off-hours, such as evenings and weekends. They are particularly insecure during holiday periods. This necessitates additional staff visits and overtime pay scales, which significantly reduce the cost-effectiveness of homecare. Furthermore, such patients are responsible for frequent readmissions to the hospital to manage complications of therapy.

Therefore, part of the physician's responsibility in structuring a homecare regimen is to develop a notion of which therapy is appropriate for each particular type of patient. There are many variables in this thought process, some of which are intangible. Some of the components are:

- Patient's interest in homecare
- Patient's willingness to be trained
- Patient's mental acumen
- Patient's dexterity
- Patient's visual acuity
- Family support
- Family trainability
- Home physical environment
- Third-party payor support for home nursing and laboratory tests
- Complexity of therapy
- Need for ongoing monitoring

To assist in this effort, a physician should look to objective criteria on such issues as the ability of the patient/family to pursue self-care. An analysis such as the ADL or Orem Self-Care Deficit Inventory (see Chapter 3) may be useful in this determination. However, it is also important to recognize that the physician's decision to utilize homecare services requires a value judgment that is not always objectively obtainable.

Developing a Therapeutic Plan

Nurses have made extensive use of the care plan concept and applied it successfully in the critical care, hospital ward, and homecare settings. Its principal value is to aid in efficient communication between various nurses on key issues regarding the patient's condition, treatment, and progress. These other nurses may not know the patient as well as the primary nurse does (or may not know the patient at all). This system has permitted greater scheduling freedom for nursing staff and improved recognition of quality standards. Physicians should consider using a similar format for homecare.

Since homecare is a team approach, it will be necessary for the physician to communicate with a variety of instructions to the team members. The development of a therapeutic plan document will assist in this process (Fig. 2.1). It is also an important step in establishing the appropriateness of vendor and professional charges for homecare.

A comprehensive homecare therapeutic plan can vary significantly, but, at a minimum, it should include the following items:

Medical Necessity Form: This is a detailed description of the patient's diagnosis; severity of illness; expected length of therapy; prognosis; requirements for therapy and special *monitoring* (including physician visits); and potential for rehabilitation.

Functional Assessment Form: This should describe the patient's capacity for self-care with objective determinations based on ADLs, Orem Self-Care Deficit Theory, or other criteria.

Prescription Form: This provides a detailed prescription of the therapy delivered and its requirements for monitoring supplies, laboratory orders, etc.

A therapeutic care plan can also include expanded areas. One plan that has been successfully implemented provides a checklist for the physician to approve specific items such as:

Specific team member functions: All team members should know who does what. This details frequency of visits, delivery schedules, etc.

Specific medical supplies: This enables the physician to define certain types or brands of supplies that he considers superior or necessary for the patient's care.

Homecare training form: This documents the patient's success at learning the necessary procedure and certifies the training process. Problems in the patient's training capacity would be noted here, and the opportunity for follow-up based on objective criteria would be established.

CORAM HEALTHCARE

PLAN OF TREATMENT
STATEMENT OF MEDICAL NECESSITY

Patient Name / I.D. Number	Certification Period From To	Start of Care Date:

Patient's Address __________________________

____

____

Primary Diagnoses: __________________________

Secondary Diagnoses __________________________

Surgical Procedures: __________________________

Allergies: __________ Diet: __________ Date of Birth: __________ Sex: Male ______ Female ______

Provider's Name / Address: __________________________

Medications (Include Oral) List Below or Attach	Dosage / Route	Infusion Time	Frequency	Duration (Or Stop Date)

ROUTE OF ADMINISTRATION
Date inserted: __________

☐ Central line (type) __________   ☐ Peripheral line (type) __________
☐ Central port (type) __________   ☐ Midline catheter (type) __________
☐ Epidural catheter/port __________   ☐ Intrathecal catheter/port __________
☐ PICC line (specify tip location, sutures, vein accessed, gauge, device name, guidewire use)

☐ Enteral Access (type) __________   ☐ Subcutaneous (type) __________
☐ Pump (type) __________
☐ Other __________

ACCESS MAINTENANCE

☐ Peripheral IV change   ☐ Every 48 to 72 hours   ☐ May leave peripheral IV cannula in place for a maximum of ______ days and change IV site for any signs or symptoms of complications.
☐ Port Access frequency: ______ using a ______ gauge ______ inch 90 degree noncoring needle.
☐ Injection cap change: ☐ weekly/PRN   ☐ Other __________
☐ Other __________

CATHETER DRESSING
☐ Use sterile dressing kit   ☐ Other __________

☐ Transparent semipermeable membrane (TSM)   ☐ Gauze
Frequency: ☐ Weekly/PRN   ☐ Three times per week/PRN   ☐ Other __________

CATHETER PATENCY MAINTENANCE

☐ Normal saline for injection ______ ml before and after each dose/PRN ______ weekly PRN
☐ Heparin flush ____ ml ____ units/ml ☐ daily ☐ after each dose ☐ Other __________
☐ Flush with ________ ml saline and ________ ml heparin ________ units/ml following catheter blood draw or if blood observed in catheter.
☐ Clamp catheter when not in use   ☐ Other __________

LAB WORK
To be obtained by: __________

☐ No labs required __________   ☐ CBC-Frequency __________
☐ Blood Chemistry-Frequency __________   ☐ Other-Frequency __________
☐ May draw labs from central line __________   ☐ Yes ☐ No

PROGNOSIS
☐ Poor   ☐ Guarded   ☐ Fair   ☐ Good   ☐ Excellent

GOALS OF THERAPY

____

____

____

REHABILITATION POTENTIAL

____

____

____

DISCHARGE PLANS

____

____

VERBAL START OF CARE DATE/NURSE'S SIGNATURE   DATE

PHARMACIST'S SIGNATURE   DATE

STANDING ORDERS

May repair Central Venous Catheter per CORAM protocol____Yes____No____N/A
May instill Urokinase 5000 I.U./ml up to 1.8 ml for clotted CVC/port____Yes____No____N/A
Nurse to carry and use emergency kit per protocols.____Yes____No____N/A
DNR Orders:____Resuscitate____Do Not Resuscitate

SKILLED NURSING VISIT ORDERS

☐ CORAM primary nursing care provider.
☐ CORAM nursing to coordinate with __________
__________(Specify other agency providing nursing support)
Standing orders for back-up: ☐ Restart peripheral IV as ordered
☐ Central catheter repair   ☐ Urokinase instillation
☐ Other __________

VISIT FREQUENCY

TREATMENT ORDERS

1. Instruct patient/caregiver in administration of home infusion therapy, infusion pump operation/troubleshooting, catheter management, and signs and symptoms of complications related to therapy.
☐ Yes ☐ No ☐ N/A ☐ Change and / or additional orders / instructions __________

2. Monitor/assess the following parameters each visit: ☐ T,P,R,BP
☐ Weight   ☐ Cardiopulmonary status   ☐ Nutritional Status
☐ Response to therapy   ☐ Medication Regime   ☐ Other __________
☐ Contact physician if temperature is __________ °F or higher.
3. RN to administer infusion therapy as ordered   ☐ Yes ☐ No
If no, infusion therapy to be administered by__________
4. Other Orders __________

MENTAL STATUS
☐ Oriented ☐ Comatose ☐ Disoriented ☐ Forgetful ☐ Depressed
☐ Lethargic   ☐ Agitated   ☐ Other __________

FUNCTIONAL LIMITATIONS

☐ Performs daily activities without difficulty   ☐ Needs assistance
☐ Amputation   ☐ Bowel/bladder incontinence   ☐ Contracture   ☐ Hearing Loss
☐ Paralysis ☐ Endurance ☐ Ambulation ☐ Speech ☐ Legally Blind
☐ Dyspnea with minimal exertion ☐ Other __________

ACTIVITIES PERMITTED

☐ Up as tol   ☐ no restrictions   ☐ bedrest   ☐ bedrest/bathroom only
☐ Other __________

SAFETY MEASURES

☐ Universal precautions   ☐ Sharps safety   ☐ IV Care/precautions
☐ Home Safety ☐ Hazardous Waste Disposal ☐ Other __________

☐ **REFER TO ADDENDUM FOR ADDITIONAL ORDERS**

PHYSICIAN'S NAME AND ADDRESS

Phone Number
DEA Number

I hereby certify that the above home infusion and home health services are medically necessary and are authorized by me with a written plan of treatment which will be periodically-reviewed by me. This patient is under my care and is in need of the services as listed on this plan of treatment.

PHYSICIAN'S SIGNATURE: DATE

CRM-0036 (Rev.2/95)   WHITE - PMR   YELLOW - PHYSICIAN

Figure 2.1. Example of Homecare Therapeutic Plan.

Caregiver plan: This is a shortened form for nonmedical family members to follow while providing care to the patient. This form would provide general guidelines for therapy, clearly state the steps to take under contingency situations (e.g., pump failure) and state whom to contact in the case of emergency.

Vendor Selection and Supervision of the Homecare Team (See Also Chapters 4 and 5)

The physician's choice of a homecare company to supply the patient's medications and/or nursing care is an important one. A well-run, accredited company will assist the physician in preparing for discharge, training, monitoring, and quality assurance. This can significantly reduce the time and effort required by the physician in the homecare process. On the other hand, a poorly run company can not only increase the physician's time requirements for treating a homecare patient but can increase the liability of doing so as well.

Physician autonomy in choosing homecare suppliers has become significantly eroded. Changes in state and federal law, the creation of alliances between hospitals and vendors, and the selection of preferred pro-viders by managed care systems have all contributed to this. An atmosphere has been created in which many physicians feel they cannot control the direction of patient referral.

However, given the importance of this decision on the patient's care and outcome, physicians should make every attempt to maintain a "veto power" on the choice of homecare suppliers. One must not forget that none of the initial steps involving homecare referral can take place without the doctor's signature. Similarly, the liability of this decision is not transferred from the physician to the discharge planner or insurance company. It rests with the physician. Therefore, physicians are well advised to maintain control over the important process of patient referral. They should make a judgment of the compa-nies based on objective criteria and reputation among other doctors.

If the physician has a preference for a particular homecare company, he should make it known to the discharge planner and case manager. They will usually comply with a physician's request, particularly if the supplier is already on a list of acceptable vendors. If not, the case manager or HMO may require that the homecare company accept reduced, out-of-network rates for their services. This means that the patient may have to pay a much larger deductible for out-of-network care. Since homecare companies are often very motivated to get the referral, they will often waive this co-payment if they can.

A similar level of control should be considered by the physician when it comes to supervising the homecare team. The physician should insist on clear and timely information from the homecare nurse and pharmacist. Similarly, he should make clear any special directions that should be followed.

Physicians need to recognize that although nurses may appear to be employees of a homecare company, they are often either independent contractors or members of a separate nursing agency. Therefore, they may require a separate evaluation to ensure adequacy of therapy.

Although homecare nurses are encouraged to act independently, they occasionally take actions without prior approval by the physician. One must permit the homecare nurse some latitude when treating the patient at home. However, the physician should make it clear when he expects to be consulted and what level of actions the nurse should take while awaiting the doctor's decision. A nurse who independently takes actions that require a physician's order can be a liability and should be replaced. On the other hand, a nurse who fails to notify the physician of a critical lab value or change in patient status should also be considered a risk.

As leader of the homecare team, the physician has legal responsibility over the team members. Since he will undoubtedly be held accountable for any errors, the physician should feel justified in exercising authority in these matters.

Adapting the Doctor-Patient Relationship to Homecare

When a physician discharges a patient to homecare, he or she must recognize that a transformation is about to occur. The distinct lines of authority and responsibility with which the doctor is familiar and comfortable are about to be redrawn.

The existing barriers between the health-care team and the patient must be dismantled so that the patient can actually participate in his own care. This is a gradual process that includes:

- Familiarizing the patient/family with dosage schedule
- Teaching administration techniques
- Teaching sterile techniques
- Teaching dressing changes
- Preparing for interaction with pharmacy and delivery staff
- Taking inventory of homecare supplies
- Learning self-monitoring techniques
- Learning about adverse reactions
- Preparing for emergencies

Not all patients are willing or able to assimilate all this information, but the closer the patient comes to awareness in these areas, the better.

The patient trained in such techniques and concepts will rightly expect to be treated in a different way by the physician than he had been treated in the hospital. Such a patient is now actively involved in his care and must be dealt with as a member of the homecare team. The same can certainly be said for family members who are involved in the caregiver role of a patient at home. For example, patients with Hickman catheters who have been thoroughly trained in homecare are apt to complain about the manner in which the hospital staff access their catheters when they are hospitalized. Knowledgeable in sterile technique, they may chide a nurse for failing

to swab an access port or for not wearing gloves. Hospital nurses are usually astonished by this interaction, surprised by the patient's assertion of independence. It then becomes necessary for the physician to instruct the hospital nursing staff of the patient's rights and responsibility in this area.

When the physician interacts with his homecare patient, he should be willing to give up some authority to the patient, so that the patient feels empowered. Using the previous example of the homecare patient admitted to the hospital, it would be appropriate in this situation to instruct the patient (to empower the patient) to be emphatic with the nurse who shows poor technique in accessing the catheter. After all, it is the patient's catheter and his own body that he is trying to protect.

However, in asserting himself, the patient is clearly stepping beyond the lines of the traditional accepted behavior for a patient in the hospital. This will likely produce consternation and discomfort on the part of the staff, some of which will feed back to the patient. The patient will then need to be reassured that he is doing the right thing, and there is no better way to accomplish this than for his own physician to inform him so.

The patient can also be permitted to share in the flow of information related to his own care. Although it is commonplace for this process to be hidden from the patient in the hospital, this is not necessary in homecare and may in fact be counterproductive.

Laboratory data, test results, and consultants' opinions can be routinely shared with the homecare patient. This helps to involve the patient in the process and provides a reasoning behind some of the duties required. For example, it may be necessary for a home TPN patient with short-bowel syndrome to infuse additional fluids or electrolytes on occasion. Obviously, it would be preferable for the patient to know the rationale behind this in specific terms. Patients can be trained about the importance of following the BUN or potassium levels, for example, and the need to treat abnormal conditions with appropriate additional fluids or electrolytes. Similarly, an AIDS patient with severe intestinal opportunistic infection and diarrhea may become dehydrated and hypernatremic. Once again, these patients can easily be taught the need to maintain fluid balance and the rationale behind taking additional infused intravenous solutions.

Not only is this information helpful in providing background, but it serves as a comfort to the patient to know that these factors are being closely monitored by the physician and homecare team. This monitoring allows for the appropriate steps to be taken to maintain the patient's health and stability so that he can remain at home. This further reaffirms the value of the monitoring process being undertaken and gives the patient positive feedback for some of the discomforts he or she may have to endure, such as additional laboratory or other testing, referrals to consultants, etc.

The patient now has an additional motivation to maintaining stability beyond the obvious need for maintenance of health. He or she is motivated to maintain care within a homecare surrounding for comfort and quality of life. Highlighting this motivation can be a useful tool in convincing the patient to undergo extra testing or therapies while at home, but certainly sharing the knowledge of the medical information is an important component in this process.

On the other hand, there are also situations in which the patient or family may go too far in asserting independence and will need to be reminded of their own limitations. For example, a cancer patient receiving intravenous morphine at home for intractable pain may complain to the family that he needs more relief. The family, seeking to comfort a loved one, may exceed the dosing limits set by the physician and thereby potentially harm the patient. The physician must remind the patient's family that while independence is the goal of homecare, it can only be independence within established standards of safe medical practice.

It may be appropriate to review concepts with the patient and to stress that while it is the goal of homecare for the patient to have flexibility in treatment scheduling and dosages to allow for an increase in the quality of life, this can only be done if it also meets the accepted norms for treatment. That is to say that by asking the patient and family to be participants in the care process, we are not permitting them to go and practice medicine on themselves.

To supervise this process effectively, the physician should have a clear concept of where the self-treatment limits exist for each patient receiving intensive homecare therapy. This will vary depending on the patient's age and capabilities, as well as on the complexity of his care. For example, a young patient with Crohn's disease who has been on home TPN for 10 years will certainly be an appropriate patient to have greater autonomy. By contrast, an elderly patient receiving a short course of home antibiotics may need to be monitored very closely within a program in which very few options are offered.

Just as the physician individualizes his decision on the appropriateness of homecare, he or she can also individualize the limits of the patient's freedom and active participation in the process. Some of the key areas regarding this concept are:

1. Instruction on when to notify the nurse or physician. This may relate to instructions given on pump or other device malfunctions, complications with catheter access, etc. Certainly, this would also include such concepts as adverse drug reactions or abnormal vital signs. The patient can be encouraged to call for any question. However, he should recognize that certain parameters *require* that he call. Therefore, he must be given clear instructions on when to notify the homecare team nurse or physician.

2. Whether or not to allow for interim steps that the patient takes before contacting the homecare nurse or physician. This would relate to system checks that the patient or family may perform on the equipment or tubing prior to calling for help. There are many activities that can be performed by the patient as a troubleshooting measure that simplify the flow of information back to the homecare nurse or physician. This will also fa-

cilitate reinstitution of therapy and reduce the amount of downtime. Another option in this category would include the use of nonprescriptive medication for fever or mild symptoms, such as itching or skin rash, and the use of prescriptive medications for anticipated side effects or reactions, such as the use of antimotility agents for diarrhea or antiemetics for nausea, etc.

3. Home charting. This includes the patient's recording of vital signs, therapy, delivery schedules, laboratory values, etc., to be available for the physician to review either during a home visit or when the patient travels to the office.

4. Permission to adjust therapy based on established parameters. This can include adjustment of flow or infusion volume, use of additional medications, changing of dosage based on symptoms or other parameters, etc.

The Physician-Patient Relationship in Homecare

Part of the physician's orientation to homecare should involve the recognition that patients and family will be more dependent on him for reassurance. The patient will often have a complex medical problem, the course of therapy may seem overwhelming, and there is a loss of security that occurs when a patient leaves the hospital. The physician must be cognizant of this, and must be willing to serve as a safety net for the patient. The physician should look for an opportunity to discuss such factors as the disease process and treatment options; the effect of homecare on the patient's and family's lifestyle; the expected course of the illness; and the psychological, emotional, and financial stresses induced by the process of homecare (5).

Just as patients and families may be expected to extend themselves beyond their normal roles in becoming part of the homecare process, physicians should expect to extend themselves from a personal perspective so as to invite dialogue with their patients receiving homecare therapeutics (6).

The Homecare Practice

Integration of the complexities of homecare therapeutics into a thriving medical practice remains a significant challenge. Existing practice patterns are ill-suited to the extra time commitments needed to appropriately manage a homecare case. Numerous telephone calls to provide direction and coordination are often required, some of which will certainly take place after hours. Activities such as patient education; development of a care plan; psychosocial assessment; consultation with the homecare nurse; telephone consultations with the patient, family, etc.; and preparation of the medical necessity forms are not reimbursable. These activities may amount to more than 10 hours per month of the physician's time in complicated cases.

Nevertheless, with sufficient planning, supervision of homecare services can be a rewarding component of a modern medical practice. We have found it useful to designate a member of our office staff as the "homecare coordinator." This individual is responsible for coordinating the flow of information to and from the office on all homecare patients. We have also instituted a system of having a separate homecare chart in the office for each homecare patient. This chart contains the homecare therapeutic plan, prescriptions, laboratory requirements, flow sheets, and nursing reports.

Physician housecalls to monitor patients who are truly homebound should also be given consideration. While this requires a significant time commitment on the part of the physician, the benefits to patient care, both medical and psychological, are invaluable.

Unfortunately, physician reimbursement for homecare services is inadequate. Current physician procedure codes and billing practices, as well as insurance reimbursement for physician activity, evolved during a period when physician housecalls were considered obsolete. The national healthcare system developed during this period heavily favored the physician who performed procedures rather than cognitive work. Housecalls were seen as having a low priority in this system. As a result, Medicare and most other health insurance carriers reimburse for housecalls at a level no different than for an ordinary office visit. Ironically, Medicare will pay substantially more for a visiting nurse to see the patient at home than a physician.

However, physician reimbursement procedures under Medicare and other carriers are in a process of review. Medicare recently began to allow billing a Current Procedural Terminology (CPT) code for "Physician Case Management." Further reform in this direction is anticipated.

Conclusion

Physicians play the pivotal role in the home-care process. They not only begin the sequence in referring the patient but remain legally and morally responsible for the standards of practice utilized by team members in caring for the patient. It is important that physicians recognize this responsibility and take on the associated duties with dedication and authority.

References

1. Kern SI. Supreme court decision on supervision. New Jersey Medicine 1992;89:495–496.
2. Council on Scientific Affairs. Educating physicians in home health care. JAMA 1991;265:769–771.
3. Weinstein M. Involving physicians in home health care. American College of Physicians Observer 1989; Jan:1–6.
4. Keenan JM. President's message. American Academy of Home Care Physicians Newsletter 1991:3(2).
5. Physicians and home care. Guidelines for the medical management of the home care patient. Chicago: American Medical Association, 1992.
6. Galloway, R. House calls [editorial]. JAMA 1991;266 (6):786.

Suggested Readings

Campion FD. A piece of my mind [editorial]. JAMA 1989; 262:556.

Doctors need larger role in home health. [editorial]. Am Med News July 1990;33:21.

Fishman S. Cancer comes home. The New York Times Magazine, June 11, 1989:70–73.

MacPherson P. Have skill, will travel. Am Med News Sept. 1990:9–10.

Position papers. Home health care. Ann Intern Med 1986; 105:454–460.

Rossman I. The geriatrician and the homebound patient. J Am Geriatr Soc 1988:348–354.

Steel K. Home care for the elderly. The new institution. Arch Intern Med 1991;151:439–442.

3

PATIENT SELECTION AND PREPARATION FOR HOMECARE

Michael M. Rothkopf

CHAPTER AT A GLANCE: Successful homecare therapeutics rely on the patient being an active participant in his or her own care. Family members or "significant others" may also be called upon to play an important supportive role. Careful patient selection and adequate training are essential. This chapter provides medical and nonmedical criteria for patient selection. It describes a process of preparation and patients' expectations. Standards for patient training and evaluation are also given.

Patient Selection for Homecare

Homecare is a patient-oriented process. It empowers the patient with medical knowledge. It provides the patient with equipment that permits him or her to continue advanced therapies while maintaining the comfort and quality of life at home. The patient is expected to become an active part of the care delivery system rather than a passive recipient.

As with all aspects of the practice of medicine, careful planning and preparation are necessary for optimal utilization of homecare. However, the active involvement of the patient as part of the medical care delivery system adds some unique aspects to the process. While it is certainly important that the physician adapt the particular therapy for homecare, the appropriate selection and preparation of the patient also deserve careful attention. The success of sophisticated medical treatment at home relies on both of these important actions.

Homecare has evolved to the point where there is virtually no disease that automatically excludes a patient from consideration. However, it is essential that the prospective homecare patient meet certain medical and nonmedical criteria. Some general guidelines useful in patient selection are presented in this chapter. More specific criteria may be found in Section II of the book, where individual therapies are covered.

It is expected that the trend in patient selection will continue toward the inclusion of greater numbers of patients. Guidelines for the selection of homecare patients are becoming less restrictive. Confidence gained through homecare experience and the development of more sophisticated, reliable, and simple-to-operate homecare technology have encouraged this progression.

As can be said for other therapeutic choices in medicine, patient selection for homecare also involves some art as well as science. In other words, there are aspects of the decision that cannot be objectively quantified. The physician should take the lead in this process, applying mechanisms of realistic logic that are integral to the practice of medicine. However, patient selection should be a collaborative effort of the homecare professional staff when the decision is difficult and additional opinions are needed to support it.

Medical Criteria

Clinical Stability

It is extremely important that the patient be medically stable prior to initiating homecare. Usually, it is not the nature of the medical condition to be treated that limits a patient's suitability for homecare but rather his or her overall medical condition.

Even seriously ill patients (e.g., those with advanced AIDS) can do well on home therapy. However, it is essential that all coexisting medical conditions be recognized and demonstrated to be under control before discharge. Monitoring practices at home will be less frequent and less rigorous. This in turn extends the time frame of management, which can lead to delayed treatment of complications.

The determination of medical stability is the responsibility of the physician and should be based on objective clinical and laboratory criteria. Generally, vital signs should be stable and within acceptable parameters. Laboratory values should be within normal limits or unchanged from baseline values. There must be no need for daily or more frequent monitoring by a physician.

Therapeutic Access

A functional, reliable access system (i.e., venous access port, artificial airway, etc.) must be in place. The access system should be simple enough to use that it facilities the homecare process. The Hickman catheter is a good example of this. It is a medical device that is well suited to long-term maintenance and to patient participation in its care. Once the catheter is inserted and properly positioned by the doctor, the patient or nurse can utilize it repeatedly for many months. The catheter

care techniques are basic and can be taught to patients with a wide range of capabilities. With proper training, even difficult patients such as children and the elderly have demonstrated proficiency in using the Hickman catheter.

Nonmedical Criteria

The following nonmedical criteria should be met before a patient is approved for homecare.

- *The patient accepts responsibility.* A key issue in homecare is the willingness of the patient to actively participate in his or her own medical care. If the patient does not wish to receive treatment at home, the outcome of home therapy is doubtful. The patient, and any other family members or friends who may be involved in the care of the patient at home, must have the ability to understand the responsibilities and risks of receiving medical therapies at home. After receiving full disclosure of costs, responsibilities, and possible complications, the patient should affirm his or her acceptance of homecare in writing.

  Initial reluctance on the part of the patient or family to accept homecare should not be a reason for exclusion. Most people are taken aback by the thought of providing their own medical care. However, a careful explanation of benefits of treatment at home, proper training, and demonstration of readily available support services can often convince the patient to attempt a course of therapy at home.

- *The patient is able to handle homecare psychologically and intellectually.* Psychosocial factors (personality traits, psychological stability, and family support) have an important influence on the success of homecare. A motivated, cooperative patient is most likely to complete a successful course of therapy at home. Patients who are known substance abusers or who have a history of medical noncompliance are usually considered poor candidates. However, the development of sophisticated data recording and tamper-proof medical equipment may allow such patients to be sent home with more confidence than in the past.

When the patient is not able to handle homecare alone, the support of a family member or friend in the role of caregiver can be instrumental in overcoming potential obstacles to home therapy (1). For example, some patients may require the assistance of a caregiver in dealing with the treatment regimen, working with the homecare nurse, or relating questions and problems to members of the homecare team. A home health aide or nurse becomes essential if there are possible serious sequelae of the disease or the treatment. Reading skills and a certain degree of learning potential are required of the homecare patient or the caregiver. The patient, perhaps with the assistance of a caregiver, must have the ability to learn how to administer the therapy, perform self-monitoring, and keep adequate records. Acceptable performance in an objective assessment of self-care training (usually administered by the homecare nurse) is required before the patient is released to homecare.

- *The patient is physically able to perform the homecare regimen.* The degrees of mobility, dexterity, and visual acuity required for homecare depend on the particular therapeutic regimen prescribed. Neurological, ophthalmological, and rheumatological problems can make compliance difficult without the reliable assistance of a caregiver.
- *A qualified homecare vendor is available.* Except perhaps in the case of the simplest therapies, homecare is not feasible without the involvement of a homecare vendor. These services take on the complex task of coordinating the homecare team and delivering medical supplies and pharmaceuticals.
- *The home environment is suitable for homecare.* The home environment should be sanitary, conducive to the performance of the therapeutic regimen prescribed. It should have adequate heating/cooling, plumbing and electrical supply. Available capacity for refrigeration is important for storage of certain medicines and supplies. Access to a telephone for communications in an emergency, and between medical visits, must be available. The home's location should be within a reasonable distance from an emergency room for access to medical care in the event of a crisis. In addition, transportation must be available between the patient's home and the physician's office or other monitoring facility, as well as to an emergency room. A plan must also be developed for home contingencies (e.g., power failure, severe weather, disruption of telephone service) that may interrupt therapy.
- *The patient is financially able to afford homecare.* The cost to the patient involved in homecare must be carefully detailed and explained to the responsible person. Reimbursement for homecare by third-party payors is not uniform. A co-pay balance may be required, and this in itself can be substantial. Secondary expenses such as physical adaptation of the home and additional personnel hired to assist with daily household duties may be incurred. It is expected that the various financial issues will be resolved as home therapy becomes more widely applied and payors participate more completely in homecare planning.

The Decision for Homecare

The physician must be the one to make the final decision regarding patient suitability for homecare, since it is the physician who bears ultimate responsibility for the outcome of home therapy. Perhaps the most dangerous situation in homecare is the premature release of the patient from the hospital. It is imperative that the physician is satisfied that his or her homecare patient is medically stable and has received proper and complete training. Any compromise in the decision process as a result of pressure from the hospital or the patient's insurance provider can expose the patient to increased medical risk and the physician to increased legal risk.

Patient Preparation for Homecare

After the physician has gone through the decision process outlined above, the preparations are made for the patient's discharge. Discharge planners, nurses, pharmacists, reimbursement specialists, case managers, delivery persons, equipment suppliers—all participate in the many orchestrated activities necessary to discharge a patient from hospital to homecare. In the midst of this workload, it is sometimes hard to remember that the patient is also a member of the homecare team. A critical component of this process is patient training for self-care.

It is the patient who will perform the basic activities previously done by the nursing staff in the hospital, such as monitoring and recording of vital signs, preparing for the infusion of homecare solutions, connecting IV tubing and/or other devices, and programming infusion pumps or other mechanical and electronic equipment. It is the patient who will be charged with the duties of interacting with the homecare supplier and the homecare nurses, and keeping the physician's office informed regarding progress.

While patients may be intimidated at first, most welcome the opportunity to become involved in their own care. It provides a form of occupational therapy for some and a liberating sense of independence for others. Similarly, family members who are at first reluctant to perform medical services for their loved one are often converted to enthusiasts. They experience a sense of satisfaction from having a role to play in the patient's care. They are proud to be able to function at a level of competence that, for this one patient, is equivalent to the services rendered by staff members with extensive training and experience.

This concept is revolutionary, since it not only employs the use of new technology but also fundamentally changes the role of the patient in his or her own healthcare delivery. Similarly, the interaction between the patient and the healthcare professionals, particularly the physician, is affected.

As described previously, the patient's role in the traditional hospital/healthcare delivery system has been that of a passive recipient of care rendered by others. Even the terms we use to describe the people involved tell us something about the psychological significance of their roles. Labels such as patient, nurse, doctor, or the more recent term *healthcare provider*, themselves offer an insight into the expected relationship. Psychologically, the patient is placed in a childlike or dependent position. The healthcare workers are put in the empowered, adult, or parent role.

The use of medical terminology is another way in which the health professional is put into a psychologically superior role. The phrases are imposing and create a curtain of secrecy that even an assertive patient may not be able to penetrate.

In a traditional care setting, such as a hospital or a doctor's office, the patient is the recipient of services rendered. The patient is not expected to participate in his or her own care. In fact, barriers are placed to prevent the patient from doing so. For example, the patient is not permitted to bring his own medications to the hospital. He must be given "privileges" to ambulate, use the bathroom, independently shower, etc. Each one of these small, independent activities requires approval by the hospital staff. Patients who are novices to the system are often amazed by this. Statements such as, "The nurse wouldn't even give me an aspirin without calling you," are common examples of the sense of bewilderment.

Certainly, these restrictions have been placed for the patient's benefit and protection. They are intended to serve as safeguards. But they are also intended to serve the needs of the hospital system and to the staff that must work within it. They are designed to accommodate scheduling and practice patterns of the physicians as well.

No one can deny that these restrictions significantly affect the perception one has as a "patient" in the hospital. The hospital system, seeking uniformity, diminishes the concept of "self" both to the individual and to the team of professionals caring for the patient. This objectification is an important part of the distinction between the patient and professional.

In their own homes, patients regain their sense of self and individuality. They do not have to conform to the standardized routine of the hospital. For example, mealtime and food selection are important components of quality of life. At home, the patient makes these choices freely. Access to friends and family members is also unrestricted. Furthermore, the patient has access to personal items such as photographs and memorabilia. At home they can enjoy the familiar views from a window or garden and the small comforts that make up the fabric of everyday life.

Given the choice, few people would want to abandon these comforts for the cold, sterile hospital room. And, when asked, most people report just that: they prefer homecare to hospital care (survey by National Resource Inc., National Association of Medical Equipment Suppliers, 1991). In a study comparing nursing home patients to homecare patients, homecare was shown to foster personal freedom. Factors such as control over one's environment, familiarity, security, individuality, and future orientation were all found to be enhanced in homecare (2). Both active and passive social contacts occurred more frequently. Patients had greater appetite, were more receptive to stimulation, and reported experiencing everyday pleasures more frequently.

With greater autonomy comes greater responsibility. Patients who are offered homecare have to realize that a powerful change is about to occur. They will now be involved in the delivery of their own health services, and they will be as responsible as the rest of the healthcare team for carrying them out.

Too often patients are told of homecare without an in-depth explanation of the primary role they will take in their treatment. This may create misunderstandings that limit the system and eventually lead to a breakdown in communication. This in turn may necessitate re-hospitalization, transfer to a nursing home, or premature discontinuation of services.

This is an issue not only for the patient but for family members involved in the process, especially the spouse. The emotional strain experienced by the spouse may be a significant burden. In a recent Scandinavian study (3), homecare spouses have fewer social interactions with friends and family and reported having less time for hobbies and other interests than spouses of nursing-home patients. Ironically, this is just the opposite of what has been reported for the patients themselves. Thus, the freedom and quality of life for the patient often comes at the expense of decreased freedom and activity of the caregiving family member.

Caregivers may be at a higher risk themselves of becoming ill. A recent study highlighted the deleterious effects on the immune system associated with the stress of providing homecare for a chronically ill relative (4). The caregivers had slower wound healing and more abnormal immune function than the control group.

On the other hand, many family members appreciate the opportunity to be of real service and care to a loved one. They see this as a chance to return the love and attention given to them in the past or, for some people, it is a tangible sign of their devotion to the patient.

Patient's Rights and Expectations

The physician or his staff should carefully explain homecare concepts—such as the patient's primary involvement in care—to the patient either prior to discharge or early in the process of homecare. The patient then also needs to recognize the change in his status and the inherent freedoms and responsibilities involved. While all homecare patients eventually come to this realization on their own, it is best that they begin homecare with realistic expectations, as explained by healthcare professionals.

The patient should also recognize that the privacy of the home will be breached by the process of homecare. Medical equipment, with its foreboding appearance, will be brought into the patient's home and appear very out of place at times. Nurses, delivery staff, physicians, and other personnel will visit the patient in the home and may, in the case of an emergency, need to enter into very private areas such as bedrooms or bathrooms within the home. This is often a source of consternation on the part of the patients, and there is sometimes a feeling that their privacy is being violated. Yet patients certainly have the right to maintain privacy and confidentiality and to set limits of their own with regard to where medical and homecare staff are permitted to traverse within the patient's home.

The patient has the right to expect prompt and professional services from every member of the homecare team. He has the right to be treated in a dignified manner, with respect to his person and property. The patient involved in homecare should have a clear understanding of the treatment options, the cost of therapies, the length of therapy, and the alternatives. Under extreme circumstances, the patient may opt to refuse therapy, which is also permissible as long as the patient is fully informed and accepts the responsibility of this action.

Patient Training/Skills Evaluation/Home Environment

Objective Determination of Skills

Standardized training and the acquisition of a body of medical knowledge is integral to the development of the healthcare professional. Rigorous criteria exist for determining adequacy of information, skills, training, etc., for nearly all fields of healthcare. This process generally culminates in the awarding of a certificate or licensure enabling an individual to practice with direct patient contact under the authority of a state board. This ensures that qualified staff are involved in patient care and that their professional activities are monitored.

When patients or family members become caregivers, how can *their* skills be assessed? Who supervises their activities? This is particularly significant in light of the discussion outlined above regarding the patient's/ family's role and responsibilities as part of the homecare team. The physician expects his or her team members to function at a specified level of proficiency. In homecare, this applies to the patient and family caregiver as well.

A number of assessment criteria have been applied to homecare patients and family members. They are generally easy to use and should be considered in each case as part of the patient preparation process. This is not to suggest that only patients who meet such rigorous criteria can be accepted for homecare. Additional home nursing or the use of specialized equipment can often compensate for the patient's limitations. However, to plan appropriately for this need, an assessment of functional capacity is necessary.

Although most of these tools have been designed with the patient in mind, they can certainly be applied to the family member serving in a caregiver role with some modifications.

The most common of these tools is the Activities of Daily Living (ADL) Index. This includes assessment of the basic ADL—ambulating, toileting, feeding, continence, bathing, dressing, and transferring—as well as the instrumental ADL (IADL)—appropriate medication use, arranging transportation, doing housework, handling finances, using the telephone, preparing meals, and shopping. Variations of ADL and IADL exist, such as the NYU Disability Index.

The Orem Self-Care Deficit is another tool for determining patient capabilities. It utilizes three components: basic conditioning, self-care requisite visits, and self-care agency. The basic conditioning factors (BCFs) are age, sex, psychosocial and cognitive status, physical abilities, cultural orientation, living conditions, and resources. The patient's self-care requisites (SCRs) involve carrying out the prescribed therapy and understanding the system under which it is delivered. An assessment of the patient's ability to perform these tasks based on knowledge, skill, and motivation is referred to as self-care agency (SCA). These three groups of factors are then used in planning, implementing, and evaluating the patient's care. Deficits in care can be monitored and corrected on this basis.

Other devices include the Bartel and

Katz Index, the Kenney Self-Care Evaluation, and the PULSES Profile. The latter is a particularly facile system involving six areas. The patient is rated on a scale of 1 to 4 corresponding to no impairment, mild impairment, moderate impairment, and severe impairment in each area. PULSES stands for *p*hysical condition, *u*pper limb function, *l*ower limb function, *s*ensory function, *e*xcretory function, and *s*upport systems. Separate assessments have been proposed for mental/cognitive area, psychosocial status, medication use and compliance, and nutritional status.

A caregiver assessment has been proposed by the Department of Geriatric Health of the American Medical Association (5). This includes an assessment of the burden of caregiving based on the number of hours of caregiving work per day, the nature of tasks to be completed, and the psychological stress related to the nature of illness and necessary care. Also included in their survey is an assessment of the caregiver based on attitude regarding the responsibility; emotional competence and stability; physical capacity; other responsibilities; and other factors. Implicit in the role of the caregiver is certainly the willingness and ability to learn and apply new knowledge as well as the willingness and ability to work with other members of the homecare team.

An important part of the physician's assessment will be determining the number and quality of the family caregivers involved in the patient's care. This may also involve a review of the family relationships and dynamics, as well as traditions based on ethnic background.

As detailed below, an environmental assessment must be performed that involves a physical safety determination for homecare, and accessibility to telephone and emergency services. Backup systems for electrical and telephone support, in the event of severe weather and power failures, need to be considered. There should be an adequate fire safety plan and appropriate plans for storage of supplies, equipment, and medications.

Finally, an assessment of the community and the economic impact of homecare should be performed. These last areas are generally performed by the discharge planner, who sends a report to the physician.

Preparing the Home Environment

Just as the patient and family dynamics may change through the process of homecare, the home environment may need to be adapted as well. Electrical outlets, telephone connections, ramps, and assistance devices such as bedside commodes may be needed to make the home environment more appropriate for the provision of homecare services. Although much of the planning in this area is usually done by the discharge planner in preparation for homecare, it is important that the physician ordering home therapy be aware of the special environmental needs of his or her patient. The process of making the transition from a hospital setting—in which the building has been designed and engineered to accommodate medical equipment, personnel, and patient access—to a home, which was designed for much less specialized use, is imposing. Nonetheless, it can be accomplished with a common-sense approach, some planning, and creativity. The key issues revolve around three major concerns for the home environment: safety, accessibility, and physical adaptations.

Safety issues include elimination of possible hazards and barriers, especially in light of the patient's possible functional limitations. A fire plan should be detailed. Clean storage of supplies and maintenance of a safe preparation area are also critical to the success and safety of homecare therapy.

Accessibility issues relate to exterior and interior doors, steps, etc. There must be sufficient space to allow for patient mobility and caregiver's access to the patient, equipment, and supplies. Access to emergency support systems via telephone must be considered in the event of a fire or the need to transport the patient urgently. Backup systems for such contingencies as power failure, ice storms, etc., must be put in place. For example, the homecare supplier could routinely oversupply by one bag any IV solution the patient must use. In this manner, should a delivery be delayed or missed because of scheduling difficulties, traffic congestion, weather considerations, etc., the patient's therapy would not be compromised.

Physical adaptation of the home is often seen as a real impediment to homecare, though it need not be. A large variety of personal assistance devices are available that can adapt the bedroom, bathroom, and kitchen into a safe and useful area for the patient. (Fig. 3.1) In our experience, physical remodeling of the home is rarely necessary.

The use of a portable IV infusion pump

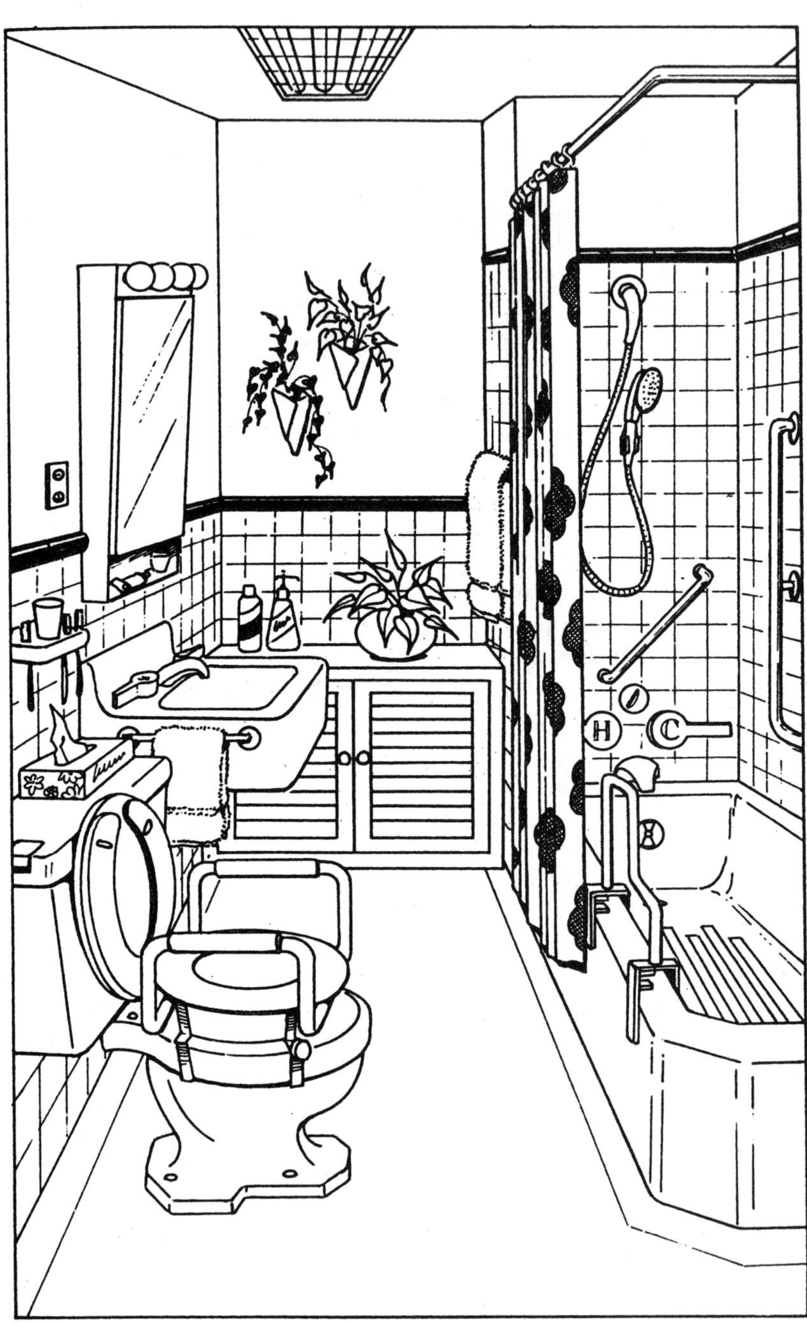

Figure 3.1.   Model bathroom.

can make a big difference with regard to whether the patient requiring infusion services feels trapped or free. The portable pump gives a measure of freedom that cannot be achieved when using a larger pump on a pole. Such freedom of movement can make a tremendous difference in morale by maximizing flexibility and control for the patient.

Summary

Patient and family involvement in homecare can be a satisfying process for everyone involved. The patient feels empowered and independent. The family has an opportunity to offer comfort and affection as well as physical assistance. Healthcare workers have an opportunity to see the patient as a complete person within his or her normal environment. The physician obtains professional fulfillment in facilitating a detailed and complicated process. To achieve these lofty goals, however, patients must be appropriately chosen and carefully trained. Once this has been accomplished, safe and effective homecare can be utilized for practically any medical condition.

References

1. Houts PS, ed. Home Care Guide for Cancer. Philadelphia: American College of Physicians, 1994.
2. Bergler R. Psychological situation of home care patients in the Federal Republic of Germany. Zentralbl Hyg Umweltmed 1993;194(1–2):33–79.
3. Lofgren AC, Bucht G, Eriksson S, Winglad B. A comparative study of the social conditions of spouses of long term patients cared for either in nursing homes or home care. Scand J Caring Sci 1992; 6(1):45–52.
4. Kiecolt-Glaser JK, Marucha PT, et al. Slowing of wound healing by psychological stress. Lancet 1995; 346:1194–1196.
5. American Medical Association, Department of Geriatric Health. Guidelines for the medical management of the home care patient. Chicago: American Medical Association, 1992.

4

THE PATIENT'S PERSPECTIVE

Fran L. Freeman and Ruth A. Elliot

CHAPTER AT A GLANCE: When a patient faces a serious illness, he or she immediately reacts on an emotional level. This chapter relates the adjustments a patient makes when facing his or her future health care and demonstrates how a patient progresses from the acceptance of his or her illness to the practical elements of preparation and support needed to receive therapy at home.

Introduction

Understanding the process of homecare is a complex endeavor with many technical and conceptual components. In this chapter, we present the viewpoint of a patient receiving medical therapy at home.

Homecare has liberated thousands of patients from hospital confinement. Although it requires much from the patient, the freedom it affords more than makes up for the added responsibilities. For some patients, it may be the only real chance at a normal life.

Home infusion, in general, and home parenteral nutrition (HPN), in particular, has been a trend setter in homecare therapeutics. Home therapy of the patient with long-term needs was envisioned in the earliest days of nutritional support, over 20 years ago. At that time, the "pioneer" patients utilized a cumbersome process in which they actually "self-mixed" their solutions under small laminar-flow hoods at home. These patients were trained in basic pharmacy techniques and were able to fare quite well for themselves. Their bedrooms became mini-pharmacies that contained stock solutions of each nutritional additive (Fig. 4.1).

Today, it is rare for patients to mix solutions. However, most patients still add one or two ingredients to their home total parenteral nutrition (TPN) bag before use. This generally relates to a multivitamin preparation or some other component that is not stable for prolonged periods. The home infusion formula has progressed to a system in which intravenous supplies and materials are delivered to the patient by the home care therapy provider. The patient connects to the infusion using sterile techniques and basic precautions. These technical aspects involve an area generally considered under hospital nursing care. Practically all home infusion patients receive some training in this area before going home. Thus, while it is no longer necessary for the patient to become his or her own pharmacist, it is still important that he or she be skilled in basic infusion therapy techniques. (Fig. 4.2)

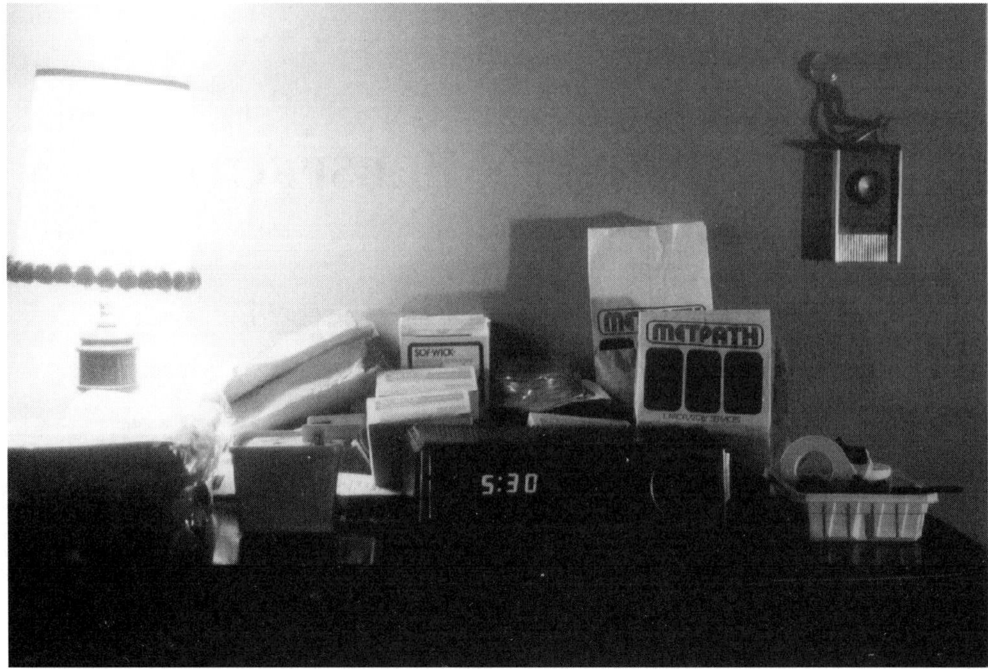

Figure 4.1. Bedroom supplies of an early homecare patient. The patient self-mixed his TPN solution from supplies delivered to him. He functioned as both pharmacist and nurse. (Photograph by Michael Rothkopf, M.D.)

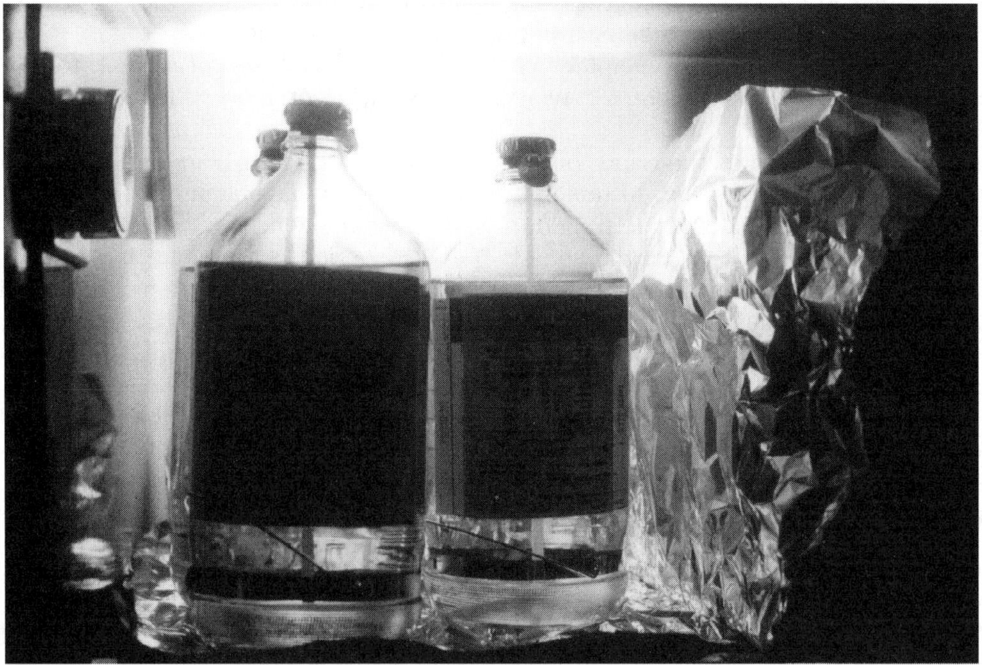

Figure 4.2. Home TPN solutions stored in a refrigerator. Most current home TPN patients add only multivitamins to their solutions before infusing. The patient is no longer responsible for "pharmacist" duties. (Photograph by Michael Rothkopf, M.D.)

Going Home

The prospect of going home can have a strong influence on the recovery of a patient. It improves the patient's mental attitude significantly and helps promote the acceptance phase of the reaction to illness, which is discussed below. Most patients would be willing to assume extra duties to facilitate discharge from the hospital. Research has found that those patients who become involved with their care achieve greater health and recovery from disease (1). At-home patients frequently recover more quickly and have better quality of life than those who remain in a hospital. However, homecare can be intimidating for some patients, and the physician should be sensitive to this issue when first approaching the patient.

Patients need to go through a process of training to become competent in the use of homecare devices. This has become easier because portable devices have been designed for simpler patient interfacing. Advancements in medical technology have produced sophisticated, portable equipment that is easy to operate by consumers.

Understanding Patients' Reactions

Until an individual suffers a serious illness, it is difficult to understand the struggles a patient must endure on a daily basis. Frustration, helplessness, and resentment are part of the routine. No matter how caring people are, the patient tends to feel isolated and severed from normal life. In some ways, the patient always remains alone because only he can go through the experience.

While physicians deal with serious illness and complex medical issues every day, the patient who has to cope with these conditions faces a significant change in lifestyle. Elisabeth Kübler-Ross described a process of adjustment for the patient facing a major illness (2). The patient progresses through stages such as denial, anger, and finally acceptance. The concept of going home with therapy may be less severe, yet it is still a major adjustment, and we believe that the Kübler-Ross stages apply (Table 4.1).

Table 4.1. Patient Reactions in Adjusting to a Major Illness

Denial
Anger
Despair
Sense of loss
Remorse
Acceptance
Control
Hope

Some people will be more affected at different stages and react more emotionally than others. The patient may initially seem attuned to what is happening and be moving forward with acceptance, but then may regress to an earlier emotional level.

Patients may be overwhelmed by the first consideration of homecare and may have trouble assimilating what is being explained. This is the denial phase. The patient may appear to be cognitive; however, the denial reaction alters his or her perception. A support person at this time can be a valuable contributor by listening to the doctor and asking questions for the patient. If the patient is alone, the physician should consider having a nurse or a sensitive member of his staff be available. This staff member could explain or answer questions once the physician has left.

Anger is the next phase of adaptation. The patient asks: "Why do I have to do this?" This anger or resentment may be directed toward the doctor, nurse, family, or others. It is amplified by the realization that the patient's activities and independence may be jeopardized. The patient will have to permit personal intrusions that will restrict him or her. If homecare is suggested at this sensitive time, it may seem overwhelming and will be rejected. It is important to understand that the patient in this phase is feeling grief. One's normal life has been interrupted. Plans and dreams may never be realized, and some of the anger the patient feels may be directed at himself.

When the anger dissipates, despair and a sense of hopelessness follow. Financial burdens and concerns about losing work because of medical absences may surface. The patient's sense of self-value is diminished. The patient can no longer care for himself or the family. A patient in this phase may express regrets for not pursuing a goal or opportunity. He may have remorse for not having enjoyed life more fully.

Once the patient gets beyond these phases, acceptance begins. The patient can develop an understanding of the problem and a positive perspective. The patient is ready to marshall reserves and attempt the process of getting better or living withthe disability—in essence, getting on with life.

At any of these stages, it is important that the patient be offered encouragement. Emotional support from others can be extremely valuable at this time. The ability to find solace from other people can help to ease the burden that the patient is facing. Anyone can be a member of the patient's emotional support team, including friends, family members, and healthcare providers.

The quality of the homecare organization is also an important component in the patient's ability to adjust to and accept the process. These companies provide supplies and services that will permit the patient to feel secure at home. They also provide an important psychological link to the health care system. The patient may have left the hospital, but he or she is still connected to a medical system that is able to respond quickly and appropriately to his or her needs.

Home infusion therapy gives a patient a great degree of control over his or her life. This would not be possible in an institutional setting. Although adjustments are needed to follow the prescribed infusion therapy, these changes are minimal when compared to the prospect of prolonged hospitalization. As long as adequate support is available, home therapy is the patient's treatment of choice.

Training and Practice

The process of training for home infusion involves learning a comprehensive model. However, these techniques are not beyond the reach of the average person and can be learned after two or three training sessions.

The patient must be able to understand very thorough verbal, hands-on, and written instructions from the nurse. To assist the patient and have him or her develop confidence in the home equipment, homecare companies provide training sessions and handbooks with step-by-step instructions to augment the training. During the teaching process, the patient must be able to demonstrate technical skill to the nurse, first with a model and then with his or her actual catheter. It must be emphasized that the success of patient proficiency is dependent on the teaching and communication skills of the homecare nurse.

Daily home nursing visits are made until the patient is confident with the home infusion process. The nurse then certifies that the patient can manage various techniques on his own. At that point, nursing visits can be decreased to once a week or less frequently. However, a nurse should continue to be available 24 hours a day for problems and emergencies. It is also important that the nurse periodically recheck the patient's techniques and certify his adequacy.

The initial prospect of performing these procedures for oneself can be somewhat intimidating (Fig. 4.3). However, the sense of independence gained is a very positive benefit, especially for a person with a chronic illness. For a patient who has undergone repeated hospitalizations, homecare is a welcome relief. After months of dealing with doctors, nurses, and technicians, the patient is finally free to make some of his own decisions.

Despite this newfound independence, a patient does come to rely on the homecare nurse. The nurse should be available to answer the many questions that arise during the course of therapy. Frequently, the nurse may become the link between the patient's medical needs and personal life. A rapport is reached and the homecare nurse becomes a critical member of the patient's support team.

The time commitment for homecare is minimal once the technical procedures become routine (Fig. 4.4). For example, a dress-

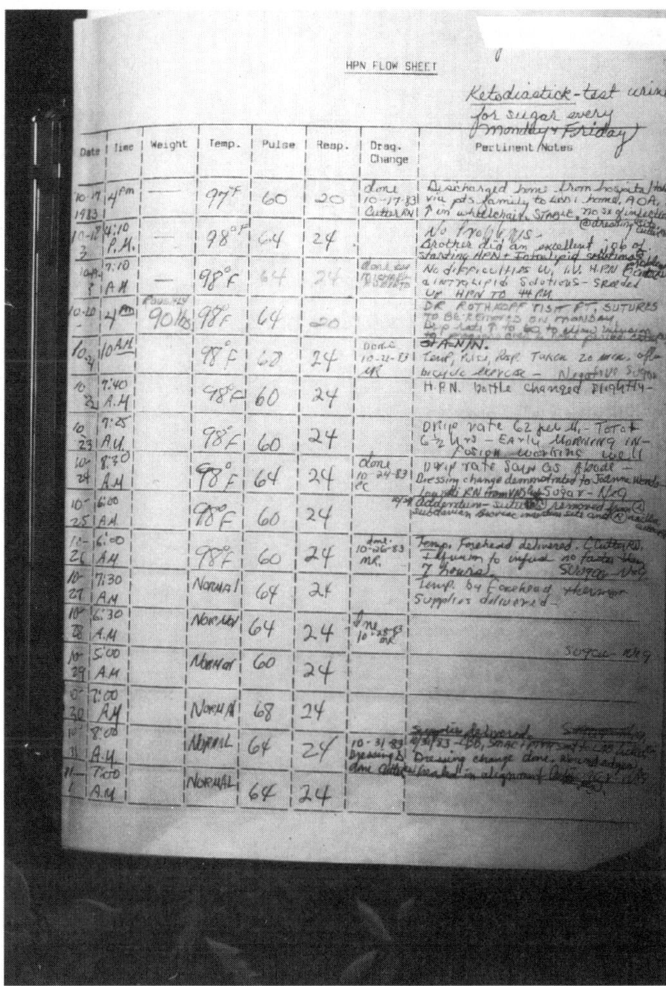

Figure 4.3. Home record of a patient—Week 1. This represents the complexity for the patient and detail required. (Photograph by Michael Rothkopf, M.D.)

ing change generally takes only 5 to 10 minutes. Similarly, the startup time for an infusion takes about 3 to 5 minutes. An experienced, trained patient prepares all the needed supplies beforehand. This minimizes the "hassle factor" and prevents surprises.

However, home infusion therapy can also complicate some seemingly simple everyday tasks. Good organization is a necessity. For example, planning for 1 or 2 nights away from home requires much attention to detail to ensure that essential supplies are not left behind and that there will be adequate refrigeration for medications and solutions. Long-distance trips require that arrangements be made in advance so the patient will know what to do and whom to call in an emergency. The homecare company can be very helpful in this regard. It usually has contacts throughout the country and very quickly can ship supplies and solutions almost anywhere.

The use of a portable pump can make a big difference between whether the patient feels trapped or independent. The portable pump gives a measure of freedom that cannot be achieved when using a larger pump on a pole. Such freedom of movement can make a tremendous difference in morale by maximizing flexibility and control for the patient.

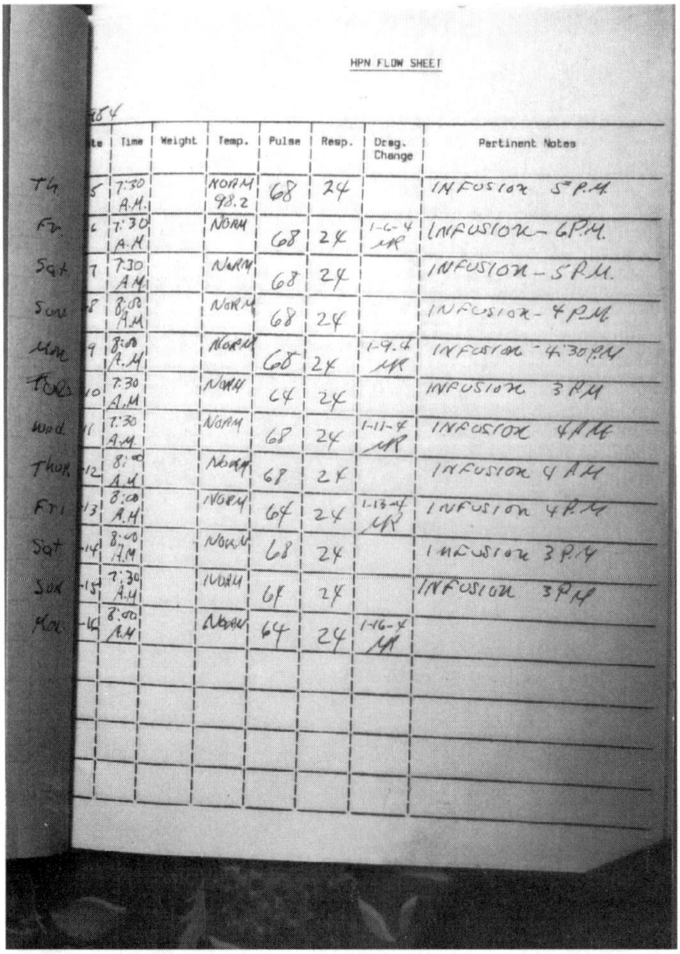

Figure 4.4. Home record of a patient—Week 10. Home TPN procedures have been incorporated into the patient's daily routine. (Photograph by Michael Rothkopf, M.D.)

Support

Home infusion therapy, while not technically difficult, can be very stressful. The type of emotional support and encouragement a patient receives is of paramount importance to his or her well-being and recovery. Caregivers play a crucial role in the outcome of a patient's recovery. When the patient and caregiver interact favorably, results are positive for both sides.

Family members are often called on to perform the role of caregiver; however, they are not always prepared to assume it. There may be reluctance in providing physical and emotional support. The family members may find it difficult to accept what is happening and may go through their own stages of adjustment. There may be resentment, embarrassment, and feelings of discomfort in the presence of the patient. Neither patient nor family member may know how to communicate their thoughts and feelings, and both patient and caregiver may feel isolated and lonely. It is important for family members to learn how to motivate each other, find coping mechanisms, and assist the patient in developing the ability to function at the highest possible level.

Sometimes friends and relatives are unsure of how to deal with the patient concerning home therapy. This may be a first encounter with intensive homecare. Since infusion therapy has long been associated with the hospital setting, it has a stigma of serious illness. Social interactions may be strained by this set of circumstances, and the patient could feel even more alienated. It is important to recognize that most people are unprepared to deal with the concept of chronic illness.

Similarly, the patient may need to talk about the change in his or her lifestyle but may be reluctant to raise the issue with friends or colleagues. This certainly is true in the workplace, where social interactions are expected to occur with some degree of professional distance. Employers need to understand the patient's special needs. On the other hand, an employee does not want to be viewed as "limited" or troublesome. A mistaken confidence might affect job security or promotional opportunities.

The homecare nurse can be very helpful in this regard, since he or she is a "safe" person with whom to talk. Through the nurse, the patient can benefit from the experience of others. By relating how other individuals using home infusion therapy have dealt with these problems, the homecare nurse also functions as a social worker. This process often translates into new insights for the patient and assures the patient that he or she is not alone.

Social behavior is affected when the patient is on nutritional support. It soon becomes apparent how many social activities revolve around eating. While a patient is not typically hungry on HPN, he or she might miss the social aspects of eating. Friends may feel uncomfortable when eating around the HPN patient and feel a need to protect the patient from his or her desire to participate in the meal.

The most difficult of the social aspects occurs around the issue of dating. This is especially true when dealing with new acquaintances. Whether to inform people right away or to conceal the problem is a dilemma that reminds the patient of the limitations of his or her disease. In an effort to protect oneself from rejection, the patient may withdraw from certain social situations.

Support groups and organizations can provide assistance to both patients and caregivers. Patients can learn more about their illness and find that there are other people struggling with similar issues. Patients should be informed of local groups and national organizations such as The Oley Foundation (Albany Medical Center, Albany, NY), which provides a newsletter on home nutrition support, as well as organizations such as the Crohn's and Colitis Foundation of America (Park Ave. South, New York, NY) and the Cystic Fibrosis Foundation (Arlington Rd., Bethesda, MD). The American Cancer Society is another important resource. In fact, the physician's office should have literature available and a contact name and number of any local group.

Lifestyle and Work Schedule

The use of homecare therapeutics and the concomitant lifestyle changes that occur can help to reorder one's priorities. The patient's schedule must be reoriented to include the time for the treatment.

Often a patient can administer therapy overnight while sleeping. In this method, interruptions of work and social activities are minimized. However, the quality of sleep may be affected. For example, the "feel" of the tubing and the sound of the infusion pump are foreign to a person's ordinary bedtime routine.

Choosing treatment during the day eradicates the concern over sleep deprivation but adds the possibility that a patient will have to take time from other activities to monitor the therapy. It also requires the patient to be able to carry equipment, solutions, and supplies with him.

One of the great advantages of homecare is that it has the potential to return an individual to the workplace. Managing a career with a chronic illness requires flexibility, but it is done, and the development of devices such as portable microcomputers has added the ability to do some work at home. When the patient is returning to the workplace, every effort should be made to allow the patient to adapt to his existing employment. Alternative work schedules can be helpful. In fact, flex hours are no longer unusual, and many companies have adopted them for personnel with various needs.

The implications of changing to a new job include new pressures and stresses, a possible loss of flexibility, and a potential change in insurance benefits. With rapidly increasing health insurance costs, many employers are cutting back in various ways, including the addition of pre-existing condition clauses and lifetime maximums. This can be a serious issue and can even preclude new employment opportunities if alternative coverage is not available. These issues are just some of the concerns facing the homecare patient in the workplace.

When one is a patient receiving homecare services, leisure time becomes very important. Unlike ordinary circumstances, this is time not only free from work but also free from the effort of home therapy. One must remember that the reason for all the effort is to enjoy more of what life has to offer. The homecare patient deserves some pampering too!

Summary

The development of portable devices for use in the home and physician willingness to treat their patients outside of the hospital have given patients new freedom. Before the patient becomes successful with home therapy, however, he must first deal with the emotional turmoil of his illness. Once he can accept his illness, he is amenable to training, accepting support people, and trying to reconstruct his life. Homecare is not for every patient, but for patients who are motivated and want to regain control over their lives, home therapy provides a worthwhile alternative.

References

1. Cousins N. Anatomy of an Illness. New York: W. W. Norton, 1979.

2. Kübler-Ross E. On Death and Dying. New York: Macmillan, 1969.

5

EVALUATING HOMECARE ORGANIZATIONS

Michael M. Rothkopf[a]

CHAPTER AT A GLANCE: Physicians have a fiduciary role in selecting and monitoring the homecare company for their patients. The choice of a vendor and nursing service can have a significant impact on the success of therapy and patient's satisfaction and confidence with care at home. For homecare therapeutics to be effective in replacing hospital-level services, a system of quality assurance and monitoring is needed. The Joint Commission on Accreditation of Healthcare Organizations provides a structure that can be applied to both hospital and homecare services. This chapter provides objective criteria to allow the physician to judge the quality of services rendered to his patient.

Introduction: The Hospital Without Walls

The concept of intensive homecare was initially developed for patients with a long-term dependence on life supportive therapy. These patients had benefited from the advances in modern medicine that enabled them to survive critical illnesses or a critical loss of function in a major organ system. Yet, although they had been given a new opportunity for life, they faced the realization that they could only survive within the confines of a modern hospital. The longer these patients lived, the less appropriate long-term hospitalization became. Gradually, patients receiving long-term mechanical ventilator support, dialysis, and par-

enteral nutrition were moved to step-down units and long-term care facilities. In a form of natural evolution, the most stable of these patients ventured homeward, taking their hospital-based equipment with them.

Thus was born the hospital without walls. It was designed to support those early pioneer patients who insisted on going home with life-support therapies. These patients needed a means of obtaining their equipment and supplies, training for the use of the machines, and techniques and support from medical professionals when complications arose.

In the beginning this was a rare event indeed. Careful planning went into each case and extensive training was given to the patient and family members. As the concept proved workable, and as the structure of intensive homecare gelled, more and more patients were given the opportunity to be treated at home

---

[a]*Barbara A. McCann wrote this chapter in the first edition.*

with a growing list of services. Today, intensive homecare is an integral part of the healthcare delivery system.

What the Homecare Organization Does

Homecare organizations are providers of medical equipment, supplies, and professional services. These are the distilled essence of what the hospital does, minus the hospital structure and its maintenance costs. "Hotel-type" services such as food service, laundry, and housekeeping are also absent from the homecare model.

For example, a patient receiving parenteral nutrition in the hospital has the use of the following equipment and supplies: hospital bed, nutrient solution, intravenous tubing, intravenous pump, intravenous catheter, catheter dressings, needles, alcohol wipes, etc. This patient receives the following services: physician visits, nursing care, pharmacist mixing of the nutrient solution, nurse hanging of intravenous solution, dietitian consultation, social services, laboratory services, food services, housekeeping, and laundry services.

By comparison, the same patient on homecare receives exactly the same array of supplies listed for the hospitalized patient except for the hospital bed. However, the homecare patient receives much more limited services than the hospital patient. Physician input is limited to writing the prescription and care plan and periodic follow-up. Nursing and pharmacist services are limited to the absolute minimum required for training and monitoring. Laboratory specimens are sent to an outside laboratory. Dietary and social service consultations are on a strictly as-needed basis. The patient or family provides much of the remaining nursing services and all of the food, housekeeping, and laundry services.

Another key activity performed by the homecare organization is the training of the patient to become a part of the homecare team. The homecare organization is also responsible for supervising the preparation of a safe home environment and for the upkeep of the equipment used by the patient receiving homecare.

While the final responsibility for outcome remains with the prescribing physician, the homecare organization is more of a partner in patient care than in most traditional healthcare models. This is because of the basic fact that the patient is at home, far from the daily contact of the physician. In fact, the homecare staff often has more direct contact with the patient than the prescribing physician. Therefore, the physician must rely more completely on statements made by members of the homecare team.

Structure of the Hospital Without Walls

Evolution and Organization

Homecare services were initially affiliated with large hospitals, particularly those with teaching services or medical school affiliations. However, in the early days, most hospitals could not provide a sufficient volume of intensive homecare patients to justify the expense and complexity of establishing their own separate homecare program.

As a result, independent homecare companies formed that could service several hospitals within a specific geographic location. This diffused the economic requirements while increasing the efficiency of the system. These organizations proved to be quite successful and soon replaced many of the hospital-based programs.

In many cases, the hospital has remained part of the homecare organization through a joint venture or partnership arrangement that makes use of hospital employees, facilities, and equipment. These affiliated hospitals generally have homecare departments that provide background work for patient referral while the patient is hospitalized. In some cases, these homecare departments train the patient and prepare the patient for home therapy.

Homecare organizations can have different structures depending on the treatments they offer and the economic conditions they operate in. They range from community-sponsored visiting nurse agencies, to homecare departments within hospitals, to free-standing homecare companies. They may be government agencies, nonprofit organizations, or for-profit corporations. They may be privately held or publicly traded.

Staffing

Establishing the necessary support system to provide intensive homecare requires specialized staffing. Motivated professional (nurses and pharmacists) and support staff (biomedical technicians, reimbursement specialists, inventory managers, and delivery persons) are needed. Each staff member must be knowledgeable of the special needs of the homecare patient and of the protocol guidelines for the tasks they perform. An on-call system with 24-hour availability of each key component must be in place.

Contingency Planning

A thorough contingency plan should exist. The homecare facility must recognize the patients' dependence on life-sustaining therapy. Adequate planning should exist to cope with such crises as severe weather conditions, fires, and power outages. The homecare facility should have alternative methods to enable preparation and delivery of solutions, equipment, materials, and continuity of care regardless of conditions. In the event that the homecare facility cannot meet the conditions, arrangements should be in place to notify other facilities or local hospitals and transfer the patient.

Licensure

Specific licensure to operate a homecare facility is generally not required or even available in most states. However, most homecare organizations maintain a pharmacy that is governed by the state board of pharmacy in each respective state. Regional or national companies often have additional requirements for out-of-state pharmacy licenses, since they may dispense prescription medications to patients across state boundaries.

Some homecare companies are licensed as nursing agencies, although this is not always a requirement. Significant variation exists from state to state on this issue. Medicare-certified visiting nursing agencies are established based on federal guidelines. These agencies are generally the only organizations that can coordinate homecare services for Medicare and other federally insured beneficiaries such as CHAMPUS. However, their availability is generally limited to one agency per county.

Choosing a Homecare Organization

The Physician's Fiduciary Responsibility

Effective planning of homecare therapeutics means that physicians now face the issue of choosing a vendor who will supply drugs and services to their patients. The referring physician should recognize the significance of this decision and evaluate care options critically. He must realize that the homecare company and nursing agency will be responsible for training and monitoring his patient. The patient often has no medical knowledge and therefore has much trepidation about the process. Therefore, the choice of homecare organization can significantly affect patient attitude.

The referring physician must be cognizant of legal liability issues should the patient suffer from an error made during homecare therapy. This liability may extend beyond medical malpractice to include issues of product liability and supervision of ancillary staff. The referring physician should be aware of these factors and satisfy himself that the referral serves the best interests of his patient. Insurance companies, HMOs, and discharge planners attempt to influence the pattern of referral based on economic issues (see Chapters 8 and 9). However, the physician bears the major liability risk and needs to satisfy himself that the referral is appropriate.

Despite the importance of their decisions, referring physicians are often poorly prepared to make such choices. The field is very new and few standards are available to allow for objectivity. Many claims regarding quality and depth of services are made without substantiation. The physician should take an active role in selecting the homecare supplier specific to his patient's needs. It is not sufficient to simply accept the statements of a vendor promising service. While these statements are generally given in earnest, the profit motive sometimes causes companies to stretch beyond their capabilities.

Physician Evaluation of Homecare Organizations

Quality of Care Provided

The quality, professionalism, and efficiency of the homecare company will determine how the patient deals with the complex task of self care. It will have a major impact on the progress and outcome of therapy. The patient's perceptions of and satisfaction with homecare (and the physician who supervises it) also rest on these issues.

It is expected that eventually market conditions and government regulation will exclude those vendors who are inadequate. In the interim, the referring physician must be vigilant. A checklist including documentation of the facility's licensure, staffing, geographic limits, and scope of services is a useful tool. Additionally, information regarding the company's experience (i.e., the number of patients treated in each category of homecare) should be made available. Evidence of a quality assurance system that checks on the operational adequacy of the homecare provider should be present. The referring physician should scrutinize the promotional literature and ask the representative for facts to back up the claims.

Cost Effectiveness

There are significant expenses associated with homecare. The patient, insurer, or government agency will rightly expect that the physician has selected a vendor who will abide by the concept of cost-effectiveness. Furthermore, the patient has the right to expect that he will not be taken advantage of by unscrupulous medical suppliers. Most patients depend on their doctor to monitor this concern.

Protocols

The homecare company often serves to educate the physician about standards of care for the home setting. Many physicians are not knowledgeable of the field and lack extensive experience with homecare. Written protocols that define appropriate monitoring and treatment can be very useful to the doctor. They provide guidelines to follow and a framework to define a standard of treatment.

Scope of Services

Just as the physician makes a conscious decision on referring a patient for a consultation, radiologic examination, or hospital admission, the referral to a homecare company should involve a value judgment based on the patient's needs and physician's expectation that those needs can be met. Every vendor is not necessarily capable of providing for all of the patient's needs, although many claim to be. The quality and scope of services an individual homecare facility can provide may vary significantly. Geographic or financial issues may also affect the referral process.

For example, a local homecare company may do a stellar job taking care of long-term adult TPN patients. They may have had extensive experience with such cases and anticipate the needs of the patients. However, this same organization may not be able to adjust its operations sufficiently to care for a pediatric home antibiotic patient or a pregnant woman on tocolytic therapy.

Geographic Service Area

The selection of a homecare organization by the physician is the selection of a team that will help him manage a patient receiving homecare therapeutics. Therefore, the team members, particularly the nurses, must have the capacity to reach the patient in a timely manner. This calls on a finite geographic reach, which is a function of the area and accessibility.

Therefore, an important part of the selection process involves questioning the homecare agency as to the geographic accessibility of nurses to the patient. A homecare nurse should be expected to reach a patient's home within 1 or 2 hours after being called. In a rural area, served by an interstate highway, this could easily equate to 50 miles or more. However, in a congested suburb or urban setting, it might be substantially less.

Reputation

The company's reputation in the community for professionalism and quick response time is another valuable factor. Reviewing a sample medical record is also helpful in assessing the appropriateness of care and adequacy of documentation. An analysis of the management and key personnel is warranted, including information on the medical background of these individuals. Similarly, the composition of a professional advisory board and its real contribution to maintaining quality standards should be evaluated.

Accreditation Status

Standards for homecare services are being implemented. The Joint Commission on the Accreditation of Healthcare Organizations (JCAHO) published homecare standards in 1988 and 1995 (1). The JCAHO has an active accreditation process that involves site visits and evaluations of each homecare facility. The National League for Nursing has also instituted a Community Health Accreditation Program (CHAP). This program is voluntary and is intended to provide an index of quality for homecare providers.

Several professional organizations have also published criteria for participation in homecare for their members. These include the American Nurses Association (2), The American Society for Parenteral and Enteral Nutrition (ASPEN) (3, 4), and the American College of Physicians (5).

JCAHO Standards for Homecare Providers

Background and Evolution

Between 1986 and 1988, the JCAHO undertook a national consensus process with homecare providers, consumers, and payers to develop standards that addressed the scope of homecare services. This included not only the services provided by the traditional home health agencies but also by private-duty companies, pediatric homecare agencies, home-infusion companies (intensive homecare), and home respiratory and durable medical equipment companies. What emerged after four national field reviews by over 5000 participants and 10 national meetings was a unique approach to standards for homecare. Knowledge of these standards can be utilized by a referring physician to objectively determine the adequacy of care rendered by a particular homecare organization.

The Eleven Standards

The national consensus reached was that regardless of the type of services provided, seven common areas must be addressed in all segments of the homecare industry. In addition, four standards should be addressed that are unique to the particular services being delivered. Together, these 11 standards form the basis of the JCAHO accreditation process (Table 5.1). These 11 principles of quality homecare are translated into the chapters in the manual of Standards for the Accreditation of Home Care (1) and the Accreditation Manual for Home Care (6).

The Accreditation Process

The accreditation process that implements these standards includes documentation review; patient, caregiver, and staff interviews; and home visits. A documentation review includes not only the entries in records, but also policies and procedures to ascertain the effectiveness of the organization's procedures. Staff members are then interviewed regarding their care and their understanding of policies and procedures. The home visits focus on observing the delivery of care and interactions between the staff and the patient or caregiver, as well as interviewing the patient and caregiver.

Organizationally, the review process considers the services offered, the organization's work in evaluation of its own effectiveness, and the long-term and short-term plan to remain viable and to respond to the needs of the population chosen to be served. The surveys are conducted by individuals whose experience and area of expertise are relevant to the type of

Table 5.1. The Eleven Standards

The seven common areas are:

1. Patient rights and responsibilities are recognized and respected.
2. There is an effective process of patient intake, assessment of needs, planning to meet those needs, coordination of care, and appropriate discharge.
3. There is effective safety management and infection control in the delivery of services.
4. Documentation represents care provided.
5. There is appropriate governance of the organization.
6. There is effective and efficient management of the organization.
7. The organization systematically monitors and evaluates the quality and appropriateness of care.

Standards that are unique to particular services being delivered relate to:

8. The delivery of services by home health professionals;
9. Personal care and support of activities in daily living;
10. Home pharmaceutical services including the compounding, dispensing, delivery, and administration of the drug or instruction in self-administration and ongoing clinical monitoring of the patient; and
11. The selection, delivery, and set-up of medical equipment in the home, including instruction in its safe and appropriate use and ongoing maintenance.

provider being reviewed. They include RNs, certified IV nurses, homecare pharmacists, and registered respiratory therapists.

The goals of the accreditation process are fourfold:

1. To provide a valid outside assessment of an organization's compliance with national standards;
2. To provide a forum for consumers, providers, and payers to develop and utilize national standards to define quality homecare as the services provided increase or change in scope;
3. To provide onsite consultation and education to providers on how to improve care; and
4. To demonstrate the credibility of an emerging industry.

In the execution of this process, the homecare standards come to life as a management process directed at delivering quality care.

At the completion of an accreditation process the homecare organization is judged by a numerical scoring system and is issued a review of its activities. The organization then receives one of five types of accreditation: Not Accredited, Provisional Accreditation, Conditional Accreditation, Accreditation, or Accreditation with Commendation (Table 5.2). An organization that is found to be in overall compliance with the standards is awarded accreditation for 3 years. The accreditation is not automatically renewed.

The following is an overview of the key areas of the standards and their intent from the perspective of the expected behavior of the organization and outcomes demonstrated in patient care. These are offered to familiarize the reader with some of the detailed analysis that goes with the accreditation process. A physician involved in providing or assessing homecare services can request a copy of the standards from JCAHO.

Appropriate Involvement of the Patient and Caregiver

A new and important player has emerged in defining the quality of healthcare: **the patient.** This is particularly evident in homecare. Without round-the-clock staff and immediate access to expertise found in a hospital, quality of care is determined by the effective interaction of the homecare staff, the patient, and his or her caregiver(s).

The patient has the right to make informed decisions regarding care. The provision of intensive homecare particularly challenges this right. It means that the staff must provide sufficient information for the patient to make decisions about care. Recognizing the complexity of this treatment, the challenge is communicating in a language or manner that patients can reasonably be expected to understand. Overlooking how one commu-

Table 5.2. Types of Accreditation Decisions

Type of Decision	*Conditions That Lead to This Type of Decision*
Accreditation with Commendation This is the highest accreditation decision. It is awarded when an organization has demonstrated exemplary performance.	An organization is eligible for accreditation with commendation if the summary grid score for all applicable services is 90 or above and no follow-up monitoring has been assigned.
Accreditation This decision means an organization is in overall compliance with applicable standards. Accreditation is awarded with or without type I recommendation. A type I recommendation(s) is a recommendation or a group of recommendations that must be resolved within a specified period of time or the organization risks losing its accreditation.	An organization in this category demonstrates overall compliance with the applicable standards but needs improvement in a specific area(s) to achieve overall compliance with standards in that area. Many times, such improvement will be monitored through the assignment of some type of follow-up monitoring, such as a focused survey or written progress report.
Conditional Accreditation This indicates that multiple substantial standards compliance deficiencies exist in an organization. Correction of deficiencies, which serve as the basis for further consideration of continuing accreditation, must be demonstrated through follow-up survey.	This accreditation is given when the survey results in the assignment of follow-up monitoring in many areas, indicating that the organization's overall performance is marginal, and when an organization has not corrected type 1 recommendations in the time frames specified. Organizations with this status must develop a plan of correction, have it approved by the Joint Commission, and demonstrate sufficient improvement in a follow-up survey within 6 months. After the follow-up survey, the organization will either be accredited (with or without type 1 recommendations) or not accredited.
Provisional Accreditation	A provisional accreditation is given when an organization has demonstrated substantial compliance with the selected structural standards surveyed in the first of two surveys conducted under the Early Survey Policy. The second survey is conducted approximately 6 months later to allow the organization time to demonstrate a track record of performance. Provisional accreditation status remains until the organization completes this second, full survey.
Not Accredited	This results when an organization has been denied accreditation, when its accreditation is withdrawn by the Joint Commission, or when it withdraws from the accreditation process. This designation also describes any organization that has never applied for accreditation.

From Accreditation Manual for Home Care. Oakbrook Terrace, IL: Joint Commission on Accreditation of Healthcare Organizations, 1994.

nicates and whether it is done in an understandable manner can result in the failure of the therapy. Providers need to be aware that the primary caregivers (the patient and family) must understand what their responsibilities are and, simply, what they are supposed to do.

The challenge of effective communication with the patient and caregiver also extends to their rights as recipients of healthcare. Providing services in the informal atmosphere of the home can lead the staff to loosen some of the professionalism associated with the institutional setting.

The following questions are posed by JCAHO to evaluate compliance with standards in the area of patients' rights and responsibilities:

1. Do we inform the patient about the nature and purpose of technical procedures performed in the home and who will perform the procedure?
2. Do we advise patients that they have the right to refuse all or part of their care and inform them of the consequences?
3. Do we obtain documented voluntary consent for a patient to receive experimental treatment or to participate in research protocols?
4. Is the patient advised at admission of the organization's charges and policy for payment of service? Critically, do they know that when the payment ends it may halt the delivery of services by some companies?

As the standards emphasize important elements of communication with the patient, they also require that the organization and staff seek effective communication with patients. This is done in two particular standards:

1. Does the organization have a process for receiving and acting on patient complaints without reprisal to the patient? Is the patient informed about this process?
2. Does the organization monitor patient satisfaction with the care as part of their ongoing quality assurance process?

For many professionals, these standards may seem basic, but they are easily forgotten amid the challenges of arriving in the home to find situations where there is no running water, the refrigerator does not work, the wrong pump was delivered, or the family does not speak English. The accreditation survey evaluates the integration of these rights into the process of treatment, and acknowledges the unique demands of care at home and the role of the patient and caregivers.

Another significant area that affects outcomes is patient and caregiver instruction. The standards address several aspects of patient instruction, including self-treatment (such as the preparation of sterile preparations in the home) and the disposition of hazardous substances such as needles, syringes, and tubing that are by-products of treatment. A primary concern in the review of instruction is its comprehensiveness relative to the patient's responsibility; an organization should have procedures for monitoring the patient's understanding of instructions.

Timely Access to Care

Intensive care in an institution relies on a myriad of staff in various departments to be available on short notice to respond to the needs of patients. The homecare standards try to emphasize the very different environment in which intensive homecare must be effectively delivered.

A homecare organization should accept a patient only if it is capable of providing care at the level of intensity required by the patient's condition. This standard considers not only an assessment of meeting the routine daily treatment needs, but also the ability to respond at off hours or to difficult conditions. For example, can the staff respond at 2:00 a.m. on Saturday morning or during an unexpected storm? Are there staff, supplies, drugs, and drug products available 24 hours a day, 7 days a week?

Associated with this issue is acknowledging when the patient has needs that the organization cannot meet. One expectation of a quality provider is that they be aware of alternative services available in the community to meet specific needs and that they will refer the patient and/or the physician to these services. In some instances, this will also mean advising patients and their physicians in a timely manner that a transfer is needed. Again, the issue of communication is tied to assuring a process that results in timely care and, consequently, continuity in meeting the patient's care needs.

Appropriate Clinical Decision Making

Quality care in any setting requires knowledge of the patient's needs and appropriate responses to them. The challenge of homecare adds the consideration not only of the patient, but also of the family or support system and the home environment. Initial and periodic assessments should identify the problems, needs, and capabilities of the patient and family.

For example, the patient's need may be home antibiotic therapy. However, beyond the immediate medical need is the environmental problem. It might be that the patient lives in a rural area and delivery of the antibiotic in a stable state may require special arrangements for transportation.

A psychosocial problem may be the issue for an elderly patient whose primary caregiver is a reluctant daughter-in-law with two preschool children at home. There may be a problem in treatment compliance because, although the daughter-in-law can be taught administration, the frequency of administration required is too demanding. Conversely, adverse home conditions can be overcome by the staff's recognition of the psychological strengths afforded by a particularly motivated patient or dedicated caregiver.

The ability to conduct a complete assessment also adds a dimension to the qualifications of the professional involved. This staff member must have not only the required clinical skills associated with the type of treatment provided, but also the skills to assess the psychological, social, and physical environment in which treatment will be delivered.

The Plan of Care

The standards distinguish between the plan of treatment, which is the physician's orders, and the plan of care, which is the organization's plan of action in response to the patient's needs and problems in accordance with the doctor's orders. The intent of the standards is to make this process and document an organizational and clinical tool in response to patient needs.

From the clinical perspective, the plan reflects a consideration of the medical needs of the patient and the environmental, psychological, and social problems associated with the process of treatment. In this regard the survey process evaluates the specific services being provided and the action being taken to respond to the needs and problems noted in the assessment. The evaluation also considers whether the action taken and services provided work toward the achievement of the goals for this patient.

Goals are a basic professional expectation—a statement of what one expects to accomplish for a specific patient and the desired outcome. The standards require that the staff state goals in reasonable and measurable terms. A goal such as "The patient will successfully complete IV antibiotic therapy" is not acceptable, as it does not define "successfully." Does this mean that therapy will be completed without any adverse outcome, such as an incidence of phlebitis or site infection? Or does it mean that the patient will be in compliance with the regimen, or that the patient will be disease-free? The challenge of quality care includes defining our goals in care and when we have achieved them.

The plan of care should also act as a document of effective management. The plan to meet a patient's needs should consider the effective and appropriate utilization of an organization's resources. Resources in this instance include staff members and their time. The care plan should include the type, frequency, and duration of services to be provided. For example, nurses should not be performing services that could more effectively be provided by a less costly but well-trained aide. The frequency should be reasonable and not reflect overutilization or underutilization of services. The duration of care should be sufficient to meet the goals of care.

A primary reason that care plans fail in meeting these expectations is that they are not kept current. The standards and survey process carefully consider whether the actions and services being provided are consistent with the plan and whether the problems and goals noted are current with what is being observed in the home. In the absence of an ongoing care planning process, interventions can become a series of reactions without direction. This can result in a wasteful use of an organization's resources and an adverse outcome for a patient.

Effectively Coordinating Care

The most qualified staff and the most comprehensive care planning can result in poor quality homecare if there is ineffective coordination. Unlike in a hospital, the team with whom communication must occur is often physically scattered. The team comprises the patient and the caregiver in the home, the physician in the office, the homecare staff (nurse, pharmacist, dietitians, etc.), and frequently other homecare organizations or contractors who are also providing services.

A second factor unique to homecare is that no single individual consistently emerges as being responsible for coordinating care. In response, the standards require that an accredited provider designate a qualified staff member to assume this role. This individual's responsibility is to facilitate communication about patient needs, services, and problems and responses to staff, physician(s), and the patient. Also, the coordinator must interact with other organizations involved in delivering care.

Finally, the standards and survey process evaluate whether the actions and goals of the services provided are complementary and reflect cooperative care planning. These standards assess yet another dimension of effective clinical and organizational utilization of resources. They focus on these critical questions:

1. Is there duplication of effort?
2. Are the instructions and/or actions and services acting at cross-purposes for the patient?
3. Is there a gap—a need that could be met being lost in the coordination of effort?

The serious problems that can result from poor coordination mandate a formal care coordination system in homecare. A more informal system may suffice in an institution by virtue of the checks and balances of multiple staff members who come in direct contact with the patient and other caregivers.

Effective Execution of the Plan of Care

The accreditation process challenges the homecare provider to demonstrate that clinical decisions are appropriate for the patient's needs. Are you stabilizing or improving the patient's clinical status? Is the care achieving the stated goals? The answers lie not only in the evaluation of individual patient outcomes but also in the evaluation of the systems put in place to ensure that quality care is provided.

Assessment begins with the staff—particularly the number, qualifications, and current competence of the staff. The Joint Commission standards require that staffing be appropriate to the treatment and the level of care provided.

The organization is expected to provide **inservice** and **continuing education** to maintain staff skills and to provide new knowledge and training as the scope of service and treatment changes. The standards also require evaluation of the qualifications of the supervisory personnel. Finally, the standards require that the competence of the staff be assessed annually and before any change in the scope of services occurs.

The next element in assessing patient outcomes is reviewing the process of care. A key factor assessed in the standards is whether correct and sufficient information is being gathered in order to make care decisions. A good example is the drug profile used by both the nursing and pharmacy staff in intensive homecare. The standards ask the following questions:

1. Is the patient's age noted and are regular weights recorded as appropriate to the therapy?
2. Are the patient's current diagnoses known? (For example, secondary diagnoses such as diabetes mellitus can affect the therapy related to a primary diagnosis.)
3. Is there a current medication list that notes the route, dose, and frequency of all pre-

scription and nonprescription drugs—not just those provided by your organization?

4. Do you know of any drug allergies or sensitivities?
5. Has the home visiting staff reported home remedies being used and, if so, what are they?
6. Do you have all necessary current laboratory values?

What is done with this information is then the next step in evaluating outcome. In many ways the standards are asking whether the care coordination addressed earlier is working. A key player on this team is the attending physician. The survey process looks not only at whether care is rendered in accordance with physician orders, but whether information is regularly exchanged with the physician. Is the physician contacted when the patient's condition changes or when an unexpected response to therapy occurs?

For example, the standards assess not only if the nurse in the home has conveyed information about the weight of a TPN patient receiving lipids, but also if the pharmacist has conveyed to the nurse the drug monitoring results that indicate that the patient may be digitalis toxic, with particular symptoms that should be assessed.

The standards require an ongoing assessment of **drug administration:**

1. Is the drug therapeutically appropriate for the patient?
2. Is there therapeutic duplication in a patient's drug regimen?
3. Are the dose, frequency, and route of administration appropriate for the patient?
4. Is there adherence to the drug regimen?
5. Are there potential drug, food, or diagnostic test interactions or disease limitations to drug use?
6. Are clinical or laboratory monitoring methods used to detect drug effectiveness, side effects, toxicity, or adverse effects?

As the variety of drugs that can be administered at home increases, providers may be faced with a referral for a drug that they have not administered before. The standards require that the organization make some decisions before accepting that referral. Specifically, it must consider the resources of the agency, the qualifications of the staff, and which drugs or drug classes the homecare staff can administer safely and appropriately, including the routes of administration.

For some providers it may be easier to respond by noting that there are particular drugs, such as amphotericin B or chemotherapeutic agents, that they either will not administer or will administer only after a first dose has been given under controlled circumstances.

Once the organization has decided which drugs they will administer, the standards require that they determine who will administer the drugs and how it can be done effectively. Homecare nurses have a variety of educational and experience backgrounds to meet the different needs of patients cared for at home. Many organizations require that nurses be certified for IV drug administration and have experience in administering different types of infused drugs. Unlike in the hospital setting, the nurse primarily acts alone in the home without immediate access to clinical supervision or backup assistance. The standards require the organization to demonstrate competence of individuals to administer the drug or to instruct the patient in self-administration.

The second element of this standard is that there are policies and procedures related to each treatment modality. The intent of the standard is to introduce and maintain standardized procedures in the process of drug administration. This may mean that the procedures are adapted from the inpatient setting to reflect the unique aspects of care in the home.

The third element in the process is to ensure that the staff members are prepared to respond to adverse drug reactions. The standards and survey process consider (*a*) the types of drugs an organization provides; (*b*) the effective response to an adverse reaction or a problem (such as a spill of a chemotherapeutic agent); (*c*) the accessibility and usability of the materials (i.e., ensuring that they are not expired or reduced in effectiveness after months of being stored in the trunk of a car); and (*d*) the training of the staff (does the nurse know when and how to use the appropriate drugs or products?).

Finally, a process should exist to ensure that the administered drug is (*a*) identified as the drug ordered for that patient; (*b*) stable (e.g., without indication of deterioration); and (*c*) not contraindicated for the patient.

These standards for drug administration apply not only to an organization that provides pharmaceutical services but also to an organization that may administer a drug that was picked up at the pharmacy or a doctor's office or was delivered by another company to the patient's home.

Infection control presents another group of challenges to a homecare organization. A range of policies are needed to address personal hygiene, isolation precautions, aseptic procedures, and the appropriate cleaning and sterilization of pumps and other equipment. The staff must be instructed in infection control processes appropriate to their responsibilities, and a monitoring system should be in place to protect the patient, caregiver, and staff from communicable infection. The standards require a system of reporting infections related to care such as (*a*) infections the patient has upon admission; (*b*) infections occurring after admission; (*c*) infections of a caregiver (such as active tuberculosis); and (*d*) infections of staff members that may be transmitted to patients or may have possibly resulted from delivering patient services. These reports then need to be maintained and used. An expectation of accreditation is that an organization be able to know, monitor, and identify its performance in the area of infection control.

Ongoing Monitoring and Evaluation

The awarding of accreditation indicates that a care provider has the organizational structure and working processes that most often result in quality patient care. A central expectation of this award is that the organization assumes the responsibility to monitor and evaluate its own performance as a care provider in the absence of an accrediting body being onsite or an upcoming survey.

The quality assurance standards contemplate a commitment of resources, time, and staff from the level of governance or owner/operator to those who implement the process. Quality assurance effectively done is expected to be an important source of management data, addressing key questions such as:

1. Did we provide quality care? Does it reflect accepted community standards of practice?
2. Was the care appropriate? Did we do the right thing at the right time for the patient?
3. Was our care effective? Did we achieve our goals?
4. Were the services adequate in quantity? Did we underutilize or overutilize our resources?
5. Should we have accepted this patient for homecare?

In a period of shrinking reimbursement and the increasing liability presented by patients receiving intensive homecare, an effective organization and management team need to have the answers to these questions.

However, an organization can be easily overwhelmed in the collection of such data and inadvertently defeat the purpose of quality assurance efforts. The standards help the organization to focus its efforts where quality assurance is most valuable:

High volume: These services usually consume the majority of the organization's resources, and it is critical to ensure that what you do the most of is done well and in the most effective manner.

High risk: These services may present risk to the patient, the staff, and/or the organization and clearly need ongoing monitoring for a variety of financial and quality reasons.

Problem-prone: These services most often represent where the organization has "stretched" itself, and an otherwise commonly delivered service becomes a source of real or potential problems, such as caring for the patient who suffers from organic brain syndrome, or who has a frail caregiver, or who lives in a rural area miles from the nearest provider.

The organization should set expected levels of performance of care in these areas, which become the pivotal point of the monitoring and evaluation efforts. This means that the organization not only indicates activities, events, occurrences, and/or outcomes for each important aspect of care, but also identifies a level of performance that is expected to demonstrate that care is effective, adequate in quantity, and provided in the best setting. The level set (e.g., 100%, 85%, etc.) also represents the point at which further evaluation is initiated.

For example, if an organization determines that effective and appropriate care is provided when 90% of all patients have an assessment completed by a registered nurse within 24 hours of admission, and monitoring indicates that 92% of admissions achieved this level, no further review is needed. It is important to emphasize that the homecare organization should identify the most critical areas of care and devote its resources to monitoring those areas. The single area of monitoring that is **mandated** by the standards is patient satisfaction.

The quality assurance (QA) process emphasizes ongoing monitoring and evaluation. The process must focus on important aspects of care as described above. The management and staff must be aware of the quality and appropriateness of these areas at all times and not solely when a problem occurs.

The QA process further requires that when care is not meeting expected levels of performance, there is evidence of action being taken. Action can be demonstrated by changes in patient services, management actions, or inservice training or continuing edu-

cation. However, any action taken also needs to be evaluated to determine if it indeed achieved the expected outcome.

The final element of the QA process emphasizes communication of the results of the organization's QA efforts. The standard requires that the results be communicated to the governing body or owner/operator, who is ultimately responsible for the quality of care. Also, just as the organization is responsible for the services provided by contractors, it is also responsible for the monitoring of the quality of those services. Therefore, the expected standards of performance should be conveyed to contractors, monitored, and results communicated.

The staff should review its QA results regularly. QA information can be used appropriately in the evaluation of a staff member's performance. From a management perspective, the aggregate individual QA results add an important dimension to evaluating competence. One is able to assess individual versus overall staff performance on key issues in quality of care. In the absence of regular on-site clinical supervision of professionals, QA results can provide important insights as to whether a staff member is performing in accordance with community standards of practice and those of the provider. QA results can also be a positive affirmation that staff members are providing quality and appropriate care and that the organization recognizes this.

Improving Homecare Through Research and Development

Homecare therapeutics is a developing process on the leading edge of healthcare reform. Much of what is done in this setting is still very new, not only because of the therapy, but also because of the location. Structured clinical research designed to make optimal use of the homecare system has been slow to emerge. Most of the work to date has focused on the modification of existing hospital equipment to make it more appropriate for out-of-hospital use. However, several investigators have begun to explore modes of therapy that are best applied in a homecare setting. Such techniques, such as the use of long-term parenteral nutrition in patients with AIDS or cancer, may prove superior to their in-hospital counterparts because the treatments must be given slowly. In some cases, therapies may be toxic when given by rapid administration, whereas the same treatment given slowly over several days or weeks may be lifesaving.

To be judged effectively, homecare research must use an appropriate time frame for reference. Therapeutic measures in the ICU or operating room are judged on a minute-to-minute basis, while most medical therapies are considered on a daily or weekly interval. Homecare therapies should be evaluated on a longer scale, possibly monthly or even less frequently.

Given the capacity to utilize current parenteral pharmaceuticals over a longer period than was originally intended, it is inevitable that new therapies will emerge that not only extend the range of hospital-type therapy, but replace it. The use of low-dose dobutamine for patients with class IV congestive heart failure is a good example of this concept. Here, the gradual use of a drug initially intended for infusion in a monitored setting has reduced the toxicity of the drug sufficiently for it to be given at home. Furthermore, the clinical effect of the low-dose infusion appears to be longer-lasting than that of its original dosage.

Eventually, new pharmaceuticals will undoubtedly emerge that are specifically designed for use in the homecare system. These will be more than adaptations of existing methods. Their use will anticipate a slow, gradual response that preempts their hospital application.

References

1. Standards for the Accreditation of Home Care. Chicago: Joint Commission on the Accreditation of Healthcare Organizations, 1988, 1995.
2. Standards for Home Health Nursing Practice. Waldorf, MD: American Nurses Publications, 1986.
3. Standards for Home Nutritional Support. Silver Spring, MD: American Society for Parenteral and Enteral Nutrition, 1985.
4. Standards of Practice for Nutritional Support Dietitians, Nurses, and Pharmacists. Silver Spring, MD: American Society for Parenteral and Enteral Nutrition, 1985–1987.
5. Home Care Guide for Cancer: How to Care for Family and Friends at Home. Philadelphia: American College of Physicians.
6. Accreditation Manual for Home Care. Oakbrook Terrace, IL: Joint Commission on the Accreditation of Healthcare Organizations, 1991, 1995.

6

THE HOMECARE TEAM

Michael M. Rothkopf and Gail S. Rothkopf

CHAPTER AT A GLANCE: The safety and success of intensive homecare relies on a team of individuals who must function together as a unit. This chapter describes how the transition from hospital to homecare alters the role of the patient, physician, and healthcare personnel. The composition of a homecare team, including core and extended members, is detailed. Deliberate overlapping of team member responsibilities is an important safeguard that allows even medically complex patients to be managed at home.

Introduction

As in the hospital, patient care at home involves not only the attending physician but also a supporting team of healthcare professionals. How well this team functions as a unit is a major determinant of the safety and success of home therapy. To ensure effective operation of the team, individual roles must be clearly defined under physician leadership, and lines of communication must be well established.

The Homecare Team in Practice

The healthcare teams assembled to provide sophisticated medical care at home are composed of basically the same professionals and paraprofessionals as in inpatient care. However, the responsibilities and autonomy of each team member are generally greater than those of their hospital-based counterparts. These adaptations are related to the fact that team members no longer perform their duties under the same roof, and direct patient contact is much less frequent. Communication requires more effort, since the closest interactions among most team members often occur by telephone. Without the supporting structure of hospital policy and routine, it is essential that each team member diligently uphold his or her responsibilities for patient care and communication of patient information. The prescribing physician maintains the leadership role and ultimate responsibility for therapeutic outcome.

Table 6.1 lists familiar members of the homecare team grouped according to their level of participation in patient care. Core team members provide essential medical services and have the greatest responsibilities for patient care. They are members of virtually every homecare team and oversee the patient from initiation to completion of therapy. Various extended team members participate in patient care only as individual needs of the patient require their involvement. When examining this list of care providers, note that

"

Table 6.1 Members of the Homecare Team

Core Team
Primary physician
Homecare organization
Homecare nurse
Pharmacist
Patient (or caregiver)

Extended Team
Physician subspecialists
Reimbursement specialist
Respiratory therapist
Physical therapist
Occupational therapist
Speech therapist
Registered dietitian
Radiology technician
Medical laboratory technician
Mental health professionals
    Medical social worker
    Clinical psychologist
    Psychiatrist
    Family services
    Disease-specific support groups
Supply and delivery personnel
Homemaker or home health aide
Education coordinator

some of the team members are unique to the homecare situation. The most notable of these is a core team member, the patient, who is not seen as being officially responsible for his or her own care in the hospital.

Keeping the team members apprised of the current status of the patient is vital. Therefore, the quality of care provided to homecare patients is directly related to the quality and timeliness of intra-team communications. The homecare team must be capable of responding immediately to emergent changes in patient status. Every effort must be made to maximize the quality and speed of communication among team members. Communication should be facilitated wherever possible by use of the telephone and fax transmission as well as other applicable communication technologies (e.g., voice mail, e-mail, and data pagers). The design of the communications network for the homecare team is a function of the homecare coordinator, who is usually an employee of the home-

care organization or the homecare primary physician.

A quality assurance measure in patient care is the deliberate overlapping of team member roles. This concept is illustrated in Table 6.2. In this example, the responsibilities of the physician, nurse, and pharmacist are detailed as members of a home intravenous antibiotic therapy team. In contrast to the more separate roles performed by inpatient care providers, homecare team members share the basic responsibilities for patient evaluation, monitoring, and treatment plan development.

Beyond performing duties specific to the team member's title, each caregiver must approach the patient in a more holistic fashion than in the hospital. This is necessary because for the homecare patient, the only direct contact with the healthcare team for days may be through a single member's visit. Each contact with the patient is treated as an opportunity to collect information useful to all the disciplines involved. No matter how incidental an interaction, it is a chance to observe the patient, identify problems, and take or recommend corrective action.

This means, for example, that a respiratory therapist visiting a patient to monitor respiratory function is expected to be conscious of the complete clinical picture. As part of the therapist's expanded role in homecare, he or she must report to the appropriate team member problems unrelated to his or her discipline; for example, a patient's apparently elevated level of anxiety, or induration at an IV site.

In other examples, a nurse visiting the patient's home may notice that a number of medication bottles are present on the patient's night table. She records these and reports to the pharmacist, who checks for possible drug interactions. Alternatively, the pharmacist may contact the patient about a delivery schedule for medications and supplies and note that the patient has a large inventory of heparin flushes. He reports this to the nurse to review catheter maintenance protocols, because he is concerned that the patient may be omitting a crucial step in the procedure.

Table 6.2. Responsibilities of Core Team Members for Home IV Antibiotic Therapy

	Physician	*Nurse*	*Pharmacist*
Establish diagnosis	X		
Authorize therapy	X		
Evaluate patient	X	X	X
Develop therapeutic plan	X	X	X
Train patient		X	X
Coordinate care	X	X	X
Establish venous access	X	X	
Prepare antibiotic			X
Provide supplies		X	X
Monitor for toxicity	X	X	X
Follow infection status	X	X	
24-Hour availability	X	X	X

Adapted from Tice AD. The team concept. In: Tice AD, ed. Outpatient parenteral antibiotic therapy: management of serious infections. Part 1: medical, socioeconomic, and legal issues. Hosp Pract 1993;28(Suppl 1):7.

Members of the Homecare Team

Core Team Members

The Homecare Primary Physician

The physician occupies the principal role on the homecare team, providing leadership for the team effort, and bearing ultimate responsibility for the outcome of therapy. He or she has the final authority for medical issues and serves as a resource for the patient and team members seeking medical information. Physician involvement begins with establishment of a diagnosis. Based on medical history, physical examination, and results of diagnostic testing, the physician prescribes an individualized therapeutic plan for the patient. When deciding upon a particular therapy for the homecare patient, the physician should take into account the patient's lifestyle, "customizing" the therapeutic regimen rather than automatically prescribing the standard therapy. Safety and convenience are of paramount importance in homecare.

Encouragement of patient input in the decision-making process is also important to the success of home therapy. The patient must take an active role in his or her own care. In fact, the patient is a member of the homecare team, with responsibilities equal in importance to some of the professional members of the team.

It is essential that the physician develop an adequate plan for monitoring therapeutic progress and follow-up care. In addition to laboratory testing as required, and regular communication with the rest of the homecare team, the monitoring schedule should include direct contact with the patient (in home or office) often enough for the physician to maintain full awareness of the patient's progress. Between office or home visits, the physician must ensure his or her accessibility to the patient. It is recommended that the physician personally certify that the patient understands how to communicate questions and problems to the physician directly or through other members of the homecare team.

Patient care at home will benefit from efforts by the physician to form a good professional relationship with the other homecare professionals. The nurse and pharmacist, for example, must feel comfortable with the notion of communicating observations and opinions to the physician. An added effort is required, since the physician may never actually meet all the other members of the team. Communication with them may be limited to telephone or written reports.

In an ideal medical world, the prescribing physician would be capable of maintaining complete control over patient care. However, the intricacies of homecare team coordination, and the additional time involved in following several patients at home (as opposed to in the hospital, where patients are in a single location), usually require the professional and management services of an established homecare organization.

The physician should be actively involved in the choice of homecare organization for his or her patient, despite insurance provider restrictions of choice (methods for evaluating homecare organizations are discussed in Chapter 5). It is extremely important that the physician strive to maintain his or her authority over patient care. To avoid any confusion, the physician should identify himself as the prescribing physician directly to the homecare company at the time of referral. The physician must participate in direction of the team effort and retain the authority to remove team members he or she considers inadequate. Chapter 2 discusses these issues more completely.

The Homecare Organization

The complex task of providing healthcare personnel, services, equipment, and pharmaceuticals to the patient at home, and securing payment from the third-party payer, is the business of homecare organizations.

The homecare organization employs nurses, pharmacists, and other healthcare professionals specifically trained in outpatient therapies. Homecare organization employees can prepare the prescription and coordinate delivery of the pharmaceuticals, medical services, supplies, and equipment as necessary. It logically follows that a homecare organization employee usually serves as the homecare coordinator under the direction of the primary physician. The primary physician, in turn, is expected to comply with established protocols and standards of care.

A valuable asset to the homecare organization is a staff physician to act as a liaison for primary physicians. Optimally, this should be an individual with knowledge and experience in the homecare field. He or she can provide clinical insight and a perspective based on first-hand knowledge. This same individual can also be an effective educator for the homecare organization staff.

The quality of the care provided by the homecare organization to the patient at home is as important as the quality of care provided to the hospital patient in realizing a successful therapeutic outcome. Before referring a patient to a homecare organization, it is important to evaluate the organization as one would a hospital, especially when the choice is dictated by the patient's insurance carrier. (Again, the physician is ultimately responsible for the outcome of the therapy he or she has prescribed.)

The most reliable evaluation is based on any previous direct experience with the homecare organization or experiences of respected colleagues who have used their services. However, more objective evidence of the organization's ability to provide quality homecare services is provided through accreditation by the Joint Commission on Accreditation of Healthcare Organizations (JCAHO).

Accreditation certifies that the homecare organization can meet the rigorous requirements necessary to fulfill minimum standards of care. However, it cannot guarantee dedication of the homecare organization to upholding these standards between accreditation surveys. Evaluation of homecare organizations is the subject of Chapter 5.

Before patient referral, it is also necessary to investigate the homecare organization's experience with the particular therapy necessary for the patient. It is best to choose a homecare organization with a proven track record for the service to be provided. For example, an organization noted for exemplary care of home intravenous therapy patients may not be capable of duplicating the same quality of care for its renal dialysis patients.

To ensure that the therapy is carried out as the prescribing physician intends, the physician should put his therapeutic goals in writing, and give written orders on how often he wishes to see the patient.

The Homecare Nurse

The homecare nurse, who is usually an employee of a homecare organization, has the most frequent direct contact with the patient, and therefore occupies a central role in homecare. It is the homecare nurse who monitors the patient for the physician between office visits. Frequently, the nurse is required to visit the patient at home on a daily basis, especially early in the therapeutic course. The nurse examines the patient, noting clinical response, looking for signs of complications, and collecting specimens for laboratory analysis as necessary. The nurse is able to verify compliance with therapy and the accuracy of communications to the physician and other team members by the patient. The nurse reports on patient progress and communicates any abnormal findings immediately to the physician. If necessary, the nurse coordinates the involvement of additional team members.

Nursing duties usually begin with a more detailed evaluation and orientation of the patient referred by a physician for home therapy. The nurse assesses the patient's physical and mental abilities, as well as the psychosocial and physical environment at home. Based on these more thorough assessments, a change in treatment protocol or monitoring schedule may be suggested.

Once it has been determined that the patient is a suitable candidate for homecare, the nurse may establish intravenous access or initiate other therapeutic preparations. In the homecare situation, a qualified nurse may even insert sophisticated therapeutic access devices such as peripherally inserted central catheter (PICC) lines. He or she then begins patient training for the self-administered components of therapy. Upon completion of instruction, it is the nurse who certifies the patient's skills in the various techniques required for self-care. For example, when the patient is to undergo infusion therapy at home, the patient must demonstrate competence in sterile technique, line flushing, disposal of needles, and proper handling of infusion solutions and equipment. The nurse also certifies that the patient can recognize early signs of therapeutic failure and complications (e.g. phlebitis, fever, and insertion site infection). It is also important that the nurse supervise patient record keeping for completeness and compliance.

A homecare nurse must possess well-developed communication skills, since he or she is the most direct link to the rest of the home-care team. Ideally, there should be a good rapport between nurse and patient, as this will ease communication between them. Since the nurse is usually the first contact for the patient in routine and emergency situations, an understanding of the structure of lines of communication with team members in routine and emergency situations is vital. The nurse usually has a central role in coordination of team efforts.

Generally, a nurse is one of the team members available to the patient by telephone 24 hours a day for technical and psychological support. The nurse is also a resource for the patient's family, supplying medical information as necessary and providing psychological support. Another function of the nurse is to serve as a source of "emergency" supplies when normal distribution channels are not available or are disrupted.

With such broad responsibilities, it is easy to understand why a competent and conscientious homecare nurse is basic to successful therapy. The physician often has to rely on the nurse's clinical judgment and problem solving skills. It is essential that the nurse assigned to the homecare patient be experienced in outpatient therapy, with certified abilities in all aspects of the particular medical regimen prescribed for the patient. It is also not surprising that patient satisfaction with homecare is largely dependent on a comfortable working relationship with the homecare nurse.

The Homecare Pharmacist

The role of the homecare pharmacist, who is usually an employee of the homecare organization or subcontracted pharmacy, goes beyond preparing prescriptions and coordinating timely delivery to the patient's home.

The initial responsibility of the homecare pharmacist is to compile and review a detailed drug history of the patient. This includes not only prescription drugs, but also over-the-counter medications, home remedies, and any unusual features of the patient's diet. The pharmacist screens for allergies, any potential drug-drug or drug-food interactions, and notes tolerance of previous prescriptions. Review of a detailed drug history is imperative for elderly or medically complex homecare patients. The pharmacist also examines the homecare patient's medical history, with special attention to intercurrent medical conditions that may have an impact on the planned course of therapy.

The experienced homecare pharmacist is an important resource to the homecare team. He or she is skilled in the evaluation of pharmaceutical therapies in the context of homecare. The analysis of therapeutic choices differs somewhat from that for the hospital patient, since homecare requires more individualized prescriptions. When necessary, the input from the homecare pharmacist can be valuable to the prescribing physician in choosing medications and developing an optimal therapeutic plan for the patient to be treated at home. The pharmacist may also evaluate the monitoring schedule and assess the safety and cost-effectiveness of selected pharmaceutical therapies. In the home environment, with less frequent medical supervision and administration of therapy by less experienced personnel (patient or caregiver), margins of safety and convenience are even more important factors in decision making than in the hospital.

Once the prescription is given final approval by the physician, the pharmacist coordinates delivery of pharmaceuticals and supplies with the homecare nurse and delivery personnel. The pharmacist may also be involved in patient training for self-administration of pharmaceuticals.

The homecare pharmacist usually continues his involvement as a member of the homecare team for the entire course of therapy. It is the duty of the pharmacist to keep abreast of the patient's progress through communications, primarily with the physician and nurse. The pharmacist reviews the latest clinical and laboratory reports with particular attention to indications of possible toxicity or other adverse reactions. Any potential need for changes in prescription or monitoring schedule is communicated immediately to the physician and homecare nurse.

The homecare pharmacist also serves as an information resource for the physician, nurse, or patient with questions or problems related to pharmaceutical services. Additional pharmaceutical consultation is often needed for specialized areas such as pharmacodynamics.

The Homecare Patient

The role of the patient changes most radically in the transition from hospital to homecare. A passive recipient of medical care as an inpatient, the patient becomes an active participant in his or her own treatment at home. Responsibilities may include self-administration of prescribed therapies, daily monitoring of vital signs, record keeping, and communication of questions and problems to other homecare team members. The patient must diligently follow protocols designed for his or her homecare and must understand the critical nature of maintaining communication with the homecare team. It is the function of other team members to prepare the patient for this expanded participation by providing training, support, and supervision.

The homecare patient is expected to take a more active role in decision making. He or she should seek information as necessary and be receptive to communications from other team members in preparation for more extensive involvement in therapeutic decisions.

When the patient is not able to take an active role on the homecare team due to physical or psychological limitations, this part of the patient's role can be fulfilled by a caregiver, usually a close friend or family member.

More detailed information on the patient's role in homecare can be found in Chapter 3.

Extended Team Members

Physician Subspecialists

Just as for the hospitalized patient, issues may arise that require an expert opinion in a discipline other than that of the physician with primary responsibility for a homecare patient. For example, a patient on home peritoneal dialysis may develop an infection that requires specialized treatment due to the infectious agent's antibiotic susceptibility profile or the patient's allergic sensitivity to certain drugs. Under these circumstances, it may be necessary to call in an infectious disease specialist to render an opinion and adjust therapy. The input of such a specialist may be very cost-effective, especially if it results in avoidance of hospitalization. It is important, however, that the primary physician explain to the consultant his role and the specific goals to be supported by his input, e.g., the avoidance of hospital re-admission or simplification of therapy for patient convenience.

A surgical consultant who is familiar with the patient should be responsible for maintenance of venous, dialysis, or airway access for the homecare patient. Surgeons who become involved in the support of such homecare patients have shown resourcefulness in modifying their procedures so that they can be performed in outpatient settings.

Other medical specialties may be called upon as the patient's needs develop. Consultations for a single patient may include disciplines as diverse as plastic surgery for non-healing wounds to gynecology and dentistry for routine care. It is prudent to inform each consultant of the special circumstances involved in the patient's homecare. For example, safe practice of even basic dental care requires administration of prophylactic antibiotics if the patient has an indwelling venous access device such as a Hickman or Port-A-Cath catheter.

Reimbursement Specialist

With the complex changes involved in third-party payment and the uneven coverage for homecare services among health plans, a reimbursement specialist has become a common member of the homecare team. This person is generally an employee of a homecare organization but may also be a hospital discharge planner or an employee of a physician group practice. The reimbursement specialist is responsible for determining the adequacy of insurance coverage for homecare. This team member has the expertise required to analyze insurance options for the individual patient and to estimate what the patient's financial responsibility will be once the third-party payment obligation is fulfilled. The reimbursement specialist may then prepare a payment plan for the patient.

When insurance coverage for homecare services is inadequate, the reimbursement specialist may negotiate on behalf of the patient and the homecare organization with the third-party payer to increase coverage. By highlighting the economic advantages of homecare over hospital care, and by agreeing to certain limits on expenses to be paid by the insurance company, the reimbursement specialist can often procure adequate coverage for homecare services. This is possible even in cases where the benefits were not specifically included in the patient's health plan.

Another common assignment for the reimbursement specialist is the negotiation of "out-of-network" coverage and support when a physician chooses a homecare organization that is not designated a "preferred provider" by the patient's HMO or other managed care plan. For a number of reasons (detailed in Chapter 5), the physician may not want his patient serviced via the HMO's preferred homecare organization. The reimbursement specialist then acts as liaison, attempting to negotiate a payment agreement among patient, managed care provider, and out-of-network homecare organization. In these cases, the patient must be informed of the difference in out-of-pocket expenses between network and out-of-network provider choices. To remain competitive, the out-of-network homecare organization may have to waive the difference in cost over the preferred homecare provider.

Respiratory Therapist

For the patient with respiratory failure, the services of home respiratory therapists are essential. In many of these cases, the involvement of a respiratory therapist supplants the need for a homecare nurse. This is certainly true for a patient on home mechanical ventilation. In some instances though, such as the patient with cystic fibrosis, home respiratory therapy occurs in concert with nursing and other services. A single patient may require, for example, an IV nurse for intravenous antibiotic therapy, and a respiratory therapist for home nebulizer therapy, chest physiotherapy, and nasal continuous positive airway pressure (CPAP). Obviously, frequent communication and cooperation between the homecare nurse and respiratory therapist are vital to successful coordination of a complex therapeutic regimen.

Physical, Occupational, and Speech Therapists

These disciplines are important components of rehabilitation for chronically ill patients. The fact that the patient has moved from hospital to homecare does not make this any less true. Physical, occupational, and speech therapists can provide invaluable coping skills for patients, allowing them to function more easily both physically and socially. Although many of these services are provided in outpatient rehabilitation centers, when the homecare patient is not ambulatory, it may be more appropriate to begin such therapy at home.

Physical and occupational therapists may also be consulted for assistance in physical adaptation of the home to accommodate the special needs of the homecare patient. This topic is covered in Chapter 3.

Registered Dietitian

Nutritional assessment is generally performed by registered dietitians (RDs) and should not be overlooked in the management of homecare patients. These services range from review of dietary requirements and utilization of special diets to assistance with specialized nutritional support such as tube feeding or total parenteral nutrition (TPN). Many homecare organizations have successfully employed dietitians as consultants to evaluate their patients. Home visits by the dietitian can be extremely helpful in establishing special nutritional programs, since the implementation of special diets can be difficult outside the hospital.

Radiology Technician

Radiographic services using x-ray machines initially designed for military field use, and capable of using household current, are available for the homecare patient. These portable units are often brought to the patient's home as part of a mobile radiology laboratory. This allows the radiographic technician to develop films on site. Consequently, if additional views are necessary, the need for a repeat visit can be avoided.

Medical Laboratory Technician

When laboratory analyses are ordered for a homecare patient, it is now possible for most routine services to be performed without requiring the patient to leave home. Specimens for basic hematology and chemistry screening, urine analyses, and drug level measurements can easily be collected by the homecare nurse or by a phlebotomist sent to the patient's home by the laboratory. If special preparation of the specimen is required, such as centrifugation or rapid freezing, portable equipment often can be brought to the patient's home.

Mental Health Professionals

Psychological counseling services can be very beneficial to the homecare patient, caregiver, and immediate family members. These services are provided by M.S.W. social workers, Ph.D. clinical psychologists, and psychiatrists. In certain communities, family counseling is available as part of municipal services. Counseling may be arranged for the patient individually or as part of a group session. Support groups have been very successful among patients with similar medical problems. Good examples include support groups sponsored by the American Cancer Society for cancer patients and their families and by the Oley Foundation for short bowel syndrome patients.

Delivery Personnel

The delivery staff, though untrained medically, can make a significant contribution to the team effort. When they make a delivery, they check the patient's refrigerator for the stock of medications and ancillary supplies. This can provide indirect evidence of the patient's compliance with the therapeutic protocol. Furthermore, since they are not professionals, some patients feel less intimidated and are more open in talking to the delivery staff. They can often provide valuable insight into the patient's satisfaction with the program.

Homemaking Services

A homemaker or home health aide can often be of assistance to the homecare patient. While these individuals are not trained medically and cannot perform specialized nursing services, they may be very helpful in unburdening the patient and family of basic care requirements. These include bathing, toileting, cleansing of ostomy sites, food preparation, and environmental maintenance. This basic assistance may permit the patient and caregiver to concentrate their efforts on the more demanding routines required for safe practice of intensive homecare.

Educational Coordinator

In the case of a homecare patient who is a school-aged child, an educational coordinator should be consulted to assess the progress of the patient's normal intellectual development. The education coordinator may recommend additional homework or tutoring to replace classes missed at school. In the event that the child is completely unable to attend school, a home study program must be implemented.

Conclusion

Intensive homecare is a cooperative effort. Personnel from various disciplines each contribute to the process of caring for the patient at home. Despite the complexity of coordinating these services, the team approach can be very successful. It requires careful preparation of team members and efficient organization of the team effort.

A basic limitation to the expansion of homecare has been the need to maintain up-to-the-minute team communication. Without the consistent capability of immediate response to a change in patient status, homecare can be routinely prescribed only for medically stable patients.

Developing communication technologies are expected to significantly expand the scope and improve the quality of homecare. Concepts such as computerized direction of communications among team members and portable communication devices are designed to prevent or decrease the frequency of communication failures, delays, and misdirection.

References

1. Tice AD. The team concept. In: Tice AD, ed. Outpatient parenteral antibiotic therapy: management of serious infections. Part 1: medical, socioeconomic, and legal issues. Hosp Pract 1993;28 (Suppl 1).
2. Rich D. Physicians, pharmacists, and home infusion antibiotic therapy. In: Poretz DM, ed. Outpatient use of intravenous antibiotics. Am J Med 1994;97(2A).
3. Standards for the Accreditation of Home Care. Chicago: Joint Commission on the Accreditation of Healthcare Organizations, 1988, 1995.

7

UNDERSTANDING HOMECARE THERAPY FAILURES

Michael M. Rothkopf and Gail S. Rothkopf

CHAPTER AT A GLANCE: Homecare therapeutics is a safe and effective modality in the management of many conditions. Nonetheless, it is a complex system that sometimes malfunctions. This chapter describes how deficiencies in homecare procedures can lead to failures of varying outcome. These are graded based on the level of expected consequences. An analysis of how individual team member deficiencies contribute to therapeutic failures is presented, as is an illustrative case report.

Introduction

The safety and success of medical treatment at home is increasingly evident as this healthcare model becomes more commonplace. This positive outcome is the result of the careful design of home therapy protocols to prevent avoidable complications and to detect unavoidable problems early.

However, despite intensive efforts to prevent therapeutic problems, homecare failures sometimes occur. To put these failures in the proper perspective, it should be noted that the frequency of failure is believed to be equal to or less than the rate of therapeutic failure in hospitalized patients (1–10).

Most published studies of homecare focus on the successful application of a therapy at home and merely mention therapeutic failures with little analytical comment. However, an understanding of the sources of failure in home therapeutics is highly relevant for day-to-day patient management decisions.

In this chapter, homecare failures are analyzed from two perspectives. First, deficiencies in patient care are organized according to the seriousness of expected therapeutic consequences. Various levels of failure are described, and appropriate responses to each are suggested. The second type of analysis examines homecare failures as they relate to individual team member performance. The objective is to detail why failures occur and to look at how they can be prevented. Lastly, a case report is presented that illustrates the practical application of homecare therapy failure analysis.

Effect of Homecare Failures on Therapeutic Outcome

The impact of homecare deficiencies on patient health varies greatly, from little or no effect on therapeutic outcome to a serious decline in medical status. To facilitate analysis of this topic, we have organized homecare failures into four levels of concern, according to the probable consequences to patient health, as shown in Table 7.1.

The consequences of home healthcare errors are determined not only by the nature of the failure itself, but also by the medical status of the individual patient at the time it occurs. Therefore, it is important to note that this table assumes that the patient's medical status is stable prior to the deficiency. For example, an error considered unlikely to result in a serious complication for a stable, long-term homecare patient may have very serious consequences for a patient whose condition is more fragile.

Level I Failures: Low Probability of Serious Consequence

Level I deficiencies carry the least significance to therapeutic outcome. Included in this category are isolated, minor errors or omissions, usually considered to be inconsequential. However, it is important to recognize these occurrences as an early indication of failure to follow homecare protocol meticulously. Level I failures are important to address because in the more autonomous environment of home healthcare, with less frequent professional supervision, sloppy performance on the part of any team member is risky and cannot be tolerated. These low-level mistakes should alert team members involved to the fact that a more conscientious approach to patient care must be taken to prevent further, more serious errors.

A good example of a Level I failure is the failure to document scheduled monitoring of vital signs, even when measurements were actually taken and were found to be within normal limits. Although no serious consequence is foreseen, careless record-keeping is a dangerous practice in the homecare situation. The completeness and accuracy of documentation is relied on by the entire homecare team.

Although this type of failure may not warrant the filing of a formal incident report, the error should be recorded on the patient's chart so that repetition of the error, should it occur, can be documented. The team members involved must recognize the mistake and understand why it occurred in order to prevent it from happening again. Supervising professionals of the team should reinforce initial training with special emphasis on the importance of attention to detail.

Another example of a Level I failure involves incomplete planning. This could include failure to plan for a specific nonmedical need, such as a minor disability or limited reading skills. Without proper preparation such issues may grow to interfere with the provision of homecare services.

Level II Failures: Moderate Probability of Serious Consequence

While the probability of serious consequence of Level I failures is considered to be low, the risk of injury or complication increases in Level II. At the second level, the probability of a serious consequence becomes significant, although the risk of adverse effects is still not high. The greater possibility of a negative impact on the patient's health makes this type of deficiency more serious than Level I.

Examples of Level II deficiencies include repeated Level I deficiencies, indicating a careless approach to patient care. Failure to diligently fulfill responsibilities can lead to serious problems in home healthcare. Another example of a Level II deficiency is a single, isolated failure or delay in administration of a dose of a prescribed medication. Generally, such an omission will not lead to serious consequence, but the possibility of compromising patient health must be recognized. For example, failure to administer a single dose of an antibiotic is usually not enough to allow an infection to become reestablished, but this may prolong the course of therapy.

In response to a Level II failure, a formal incident report should be filed. This will result in a review by the Quality Assurance Committee of the homecare organization, who will recommend the type of corrective action to be imposed. Minimally, homecare team members involved in the failure should be required to attend appropriate in-service education programs and undergo retraining in specific problem areas. An important part

Table 7.1. Analysis of Homecare Failures[a]

Level	Probability of Serious Consequence	Examples of Failures	Appropriate Responses
I	Low	Failure to document performance of task Failure to communicate normal findings	Record deficiency on patient record Reinforce training of team members involved
II	Moderate	Single recurrence of Level I failure Single failure or delay in administration of prescribed therapy Failure to perform monitoring task for stable patient Failure to obtain specimen for routine analysis Failure to keep medical appointment by stable patient	File incident report Review of error by QA committee Inservice and retraining programs in area of deficiency for team members involved Develop plan for prevention; certify effectiveness
III	High	Repeated Level I or II failure Errors in sterile technique, dosage, and equipment use or maintenance Use of outdated or substandard supplies Failure or delay in response to abnormal clinical or laboratory report	File incident report Review of error by QA committee Impose disciplinary action recommended Complete retraining of team members involved Document remedial steps taken Develop plan for prevention; certify effectiveness
IV	Actual occurrence	Intravenous line sepsis Dehydration or fluid overload Hepatic or renal impairment Severe adverse drug reaction Therapeutic device failure	Reevaluate appropriateness of homecare for patient involved Complete review of homecare protocol and homecare team performance

[a]Based on patient with stable medical condition.

of the resolution of these problems is the development and immediate implementation of strategies for prevention of recurrences. This plan should include follow-up surveys to judge the effectiveness of remedial efforts.

Level III Failures: High Probability of Serious Consequence

Level III failures are considered to be much more dangerous than Level I or II deficiencies, because Level III failures are *expected* to have serious medical consequences.

Level III failures include frequent Level I failures and repeated Level II failures. Other typical Level III deficiencies include errors in prescription dosage, sterile technique, equipment use, or equipment maintenance. The failure to respond immediately and appropriately to an abnormal laboratory or clinical finding also belongs in this category.

Level III failures are evidence of dangerous inadequacies of the homecare team, with the probability of serious medical and legal consequences. The detection of a Level III failure demands an immediate and comprehensive response. This reaction must include not only remedial action but also preventive measures.

Beyond the filing of an incident report, and other responses listed for Level II deficiencies, a Level III failure requires additional action. The homecare team members involved must be made aware of their deficiencies and participate in a formal retraining process. Other disciplinary actions may be needed depending on the individual situations, with the possibility of termination of employment.

Level IV Failures: Occurrence of Serious Consequence

When serious adverse consequences actually do result from homecare errors, it is considered to be a Level IV failure. A significant decline in patient health calls into question the most fundamental decision in homecare: the appropriateness of outpatient care for the individual patient. The adverse consequences of Level IV failures are not only medical. Legal action may be initiated by parties injured in such situations.

Level IV failures include catheter sepsis, dehydration, and drug-related complications such as renal and hepatic impairment. Obviously, these conditions require immediate medical intervention to resolve the condition or to limit damage to patient health. Usually, this results in rehospitalization of the patient and a suspension of homecare therapy.

Regardless of the cause of a Level IV failure, the response must be a complete review of the homecare process and reevaluation of the patient for home therapy. The physician who encounters resistance from the homecare organization when he or she decides to withdraw the patient from homecare must bear in mind that the organization's reluctance to release the patient can be influenced by their own economic concerns. Prior to returning the patient to homecare after a Level IV failure, the physician must have confidence that outpatient therapy will be safe and effective for this individual patient.

Deficiencies in Homecare Team Performance as a Source of Failure

Common Factors in Homecare Therapy Failures

The potential for error and oversight in homecare may seem greater than in the hospital, where there is a more formal structure and communication among healthcare providers is easier. However, safeguards against failure in homecare have proved to be effective enough to equal or improve on hospital failure rates. An important safeguard of quality patient care is the overlapping of homecare team member responsibilities. For example, the physician, the nurse, and the pharmacist are all responsible for monitoring the patient's laboratory results for signs of adverse reactions or inefficacy of medications, and for communicating with each other when abnormal results are encountered.

When homecare failures are surveyed, several common problems emerge. These deficiencies can generally be placed in one of four categories:

1. Ineffective patient and staff training and education
2. Noncompliance with therapeutic protocols and standards
3. Inadequate communication
4. Inadequate monitoring

These four categories can be used to examine the separate roles of the physician, patient, and homecare organization/team in producing a homecare failure. Each is presented in Tables 7.2, 7.3, and 7.4. For a more detailed discussion of the individual responsibilities of each component of the homecare team, please see Chapters 2, 3, 5, and 6.

CASE REPORT

MW, a 52-year-old man with pancreatic adenocarcinoma, was referred to a physician for consideration of parenteral nutrition. He had lost 50 pounds since his diagnosis. Three months earlier, he had undergone a pancreaticoduodenectomy. He was now unable to absorb adequate nutrition because of enterocutaneous and bowel fistulas. A trial of experimental chemotherapy was under consideration.

The patient appeared cachectic with a body weight of 106 pounds. This was 60 pounds below his usual weight and 75% of his ideal body weight (IBW). The physical examination revealed muscle wasting and fat depletion. A laboratory analysis revealed diminished serum proteins and cholesterol.

Table 7.2. Physician-Related Responsibilities for Homecare Failure

1. Ineffective training/education:
   - Lack of knowledge on how homecare team operates
   - Inadequate recognition of responsibilities
2. Noncompliance with therapeutic protocols/standards:
   - Faulty patient selection
   - Errors in prescription of drugs and therapeutic regimen
   - Inappropriate prescription for homecare
   - Inadequate plan of care, including clinical and laboratory monitoring schedules
   - Inadequate homecare organization selection
3. Inadequate communication:
   - Failure to respond to request for information
   - Failure to properly document patient status or changes in protocol
   - Failure to inform team of need for prescription/therapy changes
   - Inadequate interaction with other team members; lack of cooperation; failure to keep team current on patient information; improper delegation of duties
   - Failure to coordinate team activities adequately
   - Inadequate documentation
   - Failure to respond to question, problem or data follow-up
   - Failure to control patient care
4. Inadequate monitoring:
   - Inadequate monitoring schedule
   - Reliance on secondary information; homecare organization reports of patient status; relies entirely on nursing visits
   - Failure or delay in review of lab and clinical reports
   - Failure to adjust monitoring schedule when necessary
   - Failure to monitor team performance
   - Failure to adjust therapy as necessary

Table 7.3. Patient-Related Responsibilities for Homecare Failure

1. Ineffective training/education:
     Inadequate comprehension of homecare duties
     Inadequate recognition of responsibilities
2. Noncompliance with therapeutic protocols/standards:
     Failure to administer therapy
     Failure to keep physician/nurse/delivery appointments
     Failure to maintain and operate equipment safely
     Lack of adherence to protocols (e.g., sterile technique)
3. Inadequate communication:
     Incomplete or inadequate record keeping
     Failure to report change in status
     Failure to report problems with equipment or therapy
4. Inadequate monitoring:
     Failure to monitor vital signs
     Deterioration of family support system

Table 7.4. Homecare Organization/Team-Related Responsibilities for Homecare Failure

1. Ineffective training/education:
     Failure to recheck adequacy of patient training at regular intervals
     Changes in protocol not supported by additional training
     Inability to meet service needs due to inadequate experience, staffing
2. Noncompliance with therapeutic protocols/standards:
     Inadequate documentation
     Failure to maintain and service equipment safely
     Lack of adherence to therapeutic protocols
     Poor quality or outdated supplies
3. Inadequate communication:
     Inadequate patient care coordination
     Failure to report change in patient status to physician and other team members
     Delayed response to patient need
     Delayed response to abnormal laboratory data
     Delayed response to physician request for change in regimen
4. Inadequate monitoring:
     Failure to monitor for quality assurance

The physician reviewed the patient's medical records, including the results of a GI series, and decided that parenteral nutrition was appropriate. In lieu of admitting the patient to the hospital for TPN initiation, he referred the patient to a homecare company with which he had extensive experience. The company had a program in place for TPN initiation at home, which obviated the need for hospitalization.

The homecare company chosen was part of a national corporation with a reputation for providing high-quality services. They were JCAHO accredited and could provide evidence of an extensive quality assurance program.

COMMENTARY: *The case presented is appropriate for the use of home TPN. The patient is clearly incapable of adequately absorbing nutrients via the GI tract. A careful evaluation reveals moderate severe protein-calorie malnutrition. If nutritional support is not initiated it is doubtful the patient will survive, no less tolerate chemotherapy.*

The physician also appropriately selected the option of initiating TPN at home rather than admitting the patient to the hospital. This resulted in an increased convenience factor for the patient and a reduced cost to the insurer. By choosing an accredited company with which he was familiar, the physician showed good judgment and appropriately exercised his authority as leader of the homecare team.

The homecare company chosen performed an insurance evaluation in preparation for providing services. During this process, it was learned that the patient's insurance carrier had a preference for a different homecare organization. The latter was an out-of-state company that the physician had not heard of before. It was a small company whose accreditation status was pending. Despite the physician's insistence on utilizing the homecare company he selected, the insurance carrier declared that they would not cover the homecare services unless their preferred provider was used. After learning this fact, the physician reluctantly agreed to refer the patient to the homecare company specified by the insurance carrier

COMMENTARY: *This situation highlights a common problem in homecare referrals. The insurance company has made a prior selection of a preferred provider based on economic grounds. The physician is placed in a defensive position in which his judgment is subjugated to the insurance carrier's demands. The insurance carrier has encroached on the physician's autonomy and affected his control over the homecare team.*

Physicians may fail to recognize the importance of maintaining control and authority as team leader during a homecare case. Since the physician is rarely present in the patient's home, he must rely on information given to him by the various members of the homecare team. It is vital that he be included in the flow of information so that he can use his judgment to adjust therapy and avoid complications. Furthermore, he must have confidence in the source of this information.

A PICC line was placed in the physician's office. The catheter was inserted via the left antecubital vein and advanced to 50 cm without difficulty. A chest x-ray confirmed the position of the catheter tip in the superior vena cava. The catheter hub was secured to the skin using Steri-Strips and covered with a sterile bio-occlusive dressing. In addition to verbal instructions from the physician's nurse, a handbook was given to the patient detailing the catheter length, tip position, and special care requirements.

The patient was prescribed a TPN formula to be infused over a 12-hour period from 9 pm to 9 am. The formula was specific to the patient's nutritional requirements based on his IBW. To complete the infusion in 12 hours, the solution was concentrated and was therefore hypertonic. It was intended to be given only through a central venous catheter.

The patient left the physician's office and returned home. A homecare nurse arrived several hours later to begin instruction on home intravenous procedures. As was the policy of her organization, new patients were given graduated instruction for the first 3 days of therapy, during which the homecare nurse performed most of the duties herself.

In the course of instructing the patient and his wife, the nurse noted that neither had strong English verbal or reading skills. They had both emigrated from South America 15 years earlier. They appeared uncomfortable with the concept of self-administration of medications. The nurse notified her supervisor of this fact, but not the physician. The supervisor authorized daily nursing visits for 1 week.

On the third day of therapy, a new homecare nurse was assigned to assist the patient. As she prepared the infusion, she noted that the peripherally inserted central catheter (PICC) line was out of normal position. Sixteen centimeters of the catheter could be seen overlying the patient's arm, proximal to the venous insertion site. The insertion site itself remained covered with an occlusive dressing, however.

The nurse questioned the patient on the catheter's appearance and position. He insisted that it had not changed substantially and that it had protruded from the skin since insertion. The patient could not recall being given a handbook on the catheter.

The nurse accepted the patient's statement and hung the TPN solution. It infused normally and she left the patient's home. She did not notify her supervisor or the physician of the catheter position.

COMMENTARY: *The PICC line was appropriately inserted and the TPN solution appropriately prescribed. The system was intended to be used for central TPN only, given the hyperosmolarity of the concentrated solution. However, although the technical aspects of the physician's care were appropriate, he made an error in not learning more about the patient's capacity to perform homecare therapeutics. He also failed to adequately follow up on the status of the patient early in the course of the infusion. The initial homecare nurse compounded this error by not informing the physician that she felt the patient was a poor homecare candidate and would need extra supervision. This can be classified as a Level I failure.*

Despite these deficiencies, the first 2 days of therapy were uneventful. On the third day, however, a significant error occurred: the PICC line became malpositioned without being noticed. The patient misinformed the nurse as to the status of the catheter. The nurse failed to recognize this as a change in status and accepted the patient's statement as true. She did not realize that the patient was covering up for having accidentally dislodged the catheter earlier that day while shaving.

The nurse then went on to commit another error, which can be seen as separate from the issue of catheter dislodgment: she allowed infusion of a hypertonic solution into a noncentral venous catheter. This would be an error even if the patient's statement about the catheter position were true. She should not have permitted the infusion of a hypertonic solution via a catheter whose central venous position was doubtful. This last action has a high probability of resulting in a complication of therapy.

On the seventh day of therapy the catheter site began to appear reddened. By the eighth day the upper left arm had become swollen and tender. The patient's daughter called the physician, and he was seen in the office imme-diately. It was determined that the patient had suffered a venous thrombosis of the left upper arm, and he was admitted for definitive diagnosis and therapy. Doppler ultrasound on the upper extremity confirmed the presence of an occluded left brachial and axillary vein. Two sets of blood cultures were positive for *Staphylococcus aureus*. The PICC line was removed and the patient was placed on intravenous heparin and antibiotics. His arm gradually improved over the course of several days, and he was discharged on oral warfarin therapy.

COMMENTARY: *The development of a septic venous thrombosis is a serious homecare failure. The patient was admitted and treated quickly and, fortunately, suffered no long-term sequelae of the event. However, had the daughter not intervened, there might have been a further delay in notification of the physician. This could have resulted in the patient developing endocarditis or septic shock.*

A homecare failure that requires readmission calls for the physician to reassess the appropriateness of the homecare therapy. In this case, the patient's condition requires continuation of long-term TPN. However, a retraining of the patient and family should take place, with clear understandings reached regarding the patient's responsibilities and obligations. A full quality assurance process initiated by an incident report should take place.

Summary

Despite its overall safety as a therapeutic delivery system, homecare sometimes fails. Much can be learned from carefully analyzing each of these events. As the field matures, safeguards will undoubtedly develop that will further reduce the occurrence of homecare failures.

References

1. Poretz DM. Home intravenous antibiotic therapy. Clin Geriatr Med 1991;7: 749–763.
2. Baptista RJ, Mitrano FP. Experience with 211 courses of home intravenous antimicrobial therapy. Am J Hosp Pharm 1989;46:315–316.
3. Williams DN, Gibson JA, Bosch D. Home intravenous antibiotic therapy using a programmable infusion pump. Arch Intern Med 1989;149:1157–1160.
4. Poretz DM. Treatment of serious infections with cefotaxime utilizing an outpatient drug delivery device: global analysis of a large-scale, multicenter trial. Am J Med 1994; 97:34–42.

5. Brown RB. Selecting the patient. In: Tice AD, ed. Outpatient parenteral antibiotic therapy: management of serious infections. Part I: Medical, socioeconomic, and legal issues. Hosp Pract 1993;28(Suppl 1):11–15.

6. Bernstein LH. An update on home intravenous antibiotic therapy. Geriatrics 1991;46:47–54.

7. Grayson ML, Silvers J, Turnidge J. Home intravenous antibiotic therapy: a safe and effective alternative to inpatient care. Med J Aust 1995;162:249–253.

8. Howard L, Ament M, Fleming CR, et al. Current use and clinical outcome of home parenteral and enteral nutrition therapies in the United States. Gastroenterology 1995; 109:355–365.

9. Peters SG, Viggiano RW. Home mechanical ventilation. Mayo Clin Proc 1988;63:1208–1213.

10. Naef RW, Chauhan SP, Roach H, et al. Treatment for hyperemesis in the home: an alternative to hospitalization. J Perinatol 1995;15:289–292.

8

LEGAL ASPECTS OF INTENSIVE HOME HEALTHCARE SERVICES

Michael M. Rothkopf and Herve Gouraige[a]

CHAPTER AT A GLANCE: Physicians who participate in home healthcare should be aware of the various legal issues involved. These include regulatory matters, fraud and abuse, and legal liability. This chapter briefly reviews the major legal subjects that arise in relation to intensive homecare. Special emphasis is given to issues of patient referral. General principles governing liability for injuries to patients is also addressed. Relevant state and federal legislation is cited, as is substantive case law.

Introduction

Intensive homecare services raise a number of complex legal issues. These include regulatory, referral, and liability concerns. Physicians whose practices include homecare patients must become sensitive to the various laws that are unique to this area. This chapter approaches this complex subject from the physician's perspective. It is not intended to represent a comprehensive dissertation on the law. Questions on individual issues should be referred to a competent attorney with particular knowledge in healthcare law.

Preliminary Issues

Structure

Home health agencies (HHAs) may be established as nonprofit entities, sole proprietor-

ships, partnerships, limited partnerships, corporations, or limited-liability companies. An entity's business structure affects the liability of the participants and the tax liability of the venture.

For Medicare-reimbursed HHAs, the issue of physician ownership is also important. The law prohibits a physician who has a significant financial interest in a home health agency from establishing or reviewing the plan of treatment required for a patient receiving home healthcare (Social Security Act, §1814 (a)(8) et seq., 42 USC §1395f(a)(8), et seq.).

A physician has a "significant ownership interest" in an HHA if he or she (*a*) has a direct or indirect ownership of 5% or more of the capital, stock, or profits of the agency, or (*b*) has an ownership interest of 5% or more in any mortgage, deed of trust, note, or other obligation that is secured by the agency (42 CFR §424.22[d]). A physician has "a significant financial or contractual relationship" with an HHA if he or she receives compensation as an officer or director of the agency or has di-

---

rect or indirect business transactions with the HHA that, in any fiscal year, amount to more than $25,000 or 5% of the agency's total operating expenses, whichever is less. The term "business transactions" in these regulations includes contracts, agreements, purchase orders, or leases to obtain services, supplies, equipment, space, and salaried employment.[b] Some states have modified these restrictions. For example, in New Jersey physicians have a "significant ownership interest" if they or their immediate family have any financial interest.

Licensure

The scope of these licensing requirements varies from state to state. Some states, such as Maryland, require homecare providers to be licensed (Md Health-Gen Code Ann §19-401 et seq. [1987]). Other states impose special regulations on homecare providers. For example, New York has a two-tiered regulatory scheme that requires licenses for "home care services agencies." In addition, agencies that provide a certain service must also be "certified" by the state (NYS §3600.2.2-.3).[c]

Certificate-of-Need Requirements

Some states also require new healthcare providers to obtain a certificate-of-need (CON) before providing services. These allow states to ensure that a need exists for a proposed service before it is offered, thus preventing wasteful duplication of healthcare facilities and services. In some states, these CON requirements may apply to home health agencies or to any provider of medical supplies or services in the home.

Medicare Reimbursement

The Medicare program is divided into two parts, A and B. Part A benefits, or "Hospital Insurance Benefits for the Aged and Disabled" are available to most individuals who are 65 or older and who are eligible for Social Security benefits. Part A is financed through the contributions of workers and their employers. Part A generally covers services furnished by a "hospital, skilled nursing facility, comprehensive outpatient rehabilitation facility, home health agency, or hospice program" (Social Security Act, §1861[u], 42 USC §1395x[u]).[d]

Part B ("Supplementary Medical Insurance Benefits for the Aged and Disabled") is a voluntary program that covers the services of physicians and certain other suppliers. Part B is financed through premiums paid by beneficiaries and contributions of the federal government. Under Part B, beneficiaries are also responsible for payment of a deductible and, for certain services, a 20% coinsurance (Social Security Act, §1833[a]-[b], 42 USC §13951[a]-[b]). Medicare contracts with private companies, referred to as "intermediaries" for Part A and "carriers" for Part B to pay claims in accordance with instructions from the Health Care Financing Administration (HCFA), the agency within the U.S. Department of Health and Human Services (HHS) that oversees Medicare.[e]

Congress has passed several laws that affect home healthcare coverage—the Omnibus Budget Reconciliation Act of 1987 ("OBRA

---

[b]*Under recent legislation passed by Congress, some healthcare entities providing certain home healthcare services will have to provide the names and Medicare provider numbers of all physicians who are investors. In addition, whenever a referral is made by a physician, an entity providing home healthcare services will have to report the physician's name and provider number and indicate whether he or she is an investor in the entity providing the services (see Omnibus Budget Reconciliation Act of 1989 ("OBRA '89") Pub L No. 101–239, 1989 U.S. Code Cong. & Admin. News, 103 Stat 2239, 2241).*

[c]*It should also be noted that some states may require licensure of certain HHAs as pharmacies. For example, New Jersey law states that a person who is not a licensed pharmacist, pharmacist assistant, or physician may not "dispense, fill or sell prescriptions" or "sell, dispense or furnish" any prescription drug. Thus, an entity that is supplying drugs to patients as part of its home health services may also have to be licensed as a pharmacy.*

---

[d]*"Hospice Services" refers to care provided to terminally ill patients, some of which may be provided at home. The regulations covering these services, however, are beyond the scope of this chapter.*

[e]*The one distinction between Part A and Part B is that Part A does not cover home health agencies engaged primarily in the treatment of mental diseases (Social Security Act 1861[o], 42 USC §1395x[o]).*

'87"), the Omnibus Budget Reconciliation Act of 1989 ("OBRA '89") and the Omnibus Budget Reconciliation Act of 1990 ("OBRA '90").[f]

Home Healthcare Services Offered through HHAs

These agencies offer a number of different types of services, including nursing services, home health aides, physical therapy, and durable medical equipment (DME). Medicare reimburses for these HHA services if all the conditions of the Medicare statute are met. Home healthcare services are covered by both Parts A and B. If a service is eligible for reimbursement under both parts, the regulations require that payments be made under Part A8 (MIM §3122.1).

Coverage of HHA Services

"Home health services" has a specific meaning under the Medicare statute. To be covered under Medicare, these services must be furnished or coordinated by an HHA. Other sections of the statute and HCFA's regulations impose additional requirements.

These requirements can be summed up as follows: the services must be reasonable and necessary, the patient must meet certain specified conditions, the services must be those that are specifically enumerated, and none of the specified exclusions may apply.

Fraud and Abuse

Federal and state laws prohibit practices that fall under the broad rubric of "fraud and abuse." These include filing false claims; paying or receiving a kickback or rebate for the referral of patients; and paying or receiving other forms of remuneration in exchange for the referral of patients. Because these laws cover a variety of situations, it is vitally important for anyone involved in the provision of home healthcare to become familiar with the basic principles involved.

The most important laws governing fraud and abuse are federal laws governing Medicare and Medicaid payments. There are two major groups of laws in this area. The first set prohibits the making of false claims. The second bars the payment or receipt of kickbacks, bribes, rebates, or other forms of remuneration.

Fraud under the Medicare Program

The most straightforward of the fraud and abuse provisions are those that deal with false claims. Violation of Section 1128B is a felony for which one may be fined up to $25,000 and/or imprisoned for up to 5 years. In addition, HCFA may seek civil money penalties of $2,000 for each fraudulent item or service claimed (Social Security Act §1128A, 42 USC §1320a-7a). An individual may also be subject to an additional assessment of not more than twice the amount claimed for each item or service (Ibid.). Under a separate statute, the Program Fraud Civil Remedies Act (31 USC §3801–3812), HHS may seek civil money penalties of up to $5,000 for each claim and assessments of up to twice the amount claimed against any person who submits a false, fictitious, or fraudulent claim. Finally, an individual engaged in the activities noted above may also be excluded from participation in the Medicare and/or Medicaid programs (Social Security Act §1128, 42 USC §1320a-7). A state licensing authority may also use such convictions in disciplinary proceedings against the physician.

False Claims Act

The False Claims Act (31 USC §3729 et seq) applies to any person who knowingly presents any false or fraudulent claim to the government for payment or approval.[g] Persons making such false claims are liable for civil penal-

---

[f]*It is also likely that Congress and HCFA will make even more changes in the provisions applicable to providers of homecare services.*

[g]*The requisite "knowledge" under the Act may be in the form of "deliberate ignorance or reckless disregard" (United States v. Krizek 859 F. Supp.5. (D.D.C. 1994)).Violation of Act upheld where psychiatrist's wife, responsible for overseeing billing operation, was found to have acted with reckless disregard for the truth or falsity of Medicare and Medicaid submissions, where wife failed to establish the actual time the psychiatrist spent with the patients, and simply presumed that 45 to 50 minutes had been spent.*

ties in the amount of not less than $5,000 and not more than $10,000, and treble the amount of damages the government sustains as a result of the false claim. The violator is also responsible for the costs incurred by the government in bringing the action. This is a particularly punitive statute, as the penalty applies to *each* false claim presented to the government. In United States v. Diamond 667 F. Supp. 1204 (S.D.N.Y. 1987), a physician was found to have submitted 39 false Medicare claims. The court held that it was required to impose the penalty ($2,000 at the time) for each claim for a total of $78,000, despite the fact that the actual damages claimed by the government amounted to only $549. See also United States v. Killough 848 F.2d 1523 (11th Cir 1988), where a violator of the False Claims Act was required to pay the penalty amount for each of 52 fraudulent invoices submitted to the government.

Kickbacks may also be covered by the False Claims Act. In United States v. Kensington Hosp. (760 F. Supp. 1120 [E.D.Pa. 1991]), the court held that the Act applied to kickbacks, despite the fact that the level of reimbursement is fixed under Medicaid, and as such, the government suffered no loss. The court stated that the government need not show actual damage in order to prove a violation of the False Claims Act. Furthermore, the Court of Appeals for the Second Circuit has recently held that where kickbacks are involved, the False Claims Act is not preempted by the Anti-Kickback Act. (U.S. General Dynamics Corp. 19 F3d 770 [2nd Cir 1994]). While a kickback defendant is not on the hook for any treble damages, as there is no actual damage to the government, penalties for up to $10,000 per each violation can be assessed. If the kickback scheme is of a repetitive nature, as they often are, the total penalty can be staggering.

Finally, 31 USC §3730 allows private persons to bring an action under §3729 for themselves and the U.S. Government. The government is responsible for the prosecution of the case, and the plaintiff (known as the "Qui Tam" plaintiff) receives between 15 and 25% of any proceeds from the action or settlement of the claim. See, for example, United States ex rel Woodward v. Country View Care Center, Inc. (797 F.2d 888 [C.A.10 1986]). This provision obviously provides great incentive for whistle-blowers, who stand to make up to 25% of sometimes multimillion-dollar penalties and damage awards. (See 809 CCH Medicare and Medicaid Guide, July 8, 1994, where National Medical Enterprises Inc. settled a case brought under the Act for $379 million).

In sum, the False Claims Act acts as a tool to fight health care fraud above and beyond 42 USC §1320a-7. The penalties are much higher than under 42 USC §1320a-7a, and the False Claims Act allows for suits by private parties.

Administrative Remedy for False Claims

The Program Fraud Civil Remedies Act was enacted in 1986. 31 USC §3801 et seq provides Federal agencies that are the victims of false or fraudulent claims and statements with an administrative remedy to recompense the agencies for losses resulting from the claims. The act provides for a penalty of not more than $5,000 for each false, fictitious, or fraudulent claim or statement. Parties in violation of this section are also liable for double the amount of damages caused by such false claims. In actions brought by the U.S. Department of Health and Human Services, reviewing courts have upheld rulings by administrative law judges (ALJs) awarding double damages and the maximum $5,000 penalty, even when there were multiple claims or statements. The reader is referred to Orfanos v. Department of Health and Human Services (896 F. Supp. 23 [DDC 1995]), in which the court upheld an ALJ decision awarding double damages and the maximum penalty for each of 34 occasions when the defendant forged her deceased mother's signature on social security checks.

It is unclear whether this statute contemplates kickback schemes. It does not appear so from the text of the statute, and apparently no court has been presented with the issue. However, the same rationale for including kickbacks under the False Claims Act would seem to apply, as the language and purpose of the two sections are similar. Proceeding under §3802 is likely more attractive to agencies such as the Department of Health and Human Services than taking advantage of the higher penalties and damages available under the False Claims Act, as the agencies themselves retain the proceeds.

Physician Self-Referral

A number of state legislatures have enacted laws regarding physician self-referral. This is generally derived as the referral by a physician to a provider in which the physician has a financial interest. Federal law related to this issue is constructed under legislation referred to as "Stark II." There is a key difference between the laws relating to fraud and abuse detailed above and Stark II. The earlier legislation requires some degree of intent to induce referrals in order to find violation. Stark II makes proving *intent* unnecessary. The *act* of referral of a Medicare or Medicaid patient to an entity the physician has an interest in is a violation.

Stark II legislation extended a prior ban of physician self-referral to laboratory services (Stark I) to include a whole array of healthcare services covered under either Medicare or Medicaid. This includes inpatient and outpatient care, radiology, and other diagnostic services and home healthcare. The law imposes substantial monetary penalties for each prohibited referral and possible exclusion for Medicare and Medicaid participation.

Yet, despite the broad-reaching implications of federal and state law on physician self-referral, it is still unclear how these laws will apply in the environment of healthcare. Of particular importance is the issue of interpretation of exceptions and exception to these laws for such structures as integrated healthcare delivery systems (IDS). Furthermore, comprehensive health system reform, championed by both political parties, is expected to modify certain provisions of the state laws that are thought to be overly restrictive.

Medicare Anti-Kickback Prohibitions

Substantive Law

A second law prohibits paying or receiving kickbacks, bribes, or rebates in return for the referral of a patient for items or services reimbursed by Medicare or Medicaid. The statute prohibits solicitation or offering of any remuneration, directly or indirectly, overtly or covertly, in cash or in kind:

(i) In return for referring an individual for the furnishing of any item or service for which payment may be made in whole or in part under Medicare or Medicaid, or

(ii) In return for purchasing or recommending leasing, ordering, any good, facility, service, or item for which payment may be made in whole or in part under Medicare or Medicaid.

By using the term "remuneration," Congress expressed its intent to cover a broad range of activities. This ensures that decisions concerning a patient's treatment will be made on the basis of sound medical judgment rather than on the basis of a possible financial benefit.

The statute does, however, contain a number of exceptions. Thus, the following payments are not branded illegal: payments of discounts that are reported and in some instances passed on to Medicare; compensation payments by employers to bona fide employees; payments by vendors to certain group purchasing organizations; and payments sanctioned by federal "safe harbor" regulations (Social Security Act §1128B(b)(3), 42 USC §1320a-7b).

As with the false claims provision, violation of the anti-kickback law is a felony punishable by fines of up to $25,000 and/or imprisonment for up to 5 years (Social Security Act §1128B[d], 42 USC §1320a-7b[d]). In addition, HCFA may also seek to exclude the provider from the Medicare and/or Medicaid programs (Social Security Act §1128(b)(7), 42 USC §1320a-5).

Because Section 1128B's prohibition on kickbacks is so broad, it covers a wide variety of factual situations. To understand it fully, it is helpful to examine the various interpretations of the statute that have been issued by the courts and the HHS Office of the Inspector General (OIG), which is charged with enforcing it.

Judicial Interpretations

A number of recent cases have considered whether particular conduct violates the anti-kickback provisions of Section 1128B. In one important case, United States v. Greber (760 F2d 68 [3rd Cir], cert denied, 474 US 988 [1985]), the court examined payments made by a medical diagnostic company providing Holter monitor services to physicians. The company billed Medicare for the services it provided and then forwarded 40% of the amount it received to the referring physician. The defendant alleged these payments were legitimate "interpretation fees. The court stated: "If one purpose of the payment is to induce referrals, the Medicare statute has been violated" (Ibid. at 69).

In 1989, two other courts considered the reasoning of the Greber opinion and accepted it. In United States v. Kats (871 F2d 105 [9th Cir 1989]), a medical services company referred blood and urine specimens that it collected from physicians and clinics to a reference laboratory, which then "kicked back" half of its receipts to the referring entity. The court held that the anti-kickback statute was violated because one of the material purposes of the payments was to obtain money for the referral of specimens.

In United States v. Bay State Ambulance and Hospital Rental Service Inc. (874 F2d 20 [1st Cir 1989]), the First Circuit affirmed the convictions of an ambulance service and an employee of the hospital with which the service had contracted. The employee's job included administering the hospital's contracts for ambulance services. He also performed "consulting services" for the defendant ambulance company and was involved in a separate business venture with one of the principals of the ambulance company. In the course of these dealings, he received two cars and cash payments from the ambulance company. The jury found that the automobiles were merely a way for the ambulance company to ensure that it received the hospital's business. Therefore, the anti-kickback provisions of Section 1128B had been violated.

In sum, these cases hold that it is illegal to pay or receive any form of remuneration if one purpose of the payment is to induce referrals. According to the courts considering these cases, the statute is violated if inducement is only one purpose of the payment and even if the payment constitutes reasonable compensation for work actually performed. Thus, whenever a firm involved in furnishing home health services makes a payment or provides some other form of remuneration to a physician, hospital, or other individual or entity who is in a position to refer patients for services, questions may be raised under the anti-kickback law.

OIG Pronouncements and Cases

FRAUD ALERT. In April 1989, the OIG issued an unprecedented "Fraud Alert" to all Medicare providers. In it, the OIG reported on a proliferation of "joint ventures" between those in a position to refer business, such as physicians, and those providing items or services for which Medicare or Medicaid pays. The OIG specifically noted that the provision of durable medical equipment was often included in such arrangements.

The Fraud Alert expressed the OIG's concern about joint ventures in which physicians (*a*) become investors, (*b*) refer patients to the venture, and (*c*) are paid by the venture in the form of profit distributions. The OIG observed that:

These suspect joint ventures may be intended not so much to raise investment capital legitimately to start a business, but to lock up a stream of referrals from the physician investors and to compensate them indirectly for these referrals. Because physician investors can benefit financially from their referrals, unnecessary procedures and tests may be ordered or performed, resulting in unnecessary program expenditures.

The OIG stated that such arrangements often have specific features that violate the anti-kickback statute. Among them are the following: investors are chosen because they are in a position to make referrals; physicians who make a large number of referrals are offered greater investment opportunity; physicians may be actively encouraged to make referrals to the venture and may be encouraged to divest if they do not; the joint venture tracks its referrals and distributes this information to investors; investment interests may be nontransferable.

The Fraud Alert also noted that in some instances the structure of the venture itself may be suspect. For example, one such structure occurs when one of the parties to the venture is an existing company that is already in the business that the joint venture is supposedly entering. Thus, according to the OIG, the venture may in fact be little more than a "shell" designed to compensate investors for the referral of patients.

If the amount of capital invested by the physician is disproportionately small compared to the returns that are achieved, the entity may be violating the anti-kickback provisions. The Fraud Alert thus requires that all providers of home health care services exercise caution when entering into a business enterprise with individuals or entities that are also a source of referrals.[h] Advice of competent counsel is highly recommended when such arrangements are contemplated.

In June 1995, the OIG issued a Special Fraud Alert regarding home healthcare fraud. In that Special Alert, the Inspector General indicated that home health services are particularly vulnerable to fraud and abuse because:

1. Medicare covers an unlimited number of visits per patient,
2. Beneficiaries pay no co-payments except on medical equipment,
3. Patients do not receive explanations of benefits for bills submitted for home health services, and

4. There is limited direct medical supervision of home health services provided by nonmedical personnel.

The OIG further indicated that the following types of practices were subject to prosecution: claims for services that were never provided, duplicate claims for the same service, claims for services for ineligible patients, and claims for a service that the healthcare provider knows was not medically necessary.

The OIG in the June 1995 Special Alert ominously states:

"Home health agencies, as well as the physicians who order home health services, are responsible for insuring medical necessity of claims submitted to Medicare. A physician who orders unnecessary home health care services may be liable for causing false claims to be submitted by the home health agency, even though the physician does not submit the claim. Furthermore, if agency personnel believe that services ordered by a physician are excessive or otherwise inappropriate, the agency cannot avoid liability for filing improper claims simply because a physician has ordered the services."

"SAFE HARBOR" REGULATIONS. The anti-kickback statute is broad and the penalties for violation are serious. Congress therefore required the OIG to identify specific practices that, although technically unlawful, will not be subject to criminal prosecution or exclusion. In accordance with this mandate, the OIG issued "safe harbor" regulations that describe the specific situations that will not give rise to liability under §1128B (see 54 Federal Register 3088, July 29, 1991).

The regulations describe certain conduct that is not believed to be the type that the law was designed to forbid. Conduct meeting the "safe harbor" requirements is therefore immunized. These regulations spell out specific requirements that must be met to obtain immunity. They are useful in showing not only what types of arrangements are permissible, but, conversely, what activity is suspicious.

Since 1991, the OIG has also issued additional Safe Harbor regulations regarding rural joint ventures, certified ambulatory surgical

---

[h] *Of course, as noted above, there are restrictions that prevent a physician-owner of an HHA from signing a plan of treatment for a patient receiving services from the HHA.*

centers, and managed care organizations. Significantly, in July 1994, the OIG issued proposed clarification regulations concerning all of the Safe Harbor regulations. In essence, these proposed regulations would expressly deny protection to sham transactions that on their face purport to satisfy the Safe Harbor regulations while in reality do not fit those regulations. (See 59 Federal Register 37202 [July 21, 1994].)

The safe harbors relate to the following general areas: investment interests, space rental, equipment rental, personal services/ management contracts, sale of practice, referral services, warranties, discounts, employee payments, payment by group purchasing organizations, and waiver of beneficiary coinsurance and deductibles. Conduct that falls outside one of the safe harbors is not automatically illegal; it is simply not immunized from possible prosecution.

Investment Interests. The anti-kickback provision of Section 1128B is so broad that it would prohibit receiving a dividend from a company if one prescribed the company's products for a Medicare patient. The OIG determined that Congress did not mean to prevent such stock ownership, and therefore crafted a narrowly drawn safe harbor for certain investment interests.

Large Corporations. The safe harbors provide immunity for profit distributions, e.g., dividends, paid to referrers who own securities in a large corporation with which they do Medicare or Medicaid business. The OIG adopted this safe harbor because the remuneration received by investors in such an entity is so tangentially related to the investors' referrals that the potential for abuse is minimal. Thus, this safe harbor applies to a corporation that, in the previous fiscal year or previous 12-month period, had more than $50 million in undepreciated net tangible assets related to the furnishing of healthcare services.

To comply with the safe harbor, the following conditions must be met: (*a*) if the investment is in an equity security, that equity security must be registered with the Securities and Exchange Commission (SEC); (*b*) an investor who is in a position to make or influence Medicare or Medicaid referrals must have obtained his or her interest on terms equally available to the public through trading on a registered national securities exchange, such as the New York Stock Exchange, the American Stock Exchange, or the National Association of Securities Dealers Automated Quotation System (NASDAQ); (*c*) neither the company nor any investor may market or furnish services any differently to investing referrers than to noninvestors; (*d*) the company must not loan funds to or guarantee a loan for a referring investor if the investor uses any part of such a loan to obtain the investment interest; and (*e*) the amount of payment to an investor in return for the investment interest must be directly proportional to the amount of capital invested by that investor.

The OIG requirement that the security be registered with the SEC was adopted to provide a "bright line" rule. The OIG specifically declined to provide safe harbor protection for securities traded through the so-called "pink sheets" or "non-NASDAQ" securities that are traded through the OTC Bulletin Board Service. However, the interest may also be held in debt securities. Where such an interest is maintained, registration with the SEC is not required.

The requirement that the investment interest be obtained on terms equally available to the public through a registered national securities exchange was imposed to ensure that the investment was obtained by arm's-length trading, rather than by an entity selecting investors based on their status as sources of referrals.

Small Entities. The OIG has adopted a tight, specifically enumerated safe harbor for investment by Medicare and Medicaid referrers in small entities. The safe harbor establishes eight standards that must be met for immunity. Investors are classified as either passive or active. An active investor includes a bona fide general partner or an individual or entity that agrees in writing to undertake the venture's liability. Passive investors are those investors who are not active investors, including limited partners and shareholders. Some of the eight standards must be met by both passive and active investors, and some of the standards need be met only by passive investors.

The OIG adopted these eight standards in response to three general concerns: the manner in which investors are selected and retained, the nature of the business structure, and the financing and profit distributions of the venture.

Manner in Which Investors Are Selected and Retained. The first five standards require that (*a*) no more than 40% of the investment interest may be held by investors who are in a position to generate business for the entity; (*b*) the terms on which the investment interest is offered to a passive investor who is in a position to generate business for the entity must be no different than the terms offered to non–business-generating passive investors; (*c*) the terms on which the investment interest is offered to an investor who is in a position to generate business for the entity must not be related to the previous or expected volume of business generated by that investor for the entity; (*d*) there must be no requirement that a passive investor generate business for the entity as a condition for remaining an investor; and (*e*) neither the entity nor any investor may market or furnish the entity's items or services to passive investors differently than to noninvestors (thereby barring cross-referral schemes).

For purposes of the 40% test, those who provide items and services and those who refer patients are both considered to be "in a position to generate business"; thus, both are included in what the OIG calls the 40% "tainted pool." Accordingly, at least 60% of the value of the investment must be held by non–business-generating investors.

Business Structure. The sixth standard requires that no more than 40% of the gross revenues of the entity may come from referrals or business generated from investors. This provision was included because the OIG believes that entities should not exist by relying on business from investors' referrals.

In applying the two 60-40 rules, the OIG will examine the ownership structure to determine (*a*) whether the joint venture is owned by other entities, and (*b*) whether those entities are owned by physicians who are referring to the joint venture entity. In such a situation, these physicians will be considered investors in the joint venture entity.

The OIG plans to monitor compliance with these safe harbor provisions and to report to the HHS Secretary on whether compliance with the two 60-40 rules "adequately controls abusive arrangements or whether more stringent requirements are needed."

Financing and Profit Distributions. The seventh and eighth standards require that (*a*) the entity must not loan funds to or guarantee a loan for an investor who is in a position to generate business for the entity; and (*b*) the profits distributed to an investor must be directly proportional to the amount of his or her capital investment.

The purpose of these two standards is to ensure that the investors provide needed capital, that their funds are genuinely at risk, and that the joint venture is not in reality a sham to facilitate the distribution of payments for referrals.

Space Rentals. Section 1128B could also be construed to prevent an entity from renting space to or from a referrer, since the rental payment could constitute illegal remuneration. While such arrangements could be wholly innocent, they could also be vehicles for illegal kickbacks.

To protect bona fide rental arrangements, the OIG issued a safe harbor for arrangements meeting the following requirements: (*a*) the lease agreement must be written and signed by the parties; (*b*) the lease must specify the premises covered; (*c*) if the lease provides for rental on periodic intervals rather than on a full-time basis, it must specify exactly the schedule of the intervals, their length, and the exact rent for each interval; (*d*) the lease term must be for at least 1 year; and (*e*) the rental amounts must reflect the fair market value of the space involved and cannot take into account the volume or value of Medicare or Medicaid referrals.

Equipment Rentals. Agreements for the rental of diagnostic or other types of medical equipment may be subject to the same types of abuse as the space rental arrangements described above. To safeguard legitimate equipment rental arrangements, the OIG safe-harbored arrangements that meet the following special requirements: (*a*) an executed, written lease exists that specifies the equipment covered by the agreement; (*b*) the lease, if for periodic intervals of time rather than full-time, specifies exactly the schedule of such intervals, their precise length, and the exact rent for such intervals; (*c*) the term of the lease is for at least 1 year; and (*d*) the aggregate rental charge is set in advance, is consistent with fair market value, and is not determined in a manner that takes into account the Medicare and Medicaid business generated between the parties. In addition, the OIG cautions against the use of "wear and tear" clauses whereby payments are tied directly to the volume of business referred.

Nonetheless, the OIG concedes that legitimate considerations, such as the depreciation of equipment, could result in some part of the payment being computed on a percentage or "per use" basis without these payments necessarily influencing or being influenced by Medicare or Medicaid referrals. But the more the payments appear to reflect the volume of referrals from the financially interested party, the more suspect the arrangement becomes.

Personal Services/Management Contracts. Medical practitioners and providers often have agreements to perform services for each other on mutually beneficial terms. The personal services/management contract safe harbor sets forth the following conditions for immunity: (*a*) the agreement must be set out in writing and signed by the parties; (*b*) the agreement must specify the services to be provided; (*c*) if the agreement is intended to provide for the services of the agent on a part-time basis, then the agreement must specify the schedule of such intervals, their precise length, and the exact charge for such intervals; (*d*) the term of the agreement must be for at least 1 year; (*e*) compensation paid to the agent must be set in advance, must be consistent with fair market value, and must not vary with the value or volume of Medicare or Medicaid referrals; and (*f*) the services performed under the agreement do not involve the counseling or promotion of a business arrangement or other activity that violates any state or federal law.

Discounts. The provision or acceptance of discounts is eligible for safe harbor status, but only if certain conditions are met. For home health agencies and other providers who are paid on a cost basis, discounts are safe-harbored if (*a*) the discount is earned on purchases of the same good or service and is exercised within a single fiscal year; (*b*) the buyer claims the benefit of the discount in the fiscal year in which the discount is earned or in the following year; (*c*) the buyer fully and accurately reports the discount in its cost report; and (*d*) the buyer provides, upon governmental request, discount information supplied by the seller.

Health maintenance organizations (HMOs) and competitive medical plans (CMPs) operating under a risk-based contract need not report discounts, except as otherwise required under the contract.

All others must comply with the following three standards in order to obtain safe harbor status: (*a*) the discount must be made at the time of the original sale of the good or service; (*b*) where an item or service is separately claimed for payment, the buyer must fully and accurately report the discount received on that item or service; and (*c*) the buyer must provide, upon governmental request, discount information provided to it by the seller.

Waiver of Cost Sharing. Waiver of beneficiary coinsurance and deductible amounts will be safe harbored only if (*a*) they are owed to a hospital for inpatient services reimbursed under the prospective payment system and so long as the hospital meets certain prescribed standards, or (*b*) they are owed to specified federally qualified facilities by an individual who is eligible for assistance under designated federal programs.

The Hanlester Case

The OIG has recently had an opportunity to apply the principles that it enunciated in the Fraud Alert and the safe harbor regulations. In 1990, the agency charged that SmithKline BioScience Laboratories (SKBL) and the Hanlester Network had violated the anti-kickback law through relationships involving physician-owned joint venture labs. Without admitting liability, SKBL settled the matter for $1.5 million, and the OIG pursued its case against the Hanlester principals seeking to exclude them from Medicare.

In applying these principles to the Hanlester facts, the Departmental Appeals Board (DAB) found that (*a*) "every referral made by a limited partner would incrementally increase his payment, so at least some part of the payments [to] referring partners 'was conditioned on' his referrals"; and (*b*) the "limited partners were aware of the potential impact of their referral decisions on their income." Accordingly, the Hanlester structure violated the statute.

Having provided this guidance, the DAB sent the case back to the ALJ and asked him to reconsider a number of his decisions based on the Board's articulation of legal standards that differed from those the ALJ adopted. The DAB instructed the ALJ to reanalyze the case in light of the following:

1. An offer or payment of remuneration to induce referrals is unlawful even if it is not coupled with an agreement to refer.
2. The relevant question is whether the Hanlester arrangements involved the knowing and willful offer or payment of remuneration "with the intent of exercising influence over the reason or judgment of the physicians in an effort to cause them to refer."
3. Remuneration that exceeds the reasonable value of any services "openly provided" or of any investment made is "likely intended as an inducement for referrals."

4. If payments to the limited partners are excessive in relation to the risks involved and the returns of alternative investments in general (i.e., not health care ventures), the excess could act as an inducement.
5. Remuneration to induce referrals may be inferred from the venture's structure (e.g., investment is limited to referrers, use of alternative providers is discouraged, capital is not really contributed, venture's services are not needed).
6. Remuneration to induce referrals may be inferred from "the degree of nexus" between the remuneration and the referrals.
7. Remuneration to induce referrals may result in overutilization or inferior quality and thus evidence of these consequences is relevant to establishing whether the incentives offered were sufficient to induce referrals.

These standards, in combination with the recently issued safe harbors, provide meaningful guidance for assessing the legality of various business arrangements.

Scienter Requirement Under 42 USC §1320A-7B

Both the Ninth and Tenth Circuits have recently issued decisions interpreting the language of 42 USC §1320a-7b as requiring scienter, or specific intent, to be in violation of the Medicare/Medicaid anti-kickback statute. In Hanlester Network v. Shalala 51 F.3d §1390 (9th Cir 1995), the Court of Appeals for the Ninth Circuit addressed the issue of physician investments in clinical laboratories. The Court rendered a significant decision articulating new interpretations of §1320a-7b.

The Court, in discussing the alleged referral arrangement amongst the parties, reasoned that "mere encouragement would not violate the statute." Furthermore, the Court concluded that the term "inducement" in the context of the statute requires "an intent to exercise influence of the reason or judgment of another in an effort to cause the referral of program related business." Moreover, the Court found that in order to be in violation of the anti-kickback statute, the party must engage in the prohibited activity with a specific intent to contravene the law. Therefore, a defendant must have actual knowledge in the form of a subjective understanding that the conduct in question is unlawful.

Other courts have addressed the "knowingly and willfully" language in the statute. In United States v. Laughlin 26 F.3d 1523 (10th Cir 1994), the Court of Appeals for the Tenth Circuit held that jury instructions were defective where they did not specify that for a party to be convicted under the §1320a-7b, he must have known that the false statements or representations were false when the claim was submitted.

These cases announced a difficult standard for the government to prove violations under the statute and may come as a relief to providers who feared prosecution for oversights, etc. These cases also seem to say that an honest misunderstanding or ignorance of the statute will preclude prosecution thereunder.

Liabilities

Like all providers of healthcare services, individuals and entities that furnish home healthcare services may be liable if a patient to whom they are providing care is injured. There are several different possible bases for this liability. The entity may be liable if a patient is injured as a result of the entity's negligence. Second, in some cases, the entity may be strictly liable—that is, liable without regard to whether it has been negligent. And it may be liable for failing to adequately protest the limitations on care imposed by a third-party payor.

Negligence

Negligence occurs when an entity fails to act with reasonable care and injures someone to whom it owes a duty of care. For negligence to occur in the context of the provision of home health services to a patient, the individual or entity providing the services must owe a duty of care to the patient; there must be a breach of that duty; the breach of that duty must be the legal (or proximate) cause of the

injury, and the patient must have actually suffered injury or damage.

An individual or entity providing home healthcare services could breach its duty to a patient through its own actions or through the actions of its employees. In addition, it could also breach its duty by failing to take action that it is obligated to take.

Guidelines for Avoiding Negligence

There are, of course, an unlimited number of ways in which negligence can occur; thus, it is difficult to offer specific guidance. However, there are some basic guidelines for avoiding negligence.

ENSURE COMPLIANCE WITH ALL APPLICABLE LAWS AND REGULATIONS. In determining whether duty of care of a patient has been breached, courts (and plaintiffs) often look to the standards established in statutes and regulations. If a particular statute or regulation that was designed to protect the patient has been violated, a court may find that this proves that the entity has breached its duty. This determination is often referred to as negligence per se. Thus, if a patient is injured by the actions of a caregiver who was not, according to state law, permitted to furnish the care provided, this error might constitute negligence per se. In cases where there is no showing of negligence per se, the patient will have to show that the entity or its agent did not act reasonably under the circumstances.

ENSURE ADEQUATE QUALIFICATIONS OF ALL CAREGIVERS. Providers should consult the Medicare regulations and the standards established by the Joint Commission on Accreditation of Health Care Organizations (JCAHO) in determining what qualifications particular types of caregivers should have.

ESTABLISH INTERNAL PROCEDURES. All entities should establish internal policies and procedures to be followed by caregivers. These should cover those situations that are likely to arise and should clearly define the responsibilities of caregivers.

FOLLOW PHYSICIAN ORDERS. All caregivers should understand that they must follow the plan of treatment and other orders instituted by the patient's physician or therapist. No change should be made in the order or plan of treatment without consulting the physician or therapist who established them and without receiving his or her authorization. Any change in the orders should be clearly documented in the patient's record.

COMMUNICATE FREQUENTLY WITH THE PATIENT'S PHYSICIAN. Just as important as following the physician's orders is communicating with the physician concerning any change in the patient's condition or other matter affecting the patient's health. Communication with the physician should be frequent, detailed, and documented. Even unsuccessful attempts to reach the physician should be documented. Most important, if a change in the patient's condition necessitates a change in the physician's orders, it is the responsibility of the provider to contact that physician. Any attempt to do so should be well documented.

MAINTAIN CAREFUL DOCUMENTATION OF CARE PROVIDED. All care provided should be carefully documented, so that an entity can show it exercised reasonable care in treating the patient, should questions arise later. A provider's own records are often the "best evidence" of the care that was provided because the particular caregivers may not remember what happened or be available to explain it.

COMMUNICATE WITH PATIENT AND FAMILY MEMBERS. Providers should communicate often with the patient and family members concerning the patient's condition and treatment. Time should be taken to explain procedures and answer questions. Entities may wish to have patients (or, in some instances, family members) sign informed consent forms to ensure that patients or family members understand the care that will be provided and the risks involved in providing such care.

ESTABLISH PROCEDURES FOR RELATIONSHIP INITIATION AND TERMINATION. As no duty of care is owed to an individual who is not a patient, providers should establish strict procedures for establishing the patient-provider relationship. In addition, providers should establish procedures to be followed if third-party payors refuse to pay or stop paying for treatment. Mere cessation of care without adequate notice to the patient could constitute abandonment and subject the entity providing services to liability.

Strict Liability

In addition to negligence, courts have recently found liability on the basis of "strict liability," which relieves the complaining party of having to prove that the other party failed to act with reasonable care.

Courts have sometimes imposed strict liability when they find the defendant's action constituted a breach of its implied warranty. Under this theory, a manufacturer or seller of a product may be held strictly liable if the product was defective, i.e., not fit for its intended purpose, and caused the injury. This finding is based on the theory that the defendant breached an implied term of its contract to provide the item at issue.

The issue of breach of implied warranty has arisen in a medical context in cases where an entity furnishes blood that is tainted with hepatitis B virus (HBV) or, more recently, human immunodeficiency virus (HIV). The leading case in this area, however, failed to hold a hospital strictly liable for supplying blood tainted with HBV because, according to the court, the furnishing of blood is a service, rather than a sale, and as a result, there is no implied warranty. The court held, therefore, that the hospital could not be strictly liable (Perlmutter v. Beth David Hospital, 308 NY 100, 123 NE2d 792 [1954]). Many states have now adopted the reasoning of Perlmutter in statutes that specifically declare that those involved in obtaining, processing, storing, distributing, or using blood for medical purposes are engaged in a service rather than the sale of a product (see, e.g., Md Health Gen Code Ann §18–402 [1982]).

In addition, courts have also looked to tort principles in imposing strict liability. Under this approach, the service/sale distinction may be inapplicable. Thus, courts have held that strict liability may be imposed where injury results from the use of a defective product that is unreasonably dangerous to the user (Restatement Second Torts, §402A). This rule does not apply to products that are "unavoidably unsafe," including certain types of drugs and vaccines (see Restatement Second Torts, §402A, Comment k).

Liability as a Result of Insurer's Limitations

Finally, providers should be sensitive to the fact that the changing medical environment has created new forms of possible liability, especially as third-party payors become increasingly involved in managing patient care. In a well-known California case, Wickline v. California (183 Cal App 3rd 1175, 228 Cal Rptr 661, appeal dismissed, 239 Cal Rptr 805 [1987]), Mrs. Wickline, a Medicaid patient, suffered complications following surgery. The State of California authorized a limited, initial hospital stay that was then extended for 4 days, despite her physician's request for an 8-day extension. At the end of the 4-day period, the physician did not seek an additional extension, and Mrs. Wickline was discharged. At home, she suffered further complications and ultimately had to have a leg amputated. As a result, she brought suit.

Although the court did not find the state liable in this case, it did note that payors that impose restrictions on the provision of care may be liable if their policies result in a patient being prematurely discharged. The court also found, however, that providers have a "duty of protest" if they believe that a payor is making a decision that could adversely affect a patient. In a later case, Wilson v. Blue Cross of South Carolina (222 Cal App 3rd 660, 271 Cal Rptr 876 [1990]), the California court determined that a third-party payor could be liable regardless of whether or not the physician objected to the payor's decision to discharge a patient. Providers of home healthcare who are forced to make decisions that could be adverse to their patients, based on third-party payors' payment policies, should, however, still inform these payors that these policies could injure patients.

A physician may also be held liable to an injured patient for failing to supervise or train individuals under his or her control. In Tobia v. Cooper Hospital University Medical Center (136 N.J. 335, 643 A. 2d 1 [N.J. 1994]), the physicians were held potentially liable for not adequately supervising nurses and medical students who allegedly left a patient unattended in an emergency room stretcher without raised side rails, which resulted in the patient being injured as a result of a fall.

Conclusion

Despite its length, this chapter only provides a superficial review of the possible legal problems related to intensive homecare. While it can introduce the reader to some of the legal analysis that may be relevant to a particular situation, it cannot supply definitive answers to the legal issues that physicians involved in homecare may encounter. There is simply no way that a book chapter can substitute for the advice of a competent attorney who is familiar with an individual's practice and the healthcare field.

Acknowledgment

The authors are indebted to Fred Jacobs, M.D., J.D., for his contribution in reviewing the manuscript and updating several key points.

9

ECONOMIC IMPACT OF HOMECARE

Warren Balinsky

CHAPTER AT A GLANCE: These days the health care system is going through unprecedented change. To a great extent, this change is being brought about by economic factors, and this is certainly true in the area of homecare. Some of the underlying factors related to economics that are affecting homecare are population shifts, shifts in diseases and disabilities, new technology, and attempts to control cost. Numerous studies have shown that home or outpatient therapy can be significantly less expensive than hospital or institutional therapy in most cases. The dilemma for Medicare is how to provide reimbursement for home drug infusion therapy for appropriate patients and not add to the spiraling cost of healthcare.

Factors Promoting Growth of Homecare

New mothers and their babies were the traditional users of home healthcare. In recent years, however, the great bulk of services has been provided to the elderly and the chronically ill. Homecare is the fastest-growing service industry in the United States, serving rapidly increasing numbers of AIDS and hospice patients, as well as high-tech and pediatric patients. It is instructive to look at some of the major factors responsible for this growth, which include changes in population, shifts in diseases and disabilities, pressures to control spiraling medical costs, and new technology.

Population Shifts

In 1987, nearly six million Americans, or 2.5% of the population, received home health services (see Table 9.1). Of these, approximately three million were over the age of 65—a significant shift from 1980 data, in which approximately 70% were over age 65 (1). In 1987, females were twice as likely as males to use homecare services. Widowed and, to a lesser extent, separated or divorced persons were more likely to use home health services than married persons. The percentages of blacks, whites, and Hispanics who used home health care were similar. Increasing levels of functional limitation, which are associated with increasing age, were also associated with increases in the percentage of the population using home health services (2, 3).

Contrary to popular belief, the elderly, both white and nonwhite, are not typically abandoned by their families. Admission to a nursing home is usually a last resort. Most elderly persons remain in the community and are cared for by family and friends. But as the number of frail elderly persons continues to grow, so does the burden placed on those who

Table 9.1. Use of Home Health Care Services: Percent of Persons Receiving Home Health Visits and Mean Number of Visits and Providers Used, by Demographic Characteristics, United States, 1987

			Mean per Person with Visits	
	Total U.S.	Percent Receiving		
	Population	at Least One	Visits from	Particular
Population Characteristic	(in thousands)	Home Health Visit	All Providers	Providers Used
Total[a]	239,393	2.5	44.0	1.5
Age in years				
Under 40	153,128	1.1	15.0	1.2
Under 6	24,838	2.5	4.3	1.1
6–17	41,950	0.6	*	*
18–39	86,340	1.0	22.8	1.2
40–64	59,744	2.0	37.9	1.5
65–74	16,378	7.1	55.7	1.6
75–84	8,111	14.5	66.9	1.8
85 and older	2,032	30.9	70.6	1.8
Sex				
Male	115,861	1.6	30.7	1.4
Female	123,532	3.3	49.8	1.6
Ethnic/racial background				
White	183,396	2.6	44.2	1.5
Black	28,567	2.4	54.2	1.6
Hispanic	19,186	1.8	*	*
Marital status[b]				
Married	103,589	2.0	31.8	1.4
Widowed	13,762	12.6	70.0	1.7
Divorced/separated	19,542	3.4	61.1	1.8
Never married	40,881	1.5	43.5	1.4
Living arrangement				
Alone	35,230	6.2	70.4	1.7
With others	204,163	1.8	28.5	1.4
ADL/IADL difficulties[c]				
None	227,004	1.2	12.8	1.1
IADL difficulties only	4,910	17.7	43.4	1.6
1–2 ADL difficulties	4,625	22.9	61.0	1.7
3 or more ADL difficulties	2,854	41.4	102.0	2.1
Place of residence				
SMSA	178,539	2.4	42.4	1.5
Other	60,854	2.6	48.1	1.4
Census region				
Northeast	47,921	2.8	44.8	1.7
Midwest	60,478	2.8	38.5	1.4
South	83,766	1.9	47.9	1.5
West	47,227	2.7	45.4	1.5

From Agency for Health Care Policy and Research. National Medical Expenditure Survey—Household Survey, 1993.

[a] Includes persons with other or unknown ethnic/racial background and unknown marital status.

[b] Excludes persons under 18.

[c] Difficulties in activities of daily living (ADLs) resulting from a physical or mental health problem and including bathing, dressing, toileting, feeding, and transferring from bed or chair; and in instrumental activities of daily living (IADLs) including use of the telephone, shopping for personal items, transportation, managing money, light housework, and preparing meals.

*Cell size too small for reliable estimates.

care for them and the institutions that serve them.

Within the next 50 years, the number of people in the United States over the age of 65 is expected to more than double. The U.S. Bureau of the Census projects that by the year 2030, fully 20% of Americans will be 65 or older. This increase will be higher for those over 75, the "old-old." In addition, more women than men are living to older ages. In 1955, the female-to-male ratio was 115:100 for people over 65, whereas in 1985 the ratio was estimated to be about 138:100. This is important because elderly women tend to have a higher rate of utilization of all health services, including homecare. As the over-65 population continues to grow as a proportion of the total population, there will be a corresponding increase in the need for and use of home health services.

Shifts in Diseases

There has also been a shift in the nature of the dominant diseases plaguing all age groups, particularly the elderly. Acute illnesses have been largely replaced by chronic disorders that usually require either ongoing care or intermittent treatment on a regular basis. For persons aged 65 and over, the leading chronic disabling conditions are arthritis and hypertensive disease. Most visits to physicians by older persons are for circulatory problems, arthritis, and musculoskeletal ailments. The primary diagnoses presented most frequently by homecare patients are circulatory disease, neoplasm, diabetes, and musculoskeletal problems. Although a significantly higher proportion of persons 65 and older than of those under 65 experience functional limitations due to a chronic condition, it is not until age 75 that over half of the population is limited. Approximately 20% of the members of this age group are limited to the point that they cannot carry on one or more major activities of daily living. Chronic disorders that require ongoing care and treatment, and disabilities that accompany the aging process, have resulted not only in a greater number of homecare referrals but also in the referral of patients with greater needs (1).

As hospital stays were shortened in the 1980s, the percentage of Medicare patients discharged to homecare for continuing rehabilitative care increased from 8.16% in 1981 to 14.6% in 1985. The most common medical diagnoses or surgical procedures for Medicare home healthcare patients in 1988 were heart failure (DRG 127), stroke (DRG 14), and chronic obstructive pulmonary disease (DRG 88) (4).

Though the elderly have been, and continue to be, the largest consumers of home health services, we are also beginning to see an increase in the number of users under age 65, including children. It is estimated that about 10 million children in the United States are afflicted with chronic illness, and that about 1 million would be considered severe cases (5). The tremendous progress in medical and surgical technologies in the past two decades has meant that these children are now living to young adulthood. Homecare for them represents an important alternative to hospital care, assuming that their condition permits the delivery of such care in the home.

Another shift involves the AIDS epidemic, which has had its greatest impact on the nonelderly population. The first reported AIDS cases appeared in early 1981 as isolated outbreaks of opportunistic infections. Since then, the number of cases has grown exponentially, and the requirements for homecare of AIDS patients have grown accordingly. In fact, homecare has become a critical component in the continuum of care for the AIDS client.

Attempts at Cost Control

The third major factor responsible for the growth of homecare has been the attempt by payers to control soaring medical costs. Total health care expenditures in the United States have risen from about 6.6% of gross domestic product in 1967 to about 14% in 1993, creating pressure to provide services in less costly settings. Changes have been made in both Medicare and Medicaid to speed discharges from hospitals and nursing homes, as well as to prevent admissions to those institutions.

Although Medicare covered home health benefits from its beginning in 1966, Congress passed amendments in 1972 that promoted homecare by simplifying various administrative matters involving payment for services, eliminating some coinsurance provisions, and extending coverage to disabled persons and those with end-stage renal disease. Further amendments in 1980 eliminated the hundred-visit limitation (Part A), the three-day prior hospital stay requirement (Part A), and the $60 deductible for home health services (Part B). The Omnibus Reconciliation Act of 1981 allowed proprietary homecare agencies to be Medicare certified in states without licensing laws. Prior to this, proprietary agencies were permitted to provide services to Medicare patients only through a subcontract with a certified voluntary agency. Now they can compete directly with the voluntary agencies for Medicare patients.

The introduction of Medicare's Prospective Payment System in the 1980s also gave impetus to homecare growth. This system was based on a set of categorized diagnoses, diagnostic related groups (DRGs), which classified patients according to their diagnoses. Hospitals were paid a fixed dollar amount for a given diagnosis regardless of the patient's length of stay. They responded by integrating vertically so they could provide care in other than inpatient settings and continue to offer quality care while reducing inpatient costs and generating new revenues. One major component of this vertical integration was homecare. Similarly, one of the goals of Medicaid's waiver program was to control cost. This too significantly affected the growth of homecare.

New Technology

New technologies are playing an important role in the growth of homecare. For example, once-a-day long-lasting intravenous drugs delivered via new catheters and new computerized ambulatory multiport infusion pumps now allow patients who could earlier be cared for only in an institution to receive antibiotics, chemotherapy, parenteral nutrition, and pain medication as necessary at home. Other new technologies have made possible smaller, portable respiratory equipment and a host of other types of equipment.

Homecare Agencies

Homecare agencies consist of home health agencies, homecare aid organizations, and hospices. The first agencies appeared in the early 1980s. However, as of March 1994, The National Association for Home Care (NAHC) reported a total of 15,027 agencies in the United States. This number is made up of 7,521 Medicare-certified home health agencies, 1,459 Medicare-certified hospices, and 6,047 non–Medicare-certified agencies. The growth in agency numbers has been accompanied by a shift in sponsors, from primarily government agencies and visiting nurse associations (VNAs) to proprietary and hospital-based agencies (Table 9.2).

Reimbursement Sources

Various sources cover the costs of homecare. Frequently, the patient or family pays directly, out of pocket. Some costs of homecare are borne by private and public insurance; there is great variation, however, both in benefits and in eligibility requirements.

Medicare

Congress enacted the Medicare program in 1965 under Title 18 of the Social Security Act in order to provide health insurance for persons aged 65 years or older. Subsequently, coverage was extended to certain disabled persons and persons of any age with end-stage renal disease. Medicare consists of two parts. Part A, basic hospital insurance, covers hospitalization, posthospital skilled nursing facility care, home health care, hospice care, and blood replacement. Part B, supplementary medical insurance, is optional, although most recipients of Part A coverage purchase part B as well. Part B covers medical expenses, clinical laboratory services, home health care, out-

Table 9.2. Number of Medicare-Certified Home Health Agencies (HHAs), by Auspice, 1967–1994

| Year | Freestanding HHAs | | | | | | Facility-Based HHAs | | | TOTAL |
	VNA	COMB	PUB	PROP	PNP	OTH	HOSP	REHAB	SNF	
1967	549	93	939	0	0	39	133	0	0	1,753
1975	525	46	1,228	47	0	109	273	9	5	2,242
1980	515	63	1,260	186	484	40	359	8	9	2,924
1985	514	59	1,205	1,943	832	4	1,277	20	129	5,983
1986	510	62	1,192	1,915	826	4	1,341	17	117	5,984
1987	500	61	1,172	1,882	803	1	1,382	14	108	5,923
1988	496	55	1,073	1,846	766	1	1,439	12	97	5,785
1989	491	51	1,011	1,818	727	1	1,465	10	102	5,676
1990	474	47	985	1,884	710	0	1,486	8	101	5,695
1991	476	41	941	1,970	701	0	1,537	9	105	5,780
1992	530	52	1,083	1,962	637	28	1,623	3	86	6,004
1993	594	46	1,196	2,146	558	41	1,809	1	106	6,497
5/94	586	45	1,146	2,892	597	48	2,081	3	123	7,521

Source: Health Care Financing Administration, Office of Survey and Certification.

VNA: Visiting Nurse Associations are freestanding, voluntary, nonprofit organizations governed by a board of directors and usually financed by tax-deductible contributions as well as by earnings.

COMB: Combination agencies are combined government and voluntary agencies. These agencies are sometimes included with counts for VNAs.

PUB: Public agencies are government agencies operated by a state, county, city, or other unit of local government having a major responsibility for preventing disease and for community health education.

PROP: Proprietary agencies are freestanding, for-profit home health agencies.

PNP: Private not-for-profit agencies are freestanding and privately developed, governed, and owned nonprofit home health agencies.

OTH: Other freestanding agencies are agencies that do not fit one of the categories for freestanding agencies listed above.

HOSP: Hospital-based agencies are operating units or departments of a hospital. Agencies that have working arrangements with a hospital, or perhaps are even owned by a hospital but operated as separate entities, are classified as freestanding agencies under one of the categories listed above.

REHAB: Refers to agencies based in rehabilitation facilities.

SNF: Refers to agencies based in skilled nursing facilities.

patient hospital treatment, and blood replacement (Tables 9.3 and 9.4).

Medicare covers skilled nursing and home health aide services, speech therapy, physical therapy, occupational therapy, medical social work, and medical supplies and equipment. However, to qualify, the patient must be under a physician's care, must be homebound, and must require part-time or intermittent skilled nursing services or physical or speech therapy. A physician must design and periodically review the care plan. Home health services cannot be full-time, and the illness must be one that responds to treatment by a physician over a finite period of time. Medicare also pays for hospice benefits, including palliative and support services, for terminally ill patients.

The consequence of these limitations is that Medicare, in effect, pays for only a small amount of homecare, which is almost entirely short-term care following an acute illness (6, 7).

Medicaid

Medicaid, Title 19 of the Social Security Act, was passed in 1965 to cover medically needy individuals. In recent years Congress has expanded the law by means of consolidated omnibus reconciliation acts (CORAs) adding new services and new criteria for recipients.

Medicaid provides health services to very poor people who are also aged, blind, and disabled; to members of families with dependent children; and to first-time pregnant women. In 30 states and the District of Columbia, persons in these categories can also qualify for Medicaid as "medically needy" if their medical expenses are high enough to render them poor. Medicaid is normally the payer of last resort (8).

Table 9.3. Medicare (Part A): Hospital Insurance-Covered Services for 1993

Services	Benefit	Medicare Pays	You Pay
Hospitalization	First 60 days	All but $676	$676
Semiprivate room and board, general	61st to 90th day	All but $169 a day	$169 a day
nursing and miscellaneous hospital	91st to 150th day[a]	All but $338 a day	$338 a day
services and supplies	Beyond 150 days	Nothing	All costs
Skilled Nursing Facility Care	First 20 days	100% of approved amount	Nothing
You must have been in a hospital for at	Additional 80 days	All but $84.50 a day	$84.50 a day
least 3 days and enter a Medicare-approved	Beyond 100 days	Nothing	All costs
facility generally within 30 days after			
hospital discharge[b]			
Home Health Care	Part-time or	100% of approved amount;	Nothing for services;
Medically necessary skilled care	intermittent care for	80% of approved amount	20% of approved
	as long as you	for durable medical	amount for durable
	meet Medicare conditions	equipment	medical equipment
Hospice Care			
Pain relief, symptom management, and	If you elect the hospice	All but limited costs for	Limited cost sharing
support services for the terminally ill	option and as long as	outpatient drugs and	for outpatient drugs
	doctor certifies need	inpatient respite care	and inpatient respite care
Blood	Unlimited if	All but first 3 pints	For first 3 pints[c]
	medically necessary	per calendar year	

1993 Part A monthly premium: None for most beneficiaries
$221 if you must buy Part A (Premium may be higher if you enroll late)

From U.S. Department of Health and Human Services, Health Care Financing Administration. The Medicare 1993 Handbook. Publication No. HCFA 10050. Washington, DC: U.S. Government Printing Office, 1993.

[a]This 60-reserve-days benefit may be used only once in a lifetime.

[b]Neither Medicare nor private Medigap insurance will pay for most nursing home care.

[c]To the extent the blood deductible is met under Part B of Medicare during the calendar year, it does not have to be met under Part A.

Table 9.4. Medicare (Part B): Medical Insurance-Covered Services for 1993

Services	Benefit	Medicare Pays	You Pay
Medical Expenses Doctors' services, inpatient and outpatient medical and surgical services and supplies, physical and speech therapy, ambulance, diagnostic tests, and more	Medicare pays for medical services in or out of the hospital	80% of approved amount (after $100 deductible)	$100 deductible,[a] plus 20% of approved amount and limited charges above approved amount[b]
Clinical Laboratory Services Blood tests, urinalyses, and more	Unlimited if medically necessary	100% of approved amount	Nothing for services
Home Health Care Medically necessary skilled care	Part-time or intermittent skilled care for as long as you meet conditions for benefits	100% of approved amount; 80% of approved amount for durable medical equipment	Nothing for services; 20% of approved amount for durable medical equipment
Outpatient Hospital Treatment Services for the diagnosis or treatment of illness or injury	Unlimited if medically necessary	Medicare payment to hospital based on hospital cost	$100 deductible, plus 20% of billed charges
Blood	Unlimited if medically necessary	80% of approved amount (after $100 deductible and starting with 4th pint)	First 3 pints plus 20% of approved amount for additional pints (after $100 deductible)[b]

1993 Part B monthly premium: $36.60 (Premium may be higher if you enroll late)

From U.S. Department of Health and Human Services, Health Care Financing Administration. The Medicare 1993 Handbook. Publication No. HCFA 10050. Washington, DC: U.S. Government Printing Office, 1993.

[a]Once you have had $100 of expenses for covered services in 1993, the Part B deductible does not apply to any further covered services you receive for the rest of the year.

[b]To the extent the blood deductible is met under Part A of Medicare during the calendar year, it does not have to be met under Part B.

The Medicaid programs are really 54 separate state-administered programs funded jointly by state and federal governments. Eligibility requirements for Medicaid vary from state to state. Eligibility is also tied to various other welfare statutes. For example, families who are eligible for early and periodic screening, diagnosis, and treatment (EPSDT) and certain other CORA services are automatically eligible for Medicaid. Also, all persons receiving payments under the Aid to Families with Dependent Children (AFDC) program are automatically Medicaid-eligible, and all aged, blind, and disabled individuals (including children) who receive cash payments under the Supplementary Security Income (SSI) program are eligible in most states; however, states may have Medicaid eligibility requirements more restrictive than those of SSI.

Home health services available under Medicaid include part-time nursing, home health aide services, and medical equipment and supplies. The state has the option of providing physical, occupational, and speech therapy and audiology. It must provide home health services to all recipients 21 years and older who meet its eligibility criteria and to all other Medicaid recipients who are eligible for skilled nursing services (4).

Since its inception, Medicaid policy was strongly biased toward institutional long-term care. In 1981, however, in response to a family's appeal to the President and Congress for home coverage for their medically needy child, Congress included a section in the Omnibus Budget Reconciliation Act of 1981 that authorized the federal government to provide Medicaid payments for home- and community-based services to individuals who would otherwise receive Medicaid-reimbursed care in an institution. Under this program, states are required to obtain waivers of federal Medicaid rules in order to implement home-care services. Approval of a waiver requires, in part, a showing that the proposed home-care program is more cost effective than the services previously being provided.

States are not, however, required to cover homecare. Even where Medicaid home health services are provided, they vary dramatically in amount, duration, and scope. Few regular state Medicaid programs cover the full range of services that may be necessary in a nonhospital setting. Four types of waivers currently exist, each involving different eligibility requirements. A complete discussion of the Medicaid waivers, their legislative history, and their advantages and disadvantages may be found elsewhere (8–10).

Originally, the waiver program was intended for persons with conditions related to aging, disability, or mental retardation. Subsequent modifications of the law expanded waiver services to disabled children and persons with AIDS. By 1991, most states were using waivers to provide home- and community-based services to people with a variety of chronic disabilities.

Prior to the waiver program, typical Medicaid programs did not reimburse for nonmedical services. States now provide a range of these services, including case management, personal care, and adult day care. These services are often viewed as more clinically appropriate, are preferred by patients and families, and are less costly than institutional care (11).

Blue Cross/Blue Shield, Commercial Insurers, and Managed Care Organizations

Other third-party payers include Blue Cross/Blue Shield, various commercial insurers, and managed-care organizations. The difficulty in describing these payers is that each type really represents a large and diverse group of payers. For example, there are approximately 72 Blue Cross/Blue Shield programs across the United States, and they vary from group to group, state to state, and region to region. Generally speaking, however, almost all of these third-party payers cover homecare services. Their eligibility requirements, benefits, and limitations (deductible, coinsurance, type and amount of service) vary, but many follow Medicare guidelines.

HMOs provide comprehensive services—hospital, outpatient, emergency, homecare, and so on—to their subscribers at a fixed prepaid premium. An HMO contracts with either salaried staff members or independent practice associations (IPAs) to provide outpatient care. Inpatient care and homecare are provided by contractual arrangement with hospitals and with homecare agencies. Most often, ongoing homecare decisions are made by the HMO's local coordinators and discharge planners. This case management approach is proliferating beyond HMOs and other managed-care organizations to most health insurers and many health providers. The implication is that the growth of managed care and case management will further fuel the growth of homecare.

Because they act as both insurer and provider, HMOs are under financial pressure to provide service at the lowest possible cost. The major advantages for the subscriber are predictability and, usually, lower premiums. The major disadvantages are the limitations imposed by contractual arrangements and the loss of freedom to choose one's own providers of care without financial penalty (9).

Medicare and Medicaid are adopting many of the techniques of managed care organizations in their attempts to contain costs. In fact, many states are moving their Medicaid populations to Medicaid Managed Care programs by state mandate. These changes are having profound effects on homecare, and, to a large extent, are premised on the cost-effectiveness of homecare (12). Some examples of these issues follow.

Cost Effectiveness of Home Drug Infusion Therapy (HDIT)

Cost of HDIT

Data from numerous studies demonstrate that, in general, the cost of home or outpatient (administered at a clinic or doctor's office) antibiotic therapy to medical insurers is significantly less than hospital or other institutional care (13). A 1978 study showed that the cost of outpatient antibiotic therapy was less than one-third that of identical inpatient treatment, and many further studies have confirmed this (14). Table 9.5 shows the cost savings reported by various studies.

Table 9.5. Studies of Cost Savings from Home Intravenous Antibiotic Therapy, 1974–1986

Reference	Number of Patients (age range)	Average Savings per Day per Patient ($)	Days of Home Care	Average Savings per Patient ($)
Rucker (1974)	62 (7–27)	N.A.	10–12	N.A.
Antoniskis (1978)	20 (12–74)	165	2–32	3,665
Stiver (1978)	23 (12–78)	97	8–40	2,214
Kind (1979)	15 (3–61)	95	7–24	1,620
Swenson (1981)	8 (9–73)	148	5–35	2,371
Poretz (1982)	150 (3–86)	142	4–49	2,840
Stiver (1982)	95 (4–81)	135	8–46	3,228
Rehm (1983)	48 (10–77)	305	2–42	5,728
Poretz (1984)	79 (2–86)	N.A.	N.A.	B/C
Eron (1985)	80 (15–78)	280	2–49	5,125
Gainer (1985)	71 (13–80)	198	4–61	3,473
Kind (1985)	315 (N.A.)	350	1–79	4,725
Corby (1986)	36 (10–75)	345	13–42	9,114
Eisenberg (1986)	LSCS	N.A.	8	510–22,232
Graves (1986)	37 (3–77)	202	23[a]	2,790–4,651

From Balinsky, W. Home Care: Current Problems and Future Solutions. San Francisco: Jossey-Bass, Inc., 1994: 126.
Notes: N.A., not available; LSCS, Large-sample computer simulation; B/C, $6,588 in benefits and $1,768 in costs.
[a]Average.

For instance, a two-year (1983–1985) study by Gainer and Smego (15), involving 71 patients, showed a savings of $3,473 per patient course of therapy. They concluded: "Home intravenous antibiotic treatment produced the same outcome as hospitalized treatment. Adverse effects of drug or intravenous site were uncommon and were similar in frequency and type to those of hospitalized patients. . . . The emotional benefits of returning a patient to the home, and subsequently to work and school, are enormous" (p. 11).

Gainer and Smego (15) also projected an annual savings in health care dollars as follows: "If the estimated 50,000 cases of osteomyelitis and 15,000 cases of endocarditis were treated by home intravenous therapy for three weeks, approximately 273 million dollars would be saved" (p. 11). Though dollar amounts would, of course, be different today, the ratio of savings still holds.

As indicated by the quotation, recent cost-benefit analyses have addressed not only the direct costs of treatment, such as physician services and drugs, but also indirect costs. These include quality-of-life intangibles such as the pain and psychological suffering of illness as well as the patient's loss of earnings and decreased productivity during hospitalization (16, 13). For example, Poretz and others (17) found increased mobility, productivity, and quality of life among 79 patients receiving outpatient infusion therapy, and about half were able to work while receiving treatment.

The key to containing cost is the appropriate selection of patients. Often the amount of nursing service necessary to keep the patient safely at home (beyond the HDIT nursing visits) is what makes homecare more or less expensive than institutional care (18). Even in low-tech homecare, the need for extensive supportive services can make homecare more expensive for some patients. For this reason, in screening patients it is critical to consider economic factors in addition to the patient's capability for HDIT. If it appears that treating the patient at home will cost more than keeping the patient in the hospital, perhaps that patient should remain in the hospital.

Currently, the best example of this type of screening is New York State's Long Term Home Health Care Program (LTHHCP), which is targeted to Medicaid-eligible people who would otherwise be placed in a nursing home. The LTHHCP attempts to provide in the home all the services that these patients would receive in a nursing home, as well as modifications such as grab bars to make the home safe. However, the entire combination of services received cannot exceed 75% of what the same services would cost in a skilled nursing or other health-related facility (100% for particular patients).

Cost control is provided by a case manager, who adjusts the hours for each type of service rendered on an ongoing basis to keep the total under the cap. The result is that the government saves money on Medicaid patients whom it would otherwise have to place in a nursing home. Patients whose care would cost more at home or other appropriate facility are not selected for the program or are discharged from it.

This model could effectively be applied by Medicare for treating people with acute illness, to provide care they would otherwise have to receive in the hospital, using case managers who would handle not only safety and quality of care considerations but also cost.

Reimbursement of HDIT

Reimbursement policies of third-party payers reflect a variety of coverage patterns. This section focuses on Medicare, which sets the pattern for Blue Cross/Blue Shield and other insurance programs.

Although the largest potential group of homecare patients is the elderly, there are limits on Medicare coverage of homecare. In particular, there are no HDIT benefits per se, although Medicare does sometimes cover certain components of HDIT under other benefits. However, coverage of the basic services involved in providing HDIT is fragmentary, split between Medicare Part A and Part B. Part A covers homecare services deemed medically necessary by a physician. Medical equipment and supplies may be included under this coverage. Part B expands Part A to include physician services, ambulance transportation, prosthetic devices, independent laboratory tests, durable medical equipment (DME) such as reusable infusion pumps, and drugs and biological agents used by outpatients. However, drug coverage varies according to the carrier's interpretation of the DME benefit, and the drugs cannot be self-administered. Effective March 1994, four Medicare DME regional carriers with new regulations replaced the two DME regional carriers. This was an effort by Medicare to standardize and more quickly process the increasing number of claims. Under these new policy regulations, Medicare now covers administration of acyclovir, foscarnet, amphotericin B, vancomycin, and ganciclovir.

To qualify for home health care, Medicare patients must be confined to the home, be under a physician's care, and require intermittent skilled nursing services or physical or speech therapy (18, 19). Drugs, related services, and supplies must be an integral—although incidental—part of a physician's treatment. They must be delivered by a physician directly or by employees of a physician under a physician's direct supervision (20). This portion of the requirement means that the physician must be present or at hand when the patient is receiving care, whether in the office or in the patient's home. If a physician is not present at the treatment setting, Medicare will deny payment; if the patient is at home and a nurse administers intravenous antibiotics following a physician's orders, Medicare will deny payment (21, 25).

Limited coverage is available, however, in certain situations that require analgesics or chemotherapy administered by an external infusion pump. Medicare reimburses the patient for drugs that are listed under the DME benefit for certain specific diagnoses. For example, Medicare's hospice legislation, enacted in 1983, provides home treatment for patients with cancer. This legislation expanded Medicare coverage to include chemotherapy and nutritional products but did not cover intravenous antibiotics despite arguments that patients who receive such treatment are under similar physician supervision.

As for Medicaid, although each state has a different program, all the states have certain minimal requirements. In general, for the patient who qualifies because of lack of financial resources, Medicaid is broader and more generous in coverage than Medicare (4). Most prescription and some nonprescription drugs are covered; however, coverage of antibiotics may require prior approval. In the early 1980s, Medicaid added multidisciplinary case management services that use outpatient care and homecare as a cost-efficient way to provide quality care (22).

According to a 1987 survey sponsored by the Hoffmann-La Roche Company that included data from 50 Medicaid programs, 48 programs paid for intravenous antibiotic therapy in the home, although 29 of them required prior approval for coverage. (It should be pointed out, however, that reimbursement policies change frequently.)

Blue Cross/Blue Shield and commercial insurers usually cover HDIT, particularly when it is determined to be less costly than hospital care. Criteria set by health maintenance organizations for coverage vary widely, but most HMOs recognize that HDIT is cost-effective and therefore do cover it (19). In many cases, private payers require prior approval. Table 9.6 summarizes the third-party program.

HDIT and Medicare Policy Dilemmas

As noted, present Medicare guidelines are ill-defined and coverage is not specifically formulated to meet HDIT expenses. The Office of Technology Assessment found that the present system promotes coverage for the sickest patients, while healthier patients needing only simple antibiotic therapy must remain hospitalized to receive coverage (23). Coverage is also inconsistent and is open to varied interpretations by fiscal intermediaries (24). In 1988, Congress established that HDIT would be more extensively covered under the Medicare Catastrophic Coverage Act but then repealed that act the following year. As a result, various options for covering HDIT are currently under debate: the extent of future coverage, the particular HDIT categories (drugs, procedures, and conditions) to be included,

Table 9.6. Comparison of Third-Party-Payer Home Care and HDIT Programs

Payer	Eligible Recipients	Benefits	Requirements and Benefits for Home Care
Medicare, Part A	Persons over 65 years old and disabled persons	Services of hospital and skilled nursing facility	Patients who are confined to home and require intermittent and skilled care receive services primarily of RNs, PTs, STs, OTs, MSSs, and HHAs
Medicare, Part B	Elderly and other persons who may voluntarily purchase	Physician services, ambulance transportation, prosthetic devices, laboratory tests, roentgenograms, and drugs used by outpatients	Special requirements allow coverage of chemotherapy, nutrition, oxygen, and iv antibiotic therapy in the home
Medicaid	Medically indigent, blind, disabled, and certain other persons	Services of hospital, physician, nursing home, and others	Qualifying individuals may be entitled to a broad range of services and products, including most prescription and some nonprescription drugs (iv antibiotics may require prior approval for coverage)
Other (Blue Cross/Blue Shield, commercial insurers, health maintenance organizations)	Voluntary subscribers	Vary widely by payer, group, region, and plan	Most insurers cover skilled services and a wide range of physician-prescribed U.S. Food and Drug Administration-approved drugs deemed medically necessary; most insurers cover iv antibiotic therapy in the home, although many require prior approval for coverage

From Balinsky W. Reimbursement for outpatient parenteral antibiotic therapy; update. Rev Infect Dis 1991;13:S194.

Notes: RN, registered nurse; PT, physical therapist; ST, speech therapist; OT, occupational therapist; MSS, medical social service; HHA, home health aide.

who should be eligible, who should determine specific covered drugs and conditions (Congress, fiscal intermediaries, individual physicians), and how providers and physicians should be paid (18) (Table 9.7).

Although other third-party payers are also concerned with the cost effectiveness of HDIT and other high-tech therapies, it is Medicare's ultimate determination that will most affect the future development of HDIT (25). The extent to which Medicare opts to cover HDIT in the future will significantly affect the feasibility of HDIT as both a cost-effective treatment methodology and a profitable developing industry (18). The success of HDIT depends on the ability of equipment manufactures and vendors of related services to make a profit. If Medicare does not cover HDIT, new providers will not be encouraged to enter the market, and the development of new products may decline.

Numerous problems are involved in formulating guidelines for Medicare coverage of HDIT. For one thing, demographic data on the population currently using or eligible for high-tech homecare are insufficient (13). And because providers are so diverse, it is difficult to rectify this situation.

A second issue is that because HDIT requires complex coordination of multiple services, in covering it Medicare would need to develop, implement, and rigorously enforce guidelines to protect patients from substandard care. (At present, most states do not have licensing or certification requirements regarding HDIT that would aid in federal monitoring.) Whatever the eventual cost benefits, the development of these complex guidelines and the research involved therein would actually raise Medicare's expenditures in the first years of implementing HDIT coverage. In the long run, however, provided that patients are appropriately selected, an HDIT benefit is likely to lower costs (18).

Another question is to what extent regulatory intervention should determine Medicare coverage. Without effective guidelines and monitoring, it is unlikely that high-tech home treatment can be coordinated with other home health services in a way that avoids duplication or gaps in service for the patient and duplicate payments for services by insurers. Reimbursement policy decisions must address not only recipient eligibility but also who will provide services. Only providers given economic incentive to offer high-tech homecare will be able to remain in the picture.

Table 9.7. Issues and Options for Home Drug Infusion Therapy (HDIT) Under Medicare

ISSUES AND OPTIONS FOR COVERING HDIT

Basic Issue: Should Medicare cover HDIT?
Option: Enact a home drug infusion benefit under Medicare.

Issue 1: What routes of drug administration should be covered?
Option: Cover only intravenously administered drugs.
Option: Cover both intravenous and other routes of parenteral administration.

Issue 2: What drugs and conditions should be covered?
Option: Cover drugs and conditions specified on a list devised by the Health Care
Financing Administration (HCFA).
Option: Permit fiscal intermediaries to determine specific covered drugs and conditions, based on
general coverage categories and guidelines from HCFA.

Issue 3: Who should be eligible for the benefit?
Option: Cover only patients who can self-administer their therapies (after initial instruction) or who
have family caregivers to perform this service.
Option: Extend coverage to all patients who can be safely treated at home, including patients who
need assistance with their infusion-related or other home health care.
Option: Extend coverage to patients who cannot self-administer, but limit the amount of assistive
services such patients may receive.

Issue 4: Who should be able to provide and bill for HDIT?
Option: For patients needing only HDIT, permit providers of different components of this therapy (e.g.,
pharmacy and nursing services) to bill separately for their respective components.

Table 9.7—*Continued*

Option: For patients needing only HDIT, require that a single certified home infusion therapy provider bill for all services received by that patient.

Option: For patients needing both infusion and other home health services, permit a certified home infusion provider and the home health agency provider to bill separately for their respective services.

Option: Require that the primary provider for patients needing both infusion therapy and other home services—i.e., the provider who coordinates services and submits a bill to Medicare—be a certified home health agency.

Issue 5: Where should a benefit be placed in Medicare's structure?

Option: Make HDIT a Part A benefit.

Option: Make HDIT a Part B benefit.

Option: Make HDIT a benefit under both Parts A and B, depending on the patient's circumstance and concordant benefits.

Issue 6: Should benefit administration be consolidated?

Option: Require that the benefit be administered through a few regional fiscal intermediaries.

Issue 7: What level of case review should be required, and by whom?

Option: Do not require preauthorization for HDIT.

Option: Require Peer Review Organizations (PROs) to preauthorize some or all HDIT patients.

Option: Require fiscal intermediaries to preauthorize HDIT patients.

Option: Require PROs to retrospectively review some home infusion patient claims.

Issue 8: How should providers be paid for HDIT?

Option: Pay for the various components of an HDIT benefit under existing payment mechanisms that apply to home health, durable medical equipment, and other benefits.

Option: Pay for HDIT on the basis of actual costs, with a cap on the total costs allowed.

Option: Pay a prospective per-diem rate for HDIT services.

Issue 9: How should physicians be paid for HDIT-related services?

Option: Pay physicians for their additional supervisory time in HDIT cases on the basis of existing fee-for-service methods.

Option: Pay supervisory physicians a fixed rate (e.g., per patient or per day) for patients on HDIT.

Option: Do not pay physicians for supervisory and advisory activities related to oversight of HDIT.

OPTIONS FOR CONDUCTING RESEARCH AND DEMONSTRATIONS RELATING TO HDIT

Clinical studies

Option: Provide provisional or augmented coverage for drugs administered by HDIT providers in certain clinical studies.

Cost studies

Option: Examine the resource costs of providing HDIT and the economic characteristics of the HDIT industry.

Option: Examine the relative costs of providing drug infusion therapy in home and outpatient settings.

Option: Examine the use of basic home health services, and the need for infusion assistance, among elderly patients on HDIT.

Payment studies

Option: Examine different potential methods of paying for HDIT.

Option: Examine the feasibility and effects of paying hospitals less than the full inpatient rate for patients subsequently discharged to HDIT.

Option: Examine alternative methods of paying for drug infusion therapy in skilled nursing facilities and hospital swing beds.

Option: Examine the effects of an HDIT benefit on rural and inner-city hospitals.

Quality studies

Option: Examine the outcomes of HDIT under various conditions (e.g., different types of patients and therapies) to determine which measures might be appropriately used as indicators of good- or poor-quality care.

From Office of Technology Assessment, Home Drug Infusion Therapy under Medicare. Publication No. OTA-H-509. Washington, DC: U.S. Government Printing Office, 1992.

Conclusion and Recommendations

Studies have confirmed the patient preference, cost effectiveness, clinical safety, and psychological benefits of HDIT, a methodology that also addresses the squeeze on hospitals' finances and space limitations while continuing to generate revenue for them. However, its widespread implementation has outpaced Medicare's ability to respond with appropriate changes in policy and coverage. We are witnessing a complete economically driven restructuring of health care in this country. It is up to Congress to enact legislation and insurers to create guidelines that make for quick and effective implementation. The following recommendations address the issues of HDIT coverage that this chapter has described.

1. Medicare (and other third-party payers) should offer clearly defined and comprehensive coverage for all "appropriate" facets of HDIT and other high-tech therapies that qualify for home use in terms of self-administration feasibility and cost effectiveness. Where the need for supportive assistance involves unwarranted expenses, patients' benefits should be limited. Legislation on this matter should also allow for adaptability in view of future technological developments.

2. Strict federal guidelines for (and outgoing monitoring of) HDIT providers and related services should be created to determine suitability for Medicare reimbursement. These guidelines and monitoring efforts should be so formulated as to ensure quality control of every facet of HDIT. State agencies should be involved in determining initial and continuing compliance. Federal policy should establish explicit requirements for the coordination of HDIT's diverse services and procedures of communication among the patient and all participating providers and staff. It should also set standards for equipment and facilities, for staff qualifications, and for patient assessment and care and should determine which treatments are appropriate for HDIT (on a list of allowable drugs) with suitable provisions for including newly developed medications. And when all of this is in place, plausible billing procedures should be developed; at present, many providers consider Medicare's billing process to be unduly time-consuming and complicated (24).

3. Patient selection procedures for HDIT must be very carefully monitored and regulated, taking all relevant factors into account. The first dose of any infused drug (including changed dosages during a course of therapy) should be administered under appropriate medical supervision in case an adverse action occurs.

4. The pharmaceutical industry should continue to research and develop drugs that may be safely administered in multiple settings and promote cost effectiveness through single-agent therapies and longer-acting drugs (21).

5. The public must be educated in its use of healthcare providers. Every individual should be encouraged to take responsibility for his or her own health and should be aware of the availability of outpatient and homecare alternatives. In many cases, physicians also need to be made aware of these options so as to advise patients more appropriately.

6. Research and data collection should be encouraged to enhance the widespread efficacy of HDIT, to enlarge its scope where feasible, to coordinate its many facets more efficiently, and to advance its technology. Special attention should be directed to its use among elderly patients, as this segment of society will, in a few decades, constitute almost a quarter of our population and continue to use the greatest share of health services. Office of Technology Assessment options for conducting research and demonstrations relating to HDIT include clinical studies, cost studies, payment studies, and quality studies (see Table 9.7). This research might be at least partially funded by third-party payers in conjunction with the pharmaceutical and medical supply industries.

References

1. Ginzberg E, Balinsky W, Ostow M. Home Health Care: Its Role in the Changing Health Services Market. Lanham, MD: Rowman and Allanheld, 1984.
2. Balinsky W, Rehman S. Home health care: a comparative analysis of hospital-based and community-based agency patients. Home Health Care Services Quarterly 1984;5(1):45–60.
3. U.S. Department of Health and Human Services, Office of Inspector General. Medicare Home Infusion Therapy. Publication No. OEI-02–92-00420. Washington, DC: U.S. Government Printing Office, 1993.
4. Policy Analysis, Inc. Current Policies and Future Trends in Outpatient Drug Reimbursement. Brookline, MA: Policy Analysis, Inc., 1985. National Association for Home Care. Basic Statistics About Home Care. (February 1993 Supplement.) Washington, DC: National Association for Home Care, 1993.
5. Haddad AM. High Tech Home Care: A Practical Guide. Gaithersburg, MD: Aspen, 1987.
6. Balinsky W. Home Care: Current Trends and Future Prospects. New York Business Group on Health Discussion Papers, 1985;5(3):1–10.
7. Gould DA, Haslanger KD, Vladeck BC. Coming of age: home care in the 1990s. Pride Institute Journal 1992;11(1):19–28.
8. U.S. Department of Health and Human Services. Report to Congress and the Secretary by the Task Force on Long-Term Health Policies. Washington, DC: U.S. Government Printing Office, 1988.
9. Votroubek WL. Funding pediatric home care. In: McCoy PA, Votroubek WL, eds. Pediatric Home Care: A Comprehensive Approach. Gaithersburg, MD: Aspen, 1990.
10. Kaufman J. An overview of public sector financing for pediatric home care, Part I. Pediatric Nursing 1991;17(3):280.
11. Miller NA. Medicaid 2176 home and community-based care waivers: the first ten years. Health Affairs 1992;11(4):162–171.
12. Balinsky W, Blumengold J. Home care integrating into managed care. Caring 1995;14(6):36–44.
13. Balinsky W, Nesbitt S. Cost-effectiveness of outpatient parenteral antibiotics: a review of the literature. Am J Med 1989;87:301–305.
14. Antoniskis A et al. Feasibility of outpatient self-administration of parenteral antibiotics. West J Med 1978;128(3):203–206.
15. Gainer RB, Smego RA. Intravenous home antibiotic therapy. In: The Supplement, Vol. 1 (Educational Service to the Professions by HNS), Pine Brook, NJ: Health Dyne Co., 1985:3–12.
16. Milkovich G. Costs and benefits. Hospital Practice Symposium Supplement: Outpatient Parenteral Antibiotic Therapy 1993;28 (Suppl 1):39–43.
17. Poretz DM, Woolard D, Eron LJ, et al. Outpatient use of ceftriaxone: a cost benefit analysis. Am J Med 1984;77:77–83.
18. Office of Technology Assessment. Home Drug Infusion Therapy Under Medicare. Publication No. OTA-H-509. Washington, DC: U.S. Government Printing Office, 1992.
19. Tierce JC. Reimbursement. Hospital Practice Symposium. Outpatient Parenteral Antibiotic Therapy 1993; 28(Suppl 1):44–51.
20. Health Care Financing Administration. Medicare Carriers Manual. Publication No. HIM-14–3. Washington, DC: U.S. Government Printing Office, 1985.
21. Balinsky W. Home Care Prescription Drug Reimbursement: A Case for Intravenous Antibiotic. Public Issue Report, 1986.
22. Williams JL, Gaumes G. Home health services: an industry in transition. In: Home Health Agency Prospective Payment Demonstration for Health Care Financing Administration. Washington, DC: ABT Associates, 1984.
23. U.S. Department of Health and Human Services, Public Health Service. Home Health Care: Use Expenditures and Sources of Payment. AHCPR 93–0040. Rockville, MD: U.S. Public Health Service, 1993.
24. Fox DM, Anderson KS, Benjamin AE, Dunatov LJ. Intensive home health care in the United States: financing as technology. International Journal of Technology Assessment in Health Care 1987;3:561–573.
25. Balinsky W. Reimbursement for outpatient parenteral antibiotic therapy; update. Rev Infect Dis 1991;13: S193-S195.

10

LONG-TERM VASCULAR ACCESS

Michael H. Torosian

CHAPTER AT A GLANCE: Establishing long-term vascular access is a critical component in managing homecare patients requiring chronic parenteral therapy. This chapter reviews the indications, techniques, and complications of inserting and maintaining long-term vascular access. Peripheral and central access techniques, percutaneous and surgically inserted catheters, and external and indwelling catheter techniques are reviewed. Catheter complications can be minimized by adhering to strict insertion and maintenance protocols. For patients in whom the conventional access routes have been exhausted, innovative techniques for establishing central venous access are described. Critical analysis of key clinical factors is imperative to provide optimal medical management of patients requiring long-term access.

Introduction

Long-term vascular access is an important aspect of managing both hospitalized and homecare patients who require chronic parenteral therapy. Both peripheral and central venous access techniques have been described for specific clinical indications. Numerous factors must be considered when determining the optimal vascular access approach for an individual patient. Clinically relevant factors for selecting the appropriate access approach include the anatomic site of catheter insertion, the number of catheter lumens required, the duration and frequency of catheter use, and the type of therapy to be administered. Advantages and disadvantages are associated with each access technique and must be considered when selecting the access route. Peripheral access is commonly used for fluid resuscitation, administration of short-term antibiotics and other parenteral medications. Central venous access is typically used for total parenteral nutrition, chemotherapy, and long-term infusion of antibiotics or parenteral fluid. Frequently, parenteral therapy is initiated with peripheral catheters, with transition to the central venous route when peripheral access sites have been exhausted. This chapter summarizes the techniques of long-term venous access with a critical analysis of specific indications and advantages of each method.

Peripheral versus Central Venous Access

Peripheral venous access had most commonly been utilized in hospitalized patients in the past, but its use is rapidly being expanded to the outpatient setting. Peripheral venous access is suitable for fluid resuscitation and for administration of antibiotics, noncaustic chemotherapeutic agents, and other par-

"

enteral medications. Peripheral venous access is the first choice of vascular access in patients with short-term access needs and in cases where rapid establishment of parenteral access is necessary. Peripheral venous access can be readily established in ambulatory centers or home settings. Central venous catheterization is typically required for long-term parenteral use. Central venous access is used for administration of hypertonic parenteral nutrition, long-term infusion of antibiotics, and administration of caustic chemotherapeutic agents or fluids. Since peripheral venous access sites are limited, central venous access may be required in those in whom peripheral venous sites have been exhausted. The major complications of peripheral and central venous access include catheter dysfunction, infection, and venous thrombosis. Both common and innovative techniques for obtaining vascular access exist and can be used to establish parenteral access under a variety of clinical conditions.

Percutaneous Catheter Insertion

Percutaneously inserted catheters are particularly useful in patients requiring short-term central venous access (1–3). The primary advantage of percutaneous catheter insertion is the avoidance of an operative procedure to establish venous access. Percutaneous catheters can be inserted in the hospital, at ambulatory care centers, or at home. To reduce morbidity of catheter insertion, vascular access must be performed by experienced clinicians using strict aseptic technique (4, 5).

The most common sites for percutaneous catheter insertion are the subclavian, external or internal jugular, cephalic, and basilic veins (Fig. 10.1). There are several advantages for establishing central venous access with short catheters inserted into the subclavian or jugular veins compared to long catheters inserted peripherally into the central venous system. Because of the proximity to the central venous system, short venous catheters are generally associated with a decreased risk of dislodgement and thrombosis compared to long, peripherally inserted catheters (6). Subclavian vein catheterization is associated with the lowest incidence of catheter dislodgement, since the catheter can be anchored to the stable anterior chest wall. Catheter exit sites on the neck or extremity are unstable

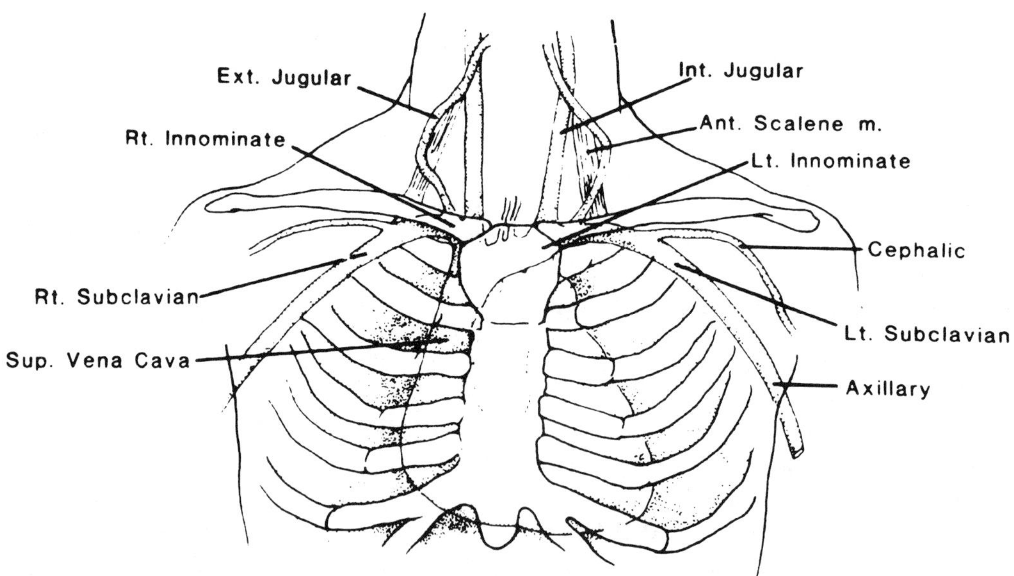

Figure 10.1.   The anatomy of the superior venous system depicts common access routes for obtaining percutaneous and surgically inserted venous catheters. (From Alexander HR, ed. Vascular Access in the Cancer Patient. Philadelphia: JB Lippincott, 1994:69.)

and are associated with an increased risk of catheter dislodgement and, perhaps, increased risk of sepsis and thrombophlebitis (7). Subcutaneous tunneling of percutaneous catheters inserted into the jugular venous system may be performed to establish an exit site on the chest wall. This technique is also used to remove catheters from potential sources of infection, such as a tracheostomy, head and neck burn, radiation therapy port, or enterocutaneous fistula site (8, 9).

Subclavian vein catheterization is the most common technique for establishing percutaneous venous access in the hospital setting. These catheters may be inserted by either an infraclavicular or a supraclavicular approach. Both techniques are acceptable and are widely used to establish central venous access. Contraindications to attempting subclavian vein catheterization include an uncorrected coagulopathy, severe pulmonary disease in a patient unable to tolerate a pneumothorax, and anatomic proximity to a tracheostomy, burn, fistula, tumor site, or radiation therapy port. Anatomic proximity to these potentially contaminated or infected sites is a relative contraindication to catheter insertion that can frequently be circumvented by percutaneously tunneling the catheter to a more distant exit site (1, 7). Subclavian vein thrombosis must be considered if attempts to catheterize this vein are unsuccessful, particularly in patients with a history of previous central venous catheterization or an underlying disease that predisposes to thrombosis (10, 11). Prior to attempting contralateral subclavian vein catheterization it is mandatory to obtain a chest x-ray to exclude the possibility of a pneumothorax caused by an unsuccessful catheterization attempt. Angiographic studies to exclude the possibility of central venous thrombosis are indicated if this diagnosis is suspected. Both the external and internal jugular veins may also be used to obtain percutaneous central venous access. Catheters inserted into the jugular veins are associated with increased patient discomfort, increased risk of catheter dislodgement secondary to cervical mobility, and, in some reports, increased catheter sepsis (12,

13). The external jugular vein is frequently tortuous, has multiple tributaries, and has competent valves that can impair catheter insertion.

The use of central venous catheters inserted at peripheral sites is becoming increasingly common. Access by peripherally inserted central catheters (PICCs) can be performed in the ambulatory or home setting. Although initial reports suggested an increased risk of thrombophlebitis and catheter dislodgement, current studies indicate that these catheters can be inserted and utilized safely. As more treatments are conducted in the outpatient and home environment, the use of these peripherally inserted catheters will increase.

Surgical Catheter Insertion

Surgically inserted central venous catheters are placed for long-term outpatient or home use. Indwelling central venous catheters are especially useful for administering total parenteral nutrition, chemotherapy, and long-term antibiotics for osteomyelitis or endocarditis (14, 15). The number of catheter lumens and type of catheter (external versus implanted) are dependent on numerous patient- and treatment-related factors.

Subclavian vein access can be obtained by surgical cutdown over the cephalic vein or by the direct puncture technique (3, 7). The technique of subclavian vein catheterization by cutdown over the cephalic vein can be performed under local anesthesia. An oblique incision is made over the deltopectoral groove and the deltopectoral fascia is incised. The cephalic vein is identified within the fat pad between the deltoid and pectoral muscles, and the catheter is inserted from the cephalic vein into the distal superior vena cava as confirmed by intraoperative fluoroscopy. Although the catheter tip may also be placed in the right atrium, this position is potentially associated with an increased risk of bacterial endocarditis and is not advocated. An exit site is chosen for the catheter just lateral to the sternal border on the side ipsilateral to the cephalic vein cutdown.

A modification of the surgical cutdown approach is the direct puncture technique (16). Catheter insertion kits are readily available to simplify the process of establishing vascular access by this technique (Fig. 10.2). This procedure is similar to that described above except that the cephalic vein is not isolated. After the catheter has been tunneled from its exit site to a small infraclavicular incision, the subclavian vein is percutaneously punctured, a Seldinger guidewire is inserted, and a dilator and peel-away sheath are introduced into the subclavian vein. The dilator is withdrawn after fluoroscopic confirmation of position and the catheter is threaded through the peel-away sheath into the central venous system. The peel-away sheath is removed and catheter position is again viewed fluoroscopically. The direct puncture technique has the advantage of reduced surgical dissection but the disadvantage of an uncontrolled venous entry site. Both the external and internal jugular veins may be catheterized by surgical cutdown and offer alternatives to the cephalic vein approach. The author recommends the external jugular vein as the preferable route because of its superficial location just beneath the platysma muscle. However, several anatomic constraints of this vein include tortuosity and the presence of valves and multiple branches that can impede catheter advancement into the central venous system. The internal jugular vein is deeper and requires retraction of the sternocleidomastoid muscle for exposure. Although this vein may be ligated, catheterization of the internal jugular vein can be achieved with venous patency by inserting the catheter through a purse-string suture in a side venotomy.

Inferior central venous access can be obtained as a primary approach for anatomic considerations (e.g., upper torso burn, bilateral radical neck surgery, or central venous thrombosis). The most common technique

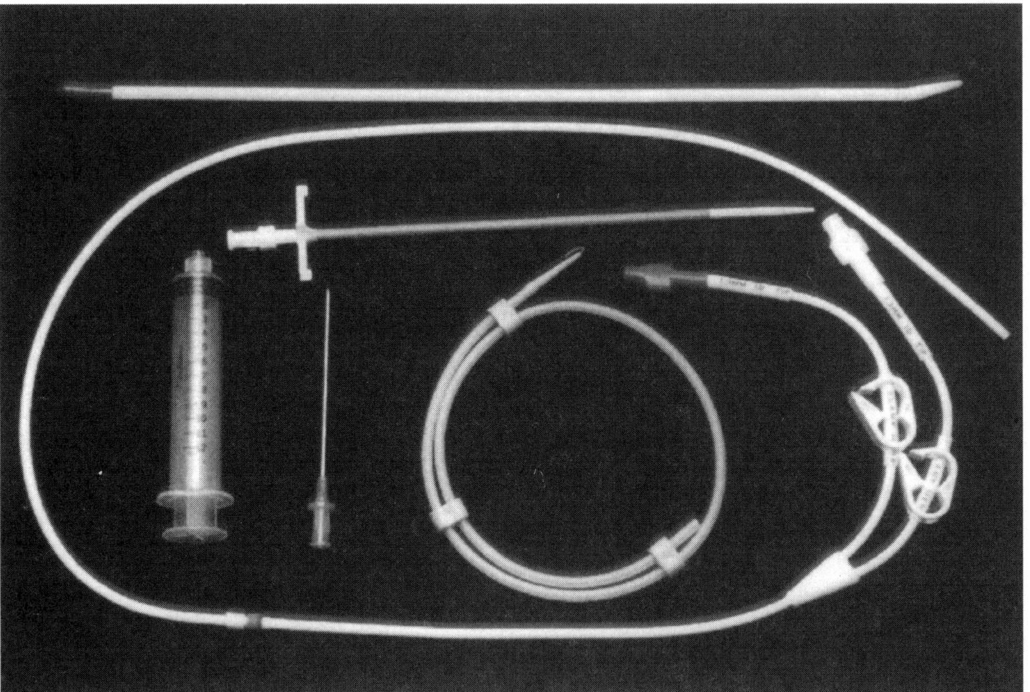

Figure 10.2.   The percutaneous venous access catheter insertion kit includes needle, syringe, flexible-tipped guide wire, soft tissue dilator, and peel-away sheath. A double-lumen Hickman catheter is also shown (From Alexander HR, ed. Vascular Access in the Cancer Patient. Philadelphia: JB Lippincott, 1994;9.)

for obtaining access into the inferior vena cava is the saphenous vein approach (17, 18). A cutdown is made over the saphenous vein, and the tip of the catheter is threaded from this site into the inferior vena cava to the level of the renal veins as determined by intraoperative fluoroscopy. The catheter is tunneled subcutaneously from the saphenous vein to exit from the low anterior abdominal wall. This long subcutaneous tunnel is necessary to provide ease of management of the catheter and to remove the catheter from potential sources of infection in the inguinal region. Fonkalsrud et al. have popularized this technique and have applied it with great success in the pediatric population (17).

Additional Surgical Considerations

Selection of an exit site for percutaneous catheters is an important surgical consideration and can significantly influence morbidity. The exit site should be chosen so that it provides easy access for sterile catheter care and minimizes risk of catheter dislodgement. Subcutaneous tunneling of the catheter is useful to establish an exit site distant from potential sources of infection, such as a tracheostomy, burn site, oropharyngoesophageal fistula, ulcerating tumor, or site of prior or future radiotherapy (8, 9). Catheters inserted into the inferior vena cava typically have an exit site on the abdomen to prevent contamination from the inguinal region. Surgically placed catheters are equipped with a Dacron cuff, which becomes densely adherent to the subcutaneous tissue by reactive fibrosis (9). To facilitate nonoperative removal of catheters, the Dacron cuff should be placed approximately 1 cm from the exit site so that limited dissection of this cuff can be performed under local anesthesia if needed at the time of catheter removal.

The method of choosing between percutaneous and surgical catheter insertion is primarily related to the anticipated duration and frequency of catheter use. Percutaneously placed catheters are useful for short-term parenteral therapy and have the primary advantage of avoiding a surgical procedure. Surgically inserted catheters are required for long-term use to provide total parenteral nutri-tion, chemotherapy, or antibiotics. In patients requiring daily or more frequent catheter access—for instance, those receiving total parenteral nutrition or antibiotics—external catheters are commonly used. In patients requiring intermittent venous access—for example, patients requiring chemotherapy—a totally implanted catheter/port system offers a convenient and useful approach (19–21).

Catheter composition is an important determinant of thrombogenicity and has been extensively investigated. Experimental and clinical studies have demonstrated a reduced incidence of thrombosis with silicone central venous catheters compared to polyethylene catheters (22, 23). McLean Ross et al. in 1982 reported a 4% incidence in central venous thrombosis in a series of 100 consecutive silicone subclavian catheters (24). The average catheter life was 19.4 days, with only one episode of pulmonary embolus in this study. Dolcourt and Bose in 1982 found no cases of clinically evident central venous thrombosis in a series of newborn infants with percutaneous silicone subclavian catheters (25). Heparin coating of central venous catheters has been tested, but no significant reduction in thrombogenicity has been demonstrated with this modification (26, 27). The process of heparin bonding increases catheter stiffness, which may be associated with increased endothelial damage following catheter insertion. Although the role of anticoagulation remains controversial, most authors advocate low-dose heparin or warfarin therapy in patients requiring long-term central venous access (28).

Vascular Access Devices

The Hickman, Broviac, and Groshong catheters are the most commonly used external, surgically inserted central venous catheters. Hickman and Broviac catheters are barium-impregnated silicone rubber catheters that are 90 cm long and can be cut to the desired length intraoperatively. Pediatric catheters are available in 2.7 and 4.2 French sizes, and adult catheters, in 6.6 and 9.6 French external diameters. A Dacron cuff is attached approximately 30 cm from the external hub for implantation in the subcutaneous tissue. Double-lumen Hickman catheters are available in 7, 9, 10, and 12 French sizes. Triple-lumen Hickman catheters are also manufactured in the 10 and 12.5 French sizes (Fig. 10.3). The Groshong catheter is an external device distinguished by a slit valve adjacent to the tip of the catheter. This tip is designed to minimize catheter thrombosis by reflux of blood into the catheter lumen and to reduce the need for daily heparin flushing. This modification alone improves ease of maintenance and reduces the cost of catheter care. Because of this specialized tip on the Groshong catheter, the catheter tip is positioned first and the external end of the catheter is cut after it has been positioned and secured at the skin exit site. Groshong catheters are available as single 3.5, 5.5, 7, and 8 French or as double-lumen catheters in sizes 5 to 9.5 French. The Groshong catheter is a silicone rubber catheter.

Implantable port devices have a housing constructed of titanium or plastic that are de-signed to be durable and have low thrombogenic potential (Fig. 10.4). The diaphragm of the port is composed of silicone rubber and is the site of venous entry with a noncoring needle. Depending on the specific model, the port is either preconnected to the catheter or attached to the catheter at the time of insertion with a flange to ensure a secure connection. Single- and double-lumen implantable devices are available for use. A modified single-lumen, low-profile device exists for use in pediatric or very cachectic adult patients. The single-lumen, adult-size implantable port has a 9.6 French catheter with a port height of 13.5 mm compared to the low-profile port with a 6.6 French catheter and a port height of 10.1 mm. The dual-lumen port devices are larger, with a height of 16.5 mm. Catheters used with the double-lumen ports include either the 9.5 French Groshong or 10–12 French Hickman-type catheters. A device has recently been designed for peripheral implantation of subcutaneous ports. These are

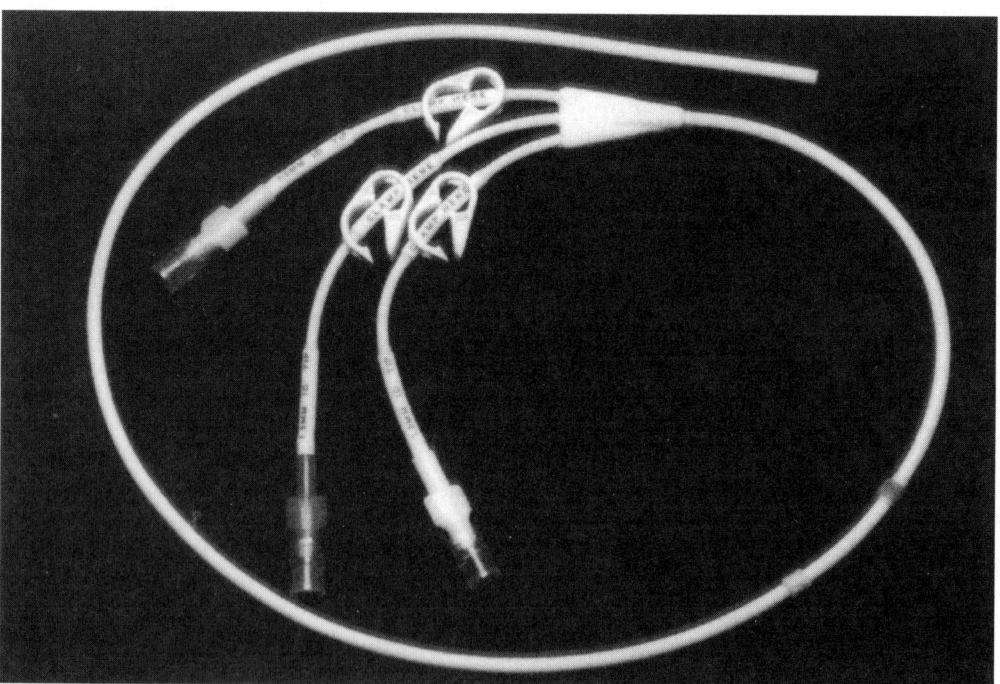

Figure 10.3.   Triple-lumen Hickman catheters are commonly used when multiple simultaneous infusions are planned, such as in bone marrow transplant recipients. (From Alexander HR, ed. Vascular Access in the Cancer Patient. Philadelphia: JB Lippincott, 1994;7.)

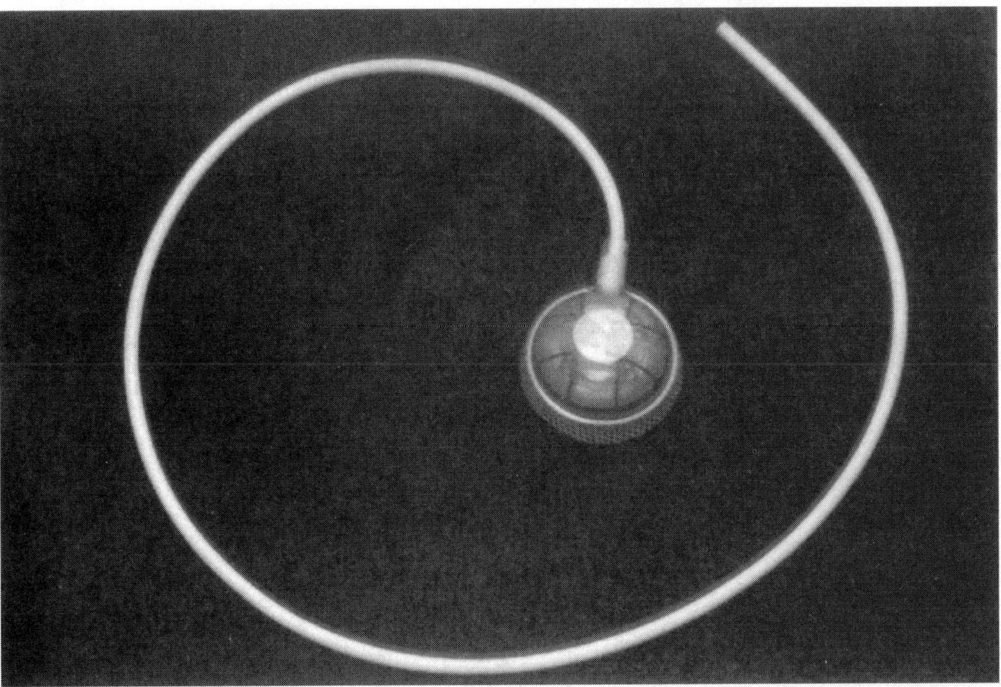

Figure 10.4. Implantable venous access devices consist of a metal or plastic port, a silicone rubber needle-entry site, and a flexible venous catheter. (From Alexander HR, ed. Vascular Access in the Cancer Patient. Philadelphia: JB Lippincott, 1994;11.)

low-profile devices that are designed to be placed in an interventional radiology suite and combine the advantages of a totally implantable device with a catheter that can be inserted by a peripheral venous route (Fig. 10.5). The availability and utilization of these peripherally implanted ports will undoubtedly increase in the future.

Because of their long-term use and the fact that they protrude continuously, Hickman, Broviac, and Groshong catheters may become damaged over time. When this occurs, it is possible to repair the catheters without removing them. Each manufacturer, and several third-party vendors, have produced repair kits for these catheters (Fig. 10.6), which can eliminate the need for a patient to undergo surgical catheter replacement.

Infusion Pumps

Various kinds of hospital equipment (such as infusion pumps) were initially used without modification in the home environment. This sometimes required that the home setting be specially prepared with the proper electrical and safety features found routinely in the hospital. Hospital equipment was not intended for use by nonprofessionals and is often more complex than is necessary for the basic use that a homecare patient requires.

Consequently, numerous infusion pumps and other mechanical support devices have been developed for use specifically by the homecare patient. Much has also been done in the area of home patient monitoring by using a central station connected to the patient's home monitor by telephone. As the field continues to grow, more adaptations of hospital-type equipment and the development of new, home-oriented systems should allow for expanded options in intensive homecare.

There are three general types of infusion pumps or assist devices: gravity flow regulators, mechanical pumps, and elastomeric and spring-loaded flow devices. Since this field is rapidly changing, it is impossible to provide a complete analysis of these products.

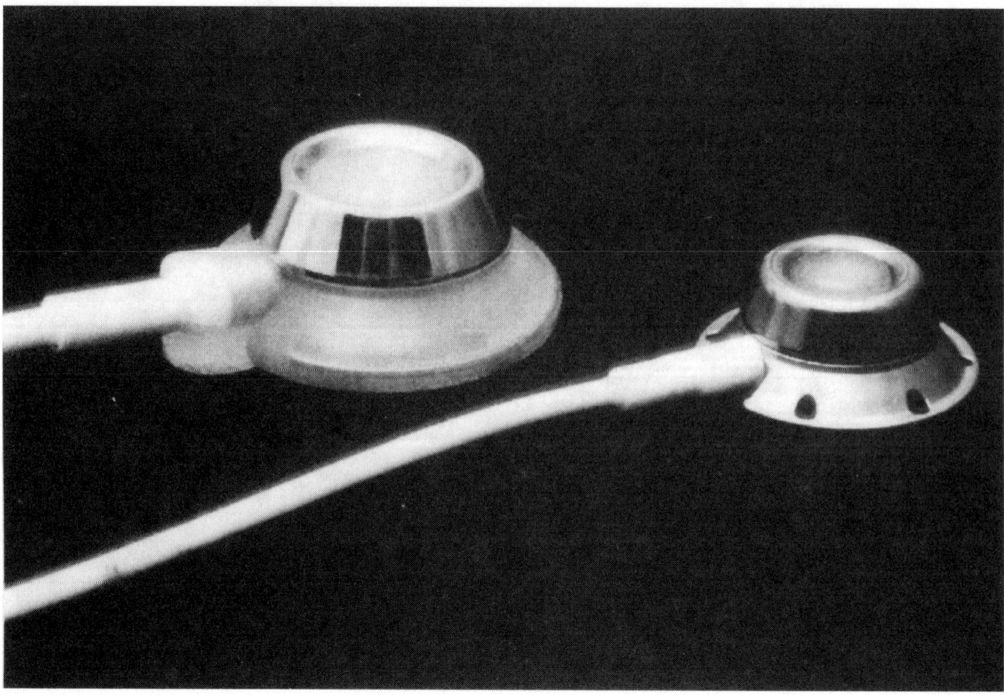

Figure 10.5.   The low-profile port (*right*) is significantly smaller and less obvious after subcutaneous implantation compared to the standard-sized port. (From Alexander HR, ed. Vascular Access in the Cancer Patient. Philadelphia: JB Lippincott, 1994;10.)

Gravity flow regulators include such devices as a "Dial-a-Flow" regulator. These are generally little more than calibrated pumping devices that reduce the diameter of the IV tubing and thereby adjust the flow rate. They are used in conjunction with a calibrated drip chamber, which permits a measurement of drops of solution per minute. A recent modification on this concept is the provision of an external pressure bag around the IV solution container to maintain constant flow.

Mechanical pumps exist in a wide variety of choices and include both pole-mounted and fully portable systems. Most are now computerized and use battery power. Some mechanical pumps can run in an automatic mode for extended periods. This can reduce the need for patient training and allow more freedom of movement.

Most mechanical infusion pumps incorporate safety systems that trigger an auditory alarm to indicate a problem with the infusion. Some also incorporate a computerized display so that the patient may correct the specific problem or contact a homecare nurse for assistance.

Elastomeric and spring-loaded flow devices utilize the stored potential energy in the stretch of elastic material or the compression of a spring to provide constant pressure and flow of infusion.

Many varieties of these concepts exist, and some hybrid products that combine them have been developed (29).

Complications

Numerous complications are associated with the use of central venous catheters. These complications can be functionally classified into categories based on insertion or maintenance of vascular access devices. Clinical studies have indicated that the incidence of complications associated with catheter insertion is directly related to the experience of the individual placing the catheter (30). Mechanical

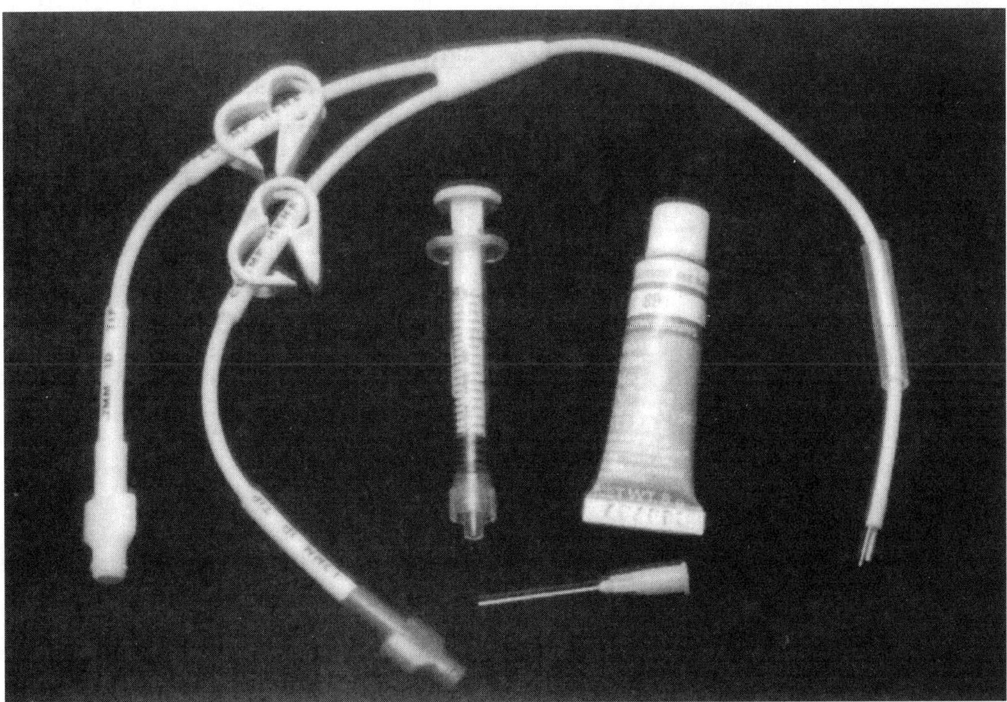

Figure 10.6.   Commercially available kits exist for repairing external portions of damaged or worn catheters. Repair of long-term access catheters can often obviate the need for catheter removal and subsequent reestablishment of vascular access at the same or a distant site. (From Alexander HR, ed. *Vascular Access in the Cancer Patient.* Philadelphia: JB Lippincott, 1994;15.)

complications associated with percutaneous insertion of subclavian vein catheters range from 4 to 13% (12) (Table 10.1). These procedure-related complications can be minimized by knowing the vascular anatomy, by avoiding technical errors during catheter insertion, and by having each access procedure strictly monitored by experienced personnel. Complications of catheter maintenance can be reduced 5- to 10-fold by adhering to established protocols of catheter management (4). The development of a nutrition support team for care of these catheters has been repeatedly shown to reduce catheter-associated morbidity (4, 5).

Early recognition and appropriate therapeutic intervention are necessary to treat catheter-related complications, some of which are life threatening. Pneumothorax is the most common complication associated with percutaneous subclavian vein catheterization and occurs by penetration of the apex of the lung during catheter insertion (6). Most pneumoth-

oraces are asymptomatic and are detected on chest x-ray following catheter insertion. However, a pneumothorax should be clinically suspected if the patient develops dyspnea or severe pleuritic chest pain. Although tension pneumothorax is an unusual complication of catheter insertion, this condition should be suspected when cyanosis and hypotension accompany dyspnea and chest pain. Tension pneumothorax is more commonly associated with mechanical ventilation and must be treated immediately by pleural aspiration followed by chest tube thoracostomy.

Three therapeutic options exist to treat asymptomatic pneumothoraces resulting from catheter insertion. Small pneumothoraces (less than 15%) typically resolve spontaneously without therapeutic intervention; close radiologic follow-up is required with frequent chest x-rays. Conservative management of small pneumothoraces generally results in a spontaneous resolution rate of approximately

Table 10.1. Mechanical Complications of Central Venous Access

Pneumothorax
Air embolus
Catheter malposition
Venous thrombosis
Catheter occlusion
Catheter embolus
Arterial puncture
Hemothorax/hemomediastinum
Hydrothorax/hydromediastinum
Thoracic duct injury
Brachial plexus injury
Subcutaneous emphysema

1% of the trapped pleural air per day. This rate may be slightly increased by administration of oxygen, thereby exchanging oxygen with nitrogen in the trapped air space. Since oxygen is more soluble than nitrogen, resolution of the pneumothorax will occur more rapidly. If the pneumothorax resulting from catheter insertion is symptomatic or is larger than 15%, tube thoracostomy should be performed as the initial therapeutic procedure. The chest tube is connected to water seal drainage and is removed when the air leak ceases. Some authors advocate an intermediate management technique of aspiration of the pleural air as therapy for small to medium-sized pneumothoraces. The author does not believe that this is a reliable therapeutic intervention; furthermore, if the pneumothorax is too large for observation, tube thoracostomy should be undertaken. Tube thoracostomy is indicated in patients with a pneumothorax who are on mechanical ventilation to prevent progression to a tension pneumothorax.

Air embolus is a potentially life-threatening complication that is evidenced by chest pain, dyspnea, and a millwheel cardiac murmur. Cyanosis, tachycardia, hypotension, and elevated central venous pressure occur following a large air embolus. Cardiac arrest may ensue and results from right ventricular outflow tract obstruction from a large air embolus. Immediate treatment of an air embolus consists of placing the patient in Trendelenburg and left lateral decubitus position to pre-vent air from blocking the right ventricular outflow tract (31–33). Placing the patient in this position allows the intracardiac air to rise into the apex of the right ventricle. Aspiration of the central venous catheter should be performed in an attempt to remove intravascular air, although this maneuver is rarely successful. Should the patient continue to clinically deteriorate, percutaneous right ventricular aspiration is performed. Rare successful resuscitation has been reported following emergency thoracotomy and direct aspiration of the right ventricle (34).

Catheter embolus is an iatrogenic complication typically caused by improper catheter insertion technique. A catheter embolus occurs when the catheter is pulled back after having been threaded beyond the tip of the needle into the intravascular space (35). A piece of the catheter is then sheared off and may travel into an intracardiac position or into a branch of the pulmonary artery. This complication can be prevented by withdrawing both the needle and the catheter as a unit in unsuccessful catheterization attempts. Removal of the embolized segment of catheter is most expeditiously performed angiographically with a transvenous snare under fluoroscopy (36).

The incidence of asymptomatic central venous thrombosis ranges from 20 to 70% as reported in the literature (10, 31). The disparity in the reported incidence of asymptomatic central venous thrombosis results from the varied definitions of this entity (ranging from fibrin sheath formation to true vascular thrombosis), differing diagnostic techniques, and variability of patient populations studied. A fibrin sheath forms around foreign bodies inserted into the venous system and should not be considered in the category of central venous thrombosis (37). Similarly, isolated catheter thrombosis should be differentiated from central venous thrombosis. Symptomatic central venous thrombosis occurs in only 1 to 5% of patients with central venous catheters (6, 38). Symptoms related to central venous thrombosis include ipsilateral arm and neck swelling; the development of collateral veins over the chest, arm, and neck; and, with extension into the internal jugular vein, symptoms of pseudotumor cerebri (39). Venous plethysmography, Doppler ultrasound, radionuclide scanning, upper-extremity venography, and magnetic resonance imaging can be used to diagnose central venous thrombosis (40, 41). Upper-extremity venography and magnetic resonance imaging are the most accurate tests to establish this diagnosis.

The treatment of catheter occlusion without central venous thrombosis consists of local instillation of urokinase or streptokinase (42, 43). Local thrombolytic therapy, however, is less successful once thrombosis has extended beyond the catheter and into the central venous system. Treatment of central venous thrombosis is dependent on the patient's clinical status and the need for continuing central venous access. If the patient no longer requires central venous access, the catheter is removed. Anticoagulation is administered as a 3-month course of warfarin. If the need for central venous access is critical and symptoms of venous thrombosis are absent or mild, the device is not removed and warfarin is continued as long as the central venous catheter remains in place (10, 24).

Catheter infection is a constant threat to patients with indwelling vascular access catheters. However, meticulous catheter care has dramatically reduced the incidence of septic complications associated with percutaneous and surgically inserted catheters. Aseptic surgical insertion techniques and the development of catheter maintenance protocols have significantly reduced catheter infection and prolonged catheter life (4). The development of nutrition support teams between the 1970s and the 1980s has been associated with a dramatic reduction in catheter-related complications. Despite optimal catheter management, catheter infection remains an important source of clinical morbidity (44). Catheter sepsis can be caused by pathogenic or opportunistic bacteria or fungi. Indwelling catheter infections can often be treated with parenteral antibiotics in a clinically stable patient—this treatment may be continued if the signs and symptoms of infection resolve. In a patient who is clinically unstable, shows signs of systemic sepsis, or fails to clinically respond to parenteral antibiotics, the infected catheter must be removed and vascular access established at a distant site for parenteral antibiotic infusion. Recent reports of sepsis with Hickman and Broviac catheters are summarized in Table 10.2 and demonstrate one septic episode per 600 days of catheter use in these collective series.

Innovative Access Approaches

Due to the prolonged use of central venous access devices, the need has arisen to develop innovative access approaches. Because of infectious and thrombotic complications, a variety of alternative, innovative venous access

Table 10.2. Summmary of Hickman and Broviac Catheter-Related Sepsis

No. of Catheters	No. of Septic Episodes	Days of Catheter Use	Ratio[a]	Reference
291	35	37,039	1 : 1,058	44
52	10	12,482	1 : 1,241	45
90	27	3,981	1 : 147	46
1,088	143	100,544	1 : 703	47
96	24	7,174	1 : 299	48
150	18	18,750	1 : 1,042	49
335	77	33,394	1 : 434	50
49	29	4,307	1 : 149	51
Totals: 2,151	363	217,671	1 : 600	

Adapted from Hurtubise MR, Bottino JE, et al. Restoring patency of occluded central venous catheters. Arch Surg 1980;115:212.
[a]Ratio indicating that one septic episode occurred for the number of days of catheter use shown.

techniques have been developed. Techniques for obtaining long-term central venous access have been devised for both the inferior and superior central venous systems. Access to the inferior vena cava is most commonly obtained by using the saphenous vein technique previously described. In addition, the femoral vein, external iliac vein, inferior epigastric vein, gonadal vein, and lumbar veins have been used for catheter insertion into the inferior vena cava (45–47). In each of these approaches, the catheter tip is positioned in the inferior vena cava at the level of the renal veins. In addition, percutaneous translumbar puncture of the inferior vena cava and catheter insertion directly into the inferior vena cava at laparotomy have been described (48). Vascular access approaches to the inferior vena cava can be achieved with low morbidity. Williard et. al. in 1991 reported 31 cases of long-term access through the inferior venous system with a complication rate of 1/254 catheter use days (49). Infections (5/31), vascular thrombosis (3/31), isolated catheter thrombosis (3/31), and catheter migration (1/31) were reported. The saphenous vein approach is typically used in nonambulating infants, while the inferior epigastric vein can be used regardless of ambulatory status (17, 47, 50).

Innovative access techniques have also been described to establish central venous access despite the presence of superior central venous thrombosis. Thoracotomy with direct insertion of an indwelling catheter into the right atrium or azygos vein has been performed (51, 52). However, this technique requires a major surgical procedure with the morbidity (e.g., atelectasis, pneumonia, respiratory insufficiency) associated with thoracotomy (53, 54). A combined angiographic/surgical technique described by Torosian et al. can be performed under local anesthesia with avoidance of thoracotomy (55). This technique requires that a patent collateral vein, such as an intercostal vein, be identified on venography. A retrograde guidewire from the femoral or basilic vein is advanced into this patent collateral vein through the thrombosed central venous system. A venous cutdown is then performed onto this collateral vein and a snare is angiographically advanced over the guide wire to the cutdown site. After the external portion of the catheter is tunneled subcutaneously to the snare, the tip of the catheter is drawn by the snare into the central venous system. The major advantage of this technique is the avoidance of a thoracotomy, and successful long-term central venous access has been achieved by this approach.

Long-term central venous access is an increasingly important aspect of the care for both hospitalized and home patients. Knowledge of the anatomic sites and available insertion techniques for obtaining central venous access is imperative. Meticulous attention to maintenance protocols and insertion techniques are essential to minimize morbidity of central venous access catheters. Innovative access techniques are an integral part of the armamentarium for establishing vascular access in the patient requiring long-term parenteral access.

Summary

Long-term vascular access has revolutionized the care of critically ill patients and patients requiring long-term parenteral therapy. Various types of catheters exist for administering antibiotics, chemotherapy, nutrition, electrolyte solutions, and hemodynamic pressure monitoring. A critical analysis of each situation will determine the optimal catheter type and vascular access route for an individual patient. The frequency of use, expected parenteral treatment duration, and availability of vascular access sites are important determinants for selecting the access device and vascular site of insertion. Strict adherence to protocols will minimize the risk of complications, and expeditious management of complications that do occur will minimize clinical morbidity. Both standard and innovative techniques for establishing long-term access exist and can be used as appropriate under a variety of clinical conditions.

References

1. Vander Salm TJ, Fitzpatrick GF. New technique for placement of long-term venous catheters. JPEN 1981;5:326–327.
2. Pollack PF, Kaddern BA, Byrne WJ, Fondkalsrud EW, Ament ME. 100 patient years' experience with the Broviac silastic catheter for central venous nutrition. JPEN 1981;5:32–36.
3. Hickman RO, Buckner CD, Clift RA, Sanders JE, Stewart P, Thomas D. A modified right atrial catheter for access to the venous system in marrow transplant recipients. Surg Gynecol Obstet 1970;148:871–875.
4. Powell-Tuck J, Lennard-Jones JE, Lowes JA, Danso, KT, Shaw EJ. Intravenous feeding in a gastroenterological unit: a prospective study of infective complications. J Clin Pathol 1979;32:549.
5. Simmons BP. CDC guidelines for the prevention and control of nosocomial infections—guideline for prevention of intravascular infections. Am J Infect Control 1983;11:183.
6. Hoshal VL Jr. Total intravenous nutrition with peripherally inserted silicone elastomer central venous catheters. Arch Surg 1975;110:644–648.
7. Grant JP. Catheter access. In: Rombeau JL, Caldwell MD, eds. Clinical Nutrition: Parenteral Nutrition. Philadelphia: WB Saunders, 1986;2:306–315.
8. Mitchell A, Atkins S, Royle GT. Reduced catheter sepsis and prolonged catheter life using a tunnelled silicone rubber catheter for total parenteral nutrition. Br J Surg 1982;69:420–422.
9. Press OW, Ramsey PG, Larson EB, Fefer A, Hickman RO. Hickman catheter infections in patients with malignancies. Medicine 1984;63:189–199.
10. Brismar B, Hardstedt C, Jacobson S. Diagnosis of thrombosis by catheter phlebography after prolonged central venous catheterization. Ann Surg 1981;194:779.
11. Nordlund S, Thoren L. Catheter in the superior vena cava for parenteral feeding. Acta Chir Scand 1964;127:39.
12. Grant JP. Subclavian catheter insertion and complications. In: Grant JP, ed. Handbook of Total Parenteral Nutrition. Philadelphia: WB Saunders, 1980.
13. Ryan JA Jr, Abel RM, Abbott WH, et al. Catheter complications in total parenteral nutrition. A prospective study of 200 consecutive patients. N Engl J Med 1974;290:757.
14. Heimbach DM, Ivey TD. Technique for placement of a permanent home hyperalimentation catheter. Surg Gynecol Obstet 1976;143:634–636.
15. Reed WP, Newman KA, DeJongh C, et al. Prolonged venous access for chemotherapy by means of the Hickman catheter. Cancer 1983;52:185–192.
16. Stellato TA, Gauderer MW, Cohen AM. Direct central vein puncture for silicone rubber catheter insertion. Surgery 1981;90:896–899.
17. Fonkalsrud EW, Ament ME, Berquist WE, Burke M. Occlusion of the vena cava in infants receiving central venous hyperalimentation. Surg Gynecol Obstet 1982;154:189–192.
18. Duffy BJ Jr. The clinical use of polyethylene tubing for intravenous therapy: a report on seventy-two cases. Ann Surg 1949;130:929–936.
19. Gyves J, Ensminger W, Niederhuber J. Totally implanted system for intravenous chemotherapy in patients with cancer. Am J Med 1982;73:841–846.
20. Lokich JJ, Bothe A Jr, Benotti P, Moore C. Complications and management of implanted venous access catheters. J Clin Oncol 1985;3:710–717.
21. Strum S, McDermed J, Korn A, Joseph C. Improved methods for venous access: the Port-A-Cath, a totally implantable catheter system. J Clin Oncol 1986;4:596–603.
22. Nejad MS. Clotting on the outer surface of vascular catheters. Radiology 1968;91:248.
23. Welch GW, McKeel DW, Silverstein P, et al. The role of catheter composition in the development of thrombophlebitis. Surg Gynecol Obstet 1974;138:421.
24. Mc Lean-Ross AH, Griffith DM, Anderson JR, Grieve DC. Thromboembolic complications with silicone elastomer subclavian catheters. JPEN 1982;6:61.
25. Dolcourt JL, Bose CL. Percutaneous insertion of Silastic central venous catheters in newborn infants. Pediatrics 1982;70:484.
26. Hoar PF, Stone JG, Wicks AE, et al. Thrombogenesis associated with Swan-Ganz catheters. Anesthesiology 1978;48:445.
27. Peters WR, Bush WH Jr, McIntyre RD, et al. The development of fibrin sheath on indwelling venous catheters. Surg Gynecol Obstet 1973;137:43.
28. Tanner WA, Delaney PV, Hennessy TP. The influence of heparin on intravenous infusions: a prospective study. Br J Surg 1980;67:311.
29. Tice A, ed. Outpatient Intravenous Therapy Source Book. Tacoma, Washington: OPIT Source Book, 1995.
30. Bernard RW, Stahle WM. Subclavian vein catheterization: a prospective study. Ann Surg 1971;173:184.
31. Flanagan JP, Gradisar IA, Gross RJ, Kelly TR. Air embolus—a lethal complication of subclavian venipuncture. N Engl J Med 1969;281:488.
32. Oppenheimer MJ, Durant TM, Lymes P. Body position in relation to venous air embolism and the associated cardiovascular respiratory changes. Am J Med Sci 1953;225:362.
33. Durant IM, Long J, Oppenheimer MJ. Pulmonary (venous) air embolism. Am Heart J 1947;33:269.
34. Shires T, O'Banion J. Successful treatment of massive air embolism producing cardiac arrest. JAMA 1958;167:1483.
35. Burri C, Krischak G. Techniques and complications of administration of total parenteral nutrition. In: Manni C, Magalini SI, Sorascia, eds. Total Parenteral Nutrition. New York: American Elsevier Scientific Publishing Co., 1976:306–315.
36. Block PC. Transvenous retrieval of foreign bodies in the cardiac circulation. JAMA 1973;224:241.
37. Hashal VL Jr, Ause RG, Hoskins PA. Fibrin sleeve formation on indwelling subclavian central venous catheters. Arch Surg 1971;102:353.
38. Fabri PJ, Mirtallo JM, Ruberg RL, et al. Incidence and prevention of thrombosis of the subclavian vein during total parenteral nutrition. Surg Gynecol Obstet 1982;155:238.
39. Sazena VK, Heilpern RJ, Murphy SF. Pseudotumor cerebri. A complication of parenteral hyperalimentation. JAMA 1976;235:2124.
40. Valerie D, Hussey JK, Smith FW. Central vein thrombosis associated with subclavian catheterization for intravenous feeding. In: Proceedings of the 2nd European Congress of Parenteral and Enteral Nutrition 1980;PJ4:72.

41. Padberg FT, Ruggiero J, Blackburn GL, et al. Central venous catheterization for parenteral nutrition. Ann Surg 1981;193:264.

42. Glynn MFX, Langer B, Jeejeebhoy KN. Therapy for thrombotic occlusion long-term intravenous alimentation catheters. JPEN 1980;4:387.

43. Hurtubise MR, Bottino JE, et al. Restoring patency of occluded central venous catheters. Arch Surg 1980;115: 212.

44. Schropp KP, Ginn-Pease ME, King DR. Catheter-related sepsis: a review of the experience with Broviac and Hickman catheters. Nutrition 1988:195–200.

45. Donahoe PK, Kim SH. The inferior epigastric vein as an alternate site for central venous hyperalimentation. J Pediatr Surg 1980;15:737–738.

46. Kenney PR, Dorfman GS, Denny DF Jr. Percutaneous inferior vena cava cannulation for long-term parenteral nutrition. Surgery 1985;97:602–604.

47. Maher JW. A technique for the positioning of permanent central venous catheters in patients with thrombosis of the superior vena cava. Surg Gynecol Obstet 1983;156:659–660.

48. Raaf JH. Vascular access in cancer patients. Cancer 1985;55:1312–1321.

49. Williard W, Coit D, Lucas A, Groeger JS. Long-term vascular access via the inferior vena cava. J Surg Oncol 1991;46:162–166.

50. Fonkalsrud EW, Berquist W, Burke M, Ament ME. Long-term hyperalimentation in children through saphenous central venous catheterization. Am J Surg 1982;143:209–211.

51. Oram-Smith JC, Mullen JL, Harken AH, Fitts WT Jr. Direct right atrial catheterization for total parenteral nutrition. Surgery 1978;83:274–276.

52. Malt RA, Kempster M. Direct azygos vein and superior vena cava cannulation for parenteral nutrition. JPEN 1983;7:580–581.

53. Bria WF, Kanarek DJ, Kazemi H. Prediction of postoperative pulmonary function following thoracic operations. J Thorac Cardiovasc Surg 1983;86: 186.

54. Shah DM, Powers SR. Prevention of pulmonary complications in high risk patients. Surg Clin North Am 1980;60:1359.

55. Torosian MH, Meranze S, McLean G, Mullen JL. Central venous access with occlusive superior central venous thrombosis. Ann Surg 1986;203:30–33.

II

Special Conditions and Therapeutics

11

HOMECARE THERAPEUTICS FOR AIDS

Gigi R. Diamond, Michael M. Rothkopf, and Rosanna Leveriza

CHAPTER AT A GLANCE: Homecare plays a significant role in the management of AIDS. It reduces hospitalization and improves quality of life. This chapter reviews the illness from the perspective of the physician's use of homecare services. The rationale, pros and cons, and patient selection criteria are discussed. Homecare approaches for treatment of opportunistic diseases and nutritional depletion are reviewed. Finally, the role of homecare in palliative treatment of the terminal patient with AIDS is presented.

Introduction

The management of acquired immune deficiency syndrome (AIDS) is a complex and dynamic challenge for the physician. This is because the caseload has been increasing while physicians must adapt to rapidly evolving treatment strategies. Antiretroviral therapy has expanded. The prophylaxis and effective treatment of opportunistic infections encompass new medications and drug regimens. A combination of these factors has yielded dramatic improvements in the survival of patients with human immunodeficiency virus (HIV) infection.

While this improved survival rate is encouraging, the financial impact of managing the epidemic using high-tech medical intervention represents an enormous potential expenditure on the healthcare system. The cost of AIDS inpatient care has been estimated to be as high as $150,000/patient (1). In the United States in 1992, there were 249,199 cases of AIDS and 1.5 million HIV-positive individuals (2). This number is expected to grow substantially as the disease spreads into the heterosexual population.

Homecare therapeutics has a critical role in HIV-related illnesses because it can decrease hospital use and improve quality of life. Not unimportantly, this also dramatically reduces the cost of AIDS care. The development of intensive homecare at a time when the incidence of HIV disease was increasing and treatment options were expanding has been one of the remarkable synergies of healthcare in the 1990s. AIDS care and intensive homecare have been evolving together since their emergence. Advances in AIDS treatments have spurred the need for homecare approaches. In a complementary fashion, developments in homecare have permitted new treatments and even AIDS clinical research to progress at a rapid pace.

This chapter reviews the complex management of AIDS with a focus on the unique opportunities available for homecare.

Epidemiology

The case definition for HIV infection has undergone several updates. Exposure categories have been broadened from homosexual/bisexual men to include heterosexual contact,

"

blood transfusion recipients (including hemophiliacs), perinatal transmission, and illicit drug users (Fig. 11.1). The list of indicator conditions used in the surveillance case definition has also been broadened. The number of new cases of HIV continues to rise, with an incidence clustered around large cities (3). There are increased cases among women, heterosexual contacts, and patients with no known risk factors (4).

Responsible estimates show the epidemic growing rapidly. Figures from the Global AIDS Policy Coalition show that some 20 million people are HIV infected worldwide. This number could be as high as 100 million by the year 2000 (5). More than 3 million humans have already developed full-blown AIDS.

HIV Pathogenesis and Natural History

The retroviruses can be divided into lymphodepletive viruses (HIV-1, HIV-2) and lymphoproliferative viruses (HTLV-I, HTLV-II). Retroviruses are enveloped viruses that contain two genomic strands of RNA and the enzyme reverse transcriptase.

After gaining entry to the host, HIV binds to the surface of CD4-positive cells, principally the CD4 (helper cell) T lymphocyte. HIV also has an affinity to other CD4-positive cells, including macrophages, monocytes, and oligodendritic cells of the brain. Once inside the cell, reverse transcriptase transcribes the viral RNA into DNA, which is then integrated into the

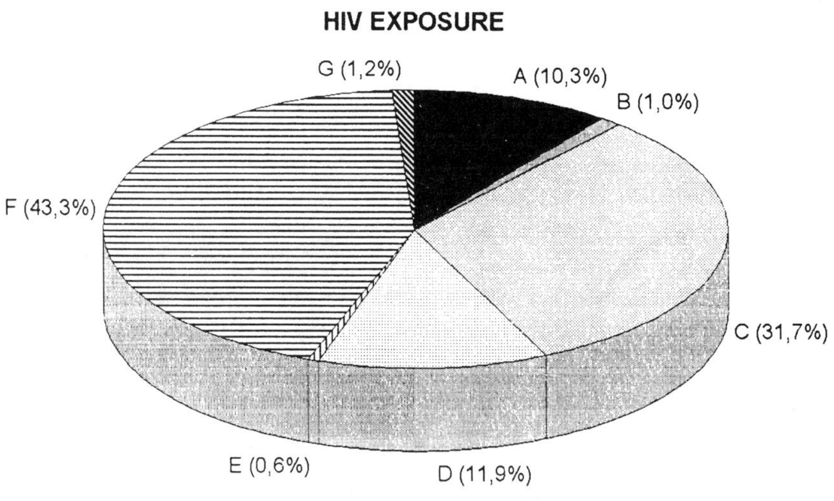

A	Heterosexual contact
B	Transfusion recipients
C	History of IV drug use
D	No risk reported
E	Persons with hemophilia
F	Male homosexual/bisexual contact
G	Perinatal transmission

Figure 11.1.   Exposure categories for HIV. Recent trends reveal change in HIV exposure from the initial predominance of male homosexual contact. (Adapted from Update: AIDS—US 1994. MMWR 1995;44(4):65. Figure prepared by Dr. Ingacio Valdes.)

host genome. The viral DNA (or provirus) is transcribed into RNA by the host's RNA polymerase. After the viral RNAs are translated into viral polypeptides, viral proteins are made, developing a virion, which can then bud from the cell surface to infect other cells (Fig. 11.2).

HIV affects the immune system at various levels. Besides depletion of T helper cells, there is T-cell functional impairment and alteration in the CD8 cytotoxic cells. HIV affects monocytes and macrophages and activates B cells, impairing specific antibody responses.

Saag and coworkers (6) have shown that HIV infection is a dynamic process. It is rapidly established in lymphoid tissue, dendritic cells, monocytes, and macrophages throughout the body. Active ongoing replication with increasing genotypic diversity of the viral population is associated with an increased viral load. This suggests that early intervention with antiretroviral drugs would be of benefit. Along these lines, Ho and colleagues (7) demonstrated that rapid HIV turnover results in high viral diversity.

The clinical spectrum of HIV infection ranges from the absence of symptoms to advanced illness. The estimated time from seroconversion to the development of full-blown AIDS is roughly 10 years (Fig. 11.3). Cofactors such as age, sex, and social conditions alter disease progression.

Oral candidiasis, fever, chronic diarrhea, disseminated herpes zoster, and hairy leukoplakia can signal immunological decline. Other surrogate markers have been used to predict the development of full-blown AIDS. Besides the widely used CD4 count, other tests such as P24 antigen, β_2-microglobulin, and neopterin levels are useful. The presence of a specific viral phenotype called syncytium inducer (SI) has been demonstrated to predict an aggressive, AZT-resistant type of illness.

Decreased serum retinol levels are associated with impaired T-cell blastogenesis and predicts more aggressive disease (8). Whether or not replacement vitamin A therapy is beneficial is currently being evaluated.

The U.S. Centers for Disease Control and Prevention (CDC) had revised the HIV classification system for adolescents and adults to emphasize the clinical importance of the CD4 count in the categorization of HIV-related illnesses (Table 11.1). However, it is expected that the reliance on CD4 counts will be superseded by the use of HIV viral load in the future.

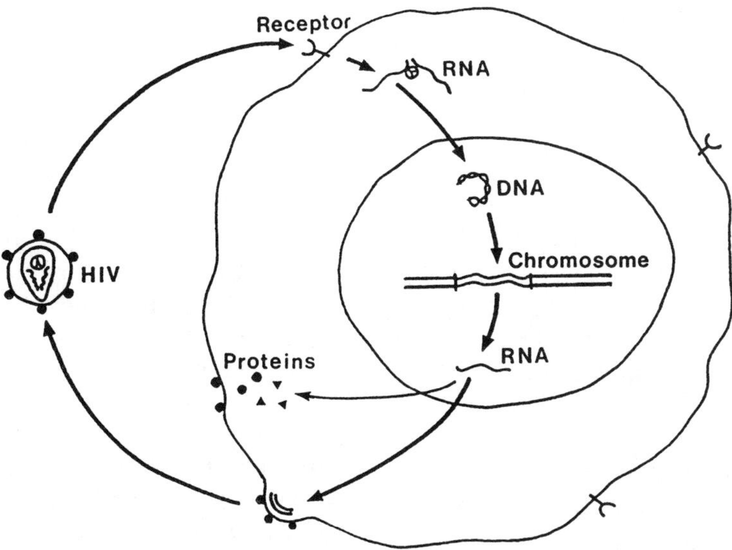

Figure 11.2. Simplified replication cycle of HIV. (Used with permission from Broder S, Merigan T Jr, Bolognesi D. Textbook of AIDS Medicine. Baltimore: Williams & Wilkins, 1994:16.)

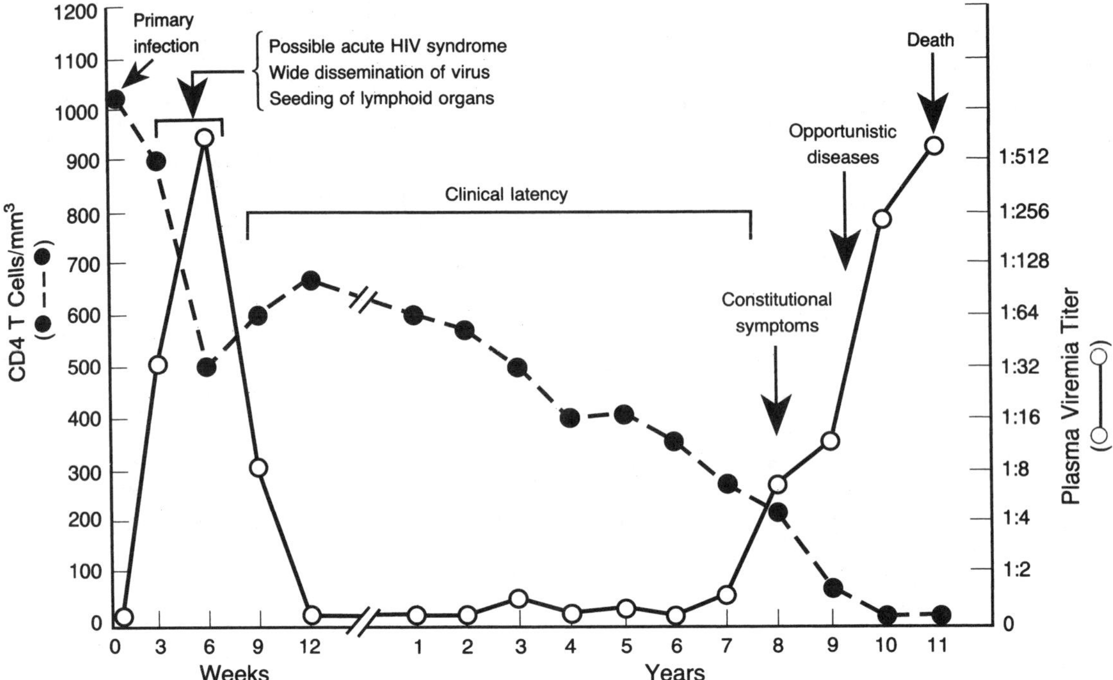

Figure 11.3. Typical course of HIV infection. Typical pattern of CD4+T cell decline and HIV plasma titers over the course of HIV infection. (Adapted from Pantaleo G, Graziosi C, Fauci AS. New concepts in the immunopathogenesis of human immunodeficiency virus infection. N Engl J Med 1993;328:327–335.)

The result of viral dynamic studies have shown that quantification of plasma HIV-1 RNA is the most accurate way to monitor a patient's disease state (9). This reflects the rate of virus production and hence the rate of CD4 cell destruction. The goal of antiretroviral therapy is to reduce the viral load level as much as possible. Viral load should be monitored frequently to determine if a change in therapy is needed.

The three tests now available for quantification of viral load are reverse transcriptase–polymerase chain reaction (RT-PCR), branched–chain DNA (bDNA), and nucleic acid sequence–based amplification (NASBA).

Homecare in AIDS

Rationale, Advantages, and Disadvantages

HIV is creating an increasing burden on hospital capacity. For example, up to one in seven New York City hospital admissions are now believed to be related to HIV (10). Janssen (11) estimated that 225,000 HIV-positive patients were admitted to U.S. hospitals in 1990. 72,000 of these patients were admitted for AIDS care. The remainder were asymptomatic HIV-positive cases. As the epidemic grows, pressure on the hospital system for the treatment of AIDS complications will become even greater.

AIDS patients require a high level of professional services to manage a complex, life-threatening illness. But the hospital setting has many disadvantages for these patients. AIDS patients are at risk of acquiring nosocomial infections with multiply resistant microorganisms that are present within the hospital population. Conversely, AIDS patients pose a risk to other immune-compromised hospital patients because they often harbor unique infectious agents. Therefore, AIDS patients themselves must often be isolated from the noninfectious patients.

Hospital personnel are fearful of AIDS patients and tend to avoid them. When the pa-

Table 11.1. Revised Classification System of HIV Disease—Centers for Disease Control and Prevention (January 1993)

CD4 Count	A	B	C
>500	A1	B1	C1
200–500	A2	B2	C2
<200	A3	B3	C3

Category A
- Asymptomatic HIV infection
- Persistent generalized lymphadenopathy
- Acute retroviral syndrome

Category B (formerly "ARC")
- Bacillary angiomatosis
- Candidiasis
  Oral
  Recurrent vaginal
- Cervical dysplasia
- Constitutional symptoms
  (e.g., fever or diarrhea)
  >1 month
- Hairy leukoplakia, oral
- Herpes zoster
- Idiopathic thrombocytopenia purpura
- Listeriosis
- Pelvic inflammatory disease
- Peripheral neuropathy

Category C (AIDS-defining conditions)
- CD4 count less than 200 cells/mm^3
- Candidiasis
  Pulmonary
  Esophageal
- Cervical cancer
- Coccidioidomycosis
- Cryptococcosis,
  extrapulmonary
- Cryptosporidiosis
- Cytomegalovirus
- Encephalopathy, HIV
- Herpes simplex
  Chronic (>1 month)
  Esophageal
- Histoplasmosis
- Isosporiasis
- Kaposi's sarcoma
- Lymphoma
- *Mycobacterium avium*
- *Mycobacterium kansasii*
- *Mycobacterium tuberculosis*
- *Pneumocystis carinii*
- Pneumonia, recurrent
- Progressive multifocal leukemia
- Salmonellosis

From Broder S, Merigan T Jr, Bolognesi D. Textbook of AIDS Medicine. Baltimore: Williams & Wilkins, 1994:46.

tient is in isolation, the only human contact permitted for the patient is through the protective barrier of gowns, gloves, and isolation masks. Furthermore, hospital staff personnel are often uncomfortable with and critical of an alternative lifestyle that an AIDS patient may profess.

There is evidence that emotional stress, such as that associated with being hospitalized, may be harmful to the immune system (12). In an already immune-compromised individual, this may be a serious detriment to management. Emotional stress has also been shown to heighten symptoms associated with reactions to toxic medications such as chemotherapy (13).

The treatment of opportunistic infection in AIDS is rarely curative. This means that repeated treatments and lifelong suppressive therapy are often needed. Given the prospect of a lifetime need for hospital-level care, homecare therapeutics seems the most logical option to satisfy the complex medical, economic, and social requirements. For this reason, AIDS practitioners often seek to integrate homecare into AIDS treatment plans early.

Homecare has been shown to reduce hospitalization and the need for hospital readmission. Greenbaum (14) discussed the use of homecare as a means of minimizing the need for critical care utilization in AIDS. Moons et al. showed that homecare could also replace outpatient center–based therapy, thereby further reducing costs and adding patient convenience (15).

Hellinger (16) and Epstein et al. (17) found that a decline in hospital utilization and more reliance on homecare resulted in a decrease in the cost burden of treating AIDS. Liekweg et al. (18) conducted a cost comparison between inpatient and outpatient/homecare methods for AIDS patients. The average costs were substantially lower for outpatient/homecare services. For example, in-hospital therapy for *Pneumocystis carinii* pneumonia (PCP) was $1023 per day versus $157 per day at home; cytomegalovirus (CMV) therapy was $615 versus $242 per day; lymphoma therapy was $891 versus $154 per day.

Homecare can have a significant value in terms of improving quality of life in AIDS patients. Bergler (19) showed that homecare encourages greater personal freedom, a higher level of social contacts, increased appetite, and a sense of well-being.

Homecare offers other advantages for AIDS patients, particularly if they live far from an advanced AIDS research center. We and others have conducted clinical trials with AIDS patients whose care was home-based rather than hospital-based. This permitted the patients to receive state-of the art therapy at home even before it was widely available in most hospitals. Many of the newer intravenous medications for opportunistic diseases were actually tested in the homecare environment during clinical trials.

Similarly, patients who travel great distances to be seen by an AIDS specialist can receive medications ordered by that physician through a local homecare service. Lockman-Samkowiak (20) reported that homecare allowed patients in rural areas access to quality care when limited hospital resources were available.

On the other hand, homecare does have some disadvantages for the AIDS patient, particularly if there is a lack of support from the family or resources are lacking. If this is the case, the patient may receive inadequate attention to his or her basic needs such as bathing and laundry. The patient may not be able to travel easily to be seen by his or her physicians for routine or even emergency care.

To address this type of problem, Milanese et al. (21) designed a multidisciplinary program that included medical, nursing, psychosocial, and homemaking support for AIDS patients, many of whom were considered not self-sufficient. They observed a decrease in hospitalization rate from 20.1% to 8% after intervention. Such programs may prove useful and cost-effective in the future.

Another problem with the homecare setting for AIDS is that it is almost invariably associated with the use of a long-term venous access catheter. AIDS patients are at a high risk for the development of infections with these devices (Fig. 11.4). We studied the infectious risks of various catheter types and found that Hickman-type catheters had less risk of infection than implanted access ports (22). However, Settle et al. (23) reported opposite findings.

It is not the home setting per se that exposes the patients to such risks. Many AIDS patients require long-term venous access while in the hospital. Poretz (24) has stated that the infectious complications of these devices are lower at home than in the hospital. But it is certainly true that the homecare patient will have less medical attention and therefore less frequent monitoring of the venous access device. The optimal management of these devices at home requires careful attention and frequent reevaluation.

Finally, there is the issue of disposal of infectious waste at home and the exposure of noninfected family members to potentially hazardous material. This also requires careful planning, although it is not an insurmountable problem.

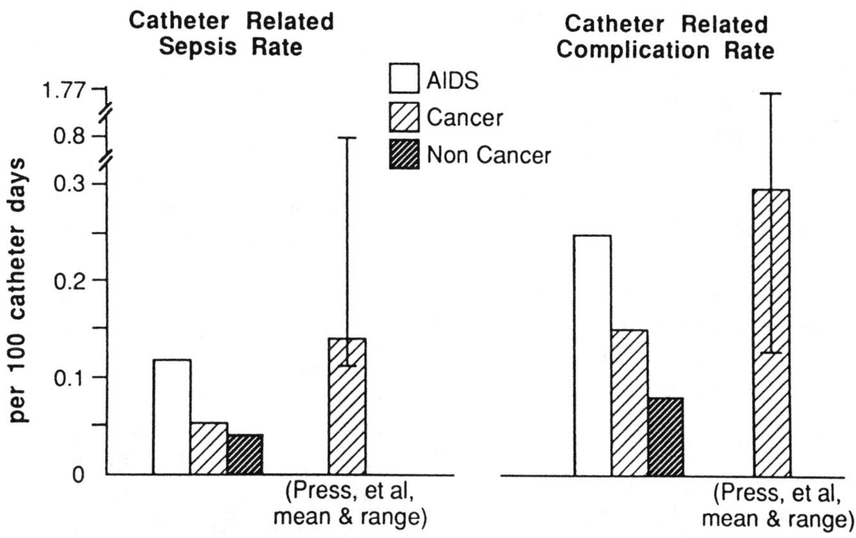

Figure 11.4. Comparison of catheter-related sepsis rate and complication rate between AIDS, cancer, noncancer patients from our group, and patients with malignancies from the literature (Press et al.). (From Singer P, Rothkopf MM, Kvetan V, et al. Risks and benefits of home parenteral nutrition in the AIDS. J Parenter Enteral Nutr 1991;15:75–79 with permission.)

Patient Selection

As is detailed elsewhere in this text (see Chapter 3), appropriate patient selection is of critical importance for homecare. Although AIDS patients are frequently more ill than other homecare patients, basic criteria still apply. These include both medical and non-medical components.

From a medical perspective, the patient should be as stable as possible. All current problems should have already been delineated and treatments should be under way. The vital signs and physical findings should be within reasonable parameters. If the patient has been repeatedly spiking fevers, for example, this should not be a new phenomenon. Laboratory values should also be unchanging from the baseline obtained in the hospital.

The nonmedical criteria are related to the patient and/or family accepting responsibility for care and agreeing to be compliant at home. The patient should be able to demonstrate the capacity to learn and master homecare techniques. He or she should also display the psychological stability to follow through with the rigors these procedures require. In addition, the home environment must be safe for homecare, with adequate storage space and access to electricity and telephone service. Preferably, there would also be nearby access to emergency medical facilities.

Opportunistic Diseases

Because of the immunodeficiency associated with HIV, HIV-related illnesses predispose the AIDS patient to a variety of opportunistic conditions. These include parasitic, bacterial, mycobacterial, and fungal infections as well as certain malignancies. This section briefly reviews the common conditions with relation to the application of homecare therapy. More detail on the treatment of infectious diseases at home can be found in Chapter 12.

This section is not intended to serve as a definitive review on the diagnosis and treatment of opportunistic diseases. For a more comprehensive analysis of this complex topic, the reader is referred to a general textbook on AIDS or infectious diseases (e.g., Broder S, Merigan TC, Bolognesi D, eds. Textbook of AIDS Medicine. Baltimore: Williams & Wilkins, 1994).

Pneumocystis carinii Pneumonia

Pneumocystis carinii pneumonia (PCP) is a parasitic infection that most often causes bilateral interstitial pneumonia. It is the first opportunistic infection in up to 60% of AIDS cases (25). It is generally seen when the CD4 count is less than 200 cells/μL.

PCP causes air-space consolidation, with numerous *P. carinii* trophozoites filling alveoli. This leads to intrapulmonary right-to-left shunting and hypoxemia. The patient presents with a history of nonproductive cough, gradually progressive shortness of breath, fevers, and general malaise. In advanced disease, these symptoms are more pronounced, resulting in respiratory distress.

The diagnosis of PCP is confirmed with greater than 90% accuracy via bronchoscopy and bronchoalveolar lavage (26). In an HIV-positive individual who was not on PCP prophylaxis, a gallium lung scan is positive in 85 to 90% of cases (27). Induced sputum is a noninvasive, cost-effective method to diagnose PCP (28). It has a high accuracy rate at institutions with personnel experienced in interpretation of these results.

The first line of therapy is trimethoprim-sulfamethoxazole (TMP-SMX), followed by pentamidine. Corticosteroids are added if the Po_2 is less than 70 mm Hg. A list of alternative therapies for PCP is provided in Table 11.2.

Intravenous therapy for PCP using TMP-SMX or pentamidine is usually continued for 14 to 21 days. Since adverse reactions are common, initial therapy should be monitored in a hospital or clinic setting. However, a stable patient can be treated successfully at home, especially to complete therapy.

An HIV-positive patient with a CD4 count less than 200 or a CD4 percentage less than 20 is at risk for developing PCP and should receive lifelong primary prophylaxis. This consists of oral TMP-SMX or dapsone; inhaled pentamidine or intravenous pentamidine given at home can also be used in patients who are intolerant of the oral medications.

Secondary prophylaxis to prevent recurrence of PCP also requires lifelong therapy. Early studies have shown that the relapse rate for PCP is approximately 5% per month and 60% at 12 months (29). Survival from each subsequent attack of pneumonia is decreased.

Cytomegalovirus

Cytomegalovirus (CMV) is a member of the herpesvirus group. As is typical of these

Table 11.2. New Therapies for *Pneumocystis* Pneumonia

Severity	Dose
Mild–Moderate Severity Episodes	
Low-dose oral TMP-SMX[a]	12–15 mg/kg/day (TMP component)
Trimethoprim + dapsone	TMP, 12–15 mg/kg/day; dapsone, 100 mg/day
Atovaquone	2250 mg/day (three 250 tablets TID)
Primaquine + clindamycin	Primaquine, 15–30 mg base/day; Clindamycin, 2400–2700 mg IV/day; 1800 mg orally/day
Aerosolized pentamidine	600 mg once daily via the Respirgard II nebulizer
Moderate–Severe Episodes	
Trimetrexate + leucovorin	45 mg/M^2/day[b] as a single IV infusion Leucovorin, 80 mg/M^2/day[b] (in four equal doses)
Adjunctive corticosteroids:	40/30 mg BID, days 1–5
(prednisone/methylprednisolone)	40/30 mg once daily, days 6–10 20/15 mg once daily, day 11 to end of course
Eflornithine	400 mg/kg/day IV (in four equally divided doses) 75 mg/kg/day orally (in four equally divided doses)

From Broder S, Merigan T Jr, Bolognesi D. Textbook of AIDS Medicine. Baltimore: Williams & Wilkins, 1994:201.
[a]Trimethoprim-sulfamethoxazole.
[b]Modified for hematological toxicity.

viruses, prolonged latency usually follows primary infection. Transmission occurs via infected body fluids, including blood products, semen, and breast milk.

Infection with CMV is common in the general population, 50% of whom are seropositive by age 50. In contrast, more than 90% of patients with AIDS are seropositive and one-third of them experience clinical manifestations of CMV infection (30). As is true with other herpes viruses, CMV causes disease by reactivation of latent virus.

CMV infection generally occurs after the sustained CD4 count is less than 50 cells/mL. It produces a systemic illness with the possibility of disseminated disease. However, its most common manifestation in chorioretinitis.

Ocular Manifestations

Between 10 and 30% of AIDS patients will develop sight-threatening CMV retinitis (31). Pathological changes from viremia can cause retinal necrosis, macular edema, optic nerve involvement, and retinal tears or detachment. Blindness will ensue if these conditions are left untreated.

The onset may be subtle or acute. The patient usually complains of visual disturbances such as blurry vision. However, the patient is sometimes asymptomatic, and early lesions are found on routine ophthalmologic examinations. Most often, the disease is bilateral. Funduscopic examination reveals granular lesions, which may coalesce. Late findings include exudates and hemorrhages denoting a vascular pattern of distribution. Left untreated, this leads to ischemic maculopathy.

Even with effective therapy, relapses of CMV retinitis will occur. Therefore, lifelong suppressive therapy is needed. Reinduction therapy may be used for recurrences. Close funduscopic monitoring of each patient is important because destruction of additional retinal tissue and progressive loss of visual function occurs with each relapse.

Extraocular Manifestations

CMV may cause neurologic, gastrointestinal, and pulmonary disease. CMV infection of the nervous system has been found in more than 20% of autopsied AIDS patients. It causes focal brain parenchymal necrosis, ventriculoencephalitis, and radiculomyelitis. Antemortem diagnosis is difficult. Polyradiculomyelitis and CSF abnormalities such as polymorphonuclear pleocytosis, hypoglycorrhachia, and elevated CMV titers have been observed.

CMV infection can occur anywhere along the GI tract. The esophagus and colon are most frequently involved. Reactivation of latent infections leads to vasculitis, submucosal ischemia, and ulceration.

CMV colitis is usually associated with fever, abdominal pain, and intermittent diarrhea. Some patients develop tenesmus, bloody stools, and small-volume bowel movements with regular frequency. CMV infection of the gastrointestinal tract has also been known to cause perforation and gangrene. Diagnosis requires a biopsy showing intracytoplasmic inclusion bodies in the submicrosal and endothelial cells (32).

CMV is a common cause of interstitial pneumonitis in immunocompromised patients. Although more common in transplant patients, it is sometimes seen with AIDS. CMV isolation from bronchoalveolar lavage fluid or lung tissue from an AIDS patient does not always correlate with pulmonary disease. Most clinicians consider the diagnosis when there is a diffuse interstitial pneumonia with hypoxemia in the absence of other pulmonary pathogens.

CMV Therapy

Treatment of CMV reactivation requires acute intervention and lifelong suppressive therapy. Since either modality calls for the use of daily intravenous administration, most patients can be expected to receive treatment via homecare.

Two drugs are currently FDA approved for the treatment of CMV: ganciclovir and foscarnet. Ganciclovir is a nucleoside analog, whereas foscarnet is an analog of inorganic pyrophosphate. Both have been shown to be effective against CMV and other herpesviruses. There is a suggestion that median survival may be longer with foscarnet (33).

Induction therapy usually consists of a 2-week course of either agent in the hospital setting. A long-term venous access catheter is placed and chronic treatment continued at home.

Both drugs are associated with side effects and must be monitored closely. Ganciclovir's major limitation is that it can produce bone marrow suppression with pancytopenia. Foscarnet has been associated with renal insufficiency and electrolyte imbalances.

Drug toxicities can be monitored and managed at home just as they are in the hospital. For example, patients receiving ganciclovir can be monitored for bone marrow suppression at home. The homecare nurse is instructed to observe for associated symptoms. Routine blood counts are obtained regularly. If marrow suppression occurs, a granulocyte colony-stimulating factor (G-CSF), such as filgrastim, can be given at home by subcutaneous injection. Other growth factors, such as erythropoietin, can also be administered at home.

The management of renal insufficiency or electrolyte imbalance secondary to foscarnet administration includes the institution of daily intravenous fluid and electrolyte replacement. Once again, this can be safely accomplished in the home setting, obviating the need for hospital readmission.

New agents and approaches are currently being tested for CMV retinitis, including nucleoside analogs, intravitreal injections of ganciclovir, and anti-CMV monoclonal antibodies. Oral ganciclovir has recently been approved as maintenance therapy for CMV retinitis only.

The treatment of extraocular manifestations of CMV is more controversial than for retinitis. Acute therapy with either agent has been used for both the neurological manifestations and CMV pneumonitis (34). However, the effect of suppressive therapy has not been studied.

CMV colitis responds to therapy with either intravenous foscarnet or ganciclovir. Dietrich et al. (35) have shown benefits from long-term maintenance therapy.

Herpes

Herpes simplex 1 and 2 (HSV-1, HSV-2) viral infections are common in the general population. It is estimated that 70% of all adults are HSV-1 seropositive. Some 16% are seropositive for HSV-2, although this figure is higher in women and homosexual men.

Herpes simplex virus causes disease in AIDS patients due to the reactivation of latent infection. This results in the eruption of painful vesicular lesions on mucocutaneous sites, usually at the point of original inoculation. The lips, mouth, and esophagus are typical areas for HSV-1, whereas the vagina and rectal mucosa may be affected by HSV-2 ulcers.

Oropharyngeal lesions produce odynophagia, which can be severe. Herpetic proctitis and vaginitis or cystitis can contribute to skin breakdown and fistula formation. The severe pain noted with defecation in patients with herpetic proctitis sometimes requires surgical diversion.

Fortunately, most HSV infections respond to acyclovir, although resistance may develop after long-term use (36). For more difficult cases, intravenous foscarnet has been successful (37).

Fungi

Candida albicans, Candida species, *Cryptococcus neoformans,* and *Histoplasma capsulatum* are frequent causes of fungal infection in AIDS. Coccidiomycosis is becoming more common in AIDS patients, particularly in the southwestern United States. Aspergillosis, blastomycosis, and sporotrichosis remain rare complications of AIDS.

Candidiasis is generally a mucosal disease, affecting areas such as the oropharynx, esophagus, GI tract, and vagina. Systemic or invasive candidiasis is rare in AIDS but may be seen in higher frequency in particular patient groups, such as IV drug abusers.

Cryptococcal meningitis and pneumonitis are common in AIDS, as is pulmonary cryptococcosis. Skin involvement is also often seen. Histoplasmosis is usually a disseminated infection in AIDS, often presenting as fever and weight loss. Respiratory symptoms are absent in 50% of cases.

The treatment of fungal opportunistic infections includes both local and systemic approaches. Topical nystatin and clotrimazole are effective first-line agents for candidiasis of the mouth or vagina. More invasive candidiasis calls for systemic therapy with either oral ketoconazole, fluconazole, or itraconazole. Systemic candidiasis generally requires intravenous therapy, usually with amphotericin B. Although it is labeled for hospital use only, amphotericin B can be given safely at home with appropriate premedication and hydration. Because of the high incidence of side effects, both the homecare team and the patient should be carefully instructed to monitor for toxicity. The serum electrolytes and complete blood counts should be monitored for any untoward effects, and adjustments should be made as necessary.

Cryptococcosis and histoplasmosis in AIDS usually require amphotericin, at least for initial therapy. There is some evidence that fluconazole and itraconazole may also have a role in the treatment of these infections (38). As with other opportunistic infections, a complete cure depends on an intact immune system. Therefore, cure is unusual in AIDS, and chronic suppressive therapy at home is usually required.

Syphilis and HIV

The natural history and pathogenesis of syphilis are complicated and still incompletely understood. Syphilis, nearly from its onset, is a systemic illness. During the primary stage, which appears clinically as a localized ulcer, *Treponema pallidum* organisms disseminate and have been shown to be present in the CSF in up to one-third of immune-competent patients.

In HIV patients, CSF syphilis may be more aggressive. Less than 5% of normal patients with primary or secondary syphilis advance to clinical neurological disease. By contrast, patients with HIV may present with neurological deficits early in the disease (39). Some clinicians feel that primary, secondary, and tertiary syphilis may occur at the same time in these individuals.

The diagnosis relies on serologic tests, including the fluorescent treponemal antibody absorption test (FTA-ABS) and the microhemagglutinin assay for antibodies to *Tre-*

ponema pallidum (MHA-TP). Some authorities have recommended a routine lumbar puncture in HIV-infected syphilis patients to diagnose tertiary syphilis. However, CSF findings may be confusing, since HIV itself can produce abnormal CSF results.

Infection with HIV can alter the course of syphilis. Although the treatment of syphilis in HIV-positive patients is still not standardized, recommendations include penicillin G benzathine with probenecid or intravenous ceftriaxone. The response to standard penicillin G benzathine injections may be insufficient. New treatment regimens have been proposed that require IV therapy for up to 3 weeks (40), usually in the homecare setting. Treatment with IV ceftriaxone can achieve high drug levels in serum and CSF. The treatment of suspected or documented tertiary syphilis mandates an intravenous approach.

Mycobacterial Diseases

Mycobacterium tuberculosis

Coinfection with HIV and *Mycobacterium tuberculosis* is common, and approximately 50% of these patients will go on to develop active tuberculosis. This is five times higher than the risk of disease progression in immunocompetent individuals. Because they produce a less aggressive immune response, AIDS patients may actually be less infectious carriers of *M. tuberculosis* than non-AIDS patients.

HIV-positive patients with *M. tuberculosis* have an increased incidence of dissemination. Most have both pulmonary and extrapulmonary disease. Constitutional symptoms, including weight loss, fever, and anorexia, are common. Chest x-ray findings are unique in that there is less cavitary disease and increased occurrences of miliary patterns. Tuberculin skin tests are often unreliable, and the definitive diagnosis rests with obtaining a positive microbiological culture from the sputum or other site.

Mycobacterium avium-intracellulare *Complex*

Mycobacterium avium-intracellulare complex (MAC) is an acid-fast organism that grows rapidly in comparison to *M. tuberculosis*. It is a ubiquitous organism and can be found in water, animals, and soil. MAC infection in the gut is usually identified with disseminated infection, although colitis can be the first sign of infection. MAC also presents as a late infection indicating a declining immune system.

Small intestine involvement is more common with associated symptoms of diarrhea, abdominal pain, fever, nausea, vomiting, weight loss, and malnutrition. Diagnosis can be established by stool examination and culture or by special staining of an intestinal biopsy.

Mycobacterial Therapy

Treatment of *M. tuberculosis* or MAC in AIDS is based on an oral multidrug regimen. For MAC, intravenous therapy may also include amikacin or ciprofloxacin (41). Therapy for MAC, like most therapies for AIDS illnesses, is usually a lifelong term process. Patients with severe gastrointestinal symptoms and/or malnutrition may require intravenous nutritional support.

Other Parasites

Microsporidia are ubiquitous spore-forming obligate intracellular parasites. There are many genera, but *Enterocytozoon bieneusi* is the most common species identified in small bowel biopsies in AIDS patients. Prevalent data are under-reported because not all AIDS patients with chronic diarrhea are biopsied, and it is difficult to detect the HIV organism microscopically. Symptoms of small bowel infection with microsporidia include multiple watery bowel movements, abdominal discomfort with flatulence, weight loss despite a good appetite, and lack of fever. The patient usually has a CD4 count of less than $50/mm^3$. Definitive treatment with albendazole is unpredictable. Therefore, aggressive symptom control with antidiarrheal agents, including octreotide acetate, and long-term intravenous home nutritional support are often the only effective measures (42).

Cryptosporidia are coccidial protozoa that infect the digestive tract epithelium. In immunocompromised hosts, it can lead to watery diarrhea, dehydration, and death. This organism is also ubiquitous and has been linked to water-borne pathogen outbreaks. The organism may also be transmitted by a fecal-oral route, by pets, and in contaminated food. Watery diarrhea, nausea, vomiting, and weight loss are typical signs. Fever is absent. Like microsporidiosis, cryptosporidiosis usually occurs once the CD4 count is less than $50/mm^3$.

Cryptosporidia may be easier to diagnose than microsporidia. Oocysts can be seen in stool samples that are stained with a modified acid-fast stain. It may also be diagnosed by intestinal biopsy. No effective therapeutic regimen is known, but paromomycin, azithromycin, letrazuril, transfer factor, and interleukin-2 have been tried with variable results. Just as in the case of microsporidiosis, the AIDS patient with cryptosporidioses usually needs aggressive symptom control and long-term hyperalimentation.

Isospora belli are protozoan parasites that invade the enterocytes of the small intestine, thereby causing protracted and watery diarrhea. Fever is usually absent, and the diagnosis can be established by stool smear (similar to *Cryptococcus*) or histologically by small bowel biopsy. *Isospora* is rare in the United States, but fortunately it responds to therapy with TMP-SMX or pyrimethamine.

Toxoplasmosis is the reactivation of a latent infection of the organism *Toxoplasma gondii*. This is almost an exclusive manifestation of immune suppression. In AIDS, the brain is most commonly affected, followed by the lung and eyes. The exact diagnosis is difficult but usually rests with the finding of high antibody titers in a patient with a suspect lesion, such as a site in the cerebral cortex. Pyrimethamine, sulfonamides, and clindamycin have been used effectively.

Neoplasms

AIDS patients are at increased risk of developing malignancy, particularly Kaposi's sarcoma, lymphomas, and carcinoma of the aerodigestive tract. These may call for the use of home intravenous chemotherapy, pain management, or nutritional support.

Nutritional Management of AIDS

Complete nutritional (i.e., nonpharmacologic) approaches to AIDS have been attempted. These are very controversial and have yielded mixed results. With the development of new, more effective AIDS therapies, they have become less common. Nonetheless, practically all AIDS care practitioners recognize the value of nutritional intervention in AIDS, to both prevent and treat malnutrition.

Many AIDS patients develop some form of malnutrition. This may include subtle vitamin deficiencies, chronic malabsorption, or protein-calorie malnutrition (PCM). The most severe manifestation of nutritional deficiency is the AIDS wasting syndrome (AWS), which can occur in up to 30% of all cases.

"Slim's disease" was first described in Uganda in the early 1980s. It was characterized by extreme weight loss, malaise, fever, maculopapular rash, oral candidiasis, and prolonged diarrhea (43). In 1987, the U.S. Centers for Disease Control (CDC) included the criteria of rapid weight loss (more than 10% or 10 kg) as an AIDS-defining illness.

The most significant relationship between malnutrition and HIV disease is that between the loss of body weight and morbidity. It has been shown that patients whose serum albumin level is below 2.5 g/dL have a poor prognosis. Cutaneous anergy has also been associated with poor nutritional states. Nutrient deficiency may be reflected by altered immune regulatory function.

Nutritional Prevention Strategies

AIDS patients should receive nutritional instruction early in the course of their illness. This should be focused on two main areas: maintaining nutritional requirements and food safety.

Most patients are unaware of even the most basic information on daily nutrient requirements. For AIDS patients, who are at a high risk of developing malnutrition, this information can be of critical importance. A simple review of normal caloric, protein, and vitamin requirements should be given to all patients. They should be counseled on the need to maintain adequate intake and to notify their doctor as soon as this becomes difficult. Early intervention with an oral supplement or appetite stimulant may delay the onset of PCM.

Avoidance of potentially contaminated food is another important instructional component for AIDS patients. Many food items contain high levels of potentially infectious material. Examples of this include *Salmonella enteropathica* in undercooked chicken and eggs, and enteropathic *Escherichia coli* in undercooked ground beef.

Even fresh salads may present a risk to a severely immunocompromised patient. These vegetables are grown in contact with the earth and may therefore contain soil organisms such as MAC. Furthermore, they may be contaminated by parasites if manure was used in soil fertilization.

Simple food safety strategies such as completely cooking fish, meats, chicken, and eggs as well as soaking vegetables in a dilute cleansing solution before eating can be effective preventive approaches.

Etiology and Diagnosis of Malnutrition in AIDS

Eating and digestion are complex processes, and AIDS is capable of interfering with them at almost every level. To make matters worse, individual nutritional defects often occur in combination. This leads to a severe and rapid form of PCM.

The normal process of assimilating nutrients from the environment involves three steps: eating (acquisition, chewing, and swallowing of food), digestion and absorption, and metabolic incorporation of nutrients into body stores. Each of these can be deranged by AIDS.

Decreased oral intake occurs because of anorexia (due to the illness, side effects of medications, or depression), odynophagia (due to lesions of the aerodigestive tract), or nausea and vomiting (due to the virus, medications, etc.). Maldigestion and malabsorption may be due to pancreatic insufficiency, rapid bowel transit, AIDS enteropathy, and opportunistic infection of the small and large bowel.

An altered metabolism with aberrant utilization of ingested nutrients may be induced by systemic response to the infection. This includes cytokine activation (i.e., interleukins and tumor necrosis factor), the neuroendocrine response (with counter-regulatory catabolic hormone release) and intermediary protein metabolism (44).

The gastrointestinal tract of AIDS patients is a prime target for infections and complications (45). Diarrhea is an important symptom of AIDS, and if chronic, usually denotes advanced illness. AIDS enteropathy produces villous atrophy and crypt hypertrophy.

Prospective studies of diarrhea in AIDS patients have identified a pathogen in up to 70% of cases. The organisms most frequently encountered are *Cryptosporidium,* microsporidia, *Cytomegalovirus, I. belli,* and *M. avium-intracellulare* (Table 11.3).

Fifteen to twenty percent of patients with diarrhea have no identifiable cause despite exhaustive workups. Some authorities believe that HIV itself might alter the gut tissue in enterocyte maturation and function. Studies on axonal density in both villi and lamina propria of patients with HIV disease have shown autonomic degeneration. Others have theorized that immune dysregulation may lead to enteropathy. T-cell activation in the lamina propria has been known to induce and release lymphokines, and studies of tumor necrosis factors in stool specimens has been linked to inflammatory bowel disease.

Several investigators have reported a high frequency of cystic secretory failure in patients with AIDS. This may lead to an overgrowth of bacteria, with subsequent diarrhea and wasting.

The diagnosis of PCM in AIDS involves a nutritionally oriented history, physical examination, and laboratory parameters. The history should include documentation of weight loss, diminished oral intake, taste alteration and problems related to chewing and swallowing. Reports of diarrhea and its frequency should be noted. A decrease in weight in relation to either the ideal body weight or usual weight should be recorded.

The physical examination focuses on the loss of lean body mass (i.e., muscle mass) and fat stores. On occasion, evidence of vitamin deficiency may also be observed. Peripheral edema is often a manifestation of diminished circulating proteins and decreased colloid osmotic pressure. Laboratory analysis often reveals low total protein and albumin levels, as well as severely decreased serum cholesterol. Paradoxically, triglyceride levels are often elevated.

Nutritional Intervention in HIV Disease

An AIDS patient who cannot maintain adequate oral intake must be assisted. Aggressive attempts at hunger stimulation with such medications as cyproheptadine, megestrol acetate, and tetrahydrocannabinol should be attempted. Even inhaled or ingested cannabis is a reasonable approach in this life-threatening situation. Oral supplementation with calorically dense liquid nutrient mixtures may also be useful.

We have had some success in the use of anabolic agents for AIDS patients with early wasting. These agents, including human growth hormone and both oral and injectable androgens, have been shown to improve nutritional status by increasing lean body mass (46).

If such measures fail, nutritional support is indicated. Enteral feeding via a nasogastric, gastrostomy, or jejunostomy tube is preferred. However, if the patient has malabsorption syndrome, this may not be sufficient. Since many AIDS patients present with malabsorption, total parental nutrition (TPN) is a commonly applied modality in AIDS (47).

TPN formulas should be specifically designed for the patient's individual nutrient requirements as delineated by energy expenditure and nitrogen balance measurement (48). A permanent intravenous catheter (peripherally inserted central catheter [PICC] line, Hickman catheter, or Port-A-Cath) should be in position with the catheter tip confirmed in the superior vena cava.

TPN is associated with significant side effects and must be monitored closely by experienced personnel. Hyperglycemia, hyperlipi-

Table 11.3. Infectious Agents that Cause AIDS Enteropathy with Chronic Diarrhea

| | | | No. (%) of Patients from Whom Indicated Agent Was Isolated | | | | | | | | | |
Location	No. of Patients	Criteria for Inclusion	Crypto-megalovirus	Crypto-sporidia	Micro-sporidia	M. avium	I. belli	E. histolytica	G. lamblia	Salmonella Species	Others[a]	No Pathogen[b]
Bethesda, Maryland	20	Diarrhea >1 w, AIDS	9 (45)	3 (15)	No examination	1 (5)	0	5 (25)	3 (15)	5 (25)	3 (15)	3 (15)[c]
Baltimore	22	Diarrhea >1 mo, negative stool examination, AIDS	1 (5)	1 (5)[d]	5 (23)	5 (23)	0	0	1 (5)	0	0	11 (50)
Brazil	23	Diarrhea >2 w, AIDS	0	5 (22)	No examination	1 (4)	1 (4)	0	0	0	1 (4)	13 (57)[c]
New York City	43	Diarrhea >1 mo, AIDS, AIDS-related complex	15 (35)	6 (14)[e]	14 (33)[e]	7 (16)	0	0	1 (2)	1 (2)	2 (5)	6 (14)

From Bartlett JG, Belhsos PC, Sears CL. AIDS Enteropathy. Clin Infect Dis 1992;15:727.

[a]*Shigella* (1 patient), *C. jejuni* (1), *Strongyloides stercoralis* (1). One patient had Kaposi's sarcoma.

[b]Numbers do not all add up because two pathogens were occasionally isolated from patients.

[c]The data from these reports may be less comparable because of the brevity of diarrhea and the inclusion of patients with pathogens that are usually detected on analysis of stool samples, which include *Salmonella, Shigella, C. jejuni,* and cryptosporidia.

[d]According to a prior report by this group, 7 (16%) of 45 patients with AIDS and diarrhea were determined to have cryptosporidiosis on stool examination.

[e]Microsporidia or cryptosporidia were detected in 19 (70%) of 27 patients with small-bowel injry and in 17 (77%) of 22 on electron microscopy.

demia, and electrolyte imbalance are common problems in the management of home TPN in AIDS. Catheter-related complications such as infection, hemorrhage, and dislodgment must also be monitored. More detail on the use of home TPN can be found in Chapter 15.

Palliative Care

As with the terminal cancer patient (see Chapter 17), an end-stage AIDS patent can benefit significantly from homecare. The prospect of an early death in a young person who may have been very productive prior to the onset of AIDS requires special social and psychological support, which may be better provided in the comfort of the home. Alternative lifestyle practices are difficult for some healthcare workers to accept, and this creates stress for the patient in the hospital. Family members of patients with AIDS may need ex-tensive counseling, particularly at the end of a loved-one's life. They may also benefit from the ability to be present with the patient at home.

Palliative measures such as hydration, supplemental oxygen, pain management, and sedation have all been utilized in the management of AIDS care. When combined with psychosocial support they can offer the terminal patient both comfort and medical care in a relaxed, familiar, and non-judgmental environment.

Conclusion

Homecare plays a valuable role in the management of AIDS. Because of the need for lifetime intravenous therapy in many cases, it is a logical solution to the complex medical, financial, and social issues that involve comprehensive AIDS care.

References

1. Green J, Oppenheimer GM, Wintfeld N. The $147,000 misunderstanding: repercussions of overestimating the cost of AIDS. J Health Polit Policy Law 1994;19(1) 69–90.
2. Balinsky W. Home Care. San Francisco: Jossey-Bass, 1994:45.
3. First 500,000 AIDS cases—United States, 1995. MMWR 1995;44(46):849–853.
4. Update: AIDS among women—United States, 1994. MMWR 1995;44(5):81–85.
5. Greene WC. AIDS and the immune system. Sci Am 1993;269:99–105.
6. Saag MS, Hammer SM, Lange JM. Pathogenicity and diversity of HIV and implications for clinical management: a review. J Acquired Immune Defic Syndr 1994;7(Suppl 2):S2–S11.
7. Ho DD, Neumann AU, Perelson AS, Chen W, Leodnard JM. Rapid turnover of plasma virions and CD4 lymphocytes in HIV-1 infection. Nature 1995;373:123–126.
8. Semba RD, Caiaffa WT, Graham NM, Cohn S, Vlahov D. Vitamin A deficiency and wasting as predictors of mortality in human immunodeficiency virus-infected injection drug users. J Infect Dis 1995;17(5):1196–1202.
9. Piatak M Jr, Saag MS, Yang LC, et al. Determination of viral load in HIV-1 infection by quantitative competitive polymerase chain reaction. AIDS 1993;7(2):S65-S71.
10. Diamond G. Personal communication.
11. Janssen, et al. Theoretical efficiency of testing in US acute care hospitals. N Engl J Med 1992;327:449.
12. Kiecolt-Glaser JK, Marucha PT, et al. Slowing of wound healing by psychological stress. Lancet 1995; 346:1194–1196.
13. Pacquement H, Rosenblatt F, Renty MC, Quintana E, Zucker JM. Experience and questions about home care on children treated for cancer. Proceedings of the First World Congress on Home Care, Rome, Italy, 1989.
14. Greenbaum DM. Influence of the acquired immunodeficiency syndrome on resource availability in critical care medicine in the coming decade [Review]. New Horizons 1994;2(3):312–320.
15. Moons M, Kerkstra A, Biewenga T. Specialized home care for patients with AIDS: an experiment in Rotterdam, The Netherlands. J Adv Nurs 1994;19(6): 1132–1140.
16. Hellinger FJ. The lifetime cost of treating a person with HIV. JAMA 1993;270(4):474–478.
17. Epstein AM, Seage G 3rd, Weissman JS, et al. Costs of medical care and out-of-pocket expenditures for persons with AIDS in the Boston Health Study. Inquiry 1995;32(2):211–221.
18. Liekweg R, Dideriksen P, Adinolfi A, Bartlett JA. Outpatient treatment of AIDS: a viable alternative that demonstrates significant cost savings [Abstract No. M.H.P.10]. Int Conf AIDS 1989 Jun 4–9;5:1040.
19. Bergler R. Psychological situation of home care patients in the Federal Republic of Germany [in German]. Zentralbl Hyg Umweltmed 1993;194(1–2): 33–79.
20. Lockman-Samkowiak J. Care of patients with acquired immune deficiency syndrome in rural areas. Journal of Intravenous Nursing 1994;17(4):206–209.
21. Milanese G, Cancelli A, Andreoni M, et al. Home care for persons with AIDS: a 15 month experience in Rome (Italy) [Abstract No. PoD 5794]. Int Conf AIDS 1992 Jul 19–24;8(2):D521.
22. Rothkopf M, Udine L, Askanazi J, Rider D. Catheter sepsis in AIDS patients on HPN. 15th Clinical Congress, ASPEN, Jan-Feb 1991.

23. Settle JT, Neff-Smith M, Wan GJ. Infections related to venous access devices in patients with AIDS. Journal of the Association of Nurses in AIDS Care 1994;5(5) 43–47.

24. Poretz DM. Treatment of serious infections with cefotaxime utilizing an outpatient drug delivery device: global analysis of a large-scale, multicenter trial. Am J Med 1994;97:34–42.

25. Centers for Disease Control. Update: acquired immunodeficiency syndrome—United States 1986. MMWR 1986;35:757–766.

26. Broaddus C, Dake MD, Stulbarg MS, et al. Bronchoalveolar lavage and transbronchial biopsy for the diagnosis of pulmonary infections in the acquired immunodeficiency syndrome. Ann Intern Med 1985;102 (6):747–752.

27. Coleman DL, Hattner RS, Luce JM, et al. Correlation between gallium lung scans and fiberoptic bronchoscopy in patients with suspected *Pneumocystis carinii* pneumonia and the acquired immune deficiency syndrome. Am Rev Respir Dis 1984;130(6):1166–1169.

28. Kirsch CM, Jensen WA, Kagawa FT, Azzi RL. Analysis of induced sputum for the diagnosis of recurrent *Pneumocystis carinii* pneumonia. Chest 1992;102(4):1152–1154.

29. Fischl MA, Parker CB, Pettinelli C, et al. and the AIDS Clinical Trials Group. A randomized controlled trial of reduced daily dose of zidovudine in patients with the acquired immunodeficiency syndrome. N Engl J Med 1990;323:1010–1025.

30. Cytomegalovirus and AIDS. HIV Hotline 1996;6(1). [Published by Foundation for Care Management, 12233 112th Way NE, Suite E309, Kirkland, WA 98034]

31. Polsky B. Combination therapy for Relapsed CMV reactivation: the cytomegalovirus retinitis retreatment trial. O.I. Interaction 1996;3(1). [Published by Health Policy & Research Foundation, P.O. Box 691458, Los Angeles, CA 90068]

32. Jacobson MA. Current management of cytomegalovirus disease in patients with AIDS. AIDS Res Hum Retroviruses 1994;10:917–923.

33. Polis A, Desmet MD, Baird BD, et al. Increased survival of a cohort of patients with acquired immunodeficiency syndrome and cytomegalovirus retinitis who received sodium phosphonoformate (foscarnet). Am J Med 1993;94:175–180.

34. McCutchan JA. Cytomegalovirus infections of the nervous system in patients with AIDS. Clin Infect Dis 1995;20:747–754.

35. Dietrich DT, Kotler DP, Busch DF, et al. Ganciclovir treatment of cytomegalovirus colitis in AIDS: a randomized, double blind, placebo-controlled multicenter study. J Infect Dis 1993;167:273–282.

36. Fletcher CV. Treatment of herpes virus infections in HIV-infected individuals [Review]. Ann Pharmacother 1992;26(7–8):955–962.

37. Hardy WD. Foscarnet treatment of acyclovir-resistant herpes simplex virus infection in patients with acquired immunodeficiency syndrome: preliminary results of a controlled, randomized, regimen-comparative trial. Am J Med 1992; 92(2A):305–355.

38. Saag MS, Powederly, WG. Comparison of Ampho B with Fluconazole in the treatment of AIDS cryptococcal meningitis. N Engl J Med 1992;326(2):83–89.

39. Musher DM, Hamill RJ. Effect of HIV on the course of syphilis and response to treatment. Ann Intern Med 1990;113:872–881.

40. Dowell ME, Ross PG. Response of latent syphilis to ceftriaxone therapy in persons with HIV. Am J Med 1992;93:481–488.

41. deLalla F, Maserati R, Scarpellini P, et al. Clarithromycin-ciprofloxacin-amikacin for therapy of *Mycobacterium avium-Mycobacterium intracellulare* bacteremia in patients with AIDS. Antimicrob Agents Chemother 1992;36(7):1567–1569.

42. Fields Newman C. The role of nutritional assessments and nutritional plans in the management of HIV/AIDS. Nutrition and HIV/AIDS, Physicians' Association for AIDS Care 1992;1:57–106.

43. Bartlett JG, Belitros PC. AIDS enteropathy [Review]. Clin Infect Dis 1992;15(4)726–735.

44. Askanazi J, Singer P, Rothkopf M, Kvetan V, Bursztein S. Energy metabolism in AIDS patients receiving TPN. Am J Clin Nutr 1990;51:7–13.

45. Singer P, Rothkopf MM, Kvetan V, Gaare J, Mello L, Askanazi J. Nutrition, the gastrointestinal tract and the acquired immune deficiency syndrome. Facts and perspectives. Clin Nutr 1989;8:281–287.

46. Berger DS, Buscher G, Wittert H, et al. Effects of growth hormone on patients with AIDS Wasting. J Am Coll Nutr 1995;14(5):529.

47. Singer P, Rothkopf MM, Kvetan V, Kirvela O, Gaare J, Askanazi J. Risks and benefits of home parenteral nutrition in the acquired immunodeficiency syndrome. J Parenter Enteral Nutr 1991;15(1):75–79.

48. Rothkopf MM, Daire M, Haverstick LP. Nutritional and metabolic assessment of patients with AIDS wasting syndrome (AWS). Submitted.

12

USE OF INTRAVENOUS ANTIMICROBIALS AT HOME

Gail S. Rothkopf

CHAPTER AT A GLANCE: Home IV antimicrobial therapy has become an option in the treatment of an expanding range of infections, from the convalescent phase of acute osteomyelitis to maintenance therapy for cytomegalovirus (CMV) retinitis. Successful treatment at home requires careful selection of patients, an individualized therapeutic regimen, and strict observance of safety precautions. An experienced homecare team that functions well as a unit is basic to the achievement of therapeutic goals.

Antibiotics developed specifically for outpatient use are now available. Their increased safety, broad antimicrobial spectra, and once- or twice-daily dosing schedule are ideal for IV therapy at home. However, when the drug of choice is more toxic or less convenient, it may be possible to improve safety and simplify dosing. With an understanding of pharmacodynamics, standard dosing recommendations can sometimes be adapted for home use.

The limited choice of antiviral and antifungal agents requires the use of toxic drugs with serious side effects. However, experience has proved that when these drugs are used with caution, viral and fungal infections can also be safely and effectively treated at home.

Introduction

The use of intravenous (IV) therapy at home was nearly unheard of until the 1970s, when consumer and economic issues created pressure for home healthcare. Early experience showed that homecare was patient-oriented and clearly cost-effective, costing roughly two-thirds of hospital-based therapy (1). The initial resistance to outpatient care was related to lack of experience, including concerns about treatment failure, complications of early discharge, and fear of litigation. But as safety and efficacy data accumulated, these concerns subsided. To date, there have been no indications of increased problems, poorer outcomes, or higher rates of litigation associated with homecare therapies (2–8). In fact, not only has homecare become increasingly accepted by physicians and preferred by their patients, in many cases it has proved to be the most rational choice for treatment.

With careful selection of the homecare patient and thoughtful design of therapeutic regimen, outpatient IV therapy provides substantial benefits to the patient, to the healthcare system, and to society in general. Treating the infection at home results in calculable savings as compared to the hospital stay. Home therapy eliminates room charges, excessive monitoring, and overuse of medical technologies. Less easily quantifiable benefits include the freeing of limited hospital space and professional services for acutely ill patients, and the avoidance of nosocomial infections. In many cases, homecare enables the patient to resume his or her daily routine with little inconvenience. This allows the patient to continue activities such as education or employment and thus remain a productive member of society.

With recent advances in antibiotic safety and convenience, and the availability of portable, programmable IV infusion systems, the scope of home antimicrobial therapy has now expanded to include nearly all infectious diseases.

Patient Selection

Successful treatment at home requires careful decision-making not only in terms of therapeutic choices, but also in selection of patients. Home IV antimicrobial therapy has evolved to the point where technically, there is no disease or antimicrobial therapy that automatically excludes a patient from consideration for homecare. However, it is essential that the patient meet certain medical and nonmedical criteria, as listed in Table 12.1 and discussed below.

Indications for IV Therapy

When considering IV antimicrobial therapy at home, it is important to establish that IV administration is required. Alternative routes of administration, including intramuscular injection or the use of newly developed oral antibiotics (e.g., advanced cephalosporins, penicillins with β-lactamase inhibitors, or fluoroquinolones), may provide adequate coverage.

Oral therapies may not be appropriate in the acute phase of a life-threatening illness. However, they can be used later in the convalescent stage to reduce the length of IV therapy when long-term antimicrobial therapy is necessary. Whenever oral therapy is a sound option, it is the preferred modality because it avoids the potential complications of intramuscular injection, venipuncture, and indwelling catheters. In addition, oral therapies are much more convenient and less costly.

Although the use of new oral antibiotics can sometimes eliminate the need for IV therapy, there remain clinical situations in which IV therapy is clearly indicated:

- when the patient has failed to respond to oral therapy;
- when there exists no oral agent that is biologically and therapeutically equivalent to parenteral therapy (e.g., vancomycin, aminoglycosides, amphotericin B and ganciclovir);
- when the patient cannot reliably absorb antimicrobials from the gastrointestinal tract due to conditions such as vomiting, diarrhea, malabsorption, or gastroparesis; or
- when an increased risk of inadequate coverage is not acceptable. The elevated tissue levels essential to the resolution of serious infection may be difficult to achieve dependably with oral administration of antimicrobials.

Table 12.1. Patient Selection Criteria for Home IV Antimicrobial Therapy

- Intravenous delivery is required.
- Patient is medically stable.
- Reliable venous access can be achieved.
- Patient has the physical, psychological, intellectual, and financial resources necessary for homecare.
- Home environment is suitable.

Medical Stability

It is not the type of infection that limits patient selection for home care, but rather the overall medical condition. It is of paramount importance that the patient be medically stable. Furthermore, the pathogenesis of the infection should be understood, and a definite therapeutic response should be documented.

Complicating factors such as deficiencies of the immune system and underlying predisposing medical conditions (e.g., diabetes) must be considered in the decision to treat the patient at home. It is essential that such coexisting medical conditions also be under control before the patient is released to homecare, where monitoring practices will be less rigorous. For some infections, notably endocarditis, the possibility of late suppurative or immunologic sequelae must factor into the decision to administer IV antimicrobial therapy at home. In cases where there are possible serious sequelae of the disease or treatment, a live-in caretaker or companion is an absolute requirement.

The determination of medical stability is the responsibility of the physician and should be based on objective clinical and laboratory criteria. Spiking fevers or chills, or other manifestations of serious infection such as organ failure, should be absent. Laboratory values for leukocyte counts and sedimentation rate should be within normal limits. There must be no need for daily or more frequent monitoring by a physician.

Reliable Venous Access

Another medical criterion for referral to homecare is the ability to achieve reliable venous access, peripheral or central. Repeated failures of venous access can complicate therapy and compromise safety, thereby excluding the patient from consideration for homecare.

Types of venous access and various delivery system models are discussed in Chapter 10.

Patient Acceptance and Abilities

A key issue in homecare is the willingness of the patient to actively participate in his or her medical care. If the patient does not wish to receive treatment at home, the outcome of home therapy is doubtful. The patient and family must have the ability to understand the responsibilities and risks of home IV antimicrobial therapy. After receiving full disclosure of costs, responsibilities, and possible complications, the patient must put his or her acceptance of home IV therapy in writing. And the patient, with a caregiver if necessary, must be able to manage the routine psychologically, physically, and intellectually.

Any previous experience the patient has had with IV therapy is helpful, making the routine of aseptic technique, drug administration, and catheter care easier to understand and implement.

A certain amount of mobility and dexterity is required for the patient to be able to take mixed solutions from storage areas, attach them to the IV tubing, flush the tubing, and then attach it to an IV catheter. Depending on the antimicrobial drug prescribed, the patient may also have to set up a programmable infusion pump, which will monitor the drug administration. Neurological, ophthalmological, and rheumatological limitations can make compliance difficult.

Homecare patients require a certain level of intelligence and literacy. They must have the ability to learn how to administer the therapy, to use aseptic technique, and to perform self-monitoring at home. It is vital that the patient be able to communicate quickly and clearly to the medical staff any changes in medical status or other problems.

In addition, the patient must be able to handle homecare financially. The costs to the patient treated at home must be carefully detailed to the person responsible for payment, because reimbursement for home IV antimicrobial therapy is erratic. Problems with reimbursement are being resolved as the safety, cost-effectiveness, and other benefits of this therapy become more widely recognized.

Home Environment

The home environment should be sanitary, be conducive to the performance of aseptic technique, and have adequate refrigerated storage for infusion materials and supplies. Access to a telephone for communications in an emergency and between medical visits is essential. In addition, the patient's home must be located within a reasonable distance to an emergency room and within the service area of a qualified homecare organization. Transportation must be available from the patient's home to the physician's office or monitoring facility as well as to the emergency room.

The Homecare Team

Intravenous antimicrobial therapy at home, as in the hospital, involves the physician and a team of healthcare professionals. The physician, nurse, and pharmacist work together for successful treatment of the infection, but in an outpatient setting their roles have undergone some redefinition. Team members no longer perform their roles in a single location, and consequently communication among the healthcare team members is more difficult. Homecare team members are more autonomous and have increased responsibilities, many of which overlap. The success of home therapy, even more than in the hospital, depends on the quality of team member interactions. Roles must be clearly defined and lines of communication well established.

Homecare Patient

The role of the patient changes most significantly in homecare, from a passive recipient of medical care in the hospital to an active participant in his or her own treatment. Responsibilities can include drug administration, daily monitoring, record keeping, and communication of medical status to other team members. Self-monitoring may include recording and evaluating pulse and temperature charts, and the ability to recognize manifestations of clinical illness (e.g., fever, chills, rigor, productive cough, inflammation), as well as signs of adverse reactions to medications. It is the role of other team members to prepare the patient for this role by providing training, support, and supervision. Because the patient is expected to take an active role in homecare, he or she should participate in decision making regarding therapy.

Primary Physician

The primary physician maintains a leadership role in homecare. The physician establishes the diagnosis, prescribes antimicrobial therapy, and performs the initial evaluation of the patient for homecare. Additional responsibilities include development of the treatment protocol, including the monitoring schedule, and adjustment of the therapeutic plan as necessary. Any changes in patient status or prescription must be communicated to the rest of the homecare team.

Ultimately, it is the physician who is responsible for the outcome of the antimicrobial therapy he or she prescribes. For this reason, it is important that the physician maintain control of patient care, beginning with the choice of homecare organization. The physician must evaluate such organizations with special attention to experience and prior results with IV antimicrobial therapy specifically. Even when members of the homecare team are employees of the homecare organization, the physician should have a role in directing their efforts. Office visits by the patient, nursing visits to the patient's home, and laboratory testing should be scheduled frequently enough that the prescribing physician remains fully aware of his or her patient's progress.

Homecare Organization

The complex task of providing healthcare personnel, prescription medications, and infusion equipment and supplies to the patient at home usually requires the involvement of a homecare organization. The homecare organization employs nurses and pharmacists specifically trained in outpatient IV therapy. It can prepare the prescription and coordinate the homecare staff and delivery of the drugs, infusion fluids, supplies, and equipment.

Homecare Nurse

The homecare nurse has the most frequent direct contact with the patient and therefore occupies a central role in homecare. Between patient office visits, the physician often has to rely on the nurse's clinical skills and judgment.

Nursing duties usually begin with a more detailed evaluation of the patient referred for home IV antimicrobial therapy. The nurse assesses the patient's psychosocial as well as physical environment at home, and begins training the patient for self-administered therapy. It is the nurse who certifies the patient's skills in sterile technique, line flushing, disposal of needles, and proper handling of infusion solutions and equipment. The nurse also certifies that the patient can recognize early signs of complications (e.g., phlebitis and fever) and adverse reactions to medications, and understands the importance of adequate record keeping. The nurse is often responsible for establishment of IV access.

The homecare nurse monitors the patient at home, noting clinical response, examining for signs of complications, and collecting specimens for laboratory analysis as necessary. He or she verifies compliance with therapy and the accuracy of communications to team members by the patient. Generally, a nurse is available to the patient by telephone 24 hours a day for technical and psychological support.

With such broad responsibilities, it is essential that the nurse be experienced in homecare, with certified abilities in all aspects of IV antimicrobial therapy.

Homecare Pharmacist

A valuable resource to the physician in the choice of antimicrobial agents and therapeutic regimens for home therapy is the homecare pharmacist. He or she can help to evaluate drugs, adapt therapies, and develop adequate monitoring schedules from the homecare perspective.

The pharmacist's expertise is also called upon to prevent adverse consequences of antimicrobial therapy. Responsibilities include the review of all patients' medications and screening of prescribed therapies for possible interactions or incompatibilities. Often the pharmacist as well as the physician monitors the patient's therapeutic progress by tracking laboratory values. Any changes detected in patient status are discussed with the physician.

For more information on the homecare team and evaluation of homecare organizations, see Chapters 5 and 6.

Antibiotic Selection

The considerations in antibiotic selection for outpatient use are the same as those applied in the hospital: efficacy, safety, convenience, and cost-effectiveness. However, emphasis is shifted when treatment occurs in an outpatient setting. At home there is less medical supervision and therapy is often administered by the patient or caregiver, who has less experience and training than hospital personnel. It follows that safety and convenience take on added significance and that cost analysis differs outside the hospital.

Antibiotics used for home therapy are often the same as those used for inpatient IV therapy. However, certain antibiotic regimens used in hospitals are difficult to comply with at home. For such cases, guidelines exist for the selection of alternative or adapted therapies. Therapeutic protocols for home IV antibiotic patients are even more individualized than for inpatients, because monitoring techniques, staffing, and environment are not as uniform as in the hospital.

The selection of antifungal and antiviral drugs is not specifically addressed in this section because choices are so limited in these categories. However, the principles involved in the selection of antibiotics apply to the selection of other anti-infective agents for homecare use.

Efficacy

The effectiveness of the antibiotic chosen is fundamentally important in avoiding complications of inadequate treatment. Ideally, pathogens should be isolated and identified, and antibiotic selection should be based on sensitivity testing. The choice of an antibiotic should also take into account the specific patient, the site of infection, and patterns of resistance in the geographic area.

When specific therapy is not possible, the same criteria for use of empiric therapy in the hospital apply to home therapy: the pathogen cannot be isolated, therapy must be started before sensitivity data is available, or a microbiologically complex infection requires expanded coverage.

Empiric therapy is based on the site of infection and the most likely pathogens. The patient's age should also be taken into account, since for some infections the assumed pathogens differ between pediatric patients and adults. Antibiotics are chosen for the appropriate antimicrobial spectrum and pattern of tissue penetration.

Antibiotic efficacy should be judged as it is in the hospital, by a favorable clinical response and laboratory evidence of resolution of the infection. Effective therapy is evidenced by patient temperature and laboratory values returning to normal, resolution of clinical signs of infection, and negative follow-up cultures.

Safety

In choosing an antibiotic for home IV therapy, the safety factor is paramount. To the greatest extent possible, potential problems with therapy must be identified and prevented. Complications resulting from therapy may be discovered later with less medical supervision, and consequently they may become more severe before treatment. Table 12.2 lists recommended precautions for home IV antibiotic therapy.

Toxic drugs should be avoided whenever possible, since frequent monitoring of serum levels or renal function is difficult at home. If peripheral delivery is planned, the parenteral antibiotic selected must be nonirritating to veins. The patient should be observed for possible side effects of therapy, both early and late.

A careful drug history is mandatory, especially for the elderly or complex patient. This information is necessary to help predict allergic reactions and to prevent problems caused by potential drug-drug interactions. Examples include the increased ototoxicity and nephrotoxicity that results from the concomitant administration of aminoglycosides and vancomycin, or aminoglycosides and diuretics, especially furosemide. The possibility of drug-food interactions should also be considered. Previous antimicrobial therapy should be noted, not only for reports of adverse reactions but also to alert the physician that the patient may harbor pathogens resistant to previously prescribed antibiotics.

The effects of the patient's age, intercurrent illnesses, and pregnancy on metabolism and excretion of the antibiotic must be recognized. Pediatric patients may show different drug distribution patterns and effective serum levels when compared to adults, and the duration of therapy may have to be altered. Very young patients usually require more frequent follow-up examinations. In elderly patients, impaired clearance of the drug could lead to toxic levels of an otherwise safe agent.

Congestive heart failure, renal insufficiency, liver disease, and malnutrition are conditions that may affect normal distribution of the antibiotic. In these illnesses, the circulation is often abnormal and can result in less than optimal delivery of the drug if standard dosages are used. Furthermore, if the patient has an abnormal serum albumin, and the antibiotic in use is extensively bound to albumin, the delivered dosage may vary significantly from what is expected. Under these circumstances, it may be necessary to do detailed pharmacokinetic studies in order to find the correct dosage. These studies are generally best performed in a hospital setting or in the physician's office, but they can be done at home if there is a trained homecare nurse available to draw drug levels at appropriate dosages and time intervals.

Prescribing physicians should also be aware of serious adverse reactions peculiar to the infection or antibiotic; for example, the Jarisch-Herxheimer reaction seen in Lyme disease and some other spirochetal infections, and the "red neck" or "red man syndrome" seen with vancomycin therapy.

Table 12.2. Safety Precautions in Home IV Antibiotic Therapy

- Avoid use of toxic drugs whenever possible. Be aware of potential adverse reactions of drugs prescribed.
- Compile a careful drug history to identify possible drug-drug interactions and to avoid predictable allergic reactions.
- Examine medical history for intercurrent illness or conditions that may affect antibiotic therapy.
- Administer first dose of antibiotic under physician supervision.
- Enforce adequate clinical and laboratory monitoring schedule.

An important precaution is the administration of the first dose of the antibiotic under medical supervision to ensure that the drug is well tolerated. A particular concern when an antibiotic is infused for the first time is the possibility of a serious anaphylactic response, especially with penicillins and β-lactam derivatives. If the patient is in the hospital, the first dose of the antibiotic can be given prior to discharge to home therapy. However, hospitalization is not necessary if the home IV therapy is prescribed for an outpatient. Approximately 50% of home IV antibiotic patients receive the initial dose in physician offices, emergency rooms, or other outpatient settings (6). Physician supervision of the first administration of the drug may not be necessary when the patient has previously been treated with the same antibiotic without any serious adverse reactions.

Convenience

Convenience is a more significant factor in homecare than in the hospital. It facilitates compliance with the prescribed therapy and expands the range of patients who can qualify for home therapy. Increased convenience results in greater safety, since there is less opportunity for error.

The most convenient antibiotic regimen employs an infrequent dosage schedule (i.e., once or twice a day) and a simple infusion system. Whenever possible, monotherapy should be used. Treatment with a single antibiotic is easier to prepare and administer and reduces the list of potential adverse effects. However, recent advances in IV pump technology have made multiple drug therapy at home practical when it is necessary to use more than one antibiotic.

Cost-Effectiveness

Cost of the antibiotic per se is a less significant factor in antibiotic selection for homecare than for inpatient use. The choice of antibiotic determines which IV delivery system can be used, and the frequency of clinical and laboratory monitoring that is required. Sometimes the increased cost of preparation, infusion, and monitoring of a less expensive antibiotic will offset any initial savings. For example, an inexpensive drug such as penicillin may be appropriate treatment for a given infection, but it may actually be a poor choice from the cost containment perspective. Penicillin has a short half-life and must be administered frequently or by continuous infusion. Consequently, pharmacy and supply costs are higher. Also contributing to the cost of penicillin therapy is the possible need for frequent laboratory monitoring of serum penicillin levels to confirm proper dosage. Use of a more expensive drug in this case may reduce the cost of therapy by eliminating the need for frequent dosing and monitoring.

Not directly calculable are savings related to scheduling and compliance. Infrequent dosing may allow a patient to maintain a normal work or school schedule, preventing financial loss to the patient. An inconvenient antibiotic regimen may lead to missed doses, which can result in the need for a longer course of therapy, or even failure of the treatment.

Dosage Management

The optimal dosing schedule for homecare patients results in safe and effective antimicrobial drug levels with the longest possible dosing interval. When prescribing antimicrobials for home IV therapy, improvements in safety, efficacy, and convenience can sometimes be achieved with manipulation of standard dosing recommendations. These alterations require an understanding of the pharmacokinetics and pharmacodynamics of antimicrobial agents.

Specific therapeutic recommendations are not within the scope of this chapter. The information provided here is intended only as a guide for the use of reference sources in the context of home therapy. Several excellent resources compiling information useful for antibiotic selection and dosage management exist. Among these are *The Sanford Guide to Antimicrobial Therapy, Facts and Comparisons,* and general textbooks of infectious diseases and pharmacology.

Pharmacodynamic and Pharmacokinetic Factors

Antimicrobial pharmacodynamics and pharmacokinetics define the range of therapeutic alterations that can be made without compromising safety or efficacy. Among the factors to consider are minimal inhibitory concentration, persistent postantibiotic effects, half-life, protein binding, and stability at room temperature.

Because extrapolation of antimicrobic effects from pharmacological data is not an entirely reliable prediction of effects in vivo, it is essential to monitor the effects of any changes in the antibiotic prescription. An infectious disease consultation is recommended for all but the least complicated infections.

MINIMAL INHIBITORY CONCENTRATION. Minimal inhibitory concentration (MIC) is the minimal serum concentration of the antimicrobial agent necessary to inhibit microbial growth. An antibiotic with an easily achievable MIC requires a lower, and therefore safer, dose from the standpoint of minimizing toxicity and adverse side effects. A related property is minimal bactericidal concentration (MBC), below which bacterial cells are not killed. It is necessary to maintain MBC in patients with neutropenia or critical infections such as endocarditis, meningitis, and osteomyelitis. Laboratory measurements of serum concentrations of the antibiotic (MIC or MBC) are necessary in serious infections or medically complex patients to confirm proper dosage.

PERSISTENT POSTANTIBIOTIC EFFECTS. Persistent postantibiotic effects (PAE's) inhibit bacterial growth beyond the period of antibiotic exposure. These residual effects can prolong antimicrobial activity when the drug levels drop below MIC. Typically, PAEs are the result of the disruption of protein or nucleic acic synthesis. The presence and persistence of PAEs are functions of the specific antibiotic and the targeted microorganism. When PAEs are present, a longer interval between does is possible.

HALF-LIFE. Biological half-life ($t_{1/2}$) is the time in which serum concentration is reduced by half. It is determined by rates of clearance from serum by metabolism and excretion of the antibiotic. A longer half-life is desirable because it requires less frequent administration and a lower dose than a drug with a short half-life.

PROTEIN BINDING. Protein binding refers to the reversible binding of antibiotic molecules to serum or tissue proteins, usually albumin. Only free drug is antimicrobially active. Therefore, if a drug is appreciably bound by serum proteins, protein binding must be taken into account when calculating total serum concentration from laboratory values of active concentration. Depending on how it is excreted, protein binding may hasten or delay clearance of the antibiotic. Protein binding is also a major dterminant of distribution of the drug beyond the circulation.

STABILITY. The stability of an antibiotic at room temperature limits how the drug can be administered and stored. High stability (greater than 12 hours) is required for continuous infusion. Less stable drugs must be administered by intermittent infusion. The stability of antibiotics at room temperature varies considerably, from less than 4 hours (imipenem) to several days (ceftriaxone) (9).

Antibacterial Agents

Antibiotics commonly prescribed for home IV therapy can be placed in one of three categories for discussion of dosage regimens. These categories are distinguished by their pharmacodynamic profiles as shown in Table 12.3, and described by Craig (9, 10).

Penicillins and Cephalosporins

Maximizing the time that serum concentrations remain above MIC is the most important parameter in determining the efficacy of these β-lactam antibiotics. When serum levels of these cell wall synthesis inhibitors fall below MIC, damaged bacterial cells are able to recover because β-lactams produce short or no PAEs. This lack of PAEs is a major distinction between this category of antibiotics and the two other categories of antibiotics described below. Persistent antibiotic effects

Table 12.3. Effects of Antibiotic Pharmacodynamics on Dosing Regimens

Antibiotic Category	Pharmacodynamics	Dosing Regimen
Penicillins Cephalosporins	Bactericidal at minimal concentration; short or no PAE	Maximize exposure time; keep serum levels above MIC
Carbapenems Vancomycin Macrolides	Bactericidal at minimal concentration; prolonged PAE	Maximize exposure time; serum levels may be allowed to drop below MIC
Aminoglycosides Quinolones Metronidazole	Bactericidal at high concentration; prolonged PAE	Maximize concentration; attain peak serum levels and area under the curve

Adapted from Craig WA. Selecting the antibiotic. In: Tice AD, ed. Outpatient parenteral antibiotic therapy: management of serious infections. Part 1: medical, socioeconomic, and legal issues. Hosp Pract 1993;28(Suppl 1):17.
PAE, Postantibiotic effect; MIC, Minimal inhibitory concentration.

are important to prolonging bacterial growth inhibition, especially against Gram-negative organisms. Consequently, penicillins and cephalosporins are more dependent on concentration for effectiveness than the other two antibiotic groups that do produce significant PAEs.

Since maintenance of adequate serum levels is essential to effective therapy with these β-lactams, minimal bactericidal concentration must be measured when treating critical infections such as osteomyelitis and endocarditis with these antibiotics.

In animal models, doses of these antibiotics are maximally effective at about four times MIC. Higher doses do not increase the rate or quality of antimicrobial activity (9, 11–14) but can unnecessarily increase the probability of adverse side effects.

β-Lactams are the most widely prescribed agents for home intravenous therapy, particularly the more recently developed cephalosporins. In hospital practice, these newer antibiotics are rarely the drug of choice for established infections. In this case, a less expensive drug with a narrower spectrum is preferred. However, with long half-lives, adequate stability at room temperature, low MICs, impressive antimicrobial spectra, and increased safety over older drugs, the new cephalosporins are well suited for home intravenous antibiotic therapy. They are especially

useful in the treatment of more serious or complex infections.

Two commonly prescribed cephalosporins for home IV therapy are ceftriaxone and ceftazidime. Ceftriaxone is often used for infections caused by *Borrelia burgdorferi,* multiply resistant Gram-negative bacteria, and viridans streptococci. Its low toxicity and once-daily dosing are ideal for home administration (15).

Ceftazidime is very active against *Pseudomonas aeruginosa,* making it important in the treatment of pulmonary infections in cystic fibrosis patients. Its 8-hour dosing interval, low toxicity, and good tissue penetration are all reasons to choose this antibiotic over the less stable imipenems and more toxic aminoglycosides.

Cefazolin offers an alternative therapy to penicillin for highly susceptible staphylococci when low toxicity and infrequent dosing are important, with the notable exception of central nervous system (CNS) infections.

Cefotaxime (interchangeable with ceftizoxime) is resistant to most β-lactamases. Its safety and utility in treating a broad range of infections in outpatient IV antibiotic therapy are outlined in a series of articles edited by Poretz (16) and are also described by Todd (17).

The usefulness of the original β-lactam, penicillin, in home IV antibiotic therapy is limited by its short half-life. However, its proven efficacy in the treatment of certain infections, its more specific antibiotic spectrum, and its low cost have been the rationale behind its prescription in homecare.

Current thought regarding administration of β-lactam antibiotics is that it is best to limit dosage to the minimum required for effective treatment. Hypersensitivity and toxic side effects such as interstitial nephritis and bone marrow suppression seem to be related to high concentration. Also, there is some evidence of decreased incidence of adverse reactions when fresh antibiotic preparations are used, suggesting that such reactions may be mediated by β-lactam breakdown products.

Carbapenems, Vancomycin, and the Macrolides

As within the first category discussed, adequate exposure time to the minimal concentration is important to bactericidal activity, but for this second category of antibiotics it is not critical that concentration remains above MIC for the entire interval between doses. The inhibitory effects of carbapenems, vancomycin, and the macrolide antibiotics are enhanced below the MIC by persistent PAEs.

The carbapenems may induce PAEs for several hours against Gram-negative bacteria. These advanced β-lactamase–resistant antibiotics are an exception to the generally weak or absent PAEs of β-lactams as noted in the first group. Imipenem, for example, maintains maximum effectiveness even when the antibiotic concentration is above MIC only 50% of the time between doses in animal studies (12). This is why a dosing interval of 6 to 8 hours can be adequate, even though the drug is unstable. Imipenem formulations include cilastatin to inhibit rapid renal hydrolysis of this antibiotic, which would otherwise decrease its usefulness. This expensive and extremely broad-spectrum antibiotic is generally reserved for use against *Pseudomonas* infections.

Vancomycin, a tricyclic glycopeptide, is possibly the most frequently prescribed antibiotic for intravenous therapy at home. It is the current drug of choice for Gram-positive infections in patients with β-lactam hypersensitivity. Vancomycin is also routinely used for treatment of infections caused by methicillin-resistant *Staphylococcus aureus* (MRSA), non-aureus β-lactam–resistant staphylococci, and enterococcus. These organisms are often implicated in infections that require long-term therapy: infections that are frequently treated at home after the acute phase of the illness. Examples include prosthetic device–associated bacteremia, peritonitis associated with continuous ambulatory peritoneal dialysis (CAPD), and multiply resistant Gram-positive infections in patients with neoplasia or on chronic hemodialysis.

Advantages of vancomycin therapy are its once- or twice-daily dosing, low MIC, high chemical stability in nonalkaline solutions, and low incidence of resistance. This drug also has the important advantage in long-term therapy of a narrow spectrum of antimicrobial activity, limited to Gram-positive cocci and bacilli.

In the past, vancomycin use has been avoided because of its association with "red neck (or red man) syndrome," vein irritation and nephrotoxicity. However, recent studies have proved vancomycin therapy to be relatively safe (18, 19). The erythematous flushing, pruritus, and hypotension of "red neck syndrome" are nonimmunologic reactions that can be avoided by infusing the antibiotic solution slowly (20). Ideally, a rate-controlling intravenous infusion device should be used, delivering no greater than 15 mg/kg per minute. This infusion technique also minimizes the chemical thrombophlebitis associated with vancomycin, although vein irritation is much less common with more highly purified vancomycin preparations available today (19, 20). The toxicity that may otherwise limit the use of vancomycin is minimized when peak and trough levels are kept within the currently recommended ranges. The dosage resulting in the safest and most effective vancomycin therapy can be estimated by using nomogram calculations. However, it is essential to confirm peak and trough serum levels directly, at least once weekly.

Also included among antibiotics with significant PAEs are the macrolides. However, because therapeutic levels of macrolide antibiotics (e.g., erythromycin) can easily be attained by oral administration, intravenous therapy with these drugs is usually limited to patients in whom oral administration in contraindicated.

Aminoglycosides, Quinolones, and Metronidazole

In contrast to the preceding two groups, the goal of dosing schedules in this category is to achieve high peak serum levels. High concentrations of these antibiotics have been demonstrated to kill faster and more extensively than low concentrations in animal models (9, 11–14, 21).

These antibiotics are inhibitors of protein and nucleic acid synthesis or processing, and consequently produce prolonged PAEs with susceptible Gram-negative bacteria and streptococci. Infrequent dosing is possible because PAEs prevent bacterial proliferation when drug levels drop below the MIC. In fact, for aminoglycosides, dosing intervals of less than 6 to 8 hours are counterproductive. This is due to the "first exposure effect," by which the uptake of drug by bacterial cells is downregulated for 6 to 8 hours after the first dose (22).

Aminoglycosides, included in this category, are not well suited for outpatient therapy. The associated ototoxicity and nephrotoxicity require close monitoring of serum drug levels, as well as renal and auditory functions. Aminoglycosides (e.g., amikacin, gentamicin, tobramycin) are reserved for severe infections by Gram-negative bacteria with multiple resistance. They are sometimes required for synergistic actions in enterococcal endocarditis and *Pseudomonas* pulmonary infections.

Administration of a single, high daily dose of aminoglycoside is considered optimal by some (23). The high peak levels necessary for maximum antimicrobial activity can be reliably attained with this regimen, and the time that the patient is exposed to elevated, more toxic levels is limited. Using infrequent high doses is advantageous because renal and auditory binding sites for aminoglycosides are saturated above 8 to 10 mg/L. Consequently, no more aminoglycoside is taken up by these

tissues at higher antibiotic levels. Another benefit of once-daily dosing is that the selection of resistant strains is less likely.

Regardless of dosing schedule, safe use of aminoglycosides requires direct measurement and monitoring of peak and trough levels of serum aminoglycoside concentration within 24 hours of initial dose, at least once a week during treatment, and after every dosage adjustment (21). Serum creatinine levels should be checked two to three times a week during the initial phase of therapy if it is stable (more frequently if it is changing).

Quinolones are bactericidal for a broad spectrum of Gram-positive and Gram-negative bacteria. They have significant PAEs and a long serum half-life, allowing once- or twice-daily dosing. These antibiotics, like aminoglycosides, show concentration-dependent activity. But in contrast to the aminoglycosides, quinolones are well suited for home administration because they have a low incidence of adverse reactions. Ciprofloxacin, a potent new 4-quinolone, has unusually good tissue penetration and an easily attainable therapeutic serum concentration. However, its high cost limits its usefulness.

Metronidazole, a nitroimidazole compound, is particularly useful in the treatment of infections due to anaerobic organisms. Its long half-life allows infrequent dosing. Side effects (peripheral neuropathy and seizures) are rare and may be dose-related. Metronidazole may by administered orally or parenterally.

Antifungal and Antiviral Agents

With increasing numbers of immunosuppressed AIDS and transplant patients, the need for treatment of mycological and viral infections is increasing. Many of these opportunistic infections require long-term or even life-long treatment.

Selecting an antiviral or antifungal agent is uncomplicated compared to selecting an antibacterial agent because there are so few choices. But since an accepted method of determining inhibitory concentrations is lacking, and there are serious potential toxicities and side effects, these therapies can be difficult to manage, especially outside the hospital. Due to the potential for serious side effects when using these drugs, extreme care must be exercised when selecting the patient and home-care staff. Nonetheless, experience shows that home therapy can be successful when the patient is medically stable and psychologically motivated and when the home environment facilitates conscientious compliance with the protocol (24–26).

Antifungals: Amphotericin B and Fluconazole

Serious fungal infections such as aspergillosis, candidiasis, and cryptococcosis generally require intravenous antifungal therapy. Two such agents are available: amphotericin B and fluconazole. Although fluconazole is a less toxic agent, amphotericin B remains the drug of choice for most serious fungal infections. Fluconazole is currently FDA approved only for candidiasis and cryptococcal meningitis.

Intravenous amphotericin B is lipid soluble and a vein irritant. When this agent is administered via peripheral catheter, it must be diluted and infused slowly to minimize phlebitis and other adverse reactions. A test dose is required to observe for reactions, which develop in 50% of patients. These include rigor, chills, fever, hypotension, and electrolyte disturbances.

Pretreatment with anti-inflammatory agents such as acetaminophen and hydrocortisone, as well as the narcotic meperidine, may block some of these reactions. Ibuprofen and dantrolene have also been used as amphotericin B pretreatment medications.

Amphotericin B should be diluted in 5% dextrose in water (not electrolyte-containing solutions) at a concentration of 0.1 mg/mL. Some clinicians have reported benefits from mixing amphotericin B in Intralipid or other lipid emulsions, which are now available premixed. This allows a higher concentration (1 to 2 mg/mL of lipid emulsion) and may reduce infusion-related side effects.

For the first 4 hours following the initial dose, blood pressure must be monitored every 15 minutes. During the remaining course of therapy, patients on amphotericin B must be monitored for renal toxicity, hypokalemia, and hypomagnesemia. The serum half-life of this drug is about 24 hours, allowing dosage intervals to be as long as 3 or 4 days. The dosage and length of therapy depend on the type of infection, the phase of treatment, and the patient's tolerance of the medication.

Although amphotericin B is still labeled as being "for hospital use only," it is commonly used in outpatient therapy. Experience has proved that use of these agents outside the hospital is safe and effective when done with caution (25–27).

Fluconazole is a water-soluble antifungal agent that is effective when administered either orally or intravenously. Its intravenous use is generally reserved for the most severe candidal infections or for cases when the oral route is not possible. It has a long half-life (22 hours), making infrequent dosing practical.

Fluconazole has a side effects profile that is much less onerous than amphotericin B. Gastrointestinal, hepatic, and epidermal toxicities have been reported, as has headache. Serious toxic reactions are rare, but drug-drug interactions are common. The usefulness of this drug is limited by the fact that it is fungistatic at therapeutic concentrations. Optimal therapy of fungal infections requires fungicidal activity when these infections occur in immunocompromised patients.

Antivirals: Acyclovir, Ganciclovir, and Foscarnet

Patients with defective immune systems are also more susceptible to serious viral infections. Since antiviral agents are not curative, these infections generally require long-term or even life-long maintenance therapy. This means that IV antiviral agents are frequently administered on an outpatient basis, since this mode of therapy has several major advantages over inpatient treatment. It is much more economical, it avoids the possibility of nosocomial infection, and the patient can better approximate a normal lifestyle. Three intravenous antiviral agents are in common use: acyclovir, ganciclovir, and foscarnet. The adult dosage of these agents varies according to diagnosis and treatment stage. In the induction phase of therapy, the dosage is two to three times daily.

Intravenous acyclovir is used for severe primary herpes simplex virus (HSV) and disseminated varicella-zoster virus (VSV) infections. It is ineffective in the treatment of cytomegalovirus (CMV) infections. This antiviral drug is a caustic agent that must be administered through a central venous line. It is associated with renal, neurological, and hepatic toxicities. The major risk of IV administration is renal failure caused by accumulation of crystalline drug in the kidney. The initial dosing schedule is one to three times daily, depending on renal function.

Ganciclovir, which has become the drug of choice for CMV infections, is also quite toxic. It is administered intravenously for retinitis or serious infections, such as CMV colitis in AIDS patients. Granulocytopenia, thrombocytopenia, and anemia are its most prominent adverse reactions. Drug-drug interactions with ganciclovir are common. For example, serious adverse effects may occur when ganciclovir is administered to patients receiving probenecid, pentamidine, trimethoprim-sulfamethoxazole, amphotericin B, zidovudine (AZT), or imipenem. Because ganciclovir may be teratogenic or carcinogenic, use of gloves and safety glasses is recommended when handling this drug.

Foscarnet, the newest intravenous antiviral agent, is generally reserved for use in ganciclovir-resistant CMV infections. However, some clinicians consider it the drug of choice for CMV retinitis. Adverse reactions are common, including nephrotoxicity and neurological effects. Foscarnet provides alternate therapy for CMV retinitis in patients who cannot tolerate ganciclovir, and for acyclovir-resistant HSV and VSV.

Laboratory Monitoring for Antimicrobial Toxicity

Once antimicrobial therapy is initiated, the continued safety and efficacy of the treatment must be confirmed by laboratory analysis. Most antibiotic therapies can be adequately monitored with weekly testing. Examples of standard monitoring schedules for toxic effects are offered in Table 12.4. Complete blood count (CBC) and differential are used to monitor hematological effects of therapy. Serum chemistry analysis is performed to obtain information on electrolyte balance and hepatic and renal function: liver enzymes, serum albumin, blood urea nitrogen, and serum creatinine. For the individual patient, the types of analyses and the frequency of testing that are appropriate depend on the antimicrobial agent prescribed, diagnosis, medical status, and response to therapy. Laboratory monitoring may be limited to every 2 weeks in a stable patient during the convalescent stage of therapy with a drug of low toxicity. A diabetic patient in the initial phase of therapy with a potentially toxic drug could require testing every 3 to 4 days.

Table 12.4. Suggested Laboratory Monitoring for Antimicrobial Toxicity

| | *Laboratory Analyses* | | |
| | | *Serum Levels* | |
Antimicrobial Agent	*CBC and Differential*	*Serum Chemistry*	*(Peak and Trough)*
β-Lactams	Weekly	Weekly	
Acyclovir	Weekly	Weekly	
Vancomycin	Weekly	Twice weekly	Weekly[a]
Aminoglycosides	Weekly	Twice weekly	Weekly[a]
Trimethoprim-sulfamethoxazole	Twice weekly	Twice weekly	
Amphotericin B	Twice weekly	Twice weekly	
Ganciclovir	Twice weekly	Twice weekly	

[a] Less frequently during late convalescent stage.
Note: This table is offered as a general guideline. Actual frequency of testing, and specific tests included, will vary according to the individual patient's prescription, stage of treatment, and medical status.

Results of monitoring tests must be available to the physician within 24 hours. Variations from the normal course of disease resolution, or signs of toxic effects, indicate the need for reevaluation and possible alteration of the therapeutic regimen. Timely response to monitoring data is the responsibility of the primary physician.

IV Access and Drug Delivery

The choice of infusion method should take into account the length of therapy, patient aptitude, system reliability, and cost-effectiveness. In most earlier studies reporting the success of home IV antibiotic therapy, the delivery system consisted of a conventional, gravity-driven IV bag or "minibag" with peripheral venous access requiring a heparin flush, or with a heparin lock. This method necessitated manipulation of the system with each dose. While the feasibility of this basic delivery method in homecare is proven, and the component parts are inexpensive, new infusion technologies have several important advantages over the IV drip method.

The most common venous access route for antibiotic delivery is peripheral. A serious disadvantage in the use of these catheters for home therapy is that they must be replaced every 2 or 3 days. For long-term therapy, central venous catheters (CVCs) or peripherally inserted central catheters (PICCs) are preferred. These catheters need less frequent replacement, providing weeks or months of reliable venous access. Although central venous access has advantages over peripheral venous access, the potential for serious complications demands consideration before its use. Central venous access may be required for administration of caustic or irritant drugs.

Mechanical infusion devices are available that have single-use, disposable components that simplify administration of the antimicrobial drug. These devices are an improvement over the gravity drip infusion method, but they still require handling with each dose.

A more significant advance in IV delivery systems is the development of computerized, motor-driven pumps. These automated pumps require changing the drug cassette just once daily. Additional advantages over older systems are ease of use, accuracy, reliability, portability, and integrated safety features. The drug delivery program is tamper-proof, and some computerized devices have a remote reporting mode that can verify compliance. In most applications, use of these advanced systems is cost-effective. The programming capabilities and easy operation of automated delivery devices has greatly expanded the scope of home infusion services.

Programmable devices can be programmed for either intermittent or continuous infusion and for single or multiple antibiotic dosing. These systems enable uncomplicated administration of complicated drug regimens.

In general, intermittent infusion is preferred, and is required for unstable antibiotics. Continuous infusion may be used in some cases to decrease the total daily dose of the antibiotic needed to maintain therapeutic levels.

For a more detailed discussion of IV access devices and drug delivery systems, see Chapter 10.

Scope of Home IV Antimicrobial Therapy

The increasingly broad range of infectious processes treatable by home IV antimicrobial therapy indicates that the type of infection is usually not an exclusionary factor in patient selection.

Infections well suited to treatment at home are those that require long-term therapy with a low probability of adverse consequence. Typically, these include chronic conditions or the convalescent stage of an acute illness. Among the most common applications of home IV therapy are treatments for the infections of immune-deficient patients (AIDS patients and transplant recipients) and serious infections of the elderly. Patients with a chronic illness that predisposes them to infection (diabetes, cystic fibrosis) are also frequently treated at home (5). The most common infections treated at home are osteomyelitis and cellulitis, followed by Lyme disease and the infectious complications of AIDS and immunosuppressive therapies (28).

Experience has proved that with careful patient selection, therapy-specific precautions, and diligent monitoring, home IV therapy is an option even for serious infections like endocarditis and meningitis in the convalescent stage. Also proven safe when cautiously applied is the outpatient use of more toxic antibacterial, antiviral, and antifungal agents.

A compilation of more recently published experience with infections treated with home IV antimicrobial therapy is found in Table 12.5. These therapies are considered to be safe and effective, provided necessary precautions are taken, as described previously in this chapter. Studies have shown that once the patient is clinically stable and afebrile, hospitalization is usually unnecessary.

Bacterial Infections

Osteomyelitis is often treated at home because it requires a prolonged course of antibiotic therapy. Intravenous therapy is frequently pre-

Table 12.5. Infections Treatable with Home IV Antimicrobial Therapy

Infections	References
Bacterial	
Bacteremia/septicemia	30, 31
Brain abscess	32
Cellulitis (skin/soft tissue)	2, 33
Endocarditis	2, 34, 35
Intraabdominal abscess	2
Lyme disease	36, 37, 38
Meningitis	39, 40
Osteomyelitis/septic arthritis	2, 41, 42, 43
PID/female genital	12, 44, 45
Pneumonia	46, 47, 48, 49, 50
Prosthetic device/catheter	2, 35
Pyelonephritis/UTI	51
Viral	24, 27, 52, 53
CMV retinitis	
CMV colitis	
CMV esophagitis	
Fungal	25, 26, 27
Fungemia	
Pneumonia	
Meningitis	

scribed to ensure that bactericidal levels are achieved and are maintained for the course of the treatment. It is critical to therapeutic success that devitalized tissue is debrided. When they are associated with osteomyelitis, cellulitis and other soft-tissue infections may be treated with IV antibiotics; otherwise effective oral therapies are prescribed.

Lyme disease is a relatively recent discovery, first described about 20 years ago. Many unanswered questions remain regarding its diagnosis and treatment. However, it is generally agreed that treatment of neurologic disease, severe carditis, and persistent arthritis requires parenteral therapy. When IV antibiotics are necessary, Lyme disease is commonly treated at home (29).

Home therapy of endocarditis is almost always reserved until late in the course of treatment due to the potentially life-threatening sequelae of antimicrobial therapy. If the patient is not in significant heart failure, and there has been no evidence of embolization, home IV antibiotic therapy is an option. Patients with penicillin-sensitive infections are considered candidates for home IV therapy. However, staphylococcal and less common types of endocarditis are not considered suitable for outpatient treatment. When associated with a prosthetic device, endocarditis requires prolonged therapy. This condition can be treated with oral antibiotics, but initial therapy is almost exclusively intravenous. Vigilant monitoring of patient status is essential for all modes of therapy for endocarditis.

Meningitis, particularly in pediatric patients, has been treated successfully with IV ceftriaxone at home. Before the transition from inpatient to outpatient therapy, the patient must be afebrile for 48 hours, show good response to therapy, and be without neurological abnormalities. Potential complications must be assessed carefully in the decision to treat the patient at home.

Pneumonia and exacerbations of chronic lung disease are treated with IV antibiotics when effective oral therapies are unavailable or contraindicated. Pneumonia, a common and potentially fatal disease of the elderly, can be treated at home if the patient is not too fragile or too sick. Hospitalization of these patients should be avoided because it increases the risk of complications. Cystic fibrosis patients are commonly treated for recurrent pulmonary infections with home IV antibiotic therapy. The course of treatment is prolonged, and in many cases it is life-long.

Pelvic inflammatory disease (PID) occasionally requires IV therapy, although good intramuscular and oral therapies are available. With prolonged treatment of recurrent or refractory infections, there is less chance for recurrence, and the patient may avoid surgical intervention.

Chronic urinary tract problems are frequently caused by pathogens susceptible only to IV antibiotics. However, acute, uncomplicated disease is treated with oral antibiotics.

Patients with acute sinusitis or severe pediatric otitis media are sometimes treated with IV antibiotics at home when the condition is unresponsive to oral therapy.

Viral Infections

The most common viral infection treated by home IV antiviral therapy is CMV retinitis. Other complications of AIDS caused by CMV have also been successfully treated on an outpatient basis, including esophagitis and colitis.

Fungal Infections

Fungemia, usually encountered as a complication of AIDS or other immunosuppressive conditions, can be successfully treated with home IV antifungal therapy. The convalescent stages of fungal pneumonia and meningitis have also been reported to be treatable on an outpatient basis. Cryptococcal meningitis and aspergillosis may require life-long treatment.

Conclusion

Experience continues to support the safety, efficacy, and cost-effectiveness of home IV antimicrobial therapy.

The scope of infections treatable by home IV therapy is expected to increase. This prediction is based in part on the pharmaceutical industry's commitment to the development of drugs designed for homecare use. Also, increasingly sophisticated and "user-friendly" infusion systems are being marketed at a reasonable cost. These improvements will allow consideration of previously unsuitable candidates for home IV therapy. Included in this group of patients are the medically complex, and the physically or intellectually disadvantaged.

Although more infections will be treatable at home, the total number of patients treated by IV therapy is not expected to increase at the present rate. Equally effective oral antimicrobial therapies are becoming available for infections that currently require the use of parenteral therapy.

References

1. Chamberlain TM, Lehman ME, Groh MJ, Munroe WP, Reinders TP. Cost analysis of a home intravenous antibiotic program. Am J Hosp Pharm 1988;45:2341–2345.
2. Poretz DM. Home intravenous antibiotic therapy. Clin Geriatr Med 1991;7:749–763.
3. Baptista RJ, Mitrano FP. Experience with 211 courses of home intravenous antimicrobial therapy. Am J Hosp Pharm 1989;46:315–316.
4. Williams DN, Gibson JA, Bosch D. Home intravenous antibiotic therapy using a programmable infusion pump. Arch Intern Med 1989;149:1157–1160.
5. Poretz DM. Treatment of serious infections with cefotaxime utilizing an outpatient drug delivery device: global analysis of a large-scale, multicenter trial. Am J Med 1994; 97:34–42.
6. Brown RB. Selecting the patient. In: Tice AD, ed. Outpatient parenteral antibiotic therapy: management of serious infections: Part I: Medical, socioeconomic, and legal issues. Hosp Pract 1993;28(Suppl 1):11–15.
7. Bernstein LH. An update on home intravenous antibiotic therapy. Geriatrics 1991;46:47–54.
8. Grayson ML, Silvers J, Turnidge J. Home intravenous antibiotic therapy: a safe and effective alternative to inpatient care. Med J Aust 1995;162:249–253.
9. Craig WA. Selecting the antibiotic. In: Tice AD, ed. Outpatient parenteral antibiotic therapy: management of serious infections. Part 1: medical, socioeconomic, and legal issues. Hosp Pract 1993;28 (Suppl 1):16–20.
10. Craig WA. Antibiotic selection factors and description of a hospital based outpatient antibiotic therapy program in the USA. Eur J Clin Microbiol Infect Dis 1995;14:636–642.
11. Vogelman B, Gudmundsson S, Leggett J, Turnidge J, Ebert S, Craig WA. Correlation of antimicrobial pharmacokinetic parameters with therapeutic efficacy in an animal model. J Infect Dis 1988;158:831–847.
12. Leggett JE, Fantin B, Ebert S, et al. Comparative antibiotic dose-effect relationships at several dosing inter-

vals in murine pneumonitis and thigh-infection models. Infect Control Hosp Epidemiol 1989;159:281–292.

13. Craig WA, Redington J, Ebert SC. Pharmacodynamics of amikacin in vitro and in mouse thigh and lung infections. J Antimicrob Chemother 1991;27 (Suppl C):29–40.

14. Leggett JE, Ebert S, Fantin B, Craig WA. Comparative dose-effect relations at several dosing intervals for beta-lactam, aminoglycoside and quinolone antibiotics against gram-negative bacilli in murine thigh-infection and pneumonitis models. Scand J Infect Dis Suppl 1991;74:179–184.

15. Tice AD. Once-daily ceftriaxone outpatient therapy in adults with infections. Chemotherapy 1991;37(Suppl 2)7–10.

16. Poretz DM, ed. Outpatient use of intravenous antibiotics. Am J Med 1994; 97(Suppl 2A):1–55.

17. Todd PA, Brogden RN. Cefotaxime: an update of its pharmacology and therapeutic use. Drugs 1990;40: 608–651.

18. Levine JF. Vancomycin: a review. Med Clin North Am 1987;71:1135–1145.

19. Farber BF, Moellering RC Jr. Retrospective study of the toxicity of preparations of vancomycin from 1974 to 1981. Antimicrob Agents Chemother 1983;23:138–141.

20. Wallace MR, Mascola JR, Oldfield EC III. Red man syndrome: incidence, etiology, and prophylaxis. J Infect Dis 1991;12:1109–1126.

21. Moore RD, Lietman PS, Smith CR. Clinical response to aminoglycoside therapy: Importance of the ratio of peak concentration to minimal inhibitory concentration. J Infect Dis 1987; 155:93–99.

22. Daikos GL, Jackson GG, Lolans VT, Livermore DM. Adaptive resistance to aminoglycoside antibiotics from first-exposure down-regulation. J Infect Dis 1990; 162:414–420.

23. Gilbert DN. Once-daily aminoglycoside therapy. Antimicrob Agents Chemother 1991;35:399–405.

24. Afheldt M, Phillips J, Rachlis A. HIV outpatient clinic: a model for delivery of treatment for HIV+ patients with CMV [abstract no. PO-B32–2265]. Int Conf AIDS 1993;9:513.

25. Walsh TJ, Gonzalez C, Roilides E, et al. Fungemia in children infected with the human immunodeficiency virus: new etiologic patterns, emerging pathogens, and improved outcome with antifungal therapy. Clin Infect Dis 1995;20:900–906.

26. Tillman K, Santos M, Lutz B. Home administration of amphotericin B [abstract no. PB0921]. Int Conf AIDS 1994;10:227.

27. Scully, BE. Home intravenous antibiotic therapy. NJ Med 1992;1:48–51.

28. Rich D. Physicians, pharmacists, and home infusion antibiotic therapy. In: Poretz DM, ed. Outpatient use of intravenous antibiotics. Am J Med 1994;97(Suppl 2A):3–8.

29. Dennis DT. Lyme disease. Dermatol Clin 1995;13: 537–551.

30. Morales JO, Von Behren L. Secondary bacterial infections in HIV-infected patients: an alternative ambulatory outpatient treatment utilizing intravenous cefotaxime. In: Poretz DM, ed. Outpatient use of intravenous antibiotics. Am J Med 1994;97(Suppl 2A): 9–13.

31. Angel JVG and the HIAT Study Group. Outpatient antibiotic therapy for elderly patients. In: Poretz DM, ed. Outpatient use of intravenous antibiotics. Am J Med 1994;97(Suppl 2A):43–49.

32. Hinkle JL. Home antibiotic therapy for brain abscesses. J Intraven Nurs 1990;1314:172–176.

33. Poretz DM et al. Treatment of skin and soft-tissue infections utilizing an outpatient parenteral drug delivery device: A multicenter trial. In: Poretz DM, ed. Outpatient use of intravenous antibiotics. Am J Med 1994; 97(Suppl 2A):23–27.

34. Stramboullian D, Bonvehi P, Arevaldo C, et al. Antibiotic management of outpatients with endocarditis due to penicillin-susceptible streptococci. Rev Infect Dis 1991;13(Suppl 2):S160–163.

35. Durack D. Endocarditis. In: Tice AD, ed. Outpatient parenteral antibiotic therapy: management of serious infections. Part II: Amenable infections and models for delivery. Hosp Pract 1993;28(Suppl 2):6–9.

36. Ismeurt RL, Wilson LW, Long CO. Lyme disease: an emerging infection with home healthcare implications. Home Healthcare Nurse 1995;13:28–33.

37. Rahn DW, Malawista SE. Lyme disease: recommendations for diagnosis and treatment. Ann Intern Med 1991;114:472–481.

38. Sigal LH. Lyme disease in New Jersey. Lawrenceville, NJ: The Academy of Medicine of New Jersey, 1993.

39. Bradley, JS. Meningitis. In: Tice AD, ed. Outpatient parenteral antibiotic therapy: management of serious infections. Part II: Amenable infections and models for delivery. Hosp Pract 1993;28(Suppl 2):15–19.

40. Arditi M, Yogev R. Convalescent outpatient therapy for selected children with acute bacterial meningitis. Semin Pediatr Infect Dis 1990;1:404.

41. Tice AD. Once-daily ceftriaxone outpatient therapy in adults with infections. Chemotherapy 1991;37(Suppl 3):7–10.

42. Mauceri AA and the HIAT Study Group. Treatment of bone and joint infections utilizing a third-generation cephalosporin with an outpatient drug delivery device. In: Poretz DM, ed. Outpatient use of intravenous antibiotics. Am J Med 1994;97(Suppl 2A):14–22.

43. Ingam C, Eron LJ, Goldberg RI, et al. Antibiotic therapy of osteomyelitis in outpatients. Med Clin North Am 1988;72:723–38.

44. Marsh PK, Tice AD, Craven PC, et al. Treatment of chronic PID with long-term home IV antibiotics [abstract no. 991]. Program and Abstracts of the 29th Interscience Conference on Antimicrobial Agents and Chemotherapy. Washington, DC, American Society for Microbiology, 1989.

45. Sweet RL. Pelvic inflammatory disease. In: Tice AD, ed. Outpatient parenteral antibiotic therapy: management of serious infections. Part II: Amenable infections and models for delivery. Hosp Pract 1993;28(Suppl 2):25–30.

46. Morales JO, Snead H. Efficacy and safety of intravenous cefotaxime for treating pneumonia in outpatients. In: Poretz DM, ed. Outpatient use of intravenous antibiotics. Am J Med 1994;97(Suppl 2A): 28–33.

47. Williams DN. Reducing costs and hospital stay for pneumonia with home intravenous cefotaxime treatment: results with a computerized ambulatory drug delivery system. In: Poretz DM, ed. Outpatient use of intravenous antibiotics. Am J Med 1994;97(Suppl 2A):50–55.

48. Trowbridge, JF. Pneumonia and chronic lung disease. In: Tice AD, ed. Outpatient parenteral antibiotic therapy: management of serious infections. Part II: Amenable infections and models for delivery. Hosp Pract 1993;28(Suppl 2):20–24.

49. Dagan R, Einhorn M. A program of outpatient parenteral antibiotic therapy for serious pediatric bacterial infections. Rev Infect Dis 1991;13(Suppl 2):S152-S155.

50. Gilbert J, Robinson T, Littlewood JM. Home intravenous antibiotic treatment in cystic fibrosis. Arch Dis Child 1988;63:512–517.
51. Millar LK. Pyelonephritis. In: Tice AD, ed. Outpatient parenteral antibiotic therapy: management of serious infections. Part II: Amenable infections and models for delivery. Hosp Pract 1993;28(Suppl 2): 31–35.
52. Baird B, Coleman P, Allen M, et al. Care requirements for AIDS patients on a trial of foscarnet for the treatment of CMV retinitis [abstract no. 2110]. Int Conf AIDS 1990;6:381.
53. Cheung TW, Fahs M, Sacks HS. Cost-effectiveness of ganciclovir (DHPG) versus foscarnet (FOS) for cytomegalovirus (CMV) retinitis in patients with AIDS [abstract no. PoD5768]. Int Conf AIDS 1992;8:D517.

Suggested Readings

Facts and Comparisons. Published monthly. St. Louis: Facts and Comparisons.
Gorbach SL, Bartlett JG, Blacklow NR, eds. Infectious Diseases. Philadelphia: WB Saunders, 1992.
Hardman JG, Gilman AG, Limbird LE, eds. Goodman & Gilman's The Pharmacological Basis of Therapeutics, 9th ed. New York: McGraw-Hill Health Professions Division, 1996.
Hoeprich PD, Jordan MC, Ronald AR, eds. Infectious Diseases: A Treatise of Infectious Processes, 5th ed. Philadelphia: JB Lippincott, 1994.
Sanford JP, Gilbert DN, Sande MA, eds. The Sanford Guide to Antimicrobial Therapy, 25th ed. Dallas: Antimicrobial Therapy, Inc., 1995.

13

LYME DISEASE MANAGEMENT:
A Homecare-Specific Therapy

Leonard H. Sigal

CHAPTER AT A GLANCE: Lyme disease occurs in various endemic areas throughout the United States. This chapter outlines the pathogenesis of the disease, the clinical findings (including early localized disease, early disseminated disease, and chronic or late disease), and laboratory findings. Management of Lyme disease is discussed, including intravenous therapy at home, the approach to chronic Lyme disease, treatment of pediatric disease, and the approach to pregnancy complicated by Lyme disease.

Introduction

Lyme disease is a multisystem infectious disease, caused by *Borrelia burgdorferi,* that potentially causes arthritis and inflammation of the skin, heart, brain, and peripheral nervous system. Lyme disease is relatively easily treated with oral antibiotics in its earliest stages. When the duration of infection is measured in years, affecting the joints or neurologic system, it may be more difficult to cure even with intravenous third-generation antibiotics such as ceftriaxone or cefotaxime. A full understanding of the pathogenesis of the disease and the proper use of testing is important before one embarks upon the management of patients with "late-stage" or "chronic" Lyme disease.

Definition

Lyme disease (LD) is a multisystem inflammatory disease affecting the skin, heart, central and peripheral nervous systems, and joints; other features—including ophthalmologic and muscle—occur, but are quite uncommon. LD was first described in studies of an outbreak of "juvenile rheumatoid arthritis" in Connecticut (Lyme arthritis). Within a few years the full spectrum of LD became clear. LD is caused by spirochetes known collectively as *Borrelia burgdorferi,* spread by the bite of *Ixodes* ticks. Days to weeks after the bite, **early, localized** LD occurs. This consists of a distinctive rash, erythema migrans (EM), at the site of the bite, and associated symptoms, often described as being compatible with a summer cold. In the same time period, or up to 9 months later, **early, disseminated** LD may occur, the spread due to spirochetemia, which includes multiple EM and cardiac and/or neurologic disease. Weeks to months or even years after infection, **chronic** or **late** LD, including arthritis and/or neurologic problems, may develop, often insidiously. Patients may present with later features of LD having never experienced an illness suggesting early infection; EM is seen in only about 70% of patients and only one-third remember "the tick bite." Two other cutaneous features of *Borrelia burgdorferi* infection may occur: lymphadenosis benigna cutis (lymphocytoma) in early disseminated LD and acrodermatitis chronica atrophicans in late LD; these are rarely seen in the United States but are more common in Europe.

A set of epidemiologic criteria for establishing the presence of LD were developed by the U.S. Centers for Disease Control and Prevention (CDC) (Table 13.1). These were not meant to be used as diagnostic criteria, but only in reporting LD; LD is a reportable disease to the CDC.

Table 13.1. CDC Epidemiologic Criteria for Lyme Disease

Presence of EM
OR
Cases with at least one late manifestation and laboratory confirmation of infection. The late manifestations include any of the following *when an alternate explanation is not found:*

- Musculoskeletal system: Recurrent brief attacks of objective joint swelling in one or a few joints, *sometimes* followed by chronic arthritis in one or a few joints. Manifestations not considered as criteria for diagnosis include chronic progressive arthritis not preceded by brief attacks and chronic symmetrical polyarthritis. Additionally, arthralgias, myalgias, or fibromyalgia syndromes alone are not accepted as criteria for musculoskeletal involvement.
- Nervous system: Lymphocytic meningitis, cranial neuritis, particularly facial palsy (may be bilateral), radiculoneuropathy or, rarely, encephalomyelitis alone or in combination. Encephalomyelitis must be confirmed by showing antibody production against *B. burgdorferi* in the cerebrospinal fluid (CSF), demonstrated by a higher titer of antibody in CSF than in serum. Headache, fatigue, paresthesias, or mild stiff neck alone are not accepted as criteria for neurologic involvement.
- Cardiovascular: Acute onset, high grade (2nd or 3rd degree) atrioventricular conduction defects that resolve in days to weeks and are sometimes associated with myocarditis. Palpitations, bradycardia, bundle-branch block, or myocarditis alone are not accepted as criteria for cardiovascular involvement.

There has been much discussion of how difficult LD is to diagnose and document. With the unbiased acquisition of a complete history and physical examination, appropriate use of testing for confirmation only, and familiarity with LD, one can arrive at the diagnosis of LD when appropriate, or reject that diagnosis and search for another. Once the diagnosis has been made, appropriate treatment and follow-up can be recommended and planned.

Teaching the patient about LD and what can be expected after therapy—e.g., the 10 to 15% incidence of the Jarisch-Herxheimer reaction or the slow resolution of complaints in over 50% of patients—will decrease anxiety and increase confidence in the physician's plan.

In many areas, LD has become a "diagnosis of exclusion"; it must be LD because the patient had "complaints compatible with LD" (other than erythema migrans, the manifestations of early LD are so nonspecific as to render this term meaningless) and no other diagnosis has made itself apparent. Reference to the LD literature clearly shows that the features of this infection are reasonably well defined and allow a diagnosis by criteria rather than by exclusion.

Etiology, Incidence, and Epidemiology

Lyme disease is caused by three closely related species included within the term *B. burgdorferi* sensu lato ("in the general sense"). The cause of LD in the United States is *B. burgdorferi* sensu stricto ("in the strict sense"), which is also found in Europe and Asia. In Europe and Asia, *Borrelia afzellii* and *Borrelia garinii* cause most cases of LD. LD has been reported in the United States, Canada, across Europe, and in Asia (e.g., Japan, Korea, and China). The differences between European and American LD (more arthritis and more multiple EM lesions in the United States) may be due to differences in the organisms. All *B. burgdorferi* isolated to date are sensitive to the standard antimicrobial agents used in LD (see below).

LD is spread by the bite of infected *Ixodes* ticks (*Ixodes scapularis* in the eastern and north-central United States [the older literature uses the name *Ixodes dammini* for the vector in the Northeast; it is now known that *I. dammini* is essentially identical with *I. scapularis,* and the latter term is preferred]; *Ixodes pacificus* in the Western United States; *Ixodes ricinus* in Europe; and *Ixodes persulcatus* in Asia).

LD is endemic in areas where ixodid ticks abound. About 90% of U.S. cases of LD are found in the following nine states: Massachusetts, Connecticut, Rhode Island, New York, New Jersey, Pennsylvania, Minnesota, Wisconsin, and California. Within each state there are hot spots of disease; the incidence is not uniform across each state, or for that matter within each endemic county. Obtaining a travel history is crucial; even if your patient does not reside in an endemic area, he or she may have traveled to an endemic area, (e.g., Nantucket, MA, Montauk Point, NY, or the north woods of Wisconsin).

Most LD is spread by infected nymphs, which emerge in the late spring and continue searching for a blood meal into the early fall; this explains the seasonal variation in incidence. Once fed, the tick drops off the host and molts to an adult in the fall. Adults seek a blood meal in the late fall, winter, and even the spring. Although their preferred host is the white-tailed deer, other mammals can be utilized, including humans. One can get LD from an infected adult in the dead of winter, although with the amount of clothing worn, the minimal time spent outside, and the easier recognition of the much larger adult, this risk is much less than in the summer and fall.

Ticks seeking a meal wait on the underside of a blade of grass or low-lying shrubs; ticks do not jump, hop, fly, or descend from trees. Ticks await a warm body exhaling carbon dioxide and then latch on as the animal brushes against the tick. Thus, areas of special risk are areas where many ticks are found.

Since nymphs are typically carried by mice, anyplace where there are many mice can represent a risk: stone walls are known as good homes for mice; the shrubs at the border between forest and lawns are also preferred homes for mice; bird feeders commonly draw mice for a free meal. If deer browse in your backyard, it is possible that they are dropping ticks on your property. If you have a pet that goes outside, it may be bringing ticks into the house. All of these items are of vastly less concern if no one in your area has ever had Lyme disease. However, if there is a neighborhood history of many cases of Lyme disease, the risk may be in your backyard, as noted above.

In unfed ticks, *B. burgdorferi* resides on the midgut wall. It takes 24 hours or more after attachment for the tick to begin ingesting blood. Shortly thereafter, the organism multiplies and disseminates, reaching the salivary glands. As the tick excretes excess water into the host throughout its meal, the organism can be passed to the host. It takes 48 hours or more after tick attachment for LD to be spread, and it is a very inefficient process. A recent study suggests that in an area where 40% of adult ixodid ticks carry *B. burgdorferi,* only 1% of people who experienced a tick bite developed LD. The risk of acquiring infection increases with duration of tick attachment and with the degree of engorgement of the tick. Thus, the same study found that the risk of developing LD increased to approximately 8% if the tick was engorged.

Pathogenesis

How *B. burgdorferi* causes LD and the persistent symptoms often ascribed to "chronic LD" is still a matter of debate. The organism does not make toxins or itself cause local tissue damage. There is evidence to suggest that the organism can activate host proteolytic enzymes, which may facilitate tissue invasion and dissemination. Using culture, polymerase chain reaction (PCR), or histologic examination, *B. burgdorferi* has been identified in skin lesions, myocardium, spinal fluid, and synovial fluid of patients with various features of LD.

Inflammation at these sites is presumably due to the immune response to the organism. If this were the only pathogenetic mechanism, persistence of live organism would be necessary for persistence of disease and all inflammation would vanish shortly after therapy. It is possible that persistence of dead or effete organism can be the focus of ongoing inflammation. The antigen-induced model of rheumatoid arthritis may be valuable in explaining persistence of inflammation. In this model, the persistence of the injected exogenous antigen, due to resistance to proteolytic degradation, allows the antigen to be a focus of ongoing inflammation. As long as the antigen persists, inflammation persists. With each "boost" in the systemic immune response to that antigen, there is a flare of arthritis. Persistence of borrelial antigen(s) may also cause ongoing production of cytokines, which may cause local and nonspecific systemic symptoms.

An intriguing potential explanation of central nervous system (CNS) complaints in LD, in the absence of CNS infection, is the extra-CNS production by activated macrophages of quinolinic acid, an excitotoxin derived from tryptophan. This compound crosses the blood-brain barrier and can have CNS effects.

Vasculitis has also been suggested as a cause of peripheral neuropathy. Furthermore, there is in vitro evidence implicating molecular mimicry as a mechanism in neurologic LD. The organism's flagellin contains an epitope that cross-reacts with human heat shock protein 60; a monoclonal antibody to the borrelial epitope modifies neural cell tumor lines in vitro, and patients with neurologic features of LD have serum antibodies to this epitope. Thus, subjective and objective clinical problems may be caused by other than live organism; the only role for antibiotic therapy is in the treatment of active infection with live *B. burgdorferi*.

Clinical Findings

Early Localized Disease

Early localized disease includes EM and associated findings. EM is recognized in 50 to 70% of patients with LD, usually within 1 month of the tick bite, although a minority of patients recall the bite. EM is often found in or near the axilla, inguina, or midriff. The lesion is usually asymptomatic, although it may burn or itch. Critical in differentiating EM from other erythemas is the fact that EM expands over the course of a few days, often with central clearing, although it may be uniform red or have a more complex "bull's-eye" appearance.

One-half of patients with EM have multiple lesions; this is the result of spirochetemia, not multiple tick bites. Early localized disease may be associated with nonspecific complaints resembling a viral syndrome.

In the absence of EM, there is nothing about this syndrome that is diagnostic of LD; further details of the syndrome are listed in Table 13.2. It can be seen that one cannot properly make a diagnosis of LD on the basis of a history of "symptoms compatible with LD."

Oral antibiotic therapy prevents progression to later features of LD in the vast majority of cases (Table 13.3); the incidence figures given for each feature of later LD are for *patients not receiving adequate therapy for early localized LD.* There is no need for intravenous therapy in early localized LD. Of note, in the first days of therapy 5 to 10% of patients with early LD experience a Jarisch-Herxheimer reaction (a worsening of many of the signs and symptoms of LD) that lasts for less than a day and is always self-limited, never fatal.

Early Disseminated Disease

Early disseminated disease (Table 13.2) occurs days to months after the tick bite, which is often not recalled. Early, disseminated LD may be the first features of *B. burgdorferi* infection, with no antecedent EM, tick bite or anything suggesting LD.

About 8% of patients with untreated LD (Table 13.2) develop carditis, which may include one or more, often variable, degrees of heart block or mild myopericarditis (including mild congestive heart failure). *B. burgdorferi* has been implicated in a few cases of chronic cardiomyopathy and in a few cases intravenous antibiotic therapy has been associated with reversal of the cardiac dysfunction. In the vast majority of cases, cardiac disease is subclinical. When symptomatic, it usually begins to resolve during or even before antibiotic therapy.

Neurologic features occur in about 10% of untreated patients (Table 13.2). The neurologic features of early, disseminated LD often

Table 13.2. Clinical Manifestations of Lyme Disease

Early localized: occurring a few days to a month after the tick bite
Erythema migrans (in 50 to 70% of patients—multiple in 50% of patients with EM)
Fatigue/malaise/lethargy
Headache
Myalgia/arthralgias
Regional/generalized lymphadenopathy

Early disseminated disease[a]: occuring days to 10 months after the tick bite
Carditis—approximately 8 to 10% of **untreated** patients
    Conduction defects
    Mild cardiomyopathy/myopericarditis
Neurologic disease—approximately 10 to 12% of **untreated** patients
    Lymphocytic meningitis
    Encephalitis
    Cranial neuropathy (most often facial, can be bilateral)
    Peripheral neuropathy/radiculoneuropathy
    Myelitis
Musculoskeletal—approximately 50% of **untreated** patients
    Migratory polyarthritis and/or polyarthralgias
    Fibromyalgia
Other—
    Skin: Lymphadenosis benigna cutis (lymphocytoma), erythema nodosum
    Lymphadenopathy: Regional and/or generalized
    Eye: Conjunctivitis, iritis, choroiditis, vitritis, retinitis
    Liver: Liver function test abnormalities, hepatitis
    Kidney: Microhematuria, proteinuria

Late/chronic disease[a]: occurring months to years after the tick bite
Musculoskeletal—approximately 50% of **untreated** patients develop migratory polyarthritis
    Approximatley 10% of **untreated** patients develop monoarthritis, usually knee
    Fibromyalgia
Neurologic disease—
    Chronic, often subtle, encephalopathy, encephalomyelitis, and/or peripheral neuropathy
    Ataxia, dementia, sleep disorder
Cutaneous—
    Acrodermatitis chronica atrophicans
    ?Morphea/localized scleroderma-like lesions

From Sigal LH, Academy of Medicine of New Jersey Lyme Disease Task Force. Lyme Disease in New Jersey: A Practical Guide for New Jersey Clinicians. Lawrenceville, NJ: Academy of Medicine of New Jersey, 1993.
[a]May occur in the absence of any prior features of Lyme disease.

resolve spontaneously; therapy is directed at prevention of progression to later features of LD and/or to hasten resolution. There are no controlled studies of therapy in LD carditis; intravenous therapy is often given, although there are many reports of successful therapy with oral agents. Likewise, there are no prospective studies of neurologic LD in the United States. A recent Swedish study suggests that oral therapy is equivalent to short-term intravenous penicillin for the treatment of neurologic features of LD. As noted above, LD in the United States is somewhat different from LD in Europe. Thus, it may not be appropriate to apply the findings of the Swedish study to American patients.

Late Disseminated Disease

Chronic or late disease may include musculoskeletal and/or neurologic problems. These occur months to years after the onset of infection and may represent the first feature of LD. About 80% of patients with untreated LD have musculoskeletal symptoms, including

Table 13.3. Current Recommendations for Therapy in Lyme Disease

Oral Therapy of Early Localized Lyme Disease		
Adults		
Doxycycline[a]	100 mg p.o. b.i.d.	3 to 4 weeks[b]
Tetracycline[a, c]	250 to 500 mg p.o. q.i.d.	3 to 4 weeks[b]
Amoxicillin[c, d]	250 to 500 mg p.o. q.i.d.	3 to 4 weeks[b]
Children		
Amoxicillin	40 mg/kg/day, divided dose	3 to 4 weeks[b]
Erythromycin	30 mg/kg/day, divided dose	3 to 4 weeks[b]
Penicillin G	25 to 50 mg/kg/day, divided dose	3 to 4 weeks[b]

Intravenous Therapy of Early Disseminated and Late (or Chronic) Lyme Disease[e]		
Adults		
Third-generation cephalosporins:		
Ceftriaxone	2 g q.d. or 1 g b.i.d.	2 to 4 weeks
Cefotaxime	3 g b.i.d.	2 to 4 weeks
Penicillin		
Penicillin G	20 million units in 6 divided doses	2 to 4 weeks
Chloramphenicol	50 mg/kg/day in 4 divided doses	2 to 4 weeks
Children		
Third-generation cephalosporins:		
Ceftriaxone	75 to 100 mg/kg/day	2 to 4 weeks
Cefotaxime	90 to 180 mg/kg/day, in 2 or 3 divided doses	2 to 4 weeks
Penicillin		
Penicillin G	300,000 U/kg/day in 6 divided doses	2 to 4 weeks

From Sigal LH. Current drug therapy recommendations for the treatment of Lyme disease. Drugs 1992;43:683–699.
[a]No studies comparing doxycycline with tetracycline have been done.
[b]There is no proof that isolated facial nerve palsy or carditis must be treated with intravenous therapy. Oral doxycycline for early Lyme neuroborreliosis has been shown to be effective in European studies. Especially in children, oral treatment for Lyme arthritis may suffice.
[c]Dosage determined by size of patient.
[d]No studies comparing amoxicillin with amoxicillin plus probenecid have been done; cefuroxime, axetil, and azithromycin have also been studied in Lyme disease.
[e]There is no proof that this is the optimal duration of therapy or, for that matter, that more than 10 to 14 days of treatment is necessary.

isolated arthralgias (in 20%), intermittent episodes of arthritis (in 50%), and chronic, usually monarthritis (in 10%)—usually affecting the knee. Many patients with arthritis describe prior arthralgia.

Antibiotic treatment is usually effective in arthritis, although synovectomy and/or disease-modifying therapy (e.g., hydroxychloroquine) has been necessary for some patients. The other feature of late LD is neurologic disease, termed "tertiary neuroborreliosis" by analogy with tertiary neurosyphilis, with which it bears some similarities. Encephalopathy, neurocognitive dysfunction, and peripheral neuropathy are features. Contrasts between the two neurologic LDs are found in Table 13.4.

Other medical problems have been ascribed to LD. Quite often the diagnosis of LD is made solely on the basis of a "positive blood test," often a false-positive ELISA. Such "proof" is not enough to ensure a linkage. Some of the less-established features of LD include ophthalmologic disease (inflammation of any of the eye structures), hepatitis (mild, occurring in early LD), splenitis, and myositis; these were well described in the National Clinical Conference on Lyme Disease, the proceedings of which appeared as a supplement to the *American Journal of Medicine* in 1995. Established cutaneous features of *B. burgdorferi* infection, more common in Europe than in the United States, are lymphocytoma and acrodermatitis chronica atrophicans.

Nonspecific complaints (e.g., headache, fatigue, arthralgia) may persist after appropriate (and ultimately successful) antibiotic treatment of LD and often linger for months

Table 13.4. Contrasts between Early Disseminated and Tertiary Neuroborreliosis

	Early Disseminated LD	*Tertiary Neuroborreliosis*
Time since ECM	Weeks to months	Months to Years
Manifestations	Facial palsy	Encephalopathy
	Peripheral nerve palsies	Myelitis
	Meningitis	Peripheral neuropathy
	Meningoencephalitis	
Associated manifestations	EM	Lyme arthritis
	Cardiac disease	
CSF	Lymphocytic pleocytosis	Intrathecal antibody production
	Intrathecal antibody production	
Serologic testing	May be positive, occasionally IgM	Routinely seropositive

with slow, spontaneous resolution. In the absence of *objective* evidence of disease, there is no reason for further antibiotic therapy in such patients. Fibromyalgia syndrome (FMS) may occur commonly as a post-LD syndrome. FMS can cause pain and mild cognitive dysfunction; the achiness of FMS should not be misdiagnosed as Lyme arthritis, and the fatigue and forgetfulness commonly reported in FMS should not be mistaken for CNS LD. FMS, related to prior LD or otherwise, does not respond to antibiotic therapy.

As noted above, *B. burgdorferi* is killed by antibiotic therapy with appropriate agents. Persistence of complaints after adequate therapy may occur, but usually resolves without further treatment. Resistance to therapy may occur but is certainly uncommon. In patients whose LD does not resolve after antibiotic treatment, the competent clinician should consider an alternate diagnosis. One must remember that all symptoms and signs that follow LD are not necessarily due to the preceding infection.

Laboratory Findings

The diagnosis of LD should be based on historical and objective physical findings; laboratory tests should serve as confirmation of the diagnosis rather than the source of the diagnosis. Currently and widely available immunologic tests used in LD are enzyme-linked immunosorbent assay (ELISA) and Western (immuno-) blot. Neither is a **diagnostic test for LD;** the detection of antibodies only suggests exposure. However, there is broad reactivity of antibodies; for example, antibodies made against the flagellin of *Escherichia coli* may cross-react with and bind to the flagellin of *B. burgdorferi*. Thus, antibodies detected in an "LD test" may not indicate infection. In fact, ELISA and Western blot should not be called "LD tests"—they both identify antibody to *B. burgdorferi* and cannot, by themselves, be viewed as making a diagnosis of LD.

False-positive testing in ELISA is relatively common and can be seen in other spirochetal diseases (e.g., syphilis and other borrelioses), in nonspirochetal infections (e.g., endocarditis and Epstein-Barr virus), and in rheumatologic diseases (e.g., rheumatoid arthritis and lupus).

Seroconversion by ELISA may not occur until 6 to 8 weeks after the onset of infection and may never occur in some patients who receive antibiotic therapy early in the course of LD. There is no proven role for testing patients who become asymptomatic following therapy; antibody levels may stay elevated for years.

A rising ELISA level or increasing numbers of bands in Western blot in the presence of persisting or expanding/evolving complaints may indicate that infection persists; such a finding should prompt further evaluation. In patients with CNS or joint inflammation, analysis of the inflammatory fluid may show higher levels of antibody (or unique reactivity by immunoblot) in the spinal or synovial fluids relative to serum. Such findings confirm that the local process is due to *B. burgdorferi* and are vital in proving that the closed-space inflammatory process is due to LD, not merely a problem present in someone who is seropositive in an anti–*B. burgdorferi* antibody assay.

Modification of the criteria published by Dressler and Steere for interpretation of Western blot (Table 13.5) are increasingly being accepted, although they may be modified in the future. It is now suggested that all positive or equivocal ELISA results be confirmed by Western (immuno-) blot, in order to identify false-positive ELISA results. Screening the general population for serologic evidence of exposure to *B. burgdorferi* will detect many more false positives than true positives and should be discouraged.

In some areas the rate of positive ELISA is 50 times greater than the rate of true LD. A false-positive ELISA is not a reason to treat, since it does not represent true exposure. As noted, the diagnosis of LD should be made on clinical grounds. There is no place for the use of ELISA as a screening tool, even in endemic areas. Given the high frequency of false-positive results in ELISA (above 5% in many endemic areas), reference should be made to Bayes' theorem: if the pretest likelihood of the diagnosis of LD is low, the predictive value of a positive ELISA is very low (approximately 7% by one recent estimate). It

is only when the pretest likelihood of LD is high that the predictive value of a positive ELISA is high; i.e., a positive test confirms the diagnosis of LD.

Recent studies suggest that polymerase chain reaction (PCR) (which identifies the nucleic acids of the organism) may be useful in documenting *B. burgdorferi* infection, although PCR positivity is not synonymous with the presence of live organism. PCR analysis is prone to false positivity and is highly dependent on the skill and care of the performing laboratory. At this time, PCR cannot be recommended for use in standard clinical practice. It remains an experimental test. Urine antigen testing is, likewise, a research tool and is of no proven value in the evaluation or confirmation of LD.

Where LD-associated organ damage is suspected, neuropsychologic testing, electrophysiologic testing (cardiac and neurologic), and brain magnetic resonance imaging may be helpful in documenting objective abnormalities. However, abnormalities in these tests are not specific for damage due to *B. burgdorferi*. Their value is in establishing that there is objective evidence of organ damage.

Optimal Management

Antibiotics are the treatment for active *B. burgdorferi* infection. Oral therapy given in a timely fashion for early LD prevents progression to later features of LD, although it may

Table 13.5. Criteria for Positive Western Blot (Immunoblot) Analysis in the Serologic Confirmation of Infection with *Borrelia burgdorferi* (Lyme Disease)[a]

Duration of Disease	Isotype Tested	Bands to Be Considered
First few weeks of infection	IgM	2 of the 8 following: 18, 21, 28, 37, 41, 45, 58, 93 2 of the 3 following: ospC (23), 39, 41[b]
After first weeks of infection	IgG	5 of the 10 following: 18, 21, 28, 30, 39, 41, 45, 58, 66, 93

[a]Criteria derived from Dressler F, Whalen JA, Reinhardt BN, Steere AC. Western blotting in the serodiagnosis of Lyme disease. J Infect Dis 1993;167:392–400.
[b]Alternate criteria for IgM reactivity, proposed at a conference sponsored by the U.S. Centers for Disease Control and Prevention. Other points noted at that conference were the need for standardization of antigen preparation and techniques used. Note that IgM criteria are to be used *only* during the first few weeks of infection.

not decrease the duration or severity of many features of early LD. Oral agents are adequate for early, localized LD in all cases, regardless of the severity of the patient's complaints or the antibody level. Suggested drug regimens for each feature of LD are given in Table 13.3.

Oral therapy is probably adequate for the treatment of isolated seventh nerve palsy (i.e., palsy not associated with other objective neurologic findings or with abnormalities of the spinal fluid); we recommend that all patients with seventh nerve palsy thought to be due to LD have a spinal fluid analysis in order to detect CNS infection or inflammation, which would then require intravenous therapy. Meningitis and other neurologic features of early, disseminated LD should probably be treated intravenously.

Some LD researchers suggest that first-degree AV block can be treated with oral therapy and that patients with more advanced degrees of block should receive parenteral therapy, although no controlled studies have ever addressed this issue. If the patient is symptomatic from the heart block, a temporary pacemaker may be needed. In such cases, admission to a hospital is warranted, and we would suggest intravenous therapy in such cases—treatment can be concluded at home once the patient is cleared for discharge.

Heart block is almost always reversible, even without antibiotics. There have been a few reports suggesting that *B. burgdorferi* infection can be the cause of a chronic congestive cardiomyopathy, which, in a few cases, has been resolved with intravenous antibiotic therapy. Heart block usually resolves entirely, although there have been a handful of cases of high-degree heart block that have not resolved after antibiotics and a number of patients whose high-degree heart block resolved, but who had first-degree atrioventricular block persist thereafter.

At least one study suggests that Lyme arthritis responds very well to oral therapy with amoxicillin with probenecid, although others have expressed concern that in such a case, oral therapy may not be adequate to treat possible subclinical dissemination to the CNS. The current recommendation for ter-tiary neuroborreliosis is intravenous therapy, although this suggestion has not been subjected to scientific testing (Table 13.3).

Management of Intravenous Therapy at Home

Intravenous therapy for LD can be given by home infusion service, although the first dose should be given in a doctor's office or emergency room to monitor for immediate adverse reactions and to properly manage a possible anaphylactic reaction. In addition, such a setting is more conducive to teaching the patient and family about how to manage the intravenous line and administer the drug. If the patient is admitted for LD, therapy can be started in the hospital and continued at home.

Intravenous therapy is given for 2 to 4 weeks, although in many communities 4 weeks is the standard. Thus, it is impractical to use a butterfly catheter, which by its very nature will require frequent changing. It is the habit of many infusion companies to use a PICC (peripherally inserted central catheter) line to minimize the number of times the line must be replaced. Our experience has been that these lines are very well tolerated and are very effective. However, there is a potential risk of thrombophlebitis. There is generally no need to use permanent indwelling catheters, since the duration of therapy is relatively short.

Axillary vein thrombosis may occur in patients with indwelling long catheters, so axillary pain and swelling must be evaluated. Pain, redness, and swelling at the site of insertion should raise the possibility of phlebitis or soft-tissue infection. If there is any doubt, evaluation by the clinician is mandated; rapid removal of any infected line is recommended.

The standard agents for intravenous therapy are the third-generation cephalosporins, ceftriaxone (Rocephin) and cefotaxime (Claforan). Home management must include weekly complete blood counts (bone marrow suppression is a known toxicity of these agents, although elevated lymphocyte or platelet counts are rarely seen). Ceftriaxone can form a sludge within the biliary system, and stone formation has been reported with this agent as well. Thus, any patient receiving ceftriaxone who reports abdominal pain must be evaluated for possible biliary disease.

Even if the patient is asymptomatic, liver function tests should be performed on a weekly basis in patients receiving home therapy with the third-generation cephalosporins. Sludging and stones from ceftriaxone both resolve upon discontinuation of ceftriaxone. There is no reason for performing cholecystectomy in such patients, although there are now many reports of such procedures being done to allow therapy for Lyme disease to continue. The unfortunate truth is that, of patients having this surgery, researchers were almost uniformly unable to confirm the diagnosis of Lyme disease! If biliary problems develop in a patient receiving ceftriaxone, one might consider completing the course of therapy with cefotaxime.

Other potential side effects or toxicities of intravenous cephalosporins include rash, headache and/or dizziness, interstitial nephritis, moniliasis, vaginitis, diarrhea (occasionally due to pseudomembranous colitis), and Coombs positivity, with occasional hemolytic anemia. All of these should be kept in mind as therapy continues. Even mild to moderate diarrhea should not be ignored—pseudomembranous colitis may be mild at first.

The current vogue in some circles of prophylactic treatment with antifungals should be strongly discouraged. Of note is the fact that prepubertal females do not experience vaginal candidiasis, even after or while receiving broad-spectrum antibiotics.

The clinician must keep in mind that some of these side effects (e.g., headache and dizziness) are often thought to be due to the underlying Lyme disease. It is crucial that the treating physician have a close working relationship with the nursing service managing the intravenous infusion. Written nursing reports as well as laboratory review are key elements of the prudent management of such patients.

Some clinicians have become convinced that patients under their care have chronic LD that has not responded to the standard care described. They then turn to the use of other agents for the treatment of "resistant LD." There is no proven role for the use of imipenem-cilastatin (Primaxin), ceftazidime (Fortaz), vancomycin (Vancocin), or ampicillin in the intravenous therapy of LD, although all have been pressed into service in the treatment of such presumed "resistant LD." Any patient not responding to standard therapy should be reevaluated and referred to an academic center doing research on LD before further therapy is given.

In cases where long-term therapy is given for vague complaints thought to be related to chronic LD, the patient experiences no long-lasting benefit, but toxicity and expense mount. None of these alternative agents has been tested and none should be used in place of the third-generation cephalosporins mentioned earlier.

If the patient has a well-described allergy to the cephalosporins, alternative drugs include intravenous ampicillin, chloramphenicol, or doxycycline. None of the other agents being touted will be discussed here in detail. One exception to this is the recent vogue of using vancomycin. There is an increasing problem with methicillin-resistant staphylococcus developing resistance to vancomycin as well. This process will only be hastened by the indiscriminate use of vancomycin in the treatment of "resistant" LD.

The major cause of lack of response to standard antibiotic therapy is that the initial diagnosis was an error or that intercurrent disease—not persistent, resistant, or chronic LD—is the cause of the ongoing problems. Administering further intravenous therapy or changing agents is usually not warranted. If a patient with LD has seemingly "failed" on intravenous therapy, we would suggest referral to an academic center where current research is being done on LD.

Some clinicians are using agents not tested for Lyme disease and of no proven efficacy. The use of these novel agents must be considered experimental. Their use should be accompanied by informed consent based on a protocol approved by the local Institutional

Review Board. Subjecting patients to such experimental regimens is unethical and should not be tolerated.

There is no evidence to suggest that oral therapy following intravenous therapy hastens the resolution of LD, nor that such practice increases the ultimate cure rate. Likewise, there is no evidence in favor of more prolonged or higher-dose treatment. One recent fad is "pulse therapy": one day of intravenous therapy per week. This practice is based on scant anecdotal evidence and is to be avoided. All of these novel approaches to the treatment of LD must be considered experimental. Their use should be accompanied by informed consent based on a protocol approved by the local Institutional Review Board. Subjecting patients to such experimental regimens is unethical and should not be tolerated.

The current recommendation in late disease is usually for 4 weeks of therapy. Some clinicians suggest more and/or longer therapy to suppress chronic infection. Implicit in their reasoning is the belief that the organism cannot be totally eradicated and the infection can never be cured. There are many examples of patients being treated by well-intentioned clinicians for LD for years when the patient had another, noninfectious explanation for the active medical problem. It is worth restating that the major cause of lack of response to standard antibiotic therapy is that the initial diagnosis was an error or that intercurrent disease, not persistent LD, is the cause of the ongoing problems.

Longer-duration therapy must also be considered to be an experimental approach to the treatment of LD and should be accompanied by informed consent based on a protocol approved by the local Institutional Review Board. If your patient is not improving after appropriate antimicrobial therapy, reconsider the diagnosis of LD. If you think that LD is the explanation, consultation as above is probably warranted.

One often overlooked side effect of such long-term therapy is the fact that these patients come to believe that they have a chronic, permanent infection that will never get better. This belief leads to anxiety, depression, despair, and the permanent assumption of "the sick role." Such crippling evades easy quantification but is nonetheless very real.

Approach to "Chronic Lyme Disease"

There is no evidence that *B. burgdorferi* is resistant to any of the standard antimicrobial agents mentioned in Table 13.3. The concerns about persisting LD are often based on:

- Persistence of seropositivity (which may continue for years and is *not* a marker of ongoing infection),
- Persistence of vague symptoms (which may indicate slow resolution of LD or intercurrent illness), or
- Onset of new complaints (which may suggest intercurrent illness—e.g., fibromyalgia or sleep disorder—but is also compatible with the possibility that prior therapy has not cured the infection). Such complaints require reevaluation of the patient.

When should the clinician be concerned about possible ongoing infection?

1. If follow-up serologic testing of a patient with later-stage disease shows an expansion of the immunologic repertoire, as demonstrated by new proteins being recognized by serum antibodies on the immunoblot.
2. If there is a new area of inflammatory disease, supported by **objective findings,** not merely new subjective complaints.
3. If there is evolution to a later feature of LD; e.g., your patient with carditis is treated with 3 weeks of intravenous antibiotics and then develops arthritis (true inflammation of a joint, not merely arthralgia, joint pain, or soreness, proven to be due to *B. burgdorferi*).
4. If there is worsening in objective markers of organ damage or dysfunction (e.g., neuropsychologic testing, brain MRI).

Pediatric Lyme Disease

Pediatric LD is somewhat different from the manifestations seen in adults. Children have a lower incidence of carditis, and in early disseminated LD neurologic disease, children more often get meningitis than radiculitis. Adults more often get radiculitis than meningitis. Treatment for children is the same as for adults, with the exception that the doses must be modified for small children and one would not use doxycycline for children below the age of 8. Children often recover faster than adults.

Pregnancy Complicated by Lyme Disease

Therapy for LD during pregnancy should be as is appropriate for the features of LD. Some clinicians treat all such women parenterally, although this practice is without proven benefit. Doxycycline obviously should not be used during pregnancy. Despite older anecdotal studies suggesting that pregnancy complicated by LD commonly results in miscarriage or fetal anomalies, there is no proof of such an association. A survey of pediatric neurologists done at the University of Connecticut was unable to identify a "congenital Lyme disease syndrome" analogous with that of congenital syphilis. Our experience and the experience of other research centers is that such pregnancies, if treated appropriately, result in normal and unaffected babies. We have yet to identify anti–*B. burgdorferi* IgM (which would indicate in utero infection) in cord blood of such infants.

Current studies suggest that the risk of contracting LD from a known tick bite is very small, especially if the tick is attached for 24 hours or less; and, if the tick is not engorged, the risk is probably as little as 1%. Thus, prophylactic therapy is not currently recommended. If the tick that bit your patient is fully engorged and has been attached for more than 48 to 72 hours, the risk of contracting LD is greater, and prophylaxis may be of value. Many clinicians will consider the degree of patient anxiety in their decision concerning prophylaxis and will offer prophylaxis with amoxicillin to any pregnant female with a tick bite.

Synopsis

LD is a tick-borne spirochetosis capable of causing many clinical problems within a well-defined clinical spectrum. Employing accepted clinical criteria and judicious use of the specific serologic tests to confirm the diagnosis allows one to make a confident diagnosis. LD almost always responds to the standard forms of therapy noted in Table 13.3, although resolution of all symptoms may be delayed. Four weeks of intravenous antibiotics is usually effective in the treatment of later features of LD, although, especially in tertiary neuroborreliosis, the response may be very gradual and delayed. There is no reason to routinely treat with a longer course of intravenous antibiotics than 4 weeks. However, on rare occasions, longer therapy may be considered.

A variety of novel approaches to the treatment of LD have been proposed by "Lyme disease experts" in the community. None of these approaches, briefly described in the text, have been subjected to scientific analysis for safety or efficacy. Often, these different approaches are based on the belief that the organism cannot be killed—that the disease can only be brought into remission, never cured. There is no evidence in favor of this belief system.

The clinician treating LD may be confronted by anxious patients prepared with educational materials, some of which are in error. It is best for the clinician to be well informed about the disease and to teach the patient and family about the disease and what to expect regarding the natural history of treated LD. Finally, if the patient does not respond as anticipated to antibiotic therapy, the astute clinician will be prepared to reconsider the veracity of the original diagnosis, rather than simply giving more antibiotics.

Suggested Readings

Dressler F, Whalen JA, Reinhardt BN, Steere AC. Western blotting in the serodiagnosis of Lyme disease. J Infect Dis 1993;167:392–400.

Karlsson M, Hammers-Berggren, Lindquist L, Stiernstedt G, Svenungsson B. Comparison of intravenous penicillin G and oral doxycycline for treatment of Lyme neuroborreliosis. Neurology 1994;44:1203–1207.

Lightfoot RW Jr, Luft BJ, Rahn DW, Steere AC, Sigal LH, Zoschke DC, Gardner P, Britton MC, Kaufman RL. Treatment of "possible Lyme disease." A practical policy position of the American College of Rheumatology and the Infectious Disease Society of America based on cost-benefit analysis. Ann Intern Med. 1993;119:503–509.

Rahn DW, Malawista SE. Lyme disease: recommendations for diagnosis and treatment. Ann Intern Med 1991;114:472–481.

Shapiro ED, Gerber MA, Holabird NB, Berg AT, Feder HM, Bell GL, Rhys PN, Persing DH. A controlled trial of antimicrobial prophylaxis for Lyme disease after deer-tick bite. N Engl J Med 1992;327:1769–1773.

Sigal LH. Current drug therapy recommendations for the treatment of Lyme disease. Drugs 1992;43:683–699.

Sigal LH, Academy of Medicine of New Jersey Lyme Disease Task Force. Lyme Disease in New Jersey: A practical guide for New Jersey Clinicians. 1993.

Sigal LH. Who should be tested and treated for Lyme disease and how? In: Sergent J, Panush R, eds. Controversies in Clinical Rheumatology—Rheumatic Disease Clinics of North America. 1993;19:79–93.

Sigal LH. Persisting complaints attributed to Lyme disease: possible mechanisms and implications for management. Am J Med 1994;96:365–374.

Sigal LH. Editorial: The polymerase chain reaction assay for *Borrelia burgdorferi* in the diagnosis of Lyme disease. Ann Intern Med 1994;120:520–521.

Sigal LH, ed. National Clinical Conference on Lyme Disease. Am J Med 1995;97(Suppl 4A):1S–91S.

Sigal LH. The Lyme disease controversy: the social and financial costs of mis-diagnosis and mis-management. Arch Intern Med 1996 (in press).

Steere AC. Lyme disease. N Engl J Med 1989;321:586–596.

14

HOME INFUSIONS OF INTRAVENOUS IMMUNOGLOBULIN

Leonard Bielory and Grace Cumming Long

CHAPTER AT A GLANCE: Intravenous immunoglobulin (IVIG) is being prescribed for an increasing number of conditions. IVIG can be given safely in the home if (*a*) medical condition warrants; (*b*) patient specificity as to dose, frequency, and rate is determined; (*c*) an adequate caregiver is available; and (*d*) the home environment is suitable. Good medical practice includes (*a*) therapeutic decisions based on knowledge of the properties of different IVIG products; (*b*) concerns about the social impact of choosing the home (rather than an ambulatory care facility) for therapy; (*c*) attention to the needs of family members or caregivers; (*d*) efforts to control costs by comparative pricing and wise negotiations; and (*e*) careful monitoring for specific patient response to therapy.

Introduction

Advances in homecare technology (1, 2) and immunotherapy, together with improvements in γ-globulin preparations, have led to increasing utilization of home administration of intravenous immunoglobulin (IVIG). IVIG was developed in 1981 as replacement therapy for patients with primary humoral immunodeficiency disorders, but currently is also being used for management of secondary immunodeficiency caused by AIDS, premature birth, chronic lymphocytic leukemia, lymphoma, bone marrow transplantation, and severe burns. In addition, IVIG is being utilized with varying degrees of effectiveness for immunomodulation in a wide array of autoimmune conditions, such as Kawasaki's syndrome and immune-mediated diseases of the nervous system (3–5). Figure 14.1 lists some of the disorders for which IVIG therapy is currently being used.

In primary and secondary immunodeficiency disorders, the principal goal of IVIG therapy is to provide sufficient antibodies to prevent life-threatening infections that often require extensive hospitalizations and aggressive antibiotic regimens (11–13). Immunomodulation therapy for autoimmune disorders moderates or interrupts the immune system's attack of host tissues. The mechanisms by which IVIG modulates autoimmune conditions are not yet fully understood (10, 12, 27, 28, 36–38).

PRIMARY IMMUNODEFICIENCY DISORDERS MANAGED BY IVIG REPLACEMENT THERAPY
INCLUDE (6–14):
    Common variable immunodeficiency (all immunoglobulins decreased)
    Severe combined immunodeficiency (all immunoglobulins decreased and T-cell dysfunction)
    X-linked agammaglobulinemia (all immunoglobulins decreased)
    Wiskott-Aldrich syndrome (IgM decreased, T-cell dysfunction, IgA and IgE elevated)
    Ataxia-telangiectasia (increased IgM and decreased IgA, IgE, and IgG)
    Immunodeficiency with elevated IgM (IgG and IgA decreased)
SECONDARY IMMUNODEFICIENCY CONDITIONS TREATED WITH IVIG PROPHYLAXIS INCLUDE
(6, 7, 11, 12, 15–26):
    Malignancies:
        Multiple myeloma
        Chronic lymphocytic leukemia (CLL)
        Small cell carcinoma of the lung
        Non-Hodgkin's lymphoma and leukemia in children
    Chemotherapy and radiation-produced immunodeficiencies
    Bone marrow transplantation
    HIV infections
    Premature births and neonatal infections
    Severe burns
AUTOIMMUNE DISORDERS MANAGED BY IMMUNOMODULATION WITH IVIG THERAPY
INCLUDE (10–12, 20, 27–35):
    Kawasaki's syndrome
    Diseases of the nervous system:
        Guillain-Barré syndrome
        Chronic inflammatory demyelinating polyneuropathy (CIDP)
        Autoimmune neutropenia
        Myasthenia gravis
    Hematological disorders:
        Idiopathic thrombocytopenia purpura (ITP)
        Autoimmune hemolytic anemia
    Recurrent spontaneous abortion (antiphospolipid antibody syndrome)

Figure 14.1.   Immunotherapy with IVIG.

The U.S. Food and Drug Administration (FDA) has approved most IVIG products marketed in the United States for use in primary immunodeficiency disorders and idiopathic thrombocytopenic purpura (ITP). Manufacturers have obtained approval of their product for other specific purposes; for example, Baxter Healthcare Corporation received FDA approval for prophylactic use of their Gammagard IVIG product for patients with chronic lymphocytic leukemia (CLL) (39).

The National Institutes of Health (NIH) have supported somewhat wider applications of IVIG therapy. An NIH Consensus Statement was issued in 1990 supporting IVIG replacement therapy for most primary immun-odeficiency diseases and for immunomodulation in selected secondary immunodeficiencies and autoimmune disorders (Table 14.1). Additional successful uses of IVIG are being reported in professional journals and conferences (5). After further studies are completed to supplement preliminary clinical information, it is likely that the scientific community will agree that additional applications of IVIG are medically indicated. The high costs and limited availability of IVIG, however, probably prohibit broadly based double-blind studies such as those required by the FDA for multiple applications of a therapeutic substance previously approved for specific purposes. For this reason, consensus conferences such as the one

Table 14.1. 1990 NIH Consensus Re: Efficacy of IVIG Therapy[a]

Immune Disorders	Supported	Need More Studies	Not Recommended
Primary immunodeficiencies	Common variable immunodeficiency Severe combined immunodeficiency X-linked agammaglobulinemia Wiskott-Aldrich syndrome Ataxia-telangiectasia Immunodeficiency with elevated IgM		
Secondary immunodeficiencies	Chronic lymphocytic leukemia (CLL) Bone marrow transplantation	HIV infections (pediatric)	Premature births and neonatal infections
Autoimmune disorders	Kawasaki's syndrome Chronic inflammatory demyelinating polyneuropathy (CIDP) Adult idiopathic thrombocytopenic purpura (ITP)	Guillain-Barré syndrome	Pediatric idiopathic thrombocytopenic purpura (ITP)

[a]Data from National Institutes of Health (NIH) Consensus Development Conference. Intravenous immunoglobulin: prevention and treatment of disease. JAMA 1990;264(24):3189–3193.

held in May 1990 by the NIH, and published reports of limited studies in refereed journals, are vitally important.

Description and Dosage of IVIG

γ-Globulin replacement therapy, utilized since 1952 (3, 39), originally required subcutaneous or intramuscular administration, which was painful and not conducive to large doses (7, 11, 13, 40–45). In 1981, intravenous γ-globulin (IVIG) was introduced. IVIG, a reduced and alkylated product with a half-life of 21 or more days, contains the antibodies produced by the humoral immune system and extracted from human plasma. Derived from healthy donors who are screened for hepatitis and human immunodeficiency virus (HIV) infections, the plasma is subjected to extraction and purification methods that isolate the antibody fraction and inactivate HIV and hepatitis B (6, 7, 9, 11–13, 42–43, 46).

Initially, IVIG was believed to be a safe therapy without hazards of infection or serious side effects (11, 13, 45). Recently, however, hepatitis C infections have been reported in patients receiving IVIG. Methods of plasma screening and IVIG preparation are being scrutinized carefully, and only further studies can ascertain the actual risks of transmitting infectious agents (47–51). IVIG may not be as free of complications as initially believed, either. Transient renal failure has been observed in patients receiving IVIG (52). Nevertheless, IVIG continues to be used with confidence and should not be neglected as a viable and safe therapy for many immune disorders. Despite present concerns that IVIG may not be free of side effects and risks, its record of more than a decade of relatively safe and largely effective use speaks for itself. As with any therapy, however, physicians should be alert to unanticipated complications.

At present, nine IVIG preparations are approved and available in the United States: Venoglobulin-I and Venoglobulin-S (Alpha), Gammar IV (Armour), Polygam (Hyland/American Red Cross), Gammagard (Hyland Division of Baxter Therapeutics), Iveegam (Immuno U.S.), Gamimune N (Miles/Cutter), Sandoglobulin (Sandoz), and Cytogram (Massachusetts Public Health Biologic Laboratories). Table 14.2 outlines pertinent information about IVIG that, for the most part, can be found in manufacturers' package inserts. γ-Globulin for intravenous use is packaged in varying doses, ranging from 0.5 to 20 g and in either liquid or lyophilized powder forms. Liquid forms need no preparation. Lyophilized IVIG requires reconstitution with accompanying sterile diluent and cannot be stored after it is reconstituted. Other variations in IVIG depend on how many donors constitute the plasma pool, the particular methods used in preparation, and the constituents of the finished product (6, 7, 9, 11–13, 42–43).

Pharmacokinetics of IVIG vary somewhat according to the product, as indicated by Table 14.2. Generally, an immediate rise in serum immunoglobulin level occurs. Thereafter, the initial serum level increase is depleted due to a distribution phase when the immunoglobulin is cleared from the intravascular space. About 72 hours after the infusion, only about half of the increased serum level remains due to redistribution, use of the globulins, clearance, catabolism, or a composite of the actions described above. Catabolism of immunoglobulin occurs largely in the plasma. IVIG manufacturers report that the half-life of their products is 21 days or more, which parallels the half-life of indigenous IgG. The actual rate of immunoglobulin elimination is relative to the immunoglobulin class/subclass, the disease state for which the immunotherapy is employed, and the patient (8, 11, 13, 53).

Specific characteristics of an IVIG product may have important therapeutic ramifications. For instance, a product with very low IgA content is needed to prevent serious allergic reactions in patients with antibodies to IgA. Diabetics may require a preparation without glucose, or even without sugar. Patients with marginal renal sufficiency or inadequate cardiac function may tolerate some IVIG products more readily than others (54). Table 14.2 provides some of the information that physicians should consider to determine the most suitable IVIG product for a particular patient; but updates in IVIG products and increasing information about possible side effects necessitate investigation into the properties and actions of a particular IVIG brand at the time of therapeutic decisions.

Dosage of IVIG is determined by the patient's body weight, disease condition, and therapeutic response. Generally, primary and secondary immunodeficiency diseases are treated with a dose of 100 to 600 mg/kg every 3 to 4 weeks. Autoimmune diseases may respond to doses ranging from 400 mg/kg to 4 g/kg administered over a period of 1 to 5 days every 2 to 12 weeks (6, 10–13, 18, 27, 28, 32–34). The patient specificity of both replacement and modulation therapy requires careful attention by healthcare personnel, patient, and family to determine the best dosage and schedule (11, 13).

Requiring equally careful attention to a specific patient's needs is the rate of infusion that can be tolerated without serious side effects. The first infusion should be given under close medical supervision, since most anaphylactic reactions—manifesting as anxiety, nausea, malaise, dyspnea, facial swelling, flushing, cyanosis, and hypotension—occur at that time. Anaphylactic reactions may be associated with IgA deficiency or common variable immunodeficiency, conditions that may result from antibodies against IgA. If no complications occur at the time of the introductory infusion, the likelihood of additional non-anaphylactic reactions (chills, nausea, vomiting, fatigue, headache, backache, and fever) accompanying IVIG infusions is usually less than 5% and can be eliminated or markedly reduced by slowing the rate of administration (7, 11, 13, 43, 55). Some patients tolerate rapid infusions of IVIG, which have been found to be safe and effective. For other patients the therapy must be given slowly, and large doses

Table 14.2. Comparison of IVIG Products[a]

Name	Venoglobulin-I	Venoglobulin-S	Gammagard	Polygam	Gamimune N	Gammar I.V.	Iveegam	Sandoglobulin	Cytogam
Manufacturer	Alpha Therapeutic Corporation		Baxter/Hyland	Hyland/ American Red Cross	Cutter/Miles	Armour	Immuno AG	Sandoz	Mass. Public Health Biologic Labs./ MedImmune
Indications	Primary immunodeficiencies, ITP		Primary immunodeficiencies, ITP, CLL		Primary immuno-deficiencies, ITP, pediatric HIV, GVHD, BMT	Primary immuno-deficiencies	Primary immuno-deficiencies, KS	Primary immuno-deficiencies, ITP	CMV prophylaxis in kidney transplanta tion
Contra-indications	IgA deficiency with antibodies to IgA		None; caution with IgA deficiency		IgA deficiency with antibodies to IgA	IgA deficiency with antibodies to IgA	IgA deficiency with antibodies to IgA	IgA deficiency with antibodies to IgA	IgA deficiency with antibodies to IgA
Plasma source	6000–9000 donors, plasmapheresis	>10,000 donors, plasmapheresis	10,000 donors, plasmapheresis	Volunteer donors via American Red Cross	>2000 donors	>8000 donors, plasmapheresis	>6000 donors, plasmapheresis	>16,000 voluntary donors	2000–5000 donors; top 5% CMV titers selected
Method of preparation	Cold alcohol fractionation, PEG, ion-exchange chromotography; Veno-S receives added solvent detergent treatment		Cohn-Oncley, ultrafiltration, ion-exchange chromatography, solvent detergent treatment		Cohn-Oncley, pH 4.25 + low salt	Cohn-Oncley, ultra-filtration	Cold ethanol, PEG, trypsin	Cold alcohol fractionation, pH 4.0 + trace pepsin	Cohn-Oncley, ultra-filtration
Immune globulin properties include:									
% Gammaglobulin	>97	≥99		>90	>98	>98	100	>96	99
% Monomers	>95			95	>95	>98	93.8	92	
IgG_1%	60.9	65.7–67.2		67	60.0	69	64.1	60.5	65
IgG_2%	29.4	23.7–25.3		25	29.4	23	30.3	30.2	28
IgG_3%	5.3	5.7–5.9		5	6.5	6	0	6.6	5.2
IgG_4%	4.4	3.0–3.4		3	4.1	2	1.5	2.8	1.7
IgA content	24 µg/mL	15.1 µg/mL		<3.7 µg/mL	270 µg/mL	25 µg/mL	<2.0%	720 µg/mL	0.03–0.20 mg/mL
IgM content	<11.1 µg/mL			<40 µg/mL	trace	<100 µg/mL	trace	<20 µg/mL	trace
Half-life	29 ± 7.6 days	33.5 ± 7 days		24 days	21 days	21 days	23–29 days	21 days	24 days[b]

Table 14.2—*Continued*

Name	Venoglobulin-I	Venoglobulin-S	Gammagard	Polygam	Gamimune N	Gammar I.V.	Iveegam	Sandoglobulin	Cytogam
Other pharmaceutical properities include:									
pH (after reconstitution)	6.8	5.2–5.8	6.8		4.25	7.0	7.0	6.6	5.5
Sugar content	2.0% D-mannitol	5.0% D-sorbitol		2% glucose	(5%) 10% maltose/ (10%) no sugar, glycine based	5.0% Sucrose	5.0% Glucose	5% Sucrose	5% Sucrose
Sodium content (at 5% concentration)	0.5%	1.3 mEq/L		0.85%	Trace	0.5%	0.3%	0%–0.9% depending on diluent	
Purchase/policies information includes:									
Supply (g)	2.5, 5.0, 10.0	2.5, 5.0, 10.0	0.5, 2.5, 5.0, 10.0	2.5, 5.0, 10.0	(5%) 0.5, 2.5, 5.0, 12.5/(10%) 5.0, 10.0, 20.0	1.0, 2.5, 5.0, 10.0, and bulk packages	0.5, 1.0, 2.5, 5.0	1.0, 3.0, 6.0, 12.0, and bulk packages	2.5
Form Storage	Lyophilized <30°C [86°F]	Liquid ≤25°C [77°F]	Lyophilized <25°C [77°F]		Liquid Refrigerate; do not freeze	Lyophilized <30°C [86°F]	Lyophilized Refrigerate 2°C–8°C	Lyophilized 25°C [77°F]	Lyophilized 2°C–8°C
Shelf life	24 months		27 months		24 months	24 months	24 months	36 months	
Return policy warranty	Shipping error, defective or damaged product; NOT out-of-date product.		No		Limited	Limited	Limited	Yes	Out-of-date product only
24-Hour Emerg. Service	Cost; unless orders >60 g, free or upon approval		Free		Cost	Free	Free	Free	

^aInformation obtained from manufacturers' package inserts and Siegel J. Intravenous immune globulins: therapeutic, pharmaceutical and cost considerations. Pharmacy Practice News, December 1994. Reprinted 1995 by the McMahon Group, New York.
^bHalf-life of Cytogam is 8 days post-op; 24 days if ≥60 days post-op.

might take up to 12 or more hours in a day (56, 57). Manufacturers advise a very slow infusion rate for 15 to 30 minutes, followed by a gradual increase to a maintenance infusion rate. Clinical experience indicates that during the first infusion a tolerable rate can be ascertained, but attention to a patient's continued symptoms may necessitate lowering the rate or allow a faster rate for the infusions.

With attention to patient response to therapy for determining dosage, frequency, and rate of infusion, follow-up IVIG can be given safely and effectively in the home by a registered nurse, a family member who has received appropriate training and initial supervision, the patient (but only if a competent care partner is available throughout the duration of the procedure), or some combination of the three. A survey of 25 home infusion companies in northern and central New Jersey, conducted primarily for reasons of comparative pricing of IVIG, revealed additional information about home infusion nursing policies. Some infusion companies require the nurse to remain with the patient for the duration of the IVIG infusion, whereas others vary nursing assistance and supervision according to patient and family needs and medical guidance (58). Due to the length of time between treatments, however, IVIG infusions rarely require an indwelling venous access device. So if nursing assistance is not available at least at the beginning of each infusion, or series of infusions, then the patient or a family member will have to become skilled in placement of a temporary venous catheter. Patient or family responsibility for the infusions has been shown to be medically prudent and cost effective, but physician liability and insurance coverage may create barriers to such measures (59–64).

In addition to medical guidance and nursing supervision, and the requirement that a competent care partner be with the patient for the duration of the therapy when a nurse is not on the site, other safety factors apply in home infusions of IVIG. If refrigerated storage of IVIG is necessary, then electricity and adequate refrigeration space and temperatures are important considerations.

Room temperatures for storage of nonrefrigerated IVIG must also be considered. Some homes without air conditioning have room temperatures near or even above 90°F during the summer, and none of the brands approved for use in the United States (see Table 14.2) can tolerate such heat. Even though IVIG can be given without an infusion pump by using a drip count method to adjust the rate, most home infusion companies prefer to use the pump. Thus electricity would be needed even if neither refrigeration nor air conditioning is an important factor. Running water, generally sanitary conditions, and—without exception—a telephone on the premises are additional requirements for safe administration of IVIG in the home.

Advantages/Disadvantages of Home Infusions

For many patients, home infusion therapy with IVIG is a viable alternative to the same therapy obtained through either hospitalization or an ambulatory care facility. Figure 14.2 lists patients who are likely to benefit from homecare for their IVIG infusions. Home infusions, however, are not the best option for every patient or family. High-tech homecare may violate the privacy of home, tether family members to the patient in ways that are socially and economically questionable, or otherwise disrupt family roles and relationships in unhealthy ways (65).

Three cases illustrate some of the advantages and disadvantages of home infusions of IVIG.

CASE REPORT 1

E.J., a 4-year-old with a primary immunodeficiency disease, was repeatedly hospitalized with life-threatening infections before his immune status was diagnosed. His mother recalls that every time he went to the doctor's office for a well-baby checkup he "caught" an infection that resulted in prolonged antibiotic therapy and frequently led to hospitalization,

> Patients with immune deficiency conditions who are at increased risk of infections from multiple contacts in hospitals or ambulatory care facilities.
>
> Children with any immune disorder if their condition warrants and a caretaker can cope.
>
> Patients with marked infirmities that make transportation painful, complex, or too expensive.
>
> Patients who do not match the above criteria but who live in communities greatly removed from ambulatory care facilities and do not need hospitalization.

Figure 14.2. Patients for whom home IVIG therapy can be beneficial.

which he grew to fear and hate. For the past 2 years a nurse has come to his home to administer IVIG replacement therapy every 3 weeks. Earlier, she simply carried the infusion around to allow the child mobility for the prolonged infusion. Now he wears his infusion paraphernalia in a backpack, and his mother is learning to take expanded responsibility for his care. He is able to maintain a relatively normal life except during the half-day infusions, and his mother is comfortable with the fact that her neighbors know about his condition due to the regular visits of the homecare personnel. He has not had to be hospitalized for an infection since soon after the infusion therapy was initiated.

CASE REPORT 2

B.K., who has myasthenia gravis, responded well to IVIG therapy during a myasthenic crisis. As a result, he completed high school and now attends the local community college with the use of his motorized wheelchair and the assistance of local transportation for persons with disabilities. His parents have a van to accommodate his wheelchair, and if he lived in a different location, he would be a good candidate for an ambulatory care infusion center. But the closest such resource is 150 miles away at the medical center where his physician practices. B.K. is exhausted by the trip he has to take every 6 months for medical evaluation, and both his parents work outside the home in hourly employment and have to lose a day's wages each time they drive him to the medical center. B.K. receives both periodic home infusions of IVIG and also nursing assessment and liaison with the medical center. Due to his parents' work schedules, nursing service must be provided for the entire length of the infusion, and this provides an optimum time for the nurse's evaluation, teaching, and planning. They are fortunate to have government-supplemented help for his care.

CASE REPORT 3

G.D., a semiretired college professor, suffered from an autoimmune demyelinating condition that had not responded to cortico-steroids. The condition rendered her essentially homebound without assistance. After an initial 4-day infusion in the hospital, she was discharged to homecare. With the arrival of the home infusion company's van her neighbors all became aware that she was "sick" and made the logical assumption that she was in the last stages of cancer. She received monthly 1-day infusions, which not only tethered her to a slow-rate infusion device but also required that her husband be on site for 8 to 10 hours after the nurse departed. After several months of home IVIG therapy, G.D. was able to resume a normally active life and began driving herself to a local ambulatory care facility for the infusions. Here the IVIG could be given safely in less time under close medical and nursing supervision so that her total time commitment to the procedure was half as much as with the home infusions. At the same time, her husband was released from the commitment to monitor her after the infusions.

These three cases illustrate that home infusion therapy has many advantages for some patients, but creates disadvantages for others. E.J. represents a category of patients who are best served in the home, where they are subjected to less chance of infections (66, 67) and they are not unnecessarily traumatized by the medicalization of their lives that results when receiving care in a medical center. Thus many children might be good candidates for home infusions. Furthermore, studies have indicated that children and their parents can be taught to assume the primary ongoing responsibility for the infusions, and when this can be accomplished without breaking the child's level of trust in the parents as protectors, the emotional and financial costs of the prolonged therapy can be reduced considerably (59, 60, 68).

B.K. represents another category of persons for whom home infusions might be the better approach. Any patient who is wasted from disease or whose location is a great distance from medical services may benefit from home infusions. If a patient's condition requires that someone else transport him, then that cost also needs to be factored into the equation when deciding whether a home or an outpatient infusion is the better choice.

Many adults with primary or secondary immunodeficiency diseases also are likely to be good candidates for home infusions of IVIG, and might well take large measures of responsibility for their own care (61–64). This would lessen their exposure to infections and also reduce the medicalization of life that comes with any chronic disease over time. For the same reasons that G.D. found more privacy and freedom for herself and her family with ambulatory care, however, adults who are not homebound due to their health status may opt not to have home healthcare until or unless absolutely necessary. For instance, because of widespread ignorance and intolerance about HIV infections, persons living with AIDS might find the anonymity of medical facilities preferable to home infusions as long as they can maintain some semblance of "health."

All three cases call to our attention the reality that chronic illnesses usually involve family members or other care partners in patient care and disease management. Therefore, decisions about when, where, and how therapy can best be accomplished must consider more than the patient and his or her medical condition. For E.J.'s mother, involvement in his infusion therapy is merely an extension of her daily commitment to his needs as a young child. Nevertheless, women are often exploited due to a family member's need for home healthcare. Wives, mothers, or daughters may have to give up a career or a social life that could have been continued if the family member did not require intensive homecare (69, 70). B.K.'s working-class parents present other issues for families with a member receiving high-tech homecare for chronic illness. They could not be expected to further jeopardize their family's limited economic status for either repeated trips to facilities located some distance from the home or for supervision of home infusions. Furthermore, there may be other children in such a family that need some of the time, energy, and resources that would be expended if the infusions were not done in the home with the nurse present. G.D.'s husband was expected to make a major commitment of time for her monthly infusions. Even though he consented to the arrangement, after she became free to go to the medical center he confessed his sense of inadequacy in taking the role of medical-nursing supervisor and resented the high cost of the care when she and he had to provide so much of it themselves.

Home infusions of IVIG can be life-saving, life-enhancing, or the only viable alternative. But they also can create family difficulties and violate the privacy of home. Even though IVIG need not be given in the hospital, neither is it necessary to provide it in the home. IVIG can be provided by physicians in their offices, by hospitals as part of their outpatient infusion services, and by infusion companies who offer both home infusions and ambulatory care infusion centers to meet diverse patient needs. Families and patients who reside near such ambulatory facilities may have multiple options.

The Cost Factors

Thus far we have considered medical, technical, and social factors involved in home infusions of IVIG. Cost factors should also be considered. Homecare for IVIG infusions is not necessarily less expensive than the same care provided in the hospital or in an ambulatory care facility. Studies have shown that the opposite is just as likely to be the case. Numerous research and analysis projects over the past three decades have evaluated costs and effectiveness of homecare compared to other alternatives and have found that for most patients home healthcare has been more costly and has not improved the well-being or life expectancy of the patient (71, 72). These studies, done largely to determine the cost-effectiveness and health impact of homecare for aging and chronically ill patients, should provoke physicians to consider carefully whether home infusions of IVIG for chronically ill patients can be justified in every instance.

Studies of IVIG home infusion costs, conducted by the authors in 1992 and 1993, showed that the primary reason IVIG home infusions may cost just as much as or more than hospital care, and more than the same therapy in an outpatient facility, is centered in exceptionally high charges for IVIG by some home infusion companies. For many patients, especially those receiving high-dose therapy for au-

toimmune disorders, the higher charges for IVIG add up to a bill that rivals or exceeds hospitalization. One patient, for example, initially received 120 g of IVIG over 4 days in a tertiary care hospital, at a cost of $14,005.30. This bill included not only the hospital's per diem, but extensive laboratory work and a minor diagnostic test for an unrelated condition. Thus the patient was shocked to receive a bill of $7,200.00 for monthly infusions of IVIG 60 g/dose in her home, where the nurse stayed for 1 to 3 hours and then left her and a care partner to monitor the situation for the 8 or more remaining hours the infusion required. Our studies comparing home infusions of IVIG with hospitalization for the same therapy demonstrated that such cases are not isolated incidences (73). Another study of IVIG charges by home infusion companies indicated that the prices set by infusion companies for IVIG have a wide range, with the highest prices being more than triple the lowest. There is also wide variation in charges for administration supplies and nursing services (58).

When a patient's particular situation seems to warrant home infusions as the most cost-effective or health-producing option, comparative pricing of IVIG, supplies, and nursing services is indicated. With such comparisons, moderately priced homecare can be arranged for persons with chronic illnesses that require lifetime management with this

Table 14.3. Procurement Costs for IVIG From One Wholesale Distributor

(Manufacturer) Brand Name	Package Size	1992 Wholesale $/gram	1992 AWP $/gram	1995 Wholesale $/gram	1995 AWP $/gram
(Alpha) Venoglobulin I	5 g	28.00	47.00	28.00	60.82
(Armour) Gammar IV	5 g	46.50	77.50	46.50	58.13
(Hyland/Baxter) Gammagard	5 g	37.00	53.60	37.00	63.60
(Miles/Cutter) Gamimune N	5 g	42.20	68.40	28.80	57.12
(Sandoz) Sandoglobulin	6 g	35.00	42.00	70.00	84.00
Averages		37.74	57.70	42.06	64.73

expensive therapy. The most important cost factor to consider is the charge for IVIG. One New Jersey wholesale drug distributor's price list has provided the information in Table 14.3 for IVIG procurement costs in 1992 and in 1995. Prices, which have risen about 9% between 1992 and 1995, are listed for comparably sized packages of the five brands this distributor carries. In Table 14.3, the "wholesale" price is the manufacturer's published charge to wholesale distributors, large pharmaceutical chains, infusion companies, and hospitals; average wholesale price (AWP) is an amount tabulated according to the average purchase price and used by Medicaid to determine coverage levels (74). Clinical practice reveals, however, that many IVIG providers purchase γ-globulin at contract prices around $25/g. This is well below the average figures shown in Table 14.3.

Knowledge of manufacturers' charges—information that some hospital pharmacies will provide to staff physicians in an effort to control healthcare costs—allows medical practitioners and their patients to compare prices of IVIG as well as quality of services in order to arrange the best homecare deal. Such investigations, together with wise negotiations, are crucial due to the high cost of IVIG, the large doses sometimes required for

immunotherapy, and often the chronic nature of the conditions for which the therapy is used. Annual limits and lifetime caps on insurance coverage and the risks of insurance cancellation due to high costs mean that physicians and their staffs should work with patients and their families to find modestly priced quality infusion services when IVIG home therapy is initiated. The high costs and high doses of IVIG offer infusion companies an unacceptable margin of profit that neither physicians nor consumers should tolerate.

Summary

Intravenous immune globulin (IVIG) immunotherapy has been found to be effective in the treatment of many primary immunodeficiencies, some secondary immunodeficiencies, and selective autoimmune disorders. When medically, socially, and financially indicated, IVIG can be given safely and effectively in the home by a professional nurse, a family member or care partner, or the patient. Due to the extraordinarily high costs of this therapy and its long-term use, however, cost factors take on particular importance, and cost control should be part of good medical practice.

References

1. Rothkopf MM, Askanazi, J, eds. Intensive Homecare. Baltimore: Williams & Wilkins, 1992.
2. Ruddick, W. Transforming homes and hospitals. Hastings Center Report 1994;24(Suppl 5):S11–S14.
3. National Institutes of Health (NIH) Consensus Development Conference. Intravenous immunoglobulin: prevention and treatment of disease. JAMA 1990;264(24):3189–3193.
4. Imbach P, ed. Immunotherapy with intravenous immunoglobulins: proceedings of a conference held at Interlaken 6–9 May 1990. San Diego: Academic Press, 1991.
5. MKSAP in the Subspecialty of Allergy and Immunology: Syllabus Review Meeting, Philadelphia, June 26–27, 1995.
6. Asselin BL. Clinical uses of intravenous immune globulin. Hospital Therapy 1990;April:479–489.
7. Berger M, Gilbert I. Role of gamma globulin. Semin Respir Infect 1989;4(4):272–283.
8. Berkman SA, Lee ML, Gale RP. Clinical uses of intravenous immunoglobulins. Ann Intern Med 1990;112:278–292.
9. Buckley RH, Schiff RI. The use of intravenous immune globulin in immunodeficiency diseases. N Engl J Med 1991;325(2):110–117.
10. Hassag A. Intravenous immunoglobulins: pharmacological aspects and therapeutic use. Vox Sang 1986;51:10–17.
11. Knapp MJ, Colburn PA. Clinical uses of intravenous immune globulin. Clin Pharm 1990;9:509–529.
12. Stiehm ER, Ashida E, Kim KS, Winston DJ, Haas A, Gale RP. Intravenous immunoglobulins as therapeutic agents. Ann Intern Med 1987;107:367–382.
13. Wordell CJ. Use of intravenous immune globulin therapy: an overview. Ann Pharmacother 1991;25:805–817.
14. Roifman CM, Lederman HM, Lavi S, et al. Benefit of intravenous IgG replacement in hypogammaglobulinemia patients with chronic sinopulmonary disease. AW J Med 1985;79:171–174.
15. Gale RP, Winston D. Intravenous immunoglobulin in bone marrow transplantation. Cancer 1991;68:1451–1453.
16. Winston DJ, Ho WG, Champlin RE. Cytomegalovirus infections after allogeneic bone marrow transplantation. Rev Infect Dis 1990;12(Suppl 7):S776–S792.

17. The National Institute of Child Health & Human Development Intravenous Immunoglobulin Study Group. Intravenous immune globulin for the prevention of bacterial infections in children with symptomatic human immunodeficiency virus infections. N Engl J Med 1991;325:73–80.

18. Yap PL, Todd AAM, Williams PE, et al. Use of intravenous immunoglobulin in acquired immune deficiency syndrome. Cancer 1991;68:1440–1450.

19. Morell A, Barandun S. Prophylactic and therapeutic use of immunoglobulin for intravenous administration in patients with secondary immunodeficiencies associated with malignancies. Pediatr Infect Dis J 1988;7: S87-S91.

20. Takeshi A, Kawasugi K. Use of intravenous immunoglobulin in various medical conditions. Cancer 1991;68:1454–1459.

21. Burgio GR. IVIG can save many preterm infants. In: Imbach P, ed. Immunotherapy with Intravenous Immunoglobulins. San Diego: Academic Press, 1991: 59–64.

22. Stiehm ER. Use of immunoglobulin therapy in secondary antibody deficiencies. In: Imbach P, ed. Immunotherapy with Intravenous Immunoglobulins. San Diego: Academic Press, 1991:115–126.

23. Munster AM. Control of infection following major burns: the immunological approach. In: Imbach P, ed. Immunotherapy with Intravenous Immunoglobulins. San Diego: Academic Press, 1991:149–163.

24. Chapel H, Griffiths H, Lee M. IVIG indication in patients with low-grade B-cell tumors. In: Imbach P, ed. Immunotherapy with Intravenous Immunoglobulins. San Diego: Academic Press, 1991:165–172.

25. Schaad UB. The role of IVIG in pediatric HIV infection. In: Imbach P, ed. Immunotherapy with Intravenous Immunoglobulins. San Diego: Academic Press, 1991:201–209.

26. Mofenson LM, Nugent R. Prophylactic immune globulin in children with HIV disease [Letter]. N Engl J Med 1995;332(11):750–751.

27. Imbach P, Barandun S, Cottier H, et al. Immunomodulation by intravenous immunoglobulin. J Pediatr Hematol Oncol 1990;12(2):134–140.

28. Schwartz SA. Intravenous immunoglobulin (IVIG) for the therapy of autoimmune disorders. J Clin Immunol 1990;10(2):81–89.

29. Ballow M. Mechanisms of action of intravenous immunoglobulin therapy and potential use in autoimmune connective tissue diseases. Cancer 1991;68: 1430–1436.

30. Shulman ST. Kawasaki disease and IVIG: what's going on here? In: Imbach P, ed. Immunotherapy with Intravenous Immunoglobulins. San Diego: Academic Press, 1991:261–268.

31. Coulam C, Peters A, McIntyre J, Faulk W. The use of IVIG for the treatment of recurrent spontaneous abortion. In: Imbach P, ed. Immunotherapy with Intravenous Immunoglobulins. San Diego: Academic Press, 1991:395–400.

32. Cook D, Dalakas M, Galdi A, Biondi D, Porter H. High-dose intravenous immunoglobulin in the treatment of demyelinating neuropathy associated with monoclonal gammopathy. Neurology 1990;40:212–214.

33. Dyck PJ. Intravenous immunoglobulin in chronic inflammatory demyelinating polyradiculoneuropathy and in neuropathy associated with IgM monoclonal gammopathy of unknown significance [Editorial]. Neurology 1990; 40:327–328.

34. van Doorn PA, Brand A, Strengers PFW, Meulstee J, Vermeulen M. High-dose intravenous immunoglobulin treatment in chronic inflammatory polyneuropathy. Neurology 1990;40:209–212.

35. van Doorn PA, Vermeulen M, Brand A, Mulder PGH, Busch HFM. Intravenous immunoglobulin treatment in patients with chronic inflammatory demyelinating polyneuropathy. Arch Neurol 1991;48:217–220.

36. Dietrich G, Rossi F, Sultan Y, Kaveri S, Nydegger UE, Kazatchkine MD. IVIG and regulation of autoimmunity through the idiopathic network. In: Imbach P, ed. Immunotherapy with Intravenous Immunoglobulins. San Diego: Academic Press, 1991:3–14.

37. Newland AC, Macey MG, Veys PA. Intravenous immunoglobulin: mechanisms of action and their clinical application. In: Imbach P, ed. Immunotherapy with Intravenous Immunoglobulins. San Diego: Academic Press, 1991:15–25.

38. Nydegger, UE. Hypothetic and established action mechanisms of therapy with immunoglobulin G. In: Imbach P, ed. Immunotherapy with Intravenous Immunoglobulins. San Diego: Academic Press, 1991:27–36.

39. Frey AM. The immune system: part 2, intravenous administration of immune globulin. J Intravenous Nursing 1991;14(6):396–405.

40. Berger M, Cupps TR, Fauci AS. Immunoglobulin replacement therapy by slow subcutaneous infusion. Ann Intern Med 1980;93:55–56.

41. Male D. Immunology, An Illustrated Outline. New York: Gower Medical Publishing, 1986;1–24.

42. Frey AM. The immune system and intravenous administration of immune globulin. Part 1, the immune response. J Intravenous Nursing 1991;14(5):315–330.

43. Drug Facts and Comparisons. St. Louis: JB Lippincott, 1990.

44. Eibl M. Treatment of defects of humoral immunity. Birth Defects: Original Article Series 1983;19:193.

45. Eibl MM, Wedgwood RJ. Intravenous immunoglobulin: a review. Immunodefic Rev 1989;1(Suppl):1–42.

46. Minnefor AB, Oleske JO. Immune globulin: efficacy and safety. Hosp Pract 1987;22:171–183.

47. Outbreak of hepatitis C associated with intravenous immunoglobulin administration—in the United States, October 1993-June 1994. MMWR 1994;43:505–509.

48. Yu MW, Mason BL, Tankersley DC. Detection and characterization of hepatitis C virus RNA in immune globulins. Transfusion 1994;34:569–602.

49. Lopez-Jiménez J, Villalón L, Mateos ML, Odriozola J. Hepatitis C virus antibody seroconversion in bone marrow transplant recipients treated with immune globulin: the impact of the problem. Blood 1994;84: 665–666.

50. Dammacco F, Sansonno D, Beardsley A, Gowans EJ. Failure to detect hepatitis C virus (HCV) genome by polymerase chain reaction in human anti-HCV-positive intravenous immunoglobulins. Clin Exp Immunol 1993;92:205–210.

51. Yu MW, Mason BL, Guo ZP, et al. Hepatitis C transmission associated with intravenous immunoglobulins [Letter]. Lancet 1995;345:1173–1174.

52. Tan E, Hajinazarian M, Bay W, Neff J, Mendell JR. Acute renal failure resulting from intravenous immunoglobulin therapy. Arch Neurol 1993;50:137–139.

53. Noya FJD, Rench MA, Garcia-Prats JA, et al. Disposition of an immunoglobulin intravenous preparation in very low birth weight neonates. J Pediatr 1988;112: 278–283.

54. Siegel J. Intravenous immune globulins: therapeutic, pharmaceutical and cost considerations. Pharmacy Practice News, December 1994; Reprint by the McMahon Group, New York, 1995.

55. Burks AW, Sampson HA, Buckley RH. Anaphylactic reactions after gamma globulin administration in patients with hypogammaglobulinemia: detection of IgE antibodies to IgA. N Engl J Med 1986;314:560–564.

56. Ippoliti C, Williams LA, Huber S. Toxicity of rapidly infused concentrated intravenous gamma globulin. Clin Pharm 1992;11;1022–1026.

57. Schiff RI, Sedlak D, Buckley RH. Rapid infusion of Sandoglobulin in patients with primary humoral immunodeficiency. J Allergy Clin Immunol 1991;88:61–67.

58. Bielory L, Long GC. Home health care costs: intravenous immunoglobulin home infusion therapy. Ann Allergy 1995;74(3):265–268.

59. Kobayashi RH, Kobayashi AD, Lee N, et al. Home self-administration of intravenous immunoglobulin therapy in children. Pediatrics 1990;85:705–709.

60. Kobayashi RH, Kobayashi ALD, Lee N, Fischer S, Ochs HD. The home administration of IVIG in children with primary immunodeficiency. In: Imbach P, ed. Immunotherapy with intravenous immunoglobulins. San Diego: Academic Press, 1991:47–56.

61. Ashida ER, Saxon A. Home intravenous immunoglobulin therapy by self-administration. J Clin Immunol 1986;6:306–309.

62. Chapel H, Brennan V, Delson E. Immunoglobulin replacement therapy by self-infusion at home. Clin Exp Immunol 1988;78:160–162.

63. Chapel H, Brennan V. Self-infusion of immunoglobulin at home. J Clin Pathol 1991;44:358–359.

64. Ochs HD, Lee ML, Fischer SH, et al. Self-infusion of intravenous immunoglobulin by immunodeficient patients at home. J Infect Dis 1987;156:652–654.

65. Arno PS, Arras JD, Bateman B, et al. The technological tether: an introduction to ethical and social issues in high-tech home care. Hastings Center Report 1994;24(Suppl 5):S1-S28

66. Sorensen RU, Kallick MD, Berger M. Home treatment of antibody deficiency syndromes with intravenous immune globulin. J Allergy Clin Immunol 1987;80:810–815.

67. Ochs HD, Fischer SH, Lee ML, et al. Intravenous immunoglobulin home treatment for patients with primary immunodeficiency diseases. Lancet 1986;1:610–611.

68. Kohrman AF. Chimeras and odysseys: toward understanding the technology-dependent child. Hastings Center Report 1994;24(Suppl 5):S4-S10.

69. Noddings N. Moral obligation or moral support for high-tech home care? Hastings Center Report 1994;24(Suppl 5):S6-S10.

70. Arras JD, Dubler NN. Bringing the hospital home: ethical and social implications of high-tech home care. Hastings Center Report 1994;24(Suppl 5):S19-S28.

71. Weissert WG. A new policy agenda for home care. Health Affairs (Millwood) 1991;10(2):67–77.

72. Arno PS, Bonuck KA, Padgug R. The economic impact of high-technology home care. Hastings Center Report 1994;24(Suppl 5):S15-S19.

73. Bielory L, Long GC. Home infusion therapy: comparison of costs for intravenous immunoglobulin. N J Med 1993;90(7):512–515.

74. Medi-Span. Prescription Pricing Guide. 1992;Mar.

15

HOME PARENTERAL NUTRITION

Bjørn Skeie[a]

CHAPTER AT A GLANCE: For patients who are unable to absorb normal food, parenteral nutrition (PN) may be a life-saving treatment. Advances in PN and delivery systems have made home PN (HPN) a useful tool in the management of these patients by which social and occupational rehabilitation can be achieved. The adaptation of hospital techniques to the home situation has allowed patients to carry out long-term parenteral therapy at home. Patients on HPN, however, are subject to medical and social problems, which require that the clinicians responsible for the treatment of these patients develop expertise in this field. When carried out appropriately, however, HPN is a valuable technique in the management of patients and may provide improved quality of life.

Introduction

Total parenteral nutrition (TPN) has for some time been employed for short-term and intermediate nutritional support of patients in hospitals. Ambulatory home TPN has been a logical and obvious outpatient extension of the successful development and clinical application of intravenous hyperalimentation in hospitalized patients. In 1968, a 36-year-old woman with extensive intraperitoneal metastatic ovarian carcinoma became the first patient to be fed entirely by vein at home. The first decade (1970–1980) of experience showed home parenteral nutrition (HPN) to be an acceptable form of nutritional support in selected patients and succeeded in returning many to their previous lifestyles out of the hospital (1–5). Since then, the indications for and ap-

plications of ambulatory home TPN have increased greatly. It has been demonstrated convincingly that patients with severe gastrointestinal dysfunction and resulting malnutrition can experience remarkable rehabilitation with a return to fully functioning life on HPN (6–12). Improvements in parenteral nutrition and home care delivery systems have made HPN a reality for many patient groups. HPN can cover all nutritional needs but requires appropriate indications, optimal technical management, and cautious ethical evaluation. The decision of who should receive home nutrition support must largely depend on what the patient and his or her family can handle. The supporting clinicians need to share with the patient reasonable information about what they can expect before deciding to initiate HPN. The right to participate in their own management decisions is especially important, because most of the day-to-day management falls on the patient and his or her family.

---

[a]Eldar Søreide and Jeffrey Askanazi contributed to this chapter in the first edition.

The provision of enteral and parenteral nutrition to patients in the home setting continues to be an expanding area of practice. As increasing knowledge, skill, and experience were gained in the long-term infusion techniques of home TPN, applications were inevitably expanded and extended. Much has already been learned regarding individual nutrient requirements in patients requiring long-term home hyperalimentation, and much more knowledge will be gained regarding clinical biochemistry, technology, and physiodynamics as an increasing number and variety of patients are studied. The typical indications for HPN include short bowel syndrome, Crohn's disease, enterocutaneous fistulas, antineoplastic therapy, and various more esoteric malnutrition and malabsorption syndromes. It is anticipated that eventually the fine interactions between normal body metabolism, pathophysiologic states, pharmacologic and other treatment modalities, and specific parenteral nutrition regimens will enhance our ability to manage patients with more specific metabolic and organ-failure disorders. In this regard, this chapter includes an overview of recent experience with HPN administered to patients with AIDS and chronic obstructive pulmonary disease.

It is clear that TPN at home is feasible and requires only a simple delivery system. However, meticulous care with the system is needed to avoid serious catheter-related and metabolic complications. As awareness of the safety and efficacy of home TPN grows, as scientific and technological advances in parenteral feeding techniques and substrates are extended, and as the emphasis on cost-effective home health programs is accentuated, it is predicted that the number of patients on home TPN will increase. Technological advances in the future will inevitably produce a system of ambulatory home TPN that is more even complete, safe, reliable, and cost effective.

Home enteral nutrition (HEN) has been used for many decades through gastrostomies or enterostomies in patients with swallowing dysfunction or upper intestinal obstruction. Such patients have traditionally received bolus doses of homemade blenderized tube diets. More recently, the commercial availability of prepackaged formula diets, soft small-bore tubes, and endoscopic percutaneous gastrostomies have expanded the feasibility of the enteral approach; indeed, it is being used increasingly as an alternative to parenteral nutrition in both the hospital and the home setting (13–15). Greater use of this less costly technique of nutritional support should be encouraged wherever possible, to stretch the use of the limited healthcare dollar.

General Aspects of HPN

Indications

HPN has become a primary or adjunctive treatment for a variety of patients who suffer from intestinal failure with nutritional and water-electrolyte deficits not correctable by the enteral route and who thus require short-term, extended, or lifelong intravenous nourishment to maintain normal nutrition and metabolism. Indications for chronic or permanent HPN include short bowel syndrome, malabsorption, motility disorders, radiation enteritis, and congenital bowel disease. Indications for acute or temporary HPN include Crohn's disease, malignancies, AIDS, gastrointestinal fistulas, ulcerative colitis, anorexia nervosa, etc. HPN avoids undue hospitalization and offers these patients the possibility of social rehabilitation (16, 17).

A multicenter survey of HPN in nine European countries reported on 27 centers and 194 patients (18). The four most common indications for HPN were inflammatory bowel disease (30%), mesenteric vascular disease (21%), malignancy (17%), and radiation enteritis (13%) (Table 15.1). The distribution of diseases varied, however, among the different countries. Inflammatory bowel disease, for example, represented only 17% of the indications in France but 45% in the United Kingdom, whereas malignancies represented 18% in France but only 5.5% in the United Kingdom. The number of patients who justify HPN has been estimated at two patients per year per 1,000,000 in the United Kingdom and France

Table 15.1. Indications for HPN in Adults

Inflammatory bowel disease	29.9%
Radiation enteritis	12.9%
Mesenteric vascular disease	21.6%
Malabsorption syndrome	7.2%
Pseudo-obstruction	5.7%
GI tract cancer	17.0%
Miscellaneous	5.7%

From Messing B, Landais P, Goldfarb B, et al. Home parenteral nutrition in adults: A multicentre survey in Europe. Clin Nutr 1989;8:3–9.

(19). In the United States, the absolute number of patients on HPN is unknown; estimates vary from 2,000 to 5,000 patients. A review by Howard et al. from 1986 (13) lists the indications for HPN taken from the U.S. National Registry (Table 15.2). From 1,581 patients registered in the OASIS (Home Nutrition Support Patient Registry) from 1985 to 1988, the diagnoses were Crohn's disease in 25%, ischemic bowel disorder in 11%, motility disorders in 11%, radiation enteritis in 8%, congenital bowel disease in 5%, neoplasm in 33% and AIDS in 6% (20, 21).

The single largest diagnosis of patients starting HPN in the United States is cancer, and the number of patients with malignancies on HPN is increasing. Evidence indicates that the number of home parenteral nutrition and enteral nutrition patients with cancer increased in the United States by about 25% each year from 1985 to 1990 (22, 23). Many oncologic patients are chronically malnourished secondary to the nature of the malignant process itself, the catabolism of previous antineoplastic therapy or post-therapy complications, and the anorexia associated with both (24–27). TPN can reduce the manifestations of alimentary tract toxicity and allow the administration of more chemotherapeutic doses without apparent deleterious effects. A consensus of opinion regarding the utility of parenteral nutrition in cancer patients still remains elusive; responses to anti-cancer therapy are adversely influenced by concurrent malnutrition, and yet, efforts to reverse this process are exceedingly difficult to document (28–32).

Among patients with cancer, HPN is likely to benefit those for whom treatment-associated toxicities precluding adequate enteral intake represents the dominant impediment to restoration of performance status. HPN may also benefit certain patients with malnutrition in whom the natural history of the underlying tumor can be expected to permit a period of nearly normal performance status. However, HPN is probably of no benefit in patients with severe malnutrition and rapidly progressive tumors that have not responded to chemotherapy or radiation therapy.

Short bowel syndrome is the clinical manifestation of a fundamental reduction in the functional intestinal absorptive surface area and malabsorption. The development of TPN has improved the natural course of this disease. TPN has also become a useful tool in the management of patients with inflammatory bowel disease (IBD). In the past, it was felt that TPN would have a therapeutic role in IBD, but experience indicates that it functions more as an adjunct to other therapeutic interventions (33). The specific roles of HPN in IBD include nutritional maintenance in short bowel syndrome and adjunctive therapy in jejunoileitis of Crohn's disease and Crohn's colitis. The use of home TPN and total bowel rest for these patients can promote restoration of positive nitrogen balance, resulting in significant symptomatic relief, and allowing quiescence of the active disease (11, 34–36). Patients with IBD on HPN are subject to the same infectious mechanical and metabolic problems as are other patients on HPN.

Table 15.2. Percentage of HPN Patients in Different Diagnostic Categories

Diagnosis	Percentage
Malignancies	44
Crohn's disease	20
Ischemic bowel	10
Motility disorder	5
Congenital bowel disorder	4
Other (includes short bowel syndrome unrelated to above, immune disorders, and hyperemesis gravidarum)	17

From Howard L, Heaphey LL, Timchalk M. A review of the current national status of home parenteral and enteral nutrition from the provider and consumer perspective. JPEN 1986;10:416–424.

Prior to the clinical application of intravenous nutrition, the management of internal fistulas of the gastrointestinal tract was accompanied by high morbidity and mortality rates (37, 38). A treatment regimen of total bowel rest and TPN has virtually eliminated the urgency for operations and has allowed spontaneous closure of about 70% of these fistulas. If sepsis is not a complicating factor, the patient can be treated as an outpatient until spontaneous closure of the fistula has been accomplished.

Prognosis

The overall prognosis of HPN patients depends on the prognosis of the underlying disease. In the European multicenter survey, 108 patients were followed for at least 1 year (18). The duration of HPN was 12 ± 2 months for the 41 patients who ceased HPN, 10 ± 1 months for the 30 patients who died, and 35 ± 5 months for the 37 patients still on HPN at the closing date of the survey. Prognosis according to underlying disease is presented in Table 15.3.

Table 15.3. Prognosis of HPN Patients Starting on HPN at Least One Year Prior to the End of the Survey

Diagnosis	On HPN	Off HPN	Deceased
Inflammatory bowel disease ($n = 37$)	13	21	3
Mesenteric vascular disease ($n = 25$)	8	10	7
Gastrointestinal malignancy ($n = 15$)	4	2	9
Radiation enteritis ($n = 15$)	4	4	7
Malabsorption syndrome ($n = 7$)	3	3	2
Pseudo-obstruction ($n = 5$)	1	2	2
Miscellaneous ($n = 4$)	4	0	0
Total ($n = 108$)	37 (34%)	41 (38%)	30 (28%)

From Messing B, Landais P, Goldfarb B, et al. Home parenteral nutrition in adults: a multicentre survey in Europe. Clin Nutr 1989;8:3–9.

The death rate was 28% in the group of the 108 patients starting HPN at least 1 year prior to the end of the study. The two highest death rates were observed in gastrointestinal malignancies (60%) and radiation enteritis (47%), representing one-half of the mortality. The mean duration of HPN was 10 months in the subgroup of those who died.

Data from the national registry in the United States showed that patients starting on HPN had over a 50% likelihood of continuing on HPN at the end of the year, a 25% chance of dying during the year, and about a 20% chance of coming off HPN. In most instances, those who came off HPN were then considered to have no further need of it (13).

Howard (23) compared the clinical outcomes for 1362 patients with active cancer managed on HPN with those of 122 patients with radiation enteritis ("cured cancer") and 416 patients with Crohn's disease. The clinical information was reported to the North American Home Parenteral and Enteral Nutrition Registry between 1985 and 1989. The annual survival rate was 25% for patients with active cancer, compared with 88% for patients with radiation enteritis and 95% for patients with Crohn's disease. Fifty percent of all active cancer patients starting HPN were dead within 6 to 9 months. However, the prognosis was somewhat better in children, and 20% of the active cancer patients did well, returning to full oral nutrition and experiencing complete rehabilitation. The mean survival time of cancer patients was 6 months after starting home parenteral or enteral nutrition (22). In a German report, the median survival of 498 cancer patients on HPN was 64 days. Most of these patients were severely malnourished before starting HPN (39).

HPN patients can be separated into two very different categories, short-term and long-term. In the American HPN survey, median survival of patients with malignancies was 6 months as opposed to 30 months in patients with short bowel syndrome (13). This difference may imply a need for different types of support. In the future, it will be important to evaluate life expectancy and rehabilitation status in terms of specific diagnostic categories. It seems reasonable to suggest that home nutritional support should be conducted differently for these short-term and long-term patients. Short-term patients may be served by more circumscribed nutritional support (mainly fluids and electrolytes) with fewer potential metabolic complications and less in-hospital learning time. Long-term patients, on the other hand, require complete nutrient infusions. However, once established at home, these patients often require more limited nursing support and encouragement to achieve independence.

Complications

In evaluating the cost and quality of HPN therapy, an important factor is the frequency of hospital readmissions, particularly readmissions for HPN complications. Howard et al. (13) listed the complications that led to HPN readmissions in the National Registry in 1983 (Table 15.4). Sepsis or suspected sepsis was by far the most common reason for readmission. Only one in 80 patients with suspected sepsis was managed as an outpatient. Adult active cancer patients have the same re-

hospitalization rate for HPN complications (once per year) as radiation and Crohn's disease patients. However, the rehospitalization rate for non-HPN complications is four times higher. In 61 patients with gynecologic cancers who received HPN between 1981 and 1990, minimal complications were noted from HPN, with 9% of hospitalizations due to HPN. Nutritional parameters initially improved in most patients on HPN but then decreased prior to death (40).

O'Keefe et al. (41) examined 41 patients on HPN to identify risk factors for catheter-related infection; the frequent-infection group included younger patients and those with Crohn's disease, jejunostomies, and central vein thrombosis. A greater proportion of the frequent-infection group had poor catheter-care technique and more were smokers. They had an average infection rate of one every 31 months, 52% caused by Gram-positive organisms (chiefly coagulase-negative staphylococci and *Staphylococcus aureus*), 30% caused by Gram-negative organisms, and 16% caused by fungus (chiefly *Candida albicans*).

In another study, in which the records of 27 pediatric patients (representing 230 patient-years of HPN) were examined, the central venous catheters (CVCs) were infected an average of once every 884 days. Unsuccessful medical treatment of the exit site or CVC infection was responsible for removal of 62% of the CVCs. Clotting of the CVC was responsible for removal of 24%, and breakage was responsible for 14% of the CVCs (42). An increased CVC survival time has been reported over the years. Factors contributing to this include improvement in self-care, greater experience, improvement in teaching, regular follow-up of patients, better management of infection, and better ability to treat CVC thrombosis or breakage.

In the European multicenter survey, complications related to the technical aspects of HPN were present in 37% of the patients (18) (Table 15.5). For a cumulative duration of 207 years of HPN, the overall incidence of catheter-related complications leading to catheter replacement was 0.74 per year of

Table 15.4. Reasons for HPN-Related Hospital Readmissions, National Registry 1983

	Admissions	
	Total Per 100	Patient-Months
Sepsis, suspected or confirmed	237	3.1
Catheter-related problems	62	0.8
Change of catheters	31	0.4
Fluid/electrolyte problems	24	0.3
Organ failure/dysfunction	11	0.1
Metabolic bone disease	8	0.1
Retraining in HPN technique	7	0.1
Patient/family unable to cope	5	0.05
Iron therapy	4	0.05
Other causes	14	0.2

From Howard L, Heaphey LL, Timchalk M. A review of the current national status of home parenteral and enteral nutrition from the provider and consumer perspective. JPEN 1986;10:416–424.

treatment. In the same survey, metabolic complications were reported in 30% of the patients. The four main metabolic complications associated with HPN were abnormal liver tests (20%), joint and bone pains (17%), gallbladder lithiasis (12%), and trace metals or vitamin deficits (12%) (Table 15.6).

Studies have suggested that patients who receive long-term TPN are at increased risk for the development of cholelithiasis (43, 44). Patients who receive intravenous nutrition undergo prolonged periods of fasting, which may alter bile composition and lead to gallbladder stasis, both important factors in gallstone formation.

Oral intake should not be discouraged in the majority of HPN patients, because fewer metabolic complications and more rapid intestinal adaptation of the short bowel accompany oral nutrition (45). Moreover, studies indicate that the absorption from normal food may approach 50% even in the extremely short gut (46).

Rehabilitation

A return to normal functioning, both socially and economically, is a critical measure of the cost-effectiveness of HPN. However, a true estimate of rehabilitation is often hard to gauge since it is not uncommon for HPN to start after a long, debilitating illness. Even if restoration of physical well-being is achieved, the HPN patient still lives with a real potential for further medical setbacks. In such circumstances a return to work may not be feasible. The American survey (13) indicated that 50 to 60% of HPN patients were able to work part or full time, 15 to 20% were retired or of preschool age, and 20 to 30% were unable to work. Forty-two percent of those responding described themselves as carrying on normal activity for their age.

Howard (23) reported the outcome of HPN patients from the OASIS registry in seven diagnostic categories and found in Crohn's disease complete rehabilitation in 70% of the patients over 2 years; The percentages with complete rehabilitation in the other groups were as follows: ischemic bowel disease, 30%; motility disorder, 35%; radiation enteritis, 40%; congenital bowel disease, 60%; neoplasm, 20%; and AIDS, 5%.

In a total of 88 patient-years, Greig et al. found that 96% of patients' time had been spent outside the hospital (47). Of 47 patients, 63% were able to return to previous employment, 6% became retired or unemployed, and 30% remained disabled by their disease.

In the European multicenter survey, social rehabilitation was evaluated on the basis of the patient's ability to manage HPN and on occupational status while in treatment (18). Sixty percent of patients undertook HPN unaided and 19% required the help of a nurse or a family member. Twenty-two percent were family or nurse dependent. Fifty-two percent of HPN patients were able to work and recovered their pre-HPN occupational status either full time (30%) or part time (22%). Forty-two percent of patients were unable to work but were able to cope with HPN unaided and

Table 15.5. Technical Complications during HPN Leading to Catheter Change[a]

	Number of Cases	Incidence per Year
Catheter sepsis		
Bacterial	72	
Mycotic	7	0.38
Blockage of catheter	38	0.18
Migration of catheter	22	0.11
Venous thrombosis	15	0.07
Total	154	0.74

From Messing B, Landais P, Goldfarb B, et al. Home parenteral nutrition in adults: a multicentre survey in Europe. Clin Nutr 1989;8:3–9.

[a] The cumulative duration of the 200 HPN periods represented 207 years.

Table 15.6. Frequency of Metabolic Complications during HPN (n = 194 Patients)

Complications	% of Patients
Hypercalcemia (>2.75 mmol/L)	10
Joint and/or bone pains	17
Pathologic bone fracture	3
Increased liver function tests	20
Jaundice	9
Gallbladder lithiasis during HPN	12

From Messing B, Landais P, Goldfarb B, et al. Home parenteral nutrition in adults: a multicentre survey in Europe. Clin Nutr 1989;8:3–9.

were able to go out. Six percent were house-bound and needed major assistance.

In a French report, 44 children with chronic digestive or extradigestive diseases with severe malnutrition submitted to home parenteral nutrition were studied. They found that HPN for these pediatric patients improved the quality of life of both children and parents compared with the preceding period in the hospital. However, before HPN is undertaken, the parents' capacity to cope with the treatment should be carefully evaluated (48).

HPN has a major effect on the lifestyles and employment of patients and their families. Patients find that their lifestyle is affected in many ways. Disturbances in sleep, leisure activities, travel, social life, family life, and employment are all common (49). However, it is difficult to determine the degree to which physical well-being is affected by the underlying disease and by HPN.

Technical and Nutritional Aspects

The route of administration for HPN is via the superior or inferior vena cava near the right atrium. Initial efforts to deliver HPN using either arteriovenous fistulas or shunts failed because of a high incidence of thrombosis (10, 50).

In 1973, the development of a permanent central venous catheter constructed of a non-thrombogenic silicone rubber elastomer was reported by Broviac et al. (51, 52). The use of this catheter resulted in a low incidence of infection because of the barrier provided by the subcutaneous tunnel and by the polyester cuff of the catheter. This catheter was later modified by Hickman et al. to have a larger internal diameter and thicker wall to increase its durability (53). The Broviac-Hickman catheter has since become the standard route of delivery for HPN. The Silastic or siliconed catheter is inserted percutaneously into the subclavian or jugular vein through a subcutaneous tunnel, or via the cephalic or basilic vein through a cutdown. The procedure must be done in a treatment room using standard sterile technique. A chest x-ray is performed to determine the appropriateness of the catheter position.

Although the Hickman catheter has been proved to be safe and efficacious for HPN, the use of subcutaneous infusion ports has recently been addressed for HPN in order to minimize the risk of septic and mechanical complications (54, 55). Subcutaneous infusion ports are currently the choice for HPN administration by some centers (56). Peripherally inserted central catheter (PICC) lines are also used for HPN and are increasing in popularity due to their ease of insertion. Home TPN is usually performed as a cyclic nocturnal infusion three to seven times a week. The use of single-container parenteral nutrition admixtures, which include lipids, dextrose, and amino acids, have simplified the therapy and is cost effective. The infusions are generally administered by pump.

The need for specialized training of patients and family members to safely administer nutrition therapies at home following hospital discharge is important. In 1993, written materials designed for this purpose were gathered from institutions throughout the United States and published by the American Society for Parenteral and Enteral Nutrition (ASPEN) (57).

Use of HPN for Some Specific Diseases

AIDS

The nutritional status of patients with AIDS is challenged throughout the progression of the illness by the manifestation of symptoms such as malabsorption, diarrhea, opportunistic infection, and fever. Anthropometric, biochemical, and body composition studies in AIDS patients have shown malnutrition to be a significant factor of the illness. Decreases in serum albumin, total iron-binding capacity, and retinol-binding protein have been reported in AIDS patients in the early stage of undernutrition (57). Body composition analysis performed in 33 AIDS patients demonstrated a depletion in total body potassium and body fat content, with increased extracellular water, as seen in chronic malnutrition (58).

As with many chronic diseases, the severe malnutrition that frequently accompanies AIDS can decrease longevity and increase morbidity (59, 60). In addition, the quality of life is compromised when AIDS is accompanied by major nutritional complications (61). Ensuring optimal nutritional status should generally improve the quality of life for malnourished AIDS patients (62).

Patients with protein calorie malnutrition and other nutrient deficiencies have a depression in cellular immunity with abnormal T cell and macrophage function (59, 63). Such changes could theoretically compound the immunodeficiency in AIDS patients and render them more susceptible to infections or exacerbate the severity of existing infections.

As yet, there is no widely accepted method for nutritional management of AIDS. However, when malabsorption syndrome and diarrhea do not permit effective oral or enteral feeding, parenteral feeding is indicated before wasting occurs. Peripheral parenteral nutrition (PPN), delivered via a peripheral vein, is appropriate when short-term (7 to 10 days) in-hospital preservation of lean body mass is needed. If longer nutritional support is needed, hyperalimentation via a central vein should be used. Because malnutrition can complicate the course of AIDS, nutritional support should be given before the patient becomes malnourished. An aggressive approach to nutritional therapy is advocated at each stage of the disease. HPN feeding regimens have been shown to be efficacious in stabilizing and reversing the evolution of wasting in undernourished patients (64) and in patients with AIDS and malnutrition. However, only when the enteral routes are not feasible should parenteral nutrition be used (62, 65).

We reviewed, retrospectively, the clinical course of 22 patients with AIDS and weight loss greater than 10% who received HPN for 56.2 patient-months (54). Fifteen of the patients gained weight, five patients maintained stable weight, and two patients lost weight during HPN. Nine patients were able to return to their normal activity, seven patients showed a stabilization of their clinical course, and six died or were considered as preterminal. Of the nine patients able to return to normal activity, four patients had a spectacular change in their quality of life and were able to return to work.

We found that HPN could be safely administered to the AIDS patients within acceptable standards. Catheter-related sepsis occurred at the rate of 0.12/100 catheter-days. Although the catheter-related sepsis in the AIDS patients was higher than that encountered in our other groups of HPN patients, it was acceptable when compared with the infection rate observed in the early use of indwelling catheters (52, 53) and with the infection rate observed in cancer patients (66). The low sepsis rate seems to be related to the meticulous monitoring ensured by the HPN nurse and the physician and to the use of lipid-based HPN in a triple admixture. Intriguing aspects of the pathophysiology of HIV infection, including lipid metabolism of the virus and infected cells, may lead to the introduction of specific formulations for AIDS patients on HPN.

Chronic Obstructive Pulmonary Disease

There is an increased incidence of nutritional depletion in patients with chronic obstructive pulmonary disease (COPD) (67, 68). Anthropomorphic measurements of nutritional status were abnormal in almost half of patients. Weight loss has been reported in over 70% of patients hospitalized with COPD. Weight loss has been found to be more prevalent in patients with emphysema than in those with chronic bronchitis (69). Examination of the large COPD population enrolled in the Intermittent Partial Pressure Breathing Trial has confirmed an independent effect of weight loss on mortality (70). When weight loss develops in a patient with COPD, the average life expectancy is only 2.9 years (71).

Although this is an unusual choice for the use of HPN, the study of nutritional support for malnourished COPD patients is highly instructive. The effects of refeeding and fuel utilization provide useful insight into the management of other patients who have compromised medical status.

Nutritional support should be considered in patients with respiratory disease and nutritional failure. However, the nutrients themselves exert effects on ventilation and pulmonary function and they may have profound physiologic and pharmacologic actions aside from improvement in whole-body metabolic status. Nutrient infusion may result in increases in CO_2 production (glucose), oxygen consumption (amino acids), and ventilatory drive (amino acids). It may also alter pulmonary vascular tone and the inflammatory response (lipids).

Effects of Refeeding in COPD Patients

Administration of nutrients can improve respiratory muscle function, whole-body metabolic status, and immune defense mechanisms in COPD patients. It can also influence the physiologic and pharmacologic properties of the respiratory system. Increasing carbohydrate intake may increase ventilatory demand because of increased CO_2 production. Intravenous lipids may alter pulmonary vascular tone and the inflammatory response. Amino acid infusion may increase oxygen consumption and stimulate ventilation by altering respiratory drive. It is important to keep these interactions in mind when setting up nutritional programs for pulmonary patients.

Fuel Oxidation

In a study by Goldstein et al. (72), nitrogen and energy relationships and fuel oxidation were investigated and related to strength and endurance tests before and after 2 weeks of hypercaloric diets with varied nonprotein energy sources (carbohydrate-or fat-based). The results showed that patients with emphysema and weight loss have a pattern of energy metabolism and fuel oxidation that is distinctly different from that of malnourished patients without lung disease. In other stress states, such as infection, it has been shown that hy-

permetabolism, hypercatabolism, and preferential fat oxidation occur concomitantly (73, 74). Patients with emphysema were found to be unusual because the hypercatabolism (i.e., a greater nitrogen breakdown than expected for a given energy expenditure) that is often associated with other hypermetabolic disease states is not present in patients with emphysema. Patients with emphysema also were found to have a lower fat oxidation and a higher carbohydrate oxidation than the control patients (Fig. 15.1). These patients may thus respond to nutritional therapy in a manner that differs from malnourished patients without chronic lung disease.

In emphysema, the hypermetabolism is believed to be primarily due to inefficient use of the respiratory system and to the increased work of breathing (75, 76). Our data suggest that glucose may be the fuel utilized by respiratory muscles under these conditions. Two weeks of nutritional support with either the carbohydrate-based or fat-based diet increased body weight, nitrogen balance, and arm muscle area and improved maximal inspiratory pressure, skeletal muscle strength, and endurance strength to a similar degree in malnourished patients with and without lung disease.

Carbohydrates

Nutritional intake influences respiratory function through alterations in metabolic demand with changes in respiratory quotient (RQ) and ventilatory drive. Due to the increased CO_2 production, increasing glucose intake is a stimulus to ventilation. Numerous researchers have reported a large increase in CO_2 production and RQ with the administration of hypertonic glucose (77, 78). As substrates shift from fat oxidation to glucose oxidation, an increase in RQ occurs; if sufficient glucose is given, lipogenesis occurs, with a dramatic rise in the level of CO_2 production. It is possible for a small patient to double his or her CO_2 production, going from 5% dextrose to 3000 kcal/day of glucose-based TPN. For normal subjects, such an increase in minute ventilation has no noticeable effect on breathing. However, this

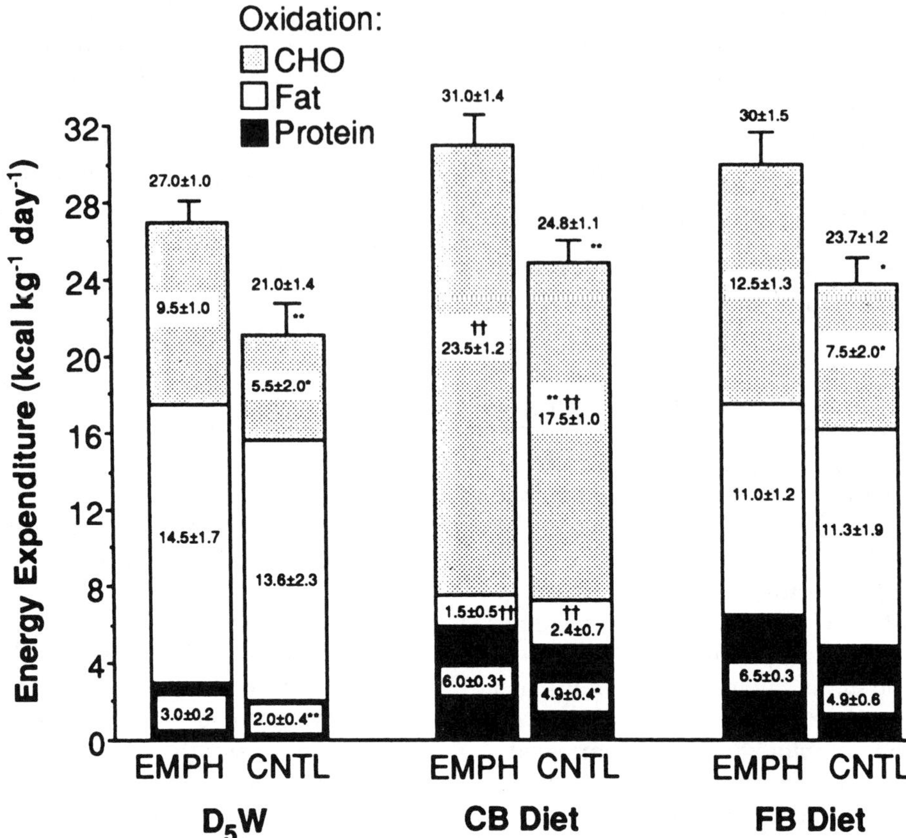

Figure 15.1. Resting energy expenditure and fuel oxidation of carbohydrate (CHO), fat, and protein in 10 emphysematous (EMPH) and six control (CNTL) patients during administration of 5% dextrose plus electrolytes (D_5W), a carbohydrate-based (CB) diet, and a fat-based (FB) diet. Legend: *, different from EMPH ($p < 0.05$); **, different from EMPH ($p < 0.01$); †, compared with FB diet, same group ($p < 0.05$);†† , compared with FB diet, same group ($p < 0.001$). (From Goldstein SA, Thomashow BM, Kvetan V, et al. Nitrogen and energy relationships in malnourished patients with emphysema. Am Rev Respir Dis 1988;138:636–644.)

can lead to respiratory distress in patients with impaired lung function.

Lipids
Substitution of fat emulsions for nonprotein calories lowers the RQ and reduces minute ventilation and ventilatory demand (79) (Fig. 15.2). Intravenous fat emulsions (IVFEs) are therefore a useful substrate in providing nutritional support for the patient with reduced pulmonary reserve.

However, numerous studies have suggested varying degrees of apparent pulmonary dysfunction when IVFEs are given.

These changes have generally not been of sufficient magnitude to carry much clinical significance, but they are of interest in understanding the relationship between IVFEs and the lung. The lung dysfunction generally consists of a decrease in Pao_2 and has been attributed to the associated hyperlipemia (80). Recent studies, however, indicate that the decrease in Pao_2 is due to ventilation/perfusion inequalities caused by an IVFE-related increase in the production of eicosanoids (prostaglandins, thromboxanes, leukotrienes), which causes alterations in the pulmonary vasomotor tone (81). The polyunsaturated fatty

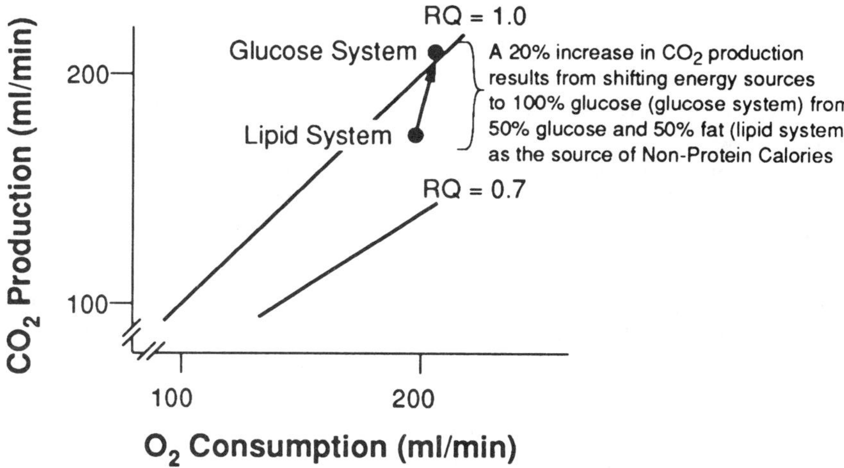

Figure 15.2.   Gas exchange and breathing patterns during TPN (glucose versus fat [$n = 5$]). Reduction of CO_2 production and RQ in substituting a part of the carbohydrate intake (glucose system) for fat intake (lipid system). (From Askanazi J, Nordenstrom J, Rosenbaum SH, et al. Nutrition for the patient with respiratory failure: glucose versus fat. Anesthesiology 1981;54:373–377.)

acids in the IVFEs serve as precursors to the eicosanoids. Experimental studies in animals have documented an increase in prostaglandin (PG) serum levels during IVFE infusion (82). Due to the varied effects of the different eicosanoids, infusion of IVFEs may have profound physiologic and pharmacologic actions aside from the provision of calories.

These effects may, in fact, be beneficial to patients suffering from pulmonary disease. In patients with cystic fibrosis, we have noticed a thinning of secretions, fewer pulmonary infections, and an overall clinical improvement after long-term TPN (83, 84). We have suggested that this may be due to an anti-inflammatory effect of Intralipid mediated via PG synthesis (85). The anti-inflammatory effects of IVFEs in cystic fibrosis may also apply to other lung disorders such as adult respiratory distress syndrome, bronchitis, and bronchiectasis.

Amino Acids

It has been shown that ventilatory drive is enhanced by progressively increasing levels of nitrogen intake. An enhanced ventilatory response to a CO_2 stimulus is reported after amino acid infusion (86). Normal subjects receiving 5% dextrose followed by intravenous

infusion of amino acids demonstrated an enhanced sensitivity to CO_2 during the amino acid infusion. Increasing protein intake to 21 g of nitrogen per day with a fixed caloric intake further enhances the ventilatory response above that observed with a lower nitrogen intake (11 g/day).

Nutritional Guidelines

Nutrition intervention programs for stable malnourished patients with COPD will require assumption of a 15 to 25% stress factor when using the Harris-Benedict equation for estimation of caloric needs. It has been suggested that caloric requirements approaching 200% of resting energy expenditure (REE) are required for effective weight gain in this patient population (87, 88). However, in patients who will receive HPN, the energy intake should be achieved gradually to avoid cardiopulmonary decompensation secondary to excessive CO_2 production and fluid overload. The effect of amino acid infusions to increase ventilatory drive and the effect of glucose infusions to increase CO_2 production suggest that both protein and glucose must be given in limited quantities. For these reasons, a high-fat diet might be beneficial for the patient with severe dyspnea or the patient being weaned from mechanical ventilation. Lipids should be administered at a slow rate to patients with respiratory failure to prevent possible pulmonary vasoconstriction.

The issue that is probably most crucial to the success of nutritional support in these patients is that of timing. It is clear that patients with decreased pulmonary reserve may not tolerate high amounts of carbohydrate or protein. Consequently, nutritional support must be instituted early in the course of the illness and in moderate quantities.

Patients should receive glucose in amounts sufficient to meet obligatory glucose needs (2 to 4 g/kg/day) without exceeding them. In an average patient this amounts to approximately 200 g/day of glucose. We prefer to use lower concentrations of dextrose (10 to 30%) to meet this requirement in order to minimize the effects of hyperosmolarity. Once minimal glucose needs are met, supplying additional calories as fat has equal nitrogen-sparing effects (88). Our recommendation is that lipids should be used to supply 50 to 60% of the daily calories in patients with respiratory failure. Lipids should be administered in a dosage of 1 to 2 g/kg/day and be infused over a minimum of 10 to 12 hours. This permits optimal uptake and utilization. Such a protocol can be achieved by means of the "triple mix" system in which IVFEs, dextrose, and amino acids are mixed together. Protein requirements may be met by the administration of 1 to 2 g of protein/kg/day.

Summary

The prevalence of HPN has been estimated to be around 2 to 4 per million in Europe and around 80 per million in the United States. The growth has been supported by health regulations favoring the discharge of patients from hospitals. Although there is common agreement about the core cases in which there is no alternative to HPN, cultural and economic differences lead to major variations in the types of disease treated. Intestinal failure due to short bowel syndrome; a relative decrease in absorptive gut mass and function due to stenosis, fistulas, or inflammation; and medical conditions such as malabsorption syndromes are clear indications for HPN. AIDS and cancer are illnesses for which the use of HPN is controversial with an overall poor prognosis, whereas for intestinal failure the outcome is good. The rehabilitation is influenced by the prognosis of the underlying disease. Problems with venous access, catheter-related sepsis, metabolic complications, and psychological adaption are often observed in HPN patients and require knowledge of the technical as well as the nutritional aspects of HPN. The management of patients on HPN thus needs the cooperation of many medical professions. HPN is expensive, and therefore the definitions of cost-effectiveness and cost versus benefit of the treatment are essential.

References

1. Dudrick SJ. A clinical review of nutritional support of the patient. Am J Clin Nutr 1981;34:1191–1198.
2. Jeejeebhoy KN, Langer B, Tsallas G. Total parenteral nutrition at home: studies in patients surviving four months to five years. Gastroenterology 1976;71:943–953.
3. Lees C, Steiger E, Hooley R, et al. Home parenteral nutrition. Surg Clin North Am 1981;61:621–633.
4. Pollack P, Kadden M, Byrne WJ, et al. 100 patient years experience with Broviac Silastic catheter for central venous nutrition. JPEN 1981;5:32–36.
5. Schneider PJ, Mirtallo JM. Home parenteral nutrition programs. JPEN 1981;5:157–160.
6. Stewart GR. Home parenteral nutrition for chronic short bowel syndrome. Med J Aust 1979;2:317–319.
7. Dudrick SJ, Jackson D. The short bowel syndrome and total parenteral nutrition. Heart Lung 1983;12:195–201.
8. Dudrick S, Speir A, Englert D. The short bowel syndrome in ambulatory home hyperalimentation. In: Deitel M, ed. Nutrition in Clinical Surgery. Baltimore: Williams & Wilkins, 1980:209–214.
9. Dudrick JD, O'Donnell JJ, Englert DM, et al. 100 patient-years of ambulatory home parenteral nutrition. Ann Surg 1984;199:770–781.
10. Scribner BH, Cole JJ, Christopher TG, et al. Long-term total parenteral nutrition. The concept of the artificial gut. JAMA 1970;212:457–63.
11. Fleming CR, McGill DB, Berkner S. Home parenteral nutrition as primary therapy in patients with extensive Crohn's disease of the small bowel and malnutrition. Gastroenterology 1977;73:1077–1081.
12. Wilmore DW, Dudrick SJ. Growth and development of an infant receiving all nutrients exclusively by vein. JAMA 1968;203:860–864.

13. Howard L, Heaphey LL, Timchalk M. A review of the current national status of home parenteral nutrition and enteral nutrition from the provider and consumer perspective. JPEN 1986;10:416–424.

14. Deetsky AS, McLaughlin JR, Abrams HB, et al. A cost-utility analysis of the home parenteral nutrition program at Toronto General Hospital: 1976–1982. JPEN 1986;10:49–57.

15. Wesley JR. Home parenteral nutrition: indications, principles and cost effectiveness. Compr Ther 1983;9:29–36.

16. Allardyce DB. Preoperative parenteral feeding in Crohn's disease: preoperatively, to reduce remission, and at home. Am Surg 1978;44:510–516.

17. Jeejeebhoy KN, Rosenberg IH. Panel report on nutritional support of patients with gastrointestinal diseases. Am J Clin Nutr 1981;34:1206–1212.

18. Messing B, Landais P, Goldfarb B, et al. Home parenteral nutrition in adults: a multicentre survey in Europe. Clin Nutr 1989;8:3–9.

19. Mughal M, Irving M. Home parenteral nutrition in the United Kingdom and Ireland. Lancet 1986 2(8503):383–387.

20. Howard L. Parenteral and enteral nutrition therapy. In: Wilson JD et al., eds. Harrison's Principles of Internal Medicine, 12th ed. New York: McGraw-Hill, 1991:428–429.

21. Howard L, Heaphey L, Claunch C, et al. Medical effectiveness of home parenteral nutrition support as judged by four years on North American registry data. JPEN J Parenter Enter Nutr 1991;15:384–393.

22. Howard L. Home parenteral and enteral nutrition in cancer patients. Cancer 1993;72:3531–3541.

23. Howard L. Home parenteral nutrition in patients with a cancer diagnosis. JPEN J Parenter Enter Nutr 1992;16:93S-99S.

24. Weiss SM, Worthington PH, Prioleau M, et al. Home parenteral nutrition in cancer patients. Cancer 1982;50:1210–1213.

25. Byrne WJ, Ament ME, Burke M. Home parenteral nutrition. Surg Gynecol Obstet 1979;149:593–599.

26. Heymsfield SB, Bethel RA, Ansley JD, et al. Enteral hyperalimentation: an alternative to central venous hyperalimentation. Ann Intern Med 1979;90:63–71.

27. Heymsfield SB. Home enteral feeding for malabsorption and weight loss. Ann Intern Med 1983;98:168–170.

28. Ng E-H, Lowery SF. Nutritional support and cancer cachexia: evolving concepts of mechanisms and adjunctive therapies. Hematol Oncol Clin North Am 1991;5:161–184.

29. Lowry SF. Cancer cachexia revisited: old problems and new perspectives. Eur J Cancer 1991;27:1–3.

30. McGeer AJ, Detsky AS, O'Rourke K. Parenteral nutrition in patients receiving cancer chemotherapy. Ann Intern Med 1989;734–736.

31. Klein S, Simes J, Blackburn GL. Total parenteral nutrition and cancer trial. Cancer 1986;58:1378–1386.

32. Weisdorf SA, Lysne J, Wind D, et al. Positive effect of prophylactic total parenteral nutrition on long-term outcome of bone marrow transplantation. Transplantation 1987;43:833–838.

33. Bodzin JH. Home hyperalimentation for inflammatory bowel disease. Nutr Clin Pract 1992;7:70–73.

34. Byrne WJ, Burke M, Fonkalsrud EW. Home parenteral nutrition: an alternative approach to the management of uncomplicated gastrointestinal fistulas not responding to conventional medical or surgical therapy. JPEN 1979;3:355–359.

35. Oakley JR, Steiger E, Lavery IC, et al. Catastrophic enterocutaneous fistulas: the role of home hyperalimentation. Cleve Clin Q 1979; 149:133–136.

36. Nance ML, Morris JB, Muellen JL. Home parenteral nutrition after near total enterectomy. J Am Coll Nutr 1993;12:281–285.

37. Dudrick SJ, MacFayden BV, Jr, Souchon EA, et al. Parenteral nutrition techniques in cancer patients. Cancer Res 1977;37:2440–2450.

38. Lavery IC, Steiger E, Fazio VW. Home parenteral nutrition in management of patients with severe radiation enteritis. Dis Colon Rectum 1980;23:91–93.

39. Schauder P, Sailer D, Muller JM. Total parenteral nutrition in the home of 498 patients with tumor disease. Med Klin 1993;88:423–426.

40. King LA, Carson LF, Konstantinides N, et al. Outcome assessment of home parenteral nutrition in patients with gynecologic malignancies: what have we learned in a decade of experience. Gynecol Oncol 1993;51:377–382.

41. O'Keefe SJ, Burnes JU, Thompson RL. Recurrent sepsis in home parenteral nutrition patients; an analysis of risk factors. JPEN J Parenter Enteral Nutr 1194;18:256–263.

42. Moukarzel AA, Haddad I, Ament ME, et al. 230 patient years of experience with home long-term parenteral nutrition in childhood: natural history and life of central venous catheters. J Pediatr Surg 1994;29:1323–1327.

43. Gerard-Boncompain M, Claudel JP, Gaussorgues P, et al. Hepatic cytolytic and cholestatic changes related to change of lipid emulsions in four long-term parenteral nutrition patients with short bowel. JPEN J Parenter Enteral Nutr 1992;16:7–83.

44. Bowyer BA, Fleming CR, Ludwig J, et al. Does long-term home parenteral nutrition in adult patients cause chronic liver disease? JPEN 1985;9:11–17.

45. Messing B, Bories C, Kunstlinger F, et al. Does total parenteral nutrition induce gallbladder sludge formation and lithiasis? Gastroenterology 1983;84:1021–1029.

46. McIntyre PB, Firchew M, Lennard-Jones JE. Patients with a high jejunostomy do not need a special diet. Gastroenterology 1986;91:25–33.

47. Greig PD, Jeejeebhoy KN, Langer B, et al. A decade of home parenteral nutrition. Gastroenterology 1981;80:1164A.

48. Loras Duclaux I, De Potter S, Pharaon I, et al. Quality of life of children with home parenteral nutrition and their parents. Pediatrie 1993;48:555–560.

49. Malone M. Home parenteral nutrition: effect on patients' lifestyle. Clin Nutr 1989;8:11–13.

50. Shils ME, Wright WL, Turnbull A, et al. Long-term parenteral nutrition through an external arteriovenous shunt. N Engl J Med 1970;283:341–344.

51. Broviac JW, Cole JJ, Schribner BH. A silicone rubber catheter for prolonged parenteral hyperalimentation. Surg Gynecol Obstet 1973;136:602–606.

52. Broviac JW, Schribner BH. Prolonged parenteral nutrition in the home. Surg Gynecol Obstet 1974;139:24–28.

53. Hickman RO, Buckner CD, Clift RA, et al. A modified right atrial catheter for access to the venous system in marrow transplant recipients. Surg Gynecol Obstet 1979;148:871–875.

54. Niederhuber JE, Ensminger W, Gyves JW, et al. Totally implanted venous and arterial access system to replace external catheters in cancer patients. Surgery 1982;92:706–712.

55. Bothe A Jr, Piccione W, Ambrosino JJ, et al. Implantable central venous access system. Am J Surg 1984;147:565–569.

56. Pomp A, Caldwell MD, Albina JE. Subcutaneous infusion ports for administration of parenteral nutrition at home. Surg Gynecol Obstet 1989;169:329–333.
57. Anonymous. Standards for home nutrition support. American Society for Parenteral and Enteral Nutrition. Nutr Clin Pract 1992;7:6569.
58. Kotler DP, Gaetz HP, Lange M, et al. Enteropathy associated with the AIDS. Ann Intern Med 1984;101:421–428.
59. Garr MA, Boles JM, Youinou PY. Current concepts in immune derangement due to undernutrition. JPEN 1987;11:309–313.
60. Jain VK, Chandra RK. Does nutritional deficiency predispose to AIDS? Nutr Res 1984;4: 537–543.
61. Singer P, Askanazi J, Rothkopf MM, Macklin E, Kvetan V. Home parenteral nutrition in AIDS. J Am Coll Nutr 1988;7:425.
62. Winick M, Andrassyre J, Armstrong D, et al. Guidelines for nutrition support in AIDS. Nutrition 1989;5:39–45.
63. Chandra RK. Nutrition, immunity and infection: present knowledge and future directions. Lancet 1982;1:688–691.
64. Starker PM, LaSala PA, Forse A, et al. Response to total parenteral nutrition in the extremely malnourished patient. JPEN 1985;9:300–302.
65. Sato SJ, Mirtalle JM. Nutritional support for the AIDS patient. US Pharmacist 1987;H:2.
66. Press OW, Ramsey PG, Larson FB, et al. Hickman catheter infection in patients with malignancies. Medicine 1984;63:189–200.
67. Hunter AMB, Carey MA, Larch HV. The nutritional status of patients with chronic obstructive pulmonary disease. Am Rev Respir Dis 1981;124:376–381.
68. Bistrain RB, Blackburn GL, Vitale J, et al. Prevalence of malnutrition in general medical patients. JAMA 1976;235:1567–1576.
69. Openbrier DR, Irwin MM, Rogers RM, et al. Nutritional status and lung function in patients with emphysema and chronic bronchitis. Chest 1983;88:17–22.
70. Wilson D, Wright E, Rogers R, et al. Body weight in COPD [Abstract]. Am Rev Respir Dis 1987;135:A144.
71. Vandenbergh E, Van de Woestije KP, Billiet L, et al. Evolution et propiostic de la bronchite an stade de la retention de CO_2. Bull Physio-Pathol Respir 1965;1:260.
72. Goldstein SA, Thomashow BM, Kvetan V, et al. Nitrogen and energy relationships in malnourished patients with emphysema. Am Rev Respir Dis 1988;138:636–644.
73. Askanazi J, Goldstein SA, Kvetan V, et al. Respiratory disease. In: Kinney JM, ed. Nutrition and Metabolism in Patient Care. Philadelphia: WB Saunders, 1988:522–530.
74. Askanazi J, Carpentier YA, Elwyn DH, et al. Influence of total parenteral nutrition on fuel utilization in injury and sepsis. Ann Surg 1980; 191:40.
75. Campbell EJM, Westlake EK, Cherniack RM. Simple methods of estimating oxygen consumption and efficiency of the muscles of breathing. J Appl Physiol 1957;11:303–308.
76. Cherniack RM. The oxygen consumption and efficiency of the respiratory muscles in health and emphysema. J Clin Invest 1959;38:494–498.
77. Askanazi J, Elwyn DE, Silverberg PA, et al. Respiratory distress secondary to a high carbohydrate load: a case report. Surgery 1980;87:596–598.
78. Covelli HD, Black JW, Olsen MV, et al. Respiratory failure precipitated by high carbohydrate loads. Ann Intern Med 1981;95:579–581.
79. Askanazi J, Nordenstrom J, Rosenbaum SH, et al. Nutrition for the patient with respiratory failure: glucose vs. fat. Anesthesiology 1981;54:373–377.
80. Greene HL, Hazlett D, Demaree R. Relationship between Intralipid-induced hyperlipemia and pulmonary function. Am J Clin Nutr 1976;29:127–135.
81. McKeen CR, Brigham KL, Bowers RE, et al. Pulmonary vascular effects of fat emulsion infusion in anesthetized sheep. J Clin Invest 1978;61:1295.
82. Hageman JR, McCulloch K, Gora P, et al. Intralipid alterations in pulmonary prostaglandin metabolism and gas exchange. Crit Care Med 1983;11:794.
83. Skeie B, Askanazi J, Rothkopf MM, et al. Improved exercise tolerance with long-term parenteral nutrition in cystic fibrosis. Crit Care Med 1987;15:960–962.
84. Askanazi J, Rothkopf MM, Rosenbaum SH, et al. Treatment of cystic fibrosis with long-term home parenteral nutrition. Nutrition 1987;3:277–279.
85. Skeie B, Askanazi J, Rothkopf MM, et al. Intravenous fat emulsions and lung function: a review. Crit Care Med 1988;16:183–184.
86. Askanazi J, Weissman C, Lasala P, et al. Effects of increasing protein intake on ventilatory drive. Anesthesiology 1984;60:106–110.
87. Donahoe M, Rogers RM, Wilson DD, et al. Oxygen consumption of the respiratory muscles in normal and in malnourished patients with chronic obstructive pulmonary disease. Am Rev Respir Dis 1989;140:385–391.
88. Wolfe BM, Culebras JM, Sim AJ, et al. Substrate interaction in intravenous feeding. Comparative effects of carbohydrate and fat on amino acid utilization in fasting man. Am Surg 1977;186: 518–540.

16

AGGRESSIVE NUTRITIONAL APPROACHES FOR CHRONIC RENAL FAILURE

Lisa P. Haverstick and Michael M. Rothkopf[a]

CHAPTER AT A GLANCE: Malnutrition has a significant impact on survival in patients with chronic renal failure. Yet, despite its importance, nutritional concepts are often given little attention in the management of patients with end-stage renal failure. This chapter reviews the metabolic functions of the kidney, nutritional considerations in chronic renal disease, and nutritional assessment of patients with chronic renal disease. Various methods of nutritional support, including enteral nutrition, nutritional dialysis, and intradialytic parenteral nutrition (IDPN) are discussed along with criteria for patient selection, administration, and complications associated with their use. Suggestions for monitoring the safety and efficacy of nutritional therapies are given, as well as formula recommendations and strategies for managing complications.

Introduction

The kidneys perform three main functions in the body: nitrogenous waste excretion; fluid, electrolyte, and acid/base regulation; and endocrine production. The kidneys are also involved in regulation of blood pressure, red blood cell production, protein homeostasis, bone metabolism, and detoxification of some drugs and poisons. Although these functions are often regarded separately, they are closely intertwined.

The kidneys maintain homeostasis within the body's internal environment despite daily fluctuations in food and fluid intake, external temperature, and physical activity. They have a large reserve capacity, and it is not until more than 60% of the nephrons are destroyed that the excretory and regulatory capacity of the kidneys diminishes. When less than 10% of functioning kidney tissue remains, renal function is severely compromised, and accumulation of waste products of metabolism (urea, creatinine, sulfate, uric acid, and organic acids) occurs.

Patients begin to experience "uremic symptoms" when the BUN is greater than 90 mg/dL (1). Restriction of dietary protein should be considered once the glomerular filtration rate (GFR) is below 25 mL/min.

The endocrine functions of the kidney are related to the production of renin and erythropoietin and to the conversion of vitamin D from food or skin to the biologically active metabolite 1,25-dihydroxyvitamin D. Derangement of these functions and other endocrine abnormalities—insulin resistance,

---

[a]*Ronald M. Abel contributed to this chapter in the first edition.*

increased levels of glucagon and parathyroid hormone (PTH), and impaired somatomedin activity—may occur in renal failure (1). These changes may, in turn, affect the nutritional status of the chronic renal failure patient. Dietary intervention can be expected to play a significant role in decreasing uremic symptoms.

Nutritional Considerations in Chronic Renal Disease

Once the kidneys are damaged, they can no longer maintain sodium, potassium, and fluid homeostasis, and restriction of the diet becomes essential. Restriction of dietary protein is also necessary to control the accumulation of urea and other protein waste products such as creatinine, uric acid, and other organic acids.

The Joint Food and Agricultural Organization/World Health Organization expert committee on protein and energy requirements has recommended a minimum of 0.55 g of protein per kilogram of body weight as the amount needed to maintain positive nitrogen balance in a healthy population. For patients with chronic renal insufficiency who are not on dialysis, similar protein intakes are recommended (i.e., 0.6 to 0.8 g/kg).

When dialysis is initiated, protein intake can be increased. The type of dialysis will affect protein intake. Patients undergoing peritoneal dialysis require more protein than those undergoing hemodialysis to due losses in the dialysate.

Guidelines for protein restriction are based on the GFR. It is important to note that with very low protein intake at least 65% of the protein consumed should be of high biological value (1–5). Nitrogen balance can be maintained and uremic symptoms controlled with diets providing 16 to 20 g/day of protein of mixed biological value. However, this is provided that these low protein intakes are supplemented with amino acids and/or ketoacids (6, 7). The latter are not widely available in the United States.

If protein intake is limited to the essential amino acids plus histidine, the body can utilize circulating nitrogen for endogenous synthesis of nonessential amino acids (8–10). The essential amino acids would be used primarily for protein synthesis, not ureagenesis. This would therefore reduce uremia. However, even though nonessential amino acids can be synthesized by the body, their availability is required for the production of various important proteins. In this respect, they may be considered "semi-essential" in certain situations. It is for this reason that a balanced amino acid formulation (essential and nonessential amino acids) is recommended in patients requiring dialysis (8–10).

Energy requirements can be determined by methods such as indirect calorimetry or estimated using a variety of formulas. The Harris-Benedict formula, which uses the patient's height, weight, age, and sex to give an estimate of resting energy needs, can then be multiplied by factors to account for the activity level of the patient and associated illnesses. For patients with renal failure, the basal energy expenditure is multiplied by 1.2 to 1.5 for maintenance calories and by 2 to arrive at repletion calorie levels (11–14). For patients on a low-protein diet, approximately 35 kcal/kg is required for nitrogen equilibrium (15).

Altered fat metabolism is frequently encountered in patients with chronic renal failure. Carnitine deficiency and reduced triglyceride clearance contribute to hypertriglyceridemia, especially in diabetic patients (16). To maintain adequate intake in patients with end-stage renal disease (ESRD), it is often necessary to increase the fat and carbohydrate content of the diet. The use of polyunsaturated and monounsaturated fats and complex, rather than simple, carbohydrates high in fiber, and regular aerobic exercise (17) may help to reduce the degree of hypertriglyceridemia.

Vitamins

Water-soluble vitamins should be supplemented in patients with chronic renal failure. However, supplementation of fat-soluble vitamins requires careful thought.

Vitamin A is transported from its main storage site (the liver) bound to retinol-binding protein. Retinol-binding protein joins with transthyretin (prealbumin), forming a complex. As this complex is metabolized by the kidney, retinol-binding protein and plasma retinol levels are increased in patients with renal failure.

Vitamin A supplementation is not routinely recommended in ESRD out of concern for toxicity. However, it is necessary to measure both retinol-binding protein and vitamin A levels to assess vitamin A status. If both retinol-binding protein and vitamin A levels are elevated, the patient probably has normal or low vitamin A status. If retinol-binding protein levels are normal but vitamin A levels are low, the patient may have vitamin A deficiency.

In ESRD, vitamin D deficiency is usually caused by impaired renal hydroxylation of 25-hydroxycholecalciferol. This state reduces intestinal absorption of calcium, which stimulates secretion of PTH, exacerbating metabolic bone disease. Hyperphosphatemia, due to inadequate clearance of dietary phosphate, reduces serum calcium and also stimulates PTH. When supplementation of vitamin D is indicated in patients with ESRD, calcitriol is the recommended form of the vitamin (11–14, 18).

Combination Dietary Management

The type of underlying nephropathy, the degree of functional impairment, the presence of hypertension, and the severity of proteinuria are some of the factors governing the progression of renal insufficiency (27–35). However, a low-protein diet (19–40) and other factors can delay the onset of diabetic nephropathy (Table 16.1) or delay the rate of progression of renal failure (32–40).

The Modification of Diet in Renal Disease (MDRD) Study evaluated the effect of two interventions in 840 patients between 1989 and 1993. The first intervention consisted of decreased dietary protein and phosphorus intake. The second intervention reduced blood pressure (41). The study indicated that dietary protein restriction has a minimal effect on the progression of renal failure. This is in direct contrast to the studies in experimental animals

Table 16.1. Factors that Can Delay the Onset of Diabetic Nephropathy

Fasting blood sugar of 100–140 mg/dL
Postprandial blood glucose of 200 mg/dL
Normal glycosylated hemoglobin
Decreased alcohol consumption
Cessation of smoking
Decreased protein intake
Maintenance of normal lipid levels
Antibiotics for control of infection when indicated
   (avoid the use of nephrotoxic agents)
Avoidance of unnecessary contrast studies
Maintenance of normal blood pressure
Angiotensin-converting enzyme inhibitors

that showed dietary protein restriction dramatically decreased the rate of progression to renal failure (42). The difference in results may be related to the control of variables in the study groups (age, duration of disease, antihypertensive treatment, etc). Such variables are difficult to control when doing human studies.

A meta-analysis of studies on protein restriction and the progression of renal disease has recently been published (86). This paper reviewed five studies of nondiabetic subjects and five other studies of Type I diabetic subjects. A total of 1413 nondiabetic and 108 diabetic patients were studied for 9 to 36 months. Pooled results showed that dietary restriction of protein to between 0.4 and 0.6 g/kg significantly reduced the risk for renal failure or death (relative risk = 0.67) in nondiabetics. Similarly, pooled results in Type I diabetes showed that restriction of dietary protein to between 0.6 and 0.85 g/kg significantly reduced the risk for the decline in glomerular filtration rate (relative risk = 0.56).

Malnutrition

Various studies (1, 34, 44–54) have documented the incidence of malnutrition in hemodialysis patients. Coexisting malnutrition in patients with ESRD increases the need for hospitalization and shortens survival (3). A study of 613 hemodialysis patients conducted over a 3-month period revealed that patients with a 5% weight loss required hospitalization twice as often as patients who either maintained or gained weight (43, 44). Such studies have increased awareness of the need for monitoring and instituting appropriate nutritional measures when indicated.

Decreased dietary intake in dialysis patients may be caused by the dietary restrictions necessary to control symptoms of uremia, especially in patients placed on severely restrictive diets to delay initiation of dialysis. Anorexia, depression, intercurrent illnesses, and dialysis scheduling conflicts all contribute to a decreased calorie intake. Fatigue and an altered sense of taste are also characteristic symptoms in patients with chronic renal failure.

Metabolic acidosis increases the activity of proteolytic enzymes and may stimulate amino acid oxidation and protein degradation. Other metabolic changes also occur in renal failure that affect the patient's ability to utilize substrate (55, 56). Alterations in the levels of glucagon, insulin, somatomedins, parathyroid hormone, and vitamin D significantly alter glucose, lipid, and protein metabolism. For example, elevated glucagon levels due to lack of renal neutral peptidase, an enzyme responsible for glucagon degradation, can enhance the deamination of amino acids to glucose and urea, which promotes malnutrition and contributes to azotemia (56).

The nutritional status of patients with ESRD may be affected further by dialysis. Paradoxically, close control of uremia may worsen nutritional status because of significant amino acid, peptide, glucose, and vitamin losses during aggressive dialysis.

In general, peritoneal dialysis leads to more substantial protein losses than does hemodialysis, due to the permeability of the peritoneal membrane. Patients on continuous ambulatory peritoneal dialysis (CAPD) can lose an average of 9 to 12 g of protein per treatment. Patients on intermittent peritoneal dialysis (IPD) lose an average of 12 to 14 g of protein per treatment. These losses are increased up to 15 to 20 g/day if the patient has peritonitis (57–59). Hemodialysis patients lose an average of 6 to 8 g of protein per treatment. Persistent proteinuria in patients still urinating can further depress serum protein levels (57, 58).

The amino acid profile of uremic patients is characterized by decreased concentrations of some essential amino acids (including tyrosine and histidine), decreased concentrations of the branched-chain amino acids, and increased concentrations of several nonessential amino acids. The ratio of essential to nonessential amino acids is decreased significantly.

This abnormal amino acid profile is caused by the metabolic alterations associated with uremia, including impaired degradation and/or decreased urinary excretion (58, 60). Regular dialysis treatments do not normalize concentrations of all amino acids and may lead to persistent losses of amino acids with each dialysis treatment (57, 58). Deficiencies of vitamins may also contribute because of their role as cofactors for various enzyme systems involved in amino acid metabolism. For example, folic acid is required for the remethylation of homocysteine to methionine, while pyridoxine serves as a cofactor in the conversion of methionine to cysteine and taurine.

The decreased activity of anabolic hormones such as insulin and somatomedins combined with increased circulating levels of catabolic hormones such as glucagon and parathyroid hormone result in protein depletion. Uremia itself is a catabolic stimulus that promotes amino acid oxidation, increases protein breakdown, and decreases protein synthesis. The catabolic nature of dialysis causes an increase in gluconeogenesis with an increased degradation of body protein for an energy source.

There are 27 important metabolic enzymes that exist primarily in kidney tissue (56). Most are also found elsewhere in the body, so the renal loss is compensated for by other tissues. However, when the enzyme is predominant in the kidney or when the rate at which the reaction occurs is dependent on substrate delivery to the kidney, compensation is inadequate. In this scenario, either loss of enzyme activity or decreased renal blood flow may lead to decreased enzyme function.

For example, the loss of renal 25-hydroxy-cholecalciferol-1-monooxygenase has a major impact on calcium metabolism (56). Hyperglucagonemia, which contributes to catabolism, is present in patients with renal disease who lack the degrading enzyme renal neutral peptidase. Low levels of phosphoglycerate dehydrogenase and phosphoserine transaminase secondary to a low protein intake may cause decreased synthesis of serine (39). Similarly, loss of arginine:glycine amidinotransferase may cause reduced synthesis of creatine and contribute to the myopathy seen in patients with ESRD (61). The decreased insulin requirements in diabetics with ESRD may be due to the decreased renal blood flow, which reduces insulin delivery to the renal insulin-degrading enzyme system.

Thus, the nutrient requirements of dialysis patients are influenced by many factors. The underlying disease process, associated medical conditions, diminished intake, effects of dialysis itself, and the loss of renal enzyme systems alter the patient's capacity to absorb and/or utilize essential nutrients. Changes in endocrine function may lead to further metabolic impairment and must be taken into consideration in the management of the patient undergoing chronic hemodialysis.

Nutritional Evaluation of Patients with ESRD

Assessment of nutritional status in ESRD patients can identify patients who need nutritional intervention and establish a baseline to evaluate the effectiveness of nutritional management (11, 43, 45–50, 62). This includes a nutritional focus at history and physical examination, including height and weight, percentage of ideal body weight, and anthropometric measurements. An analysis of serum chemistry and special testing for specific nutrients should be considered.

Review of the medical history may reveal conditions such as alcoholism, diabetes mellitus, congestive heart failure, trauma, infection, fever, or gastrointestinal disorders (45–50, 62). The weight history should compare the current weight to the established dry weight and include interdialytic changes. The diet history assesses nutrient intake. Dietary interviews and/or diet diaries provide insight to the patient's normal intake. Be sure to include both dialysis and non-dialysis days, since intake may differ. Family members may also contribute information here. The use of food models and food scales helps to increase the accuracy of the information.

Anthropometric examination includes measurement of arm circumference and skinfold thickness. Reduction in triceps skinfold measurement has been found in ESRD patients (51). However, measurement of mid-arm circumference and calculation of mid-arm muscle circumference have not always correlated with other parameters in assessing nutritional status. In light of the problems encountered in comparing renal patients with age- and sex-matched normal patients, it is recommended that the patient serve as his or her own control. Tracking changes in a single patient over time is generally a sensitive indicator of an altered nutritional state. Malnutrition in chronic hemodialysis patients is usually marasmic in type, characterized by wasting of body fat and muscle with preservation of serum protein concentrations (45–50, 60, 62).

Biochemical parameters may be of value in assessing the nutritional status in ESRD. These include blood urea nitrogen, creatinine, albumin, prealbumin, transferrin, and retinol-binding protein. They have been used to diagnose nutritional deficiencies and are also useful in monitoring the efficacy of nutritional intervention. However, they must be analyzed in conjunction with the patient's underlying disease process, since it may be the disease rather than malnutrition that is producing abnormal values.

The blood urea nitrogen (BUN)/serum creatinine ratio can be used to estimate the average protein intake of patients with ESRD, although it does have limitations. However, it has been found to be useful in nondialyzed, clinically stable, chronically uremic men (45–50, 62). A BUN/creatinine ratio greater than 15 indicates catabolism or excessive protein intake (62).

Edema and overhydration can affect the accuracy of serum albumin levels and anthropometric measurements. Lowrie and Low documented that a low serum albumin is an important predictor of mortality and an independent risk factor for death (63). But albumin, which has a half-life of 21 days, does not reflect the current nutritional status of the patient. The hydration status of the patient also affects albumin serum levels.

Other parameters used in the diagnosis of malnutrition are also difficult to interpret in renal disease patients. Thyroxine-binding prealbumin is falsely elevated in chronic renal failure. Serum transferrin level may be erroneous due to iron deficiency or overhydration. Retinol-binding protein levels are increased. Therefore, new parameters and/or standards need to be developed to accurately assess the nutritional status of the patient with chronic renal failure who is on maintenance hemodialysis (62).

Urea kinetic modeling, as described in the National Cooperative Dialysis Study by Sargent and Gotch (64), can be used to assess the adequacy of dialysis and protein intake. The protein catabolic rate (PCR) is a reflection of the amount of protein catabolized per kilogram of body weight in 24 hours and is usually equal to the dietary protein intake in nutritionally stable patients (65). The PCR should be similar to the amount of dietary protein prescribed for the patient. An elevated PCR may reflect inadequate kilocalorie and protein intake or excessive protein intake, while a decreased PCR may indicate insufficient protein in the diet or anabolism (66).

Delayed cutaneous hypersensitivity tests are not considered useful in assessing the nutritional status of maintenance hemodialysis patients. In a study of 52 patients on maintenance hemodialysis (53, 54), 60% failed to respond to intradermal skin antigens. The researchers were unable to document a correlation between cutaneous anergy and protein calorie malnutrition, although the incidence of anergy increased with the length of time patients were on dialysis. Renal failure apparently affects immunocompetence, altering cutaneous anergy panels and total lymphocyte count. However, reversal of skin test anergy has been shown in hemodialysis patients who are receiving nutritional supplements (54).

Nutritional Support

Enteral and parenteral support regimens have been used to improve the nutritional status of hemodialysis patients. "Failure to thrive" describes the well-dialyzed ESRD patient who, despite intensive diet counseling and aggressive enteral supplementation, fails to improve nutritionally. Once a patient is considered to have failure to thrive, every effort must be taken to increase the patient's intake.

Diet counseling in some patients will require supplementation with a commercially prepared formula to achieve energy or protein goals. A number of commercial formulas exist that are palatable, relatively low in cost, and easy to incorporate into the patient's diet pattern. Unfortunately, oral supplemental feeding regimens often fail due to decreased appetite, altered taste acuity, and early satiety (52, 67, 68).

Tube feedings are not a popular alternative because of the adverse psychological reaction and the risk of aspiration. Chronic debilitation makes these patients poor surgical candidates for tube enterostomies (i.e., gastrostomy or jejunostomy) (51, 67, 68). Furthermore, gastrostomies are generally avoided in patients on peritoneal dialysis because of concern about the sterility of the peritoneal site. However, gastrostomies could be considered for hemodialysis patients.

When tube feedings are used, the electrolyte content of the formula and the fluid volume required to meet nutritional goals must be considered in conjunction with the patient's primary medical diagnosis. For example, products that provide 2 calories per milliliter are available for use in cases when fluid volume must be restricted. Feeding modules of protein, fat, and carbohydrate are available for addition to foods already consumed by the patient to enhance the nutrient density.

If the patient fails to respond to aggressive enteral support, parenteral feedings may be necessary. Total parenteral nutrition (TPN) is indicated as the sole source of nutritional support when the patient has a nonfunctioning gastrointestinal tract.

Intravenous administration of nutrients during dialysis is a recent trend in the nutritional management of malnourished chronic hemodialysis patients. "Nutritional dialysis," in which amino acids and glucose are used as the dialysate for patients on peritoneal dialysis, and intradialytic parenteral nutrition (IDPN), in which nutrients are administered into the venous return line for hemodialysis patients, are two methods that have been used with some success in this patient population.

Amino Acid Dialysate

Nutritional dialysis has been attempted for patients when other methods of nutritional support have failed (59, 69). The cost of 2 liters of amino acid solution is considerably more than that of a dextrose dianeal solution, but it may be a cost-effective means of nutritional support. A standard 2-L bag of amino acid dialysate contains 22 g of amino acid, of which 16 to 18 g is absorbed (59). The amino acid dialysate has twice the osmotic pull of an equivalent amount of dextrose. It is recommended that two exchanges of amino acid dialysate be used, alternating with a dextrose-based dialysate.

Improved nutritional status, total body nitrogen, and increased transferrin levels have been reported with amino acid dialysis. An increase in high-density lipoprotein (HDL) cholesterol level and a decrease in low-density lipoprotein (LDL), very low-density lipoprotein (VLDL), and triglyceride levels have also been seen (59, 69). Increased ultrafiltration has been shown due to the amino acid dialysate osmotic pull.

Because of the cost associated with the use of an amino acid dialysate, criteria for the use of CAPD with amino acids have been established. Patients must have a serum albumin of less than 3.0 g/dL, poor oral intake despite aggressive diet counseling, protein intake of less than 0.9 g/kg/day despite the use of supplements, and a nonfunctional gut. Additionally, the patient should not be a candidate for parenteral nutrition (69).

Prolonged use of an amino acid dialysate may be necessary until an alternate form of nutritional support is feasible. Biochemical monitoring is mandatory to assess the efficacy of CAPD with amino acids. Serum transferrin determinations should be obtained weekly and a serum chemistry performed monthly to check serum albumin, creatinine, BUN, cholesterol, and triglyceride levels. A lipid profile should also be performed monthly to determine HDL, LDL, and VLDL levels.

IDPN

If the patient is malnourished due to the underlying renal condition, the catabolic effects of dialysis, and dietary constraints placed on the patient's normal eating pattern, IDPN can be used to help improve quality of life. Although IDPN provides an adequate nutritional intake, it is important to recognize that its intermittent nature requires that the patient be capable of consuming nutrients on nondialysis days. In this light, IDPN can best be viewed as a supplement to either oral intake or, in extreme cases, daily TPN. Approximately 50 to 75% of the patient's estimated needs must be provided outside of IDPN therapy (70). Patients who require more support should be considered for daily TPN.

IDPN refers to the provision of amino acids, glucose, and lipids directly into the venous drip chamber of the dialysis tubing. Time constraints dictate that the nutrient solution be concentrated to maximize the delivery of calories and protein during the dialysis treatment. A 4-hour dialysis minimum has been recommended when lipid is infused in order to prevent complications due to too rapid an infusion of lipid (67, 68, 71, 72).

IDPN is a concept that has been in existence since 1975 when Heidland and Kult demonstrated an improvement in visceral protein status, weight, and appetite after 30 weeks of treatment (73). In 1977, Hecking et al. evaluated the use of 17.25 g of essential amino acids given for 6 months during the last 90 minutes of dialysis (74). Guarnieri et al. in 1980 compared different solutions given for 8 weeks during the last 90 minutes of the dialysis on patients who received the essential amino acids plus histidine and demonstrated weight gain as a result of treatment (45). Thunberg et al. in 1980 administered solutions of varying composition based on patient need and demonstrated positive nitrogen balance and improved serum albumin (75). Piraino et al. in 1981 reported benefits with the provision of amino acids and glucose in 16 patients for 20 weeks (76).

Wolfson et al. (77, 78) evaluated the effects of intravenous infusion during hemodialysis of amino acids and dextrose. They demonstrated that intravenous infusion of amino acids and dextrose during hemodialysis prevented a decrease in plasma amino acid and dextrose levels with only a slight increase in the loss of free amino acids into the dialysate. Since most of the infused amino acids are retained, IDPN can be considered an effective form of nutritional support in chronic hemodialysis patients.

Olshan et al. (79) reported experiences with IDPN administration in an outpatient hemodialysis unit. Eight of ten patients demonstrated an average weight gain of 5.1 lb (range 2 to 9 lb) and improved appetite. Nine patients showed an improved serum albumin after 2 months of therapy. Moore et al. showed a significant increase in serum albumin levels at the end of a 3-month treatment period (80). Madigan et al. (81) evaluated the effectiveness of IDPN in nine diabetic patients with ESRD. IDPN was not as favorable in this subset as in a general ESRD population, but the improvement in serum albumin was statistically significant.

Application of IDPN

Patient Selection

Since IDPN is a complex process, its use should be limited to those patients most likely to benefit from it. Evidence of a nonfunctioning gastrointestinal (GI) tract and/or the presence of a GI abnormality that precludes ade-

Table 16.2. Indications for Use of IDPN

1. Weight loss of >10% of usual weight
2. Failure of enteral feeding regimens to improve nutritional status as documented by diet history
3. Uremic malabsorption
4. Diabetic gastroparesis
5. Uremic gastroparesis
6. Hypoalbuminemia (<3.5 g/dL)
7. Coexistent liver disease
8. Obstruction of the GI tract or pseudo-obstruction
9. Radiation enteritis
10. Short gut syndrome
11. Inflammatory bowel disease
12. Failure to thrive

quate oral intake is usually required. Table 16.2 lists suggested criteria for determining when IDPN is most appropriate (71, 82, 83).

Administration

Various methods of administration have been applied to IDPN. For example, IDPN has been infused during the entire dialysis treatment or near the end of the treatment. Infusion of nutrients immediately after dialysis is not recommended.

Nutritional hemodialysis, in which the nutrients are added directly to the dialysate, is also not recommended because of the increased length of the dialysis treatment time (8 to 10 hours). Furthermore, this method is more costly due to the volume of solution required to achieve nutritional goals (52, 53).

Nutrient infusion during the last 60 to 90 minutes of dialysis may be an interesting alternative to standard IDPN therapy. Some researchers feel that chronic dialysis patients utilize nutrients more efficiently during the end of the dialysis treatment. Protein synthesis is reported to be accelerated during this time as well (54, 67, 73). However, there are objections to this approach. Glucose and amino acid levels may vary considerably, and metabolic utilization of the nutrients may be abnormal (54, 67, 73). In addition, the potential for fluid overload and rebound hypoglycemia is also increased. Finally, postinfusion monitoring may need to be extended, which increases time in the dialysis unit.

Infusion of nutrients during the entire dialysis treatment has several advantages. From a practical viewpoint, it does not increase staff or patient dialysis time. The catabolic stress of dialysis is reduced by replacing nutrient losses as they occur. The danger of fluid overload is minimized since the additional volume can be removed readily. Furthermore, additional vascular access is unnecessary. Phlebitis is also avoided since long-term use of peripheral veins is eliminated (51, 54, 59, 67–73, 76).

Solutions of a mixed amino acid source are recommended to help normalize plasma aminograms. Approximately 90% of the amino acids given via IDPN are retained, which negates the losses that normally occur with dialysis (16). Calorie goals can be achieved with the use of a mixture of dextrose or dextrose and lipid depending on the patient's requirements and tolerance of the substrates and volume. Glucose is usually limited to 3 to 5 mg/kg/minute and fat to less than 60% of total kilocalories. Standard vitamin and electrolyte preparations are not recommended for the patient with renal failure due to the metabolic alterations associated with a diseased

Table 16.3. Initiating IDPN Infusion

1. Calculate the volume of IDPN solution into the total membrane pressure (TMP).
2. Obtain predialysis blood work, including glucose, sodium, potassium, phosphorus, magnesium, and triglycerides.
3. Prime IDPN tubing and insert extension tubing into the venous drip chamber. Set volume to be infused as per MD's order.
4. Infuse at determined rate.
5. Obtain postdialysis blood work.
6. Observe the patient for 30–60 minutes after the first treatment for rebound hypoglycemia. Have patient consume snack prior to the end of the dialysis treatment.
7. Fat emulsion. Administer test dose of 1 mL/min for 30 minutes and observe patient tolerance. Monitor for dyspnea, cyanosis, nausea, vomiting, headache, sweating, increased temperature, chest pain, or abdominal pain.

kidney. It is often necessary to individualize each treatment regimen based on the individual requirements of each patient selected for this mode of therapy (Table 16.3)

Complications

Although published data are limited, IDPN is generally well tolerated. Communication between team members, documentation, and close monitoring can help to prevent problems from occurring or help to reduce the severity of a problem (Table 16.4).

Hypoglycemia may result if IDPN is abruptly discontinued. This can be managed easily by the provision of a carbohydrate-rich snack or, in severe cases, the infusion of 50% dextrose.

Hyperglycemia can result from provision of excess glucose in the parenteral nutrition solution. It may be necessary to add insulin to the parenteral nutrition solution if the serum glucose remains elevated during treatment.

Electrolyte imbalances can occur with any intravenous nutritional regimen. This is heightened in IDPN by the changes in electrolyte clearance and by the use of dialysis. Shifts of potassium, magnesium, and phosphorus commonly occur when refeeding malnourished patients (78). Hyponatremia is also frequently seen due to alterations in sodium and water exchange.

Hyperlipidemia can occur when lipid is substituted for glucose as an energy source. For this reason, it is important to check serum lipid levels prior to administration of the lipid emulsion. Lipids should not be administered if the serum triglyceride level is above 200 mg/dL. Triglyceride levels should also be checked 6 to 8 hours after lipid infusion to ensure adequate clearance of the lipid.

Fluid overload can occur if the volume of infusion exceeds the patient's needs and the excess fluid is not removed during the dialysis treatment. Monitoring interdialytic weight gains carefully will help to avoid this problem.

Azotemia can occur if the protein load received by the patient is greater than needed. Nitrogen balance, assessed by calculating urinary nitrogen appearance, can be used to assess the patient's tolerance of the amino acid load.

Table 16.4. Complications and Interventions during Intradialytic Parenteral Nutrition (IDPN)

Complication	Usual Cause	Symptoms	Intervention
Hyponatremia	Low Nal concentration of IPN solution.	Cramps during and after dialysis. 2. Hypotension during and after dialysis.	1. Notify the MD and RD. 2. Obtain post-dialysis Nal level. 3. If necessary add 75 MEQ of Nal to 1 liter of formula. 4. Monitor post-dialysis Nal level for at least 1 week.
Post IPN infusion hypotension	1. Anemia—low hct. 2. High glucose load.	Weakness, dizziness, confusion, disorientation, SOB, imbalance.	1. Keep hct greater than 25%. 2. Lower the dextrose concentration. 3. Make sure to check glucose level in order to give insulin.
Loss of infused vitamins	Water-soluble vitamins are dialyzed out when infused during the treatment.	1. Short- and long-range water-soluble vitamin deficiencies. 2. If given directly into a vein, may cause irritation at the infusion site.	If using, infuse water-soluble vitamins with 50–100 mL IPN solution at the last 0.5 hr of dialysis to prevent vitamin loss.
Uremic/metabolic acidosis	1. Increased amino acids in IPN formula. 2. High dietary protein.	Higher pre-dialysis BUN.	1. Lower the amount of amino acids in IPN formula to balance it with recommended P.O. protein intake
Fluid overload	1. Additional fluid infusion with IPN. 2. Inability to remove fluid. 3. Poor tolerance (heart condition).	SOB, edema, and/or puffy face.	1. Consult MD and RD. 2. Taper the infused volume to a level the patient can tolerate.
Elevated liver enzymes	1. Amino acid imbalance. 2. Excessive fat and glycogen deposition in the liver.	Elevated SGOT, SGPT, and/or alkaline phosphatase.	Monitor levels and discuss with M.D.
Hypoglycemia (low blood sugar)	1. Abrupt ending of infusion with high glucose concentration. 2. Glucose intolerance.	Headache, dizziness, weakness, tremors, cold sweat, confusion, faintness.	*Prevention:* 1. Monitor patient's B.S. during last 1 hr of infusion for symptoms. 2. Give a few graham crackers, apple juice, piece of hard candy, or small glass of soda pop to avoid rebound hypoglycemia. 3. Diabetics may need insulin added to the IPN—check with the MD.

Table 16.4—Continued

Complication	Usual Cause	Symptoms	Intervention
			Treatment: 1. If patient is symptomatic, give something with dextrose as mentioned above. 2. Observe patient at least 45–60 minutes post-infusion for resolution of symptoms. 3. Notify MD.
Hyperglycemia (high blood sugar)	1. Too rapid infusion of dextrose/amino acid solution (i.e., faulty pump speed). 2. Infection. 3. Insulin resistance.	Nausea, thirst, headache, vomiting, weakness.	*Prevention:* 1. Monitor IV line and patient throughout infusion. Do not rely solely on the pump. Check pump over 30 min. 2. Educate patient on symptoms. *Treatment:* 1. Notify MD. 2. Obtain blood sugar via finger-stick. 3. Use the following sliding scale as a guide to administer insulin if needed (get MD order): BS: 200–250 give 5 u Reg BS: 250–300 give 10 u Reg BS: 300–350 give 15 u Reg BS: 350–400 give 20 u Reg 4. At least 1 hr after infusion, monitor patient's symptoms. 5. Follow-up with patient by phone next day for symptom resolution.
Reaction to IV fat emulsions	1. Allergic reaction. 2. Inability to tolerate (i.e., hyperlipdemia). 3. Rapid infusion of lipids.	Nausea, vomiting, sweating, pressure over eyes, flushing, high temperature, pain in chest and back.	*Prevention:* 1. Administer first lipid infusion slowly (1–5 mL/min) for the first 30 min to monitor for reaction.

Table 16.4—Continued

Complication	Usual Cause	Symptoms	Intervention
			2. Do baseline serum triglyceride level prior to first administration of lipid. 3. Repeat serum triglyceride level prior to next infusion of lipids to see how well patient is tolerating lipid. *Treatment:* Stop infusion if reaction is suspected.
Post-IPN infusion hypoglycemia	Persistence of endogenous insulin production due to high carbohydrate infusion.	Confusion, headache, disorientation, dizziness, lethargy, cold sweat faintness.	1. Give 1/2 sandwich, a few graham crackers, or 1/2 cup cranberry juice during last 0.5 hr to prevent hypoglycemia. 2. Diabetics may need insulin added to the bag—check with M.D. 3. Observe the patient.

Note: DFO and IPN can be infused during dialysis at the same time using two separate AVI pumps. DFO doesn't seem to have reaction with any of the IPN solutions. Try to separate DFO complications from IPN complications.

Monitoring

To ensure the efficacy and safety of IDPN, close monitoring is essential. Periodic checks on serum chemistry including glucose, electrolytes, and liver enzymes are recommended. Dyspnea, cyanosis, nausea, vomiting, headache, sweating, increased temperature, chest pain, and abdominal pain have been observed when lipids are infused too rapidly. Therefore, the onset of these symptoms during IDPN should lead to further evaluation.

Part of the monitoring process should also include an evaluation of patient progress. The patient's weight should be recorded with every treatment, both before and after dialysis. A weight gain should become evident after 2 weeks. If not, consideration should be given to increasing the nutrient content of the formula.

An ongoing determination must be made regarding the patient's ability to tolerate the additional fluid load of IDPN. This may vary due to other aspects of the patient's condition or dialysis. Changes in the dialysis protocol may permit the patient to tolerate larger volumes of IDPN, allowing for a greater degree of nutritional support.

Serum proteins, such as albumin, should be checked on a regular basis. These will generally respond to adequate nutritional support in 3 or 4 weeks. If this is not the case, changes in the caloric and/or protein content of the formula should be considered.

Clinicians involved in the management of IDPN should be reminded that nutritional recovery is a gradual process. Despite the slowness of patient response, it is incorrect to attempt to accelerate this process by overfeeding the patient. Too much nutritional therapy may be as harmful as too little (73, 76–79, 82, 83). Improvement in nutritional status will usually occur in 10 to 12 weeks of therapy.

Lastly, the patient should be monitored for quality-of-life issues such as appetite, activity level, and a sense of well-being. These can also be expected to improve while the patient is receiving IDPN, although results are highly variable.

Formula Recommendations

Standard amino acid solutions of 8.5 to 10% are generally used, but a 15% solution is also available if the volume needs to be further restricted. The dextrose concentrations used will vary depending on individual glucose tolerance, caloric goals, and volume tolerance. Dextrose concentrations of 50 to 70% are the most frequently used.

The addition of intravenous lipid emulsions can serve as a good source for additional calories. Lipids are calorically dense, containing approximately 9 kcal/g (compared to 4 kcal/g for protein, and 3.4 kcal/g for intravenous dextrose solutions). Commercially prepared lipid emulsions are available in concentrations of 10 and 20%. These contain 10 and 20 g of lipid per 100 mL, respectively. Glycerol and phospholipids are also part of the emulsion mix. In general, the 20% concentration is used to maximize the caloric density of the IDPN solution. In most cases, the lipid emulsion may be mixed directly into the bag containing the amino acids and dextrose (triple mixing). This permits an added degree of simplicity with the IDPN administration since an additional piggybacked line is no longer required.

Standard, commercially available vitamin preparations for parenteral use are not recommended for IDPN. Vitamin A may be contraindicated for use in the patient with ESRD due to increased serum levels. Similarly, the vitamin D contained in the parenteral vitamin preparation is not effectively utilized in patients with chronic renal failure because of the impaired conversion of 25-hydroxycholecalciferol to 1,25-dihydroxycholecalciferol (18). Water-soluble vitamins are lost with each dialysis treatment, making replacement of these losses mandatory in this patient population. Special vitamin preparations are available for patients with renal failure; otherwise, the clinician can use a vitamin B complex with additional folic acid.

Carnitine, an amino acid derivative found in the serum and in cytosol, plays an important role in lipid metabolism. As a component of the enzyme carnitine acyltransferase, it serves as a transport system for fatty acids into the mitochondria. Serum levels of carnitine are low in ESRD patients. The hypertriglyceridemia frequently found in these patients may be a manifestation of carnitine deficiency. Carnitine deficiency in this patient group may be caused by low dietary intake of carnitine and lysine, reduced absorption in the gut, reduced liver synthesis, and loss of carnitine into the dialysate. Loss of the enzyme renal butyrobetaine hydroxylase decreases synthesis of carnitine in the kidney (56, 84, 85).

The decrease in carnitine synthesis highlights the concept of renal enzyme loss in ESRD. Other important regulatory enzyme functions are significantly altered by renal disease (56, 84, 85). This induces a change in metabolism that has been implicated in the development of malnutrition in chronic hemodialysis patients because of impaired synthesis, utilization, and degradation of certain nutrients (41).

The addition of standard electrolytes and trace elements, usually a fundamental part of TPN, is often avoided in IDPN. Patients in renal failure on dialysis have unique electrolyte requirements and may not tolerate any of the trace metals such as zinc. There are no guidelines available on the quantities of electrolytes or trace metals for IDPN. These must be individualized according to the patient's laboratory values and dialysis procedure.

Several standardized formulations have been developed for IDPN (Table 16.5). These range from initial formulas of low volume and low caloric content to stable therapy formulas that infuse 1000 to 1500 mL and provide as much as 2000 kcal per treatment. In addition, some centers have developed special formulas for patients on high flux or other forms of dialysis.

Access

IDPN is usually administered via the venous drip chamber of the hemodialysis machine. This route of administration bypasses the need for insertion of a central line to provide therapy. The rapid blood flow at this site quickly reduces the osmolality of the solution to one that is safely tolerated by the veins.

Table 16.5. Standardized Formulas for IDPN

Formula 1
  11.4% Amino acids 500 mL (57 g) 228 kcal
  70% Dextrose 200 mL (140 g) 476 kcal
  20% Lipids 100 mL (20 g) 200 kcal
  B-complex with C and B_{12}[a] 1 mL
  Folic acid 0.2 mL

  801.2 mL Total calories: 904
Formula 2
  11.4% Amino acids 500 mL (57 g) 228 kcal
  70% Dextrose 250 mL (175 g) 595 kcal
  20% Lipids 200 mL (40 g) 400 kcal
  B-complex with C and B_{12}[a] 1 mL
  Folic acid 0.2 mL

  951.2 mL Total calories: 1223
Formula 3
  11.4% Amino acids 500 mL (57 g) 228 kcal
  70% Dextrose 300 mL (210 g) 714 kcal
  20% Lipids 300 mL (60 g) 600 kcal
  B-complex with C and B_{12}[a] 1 mL
  Folic acid 0.2 mL

  1101.2 mL Total calories: 1542

[a]B-complex with vitamin C and B_{12} (Lyphomed).

Studies have been done that have shown little or no damage to the walls of the blood vessels during IDPN therapy when it is administered through the venous drip chamber. If another route of access is chosen, the osmolality of the solution must be considered in order to prevent thrombophlebitis, especially if the rate of blood flow is not as rapid as it is in a central vein. Peripheral administration of the parenteral nutrition solution is not generally recommended because of the large volume of fluid that must be infused to even remotely approach caloric goals.

Summary

The patient with ESRD has unique nutritional needs. Loss of functioning nephrons leads to accumulation of waste products of metabolism and endocrine abnormalities, which affect the nutritional status of the patient.

Nutritional management of the patient with chronic renal disease varies depending on the underlying diagnosis, the type of dialysis treatment, and the presence of other medical problems (i.e., diabetes or AIDS). Macronutrient and micronutrient intake needs to be carefully balanced to prevent accumulation of toxic waste products while meeting nutritional requirements.

Malnutrition, a frequently encountered problem in the dialysis population, can have an adverse effect on patient outcome. Aggressive nutritional support can improve the nutritional status of such patients. IDPN and other nutritional strategies have produced a modest degree of success in malnourished renal patients. Further study of this important area is warranted.

References

1. Burton BT. Nutritional implications of renal disease. 1. Current overview and general principles. J Am Diet Assoc 1977;70:479.
2. Kopple JD. Nutritional therapy in kidney failure. Nutr Rev 1981;39:193.
3. Swenseid ME. Nutritional implications of renal disease. 3. Nutritional needs of patients with renal disease. J Am Diet Assoc 1971;70:488.
4. Wineman RJ, et al. Nutritional implications of renal disease. 2. The dietitian's key role in studies of dialysis therapy. J Am Diet Assoc 1977;70:483.
5. Burton BT. Current concepts of nutrition and diet in diseases of the kidney. J Am Diet Assoc 1974;65:623.
6. Borah MF. Nitrogen balance during intermittent dialysis therapy for uremia. Kidney Int 1978; 14:491.
7. Walser M. Rationale and indications for the use of alpha ketoanalogues. J Parenter Enteral Nutr 1983;8:37.
8. Mirtallo JM, et al. A comparison of essential and general amino acid infusions in the nutritional support of patients with compromised renal function. J Parenter Enteral Nutr 1982;6:109.
9. Blackburn GL, et al. Criteria for choosing amino acid therapy in acute renal failure. Am J Clin Nutr 1978; 31:1841.
10. Kopple JD. Amino acid and protein metabolism in renal failure. Am J Clin Nutr 1978;31:1532.
11. Weinser RL, Heimburger DC, Butterworth CE. Handbook of Clinical Nutrition. St. Louis: CV Mosby, 1989.
12. Monteon FJ, et al. Energy expenditure in patients with chronic renal failure. Kidney Int 1980; 30:741.
13. Feinstein EI. Nutritional therapy in maintenance hemodialysis patients. In: Nissenson AR, Fine RN, eds. Dialysis Therapy. St. Louis: CV Mosby, 1986.
14. Kopple JD. Nutrition therapy in kidney failure. In: Olson RE, ed. Present Knowledge in Nutrition. Washington, DC: The Nutrition Foundation, 1984.
15. Kopple JD, Monteon RJ, Sharb JK. Effect of energy intake on nitrogen metabolism in nondialyzed patients with chronic renal failure. Kidney Int 1986;29:734.
16. Davis M. Nutrition management of the patient with diabetes and renal disease. In: Stover J, ed. A Clinical Guide to Nutrition Care in End Stage Renal Disease, 2nd ed. Chicago: American Dietetic Association, 1994.
17. Goldberg AP. A potential role for exercise training in modulating coronary risk factors in uremia. Am J Nephrol 1984;4:132.
18. Pietrek J, Kokot F, Kuska J. Kinetics of serum 25-hydroxy-vitamin D in patients with acute renal failure. Am J Clin Nutr 1978;31:1919.
19. Brenner BM, Meyer TW, Hostetter TH. Dietary protein intake and the progressive nature of kidney disease: The role of hemodynamically mediated glomerular injury in the pathogenesis of progressive glomerular sclerosis in aging, renal ablation, and intrinsic renal disease. N Engl J Med 1982;307:652.
20. Parving HH, Anderson AR, Smidt UM, et al. Effect of antihypertensive treatment on kidney function in diabetic nephropathy. Br Med J 1987;294:1443.
21. Parving HH, Hammel E, Smidt UM. Protection of kidney function and decrease in albuminuria by Captopril in insulin dependent diabetics with nephropathy. Br Med J 1988;297:1086.
22. Marre M, Chatellier G, Leblanc H, et al. Prevention of diabetic nephropathy with enalapril in normotensive diabetics with microalbuminuria. Br Med J 1988;297:1092.
23. Marre M, Leblanc H, Suarez L, et al. Converting enzyme inhibition and kidney function in normotensive diabetic patients with persistent microalbuminuria. Br Med J 1987;294:1446.
24. Walker JD, Dodds RA, Murrels TJ, et al. Restriction of dietary protein and progression of renal failure in diabetic nephropathy. Lancet 1989;1411.
25. Davis M, Comty C, Shapiro F. Management of patients with diabetes treated by hemodialysis. J Am Diet Assoc 1979;75:265.
26. Ciavarelo A, Dimizio G, Stefoni S, Borgnino L, Vannini P. Reduced albuminuria after dietary protein restriction in insulin dependent diabetic patients with clinical nephropathy. Diabetes Care 1987;10:407.
27. Viberti G. Recent advances in understanding mechanisms and natural history of diabetic renal disease. Diabetes Care 1988;11(Suppl):3.
28. Schafer R. Implementation of low protein diets for treatment of persons with early diabetic nephropathy. Diabetes Educator 1989;15:231.
29. Evanoff G, Thompson C, Brown J, Weinman E. The effect of dietary protein restriction on the progression of diabetic nephropathy. Arch Intern Med 1987; 147:492.
30. Viberti G. Interventions based on microalbuminuria screening and low protein diet in the treatment of kidney disease of diabetes mellitus. Am J Kidney Dis 1989;13:41.
31. Morgensen CE. Management of diabetic renal involvement and disease. Lancet 1988;1:867.
32. Klahr S, et al. The progression of renal disease. N Engl J Med 1988;318:1657.
33. Klahr S, Purkerson ML. Effects of dietary protein on renal function and on the progression of renal disease. Am J Clin Nutr 1988;47:146.
34. El Nahas AM, Coles GA. Dietary treatment of chronic renal failure: Ten unanswered questions. Lancet 1986; 597.
35. Maschio G, Oldrizzi L, Tessitore N, et al. Effect of dietary protein and phosphate restriction on the progression of early renal failure. Kidney Int 1982;22:371.

36. Giordano C. Protein restriction in chronic renal failure. Kidney Int 1982;22:401.

37. Adler SG, Kopple JD. Dietary factors influencing the progression of renal failure. Nutr MD 1984;April:4.

38. Brenner BM, et al. Dietary protein intake and the progressive nature of kidney disease. N Engl J Med 1982;307:652.

39. Ihle BU, Becker GJ, Whitworth JA, et al. The effect of protein restriction on the progression of renal insufficiency. N Engl J Med 1989;321:1773.

40. El Nahas AM, Masters-Thomas A, Brady SA, et al. Selective effect of low protein diets in chronic renal diseases. Br Med J 1984;289:1337.

41. The fifth report of the Joint National Committee on Detection, Evaluation and Treatment of High Blood Pressure. Arch Intern Med 1993;15:154.

42. Brenner BM. Nephron adaptation to renal injury or ablation. Am J Physiol 1985;249:F-324.

43. Blackburn GL, Bistrian BR, et al. Nutritional and metabolic assessment of the hospitalized patient. J Parenter Enteral Nutr 1977;1:11.

44. Acchiardo SR, Moore LW, Latour PA. Malnutrition as the main factor in morbidity and mortality of hemodialysis patients. Kidney Int 1983;24(Suppl 16):S199.

45. Guarnieri G, Faccini L, Lipartiti T, et al. Simple methods for nutritional assessment in hemodialyzed patients. Am J Clin Nutr 1980;33:1598.

46. Blumenkrantz MJ, Kopple JD, Gutman RA, et al. Methods for assessing nutritional status of patients with renal failure. Am J Clin Nutr 1980;33:1567.

47. Kelly MP, Gettel S, Gee C, et al. Nutritional and demographic data related to the hospitalization of hemodialysis patients. CRN Q 1987;11:16.

48. Harvey KB, Blumenkrantz MJ, Levine SE, et al. Nutritional assessment and treatment of chronic renal failure. Am J Clin Nutr 1980;33:1586.

49. Schoenfeld PY, Henry RR, Laird NM, et al. Assessment of nutritional status of the National Cooperative Dialysis Study Population. Kidney Int 1983;23 (Suppl):S-80.

50. Harter HR. Review of significant findings from the National Cooperative Dialysis Study and Recommendations. Kidney Int 1983;23(Suppl 13):S-107.

51. Wolfson MW, Strong CJ, Minturn D, Gray DK, Kopple JD. Nutritional status and lymphocyte function in maintenance hemodialysis patients. Am J Clin Nutr 1984;37:547.

52. Richards V, Hobbs C, Murray T, Mullen J. Incidence and sequelae of malnutrition in chronic hemodialysis patients. Kidney Int 1978;14:683.

53. Bansal VK, Popli S, Pickering J, et al. Protein calorie malnutrition and cutaneous anergy in hemodialysis maintained patients. Am J Clin Nutr 1980;33:1608.

54. Hak LT, Liffell MS, Lamanna RW, et al. Reversal of skin test anergy during maintenance hemodialysis by protein and calorie supplementation. Am J Clin Nutr 1982;36:1089.

55. Rubenstein AH, Spitz I. Role of the kidney in insulin metabolism and excretion. Diabetes 1968;17:161.

56. Dixon M, Webb E, eds. Enzymes, 3rd ed. New York: Academic Press, 1979.

57. Lindholm B, Bergstrom J. Nutritional aspects of CAPD, In: Gokal R, ed. Chronic Ambulatory Peritoneal Dialysis. New York: Churchill Livingstone, 1979.

58. Schoenfeld P. Care of the patient between dialysis. In: Cogan MG, Garovay MR, eds. Introduction to Dialysis. New York: Churchill Livingstone, 1985.

59. Zlomke A. Use of amino acid dialysate for CAPD in hypoalbuminemic patient. Renal Nutr Forum 1988; Spring:7.

60. Smolin LA, Laidlaw SA, Kopple JD. Altered plasma free and protein bound sulfur amino acid levels in patients undergoing maintenance hemodialysis. Am J Clin Nutr 1987;45:737.

61. Goldman R, Moss JX. Creatine synthesis after creatine loading and after nephrectomy. Proc Soc Exp Biol Med 1960;105:450.

62. Matarese LE. Nutritional support in renal failure. In: Shronts EP, ed. Nutrition Support Dietetics Core Curriculum. Silver Spring, MD: ASPEN Publications, 1989.

63. Lowrie EC, Lew NL. Death risk in hemodialysis patients: the predictive value of commonly measured variables and an evaluation of death rate differences between facilities. Am J Kidney Dis 1990;15:458.

64. Sargent J, Gotch F. Mathematical modeling to dialysis therapy. Kidney Int 1980;18(Suppl 10):2.

65. Johnson J, Schneipp F. Comparison of urea kinetic modeling with other approaches to dietary prescription. Dial Transplant 1981;10:280.

66. Goldstein D, Frederico C. The effects of urea kinetic modeling on the nutritional management of hemodialysis patients. J Am Diet Assoc 1987;87:474.

67. O'Shea RA. Intradialytic parenteral nutrition. Renal Dietitians Newsletter 1987;Fall:6.

68. Enteral Parenteral Handbook—A Screening Tool for Nutritional Replacement in the Hemodialysis Patient. Redwood City, CA: Satellite Dialysis Centers, Inc., 1989.

69. Oren A, et al. Effective use of amino acid dialysate over four weeks in CAPD patients. Peritoneal Dial Bull 1983;3:66.

70. Rudman D, Millikan WJ, Richardson TJ, et al. Elemental balances during intravenous hyperalimentation of underweight adult subjects. J Clin Invest 1985;55:94.

71. Rogan M, Pulles J. Intradialytic parenteral nutrition. In: Nutrition Support of the Renal Patient. Chicago: National Renal Dietitians Practice Group, American Dietetic Association, 1988:44–50.

72. Hagelshaw CM. Protocol for parenteral nutrition therapies in dialysis patients. CRN Q 1984; 8:10.

73. Heidland A, Kult J. Longterm effects of essential amino acid supplementation in patients on regular hemodialysis treatment. Clin Nephrol 1975;5:238.

74. Hecking E, Post F, Bilhym R, et al. A controlled study on the value of amino acid supplementation with essential amino acids and ketoanalogues in chronic hemodialysis. Proc Eur Dial Transplant Forum 1977;7:157.

75. Thunberg B, Jain V, Patterson P, et al. Nutritional measurements and urea kinetics to guide intradialytic hyperalimentation. Proc Dial Transplant Forum 1980;10:22.

76. Piraino AJ, et al. Prolonged hyperalimentation in catabolic chronic dialysis therapy patients. J Parenter Enteral Nutr 1981;5:17.

77. Wolfson M, Jones MR, Kopple JD. Amino acid losses during hemodialysis with infusion of amino acids and glucose. Kidney Int 1982;21:500.

78. Wolfson M. Use of parenteral supplements in chronic dialysis patients. In: Nissenson AR, Fine RN, eds. Dialysis Therapy. St. Louis: CV Mosby, 1986.

79. Olshan AR, Bruce J, Schwartz AB, et al. Intradialytic parenteral nutrition administration during outpatient hemodialysis. Dial Transplant 1987;16:455.

80. Moore L, Archiardo S. Aggressive nutritional supplementation in chronic hemodialysis patients. CRNQ 1987;11:114.
81. Madigan KM, Olshan A. Effectiveness of intradialytic parenteral nutrition in diabetic patients with end stage renal disease. J Am Diet Assoc 1990;90:861.
82. Powers DV. Prolonged experience with intradialytic hyperalimentation in marasmic chronic hemodialysis patients. Contemp Dial Nephrol 1989;22.
83. Teti SP. Intradialytic TPN—An Update. Media, PA: PenTech Infusions, Inc., 1989.
84. Guarnieri G, Toigo G, Crapesi L, et al. Carnitine metabolism in chronic renal failure. Kidney Int 1987;32 (Suppl 22):S-116.
85. Bertoli M, Battistella PA, et al. Carnitine deficiency induced during hemodialysis and hyperlipidemia: Effect of replacement therapy. Am J Clin Nutr 1981; 34:1496.
86. Pedrini MT, Levey AS, Lau J, et al. The effect of dietary protein restriction on the progression of diabetic and nondiabetic renal diseases: A meta-analysis. Ann Intern Med 1996;124:627–632.

17

HOMECARE FOR THE ONCOLOGY PATIENT

Monica Bais and Michael M. Rothkopf

CHAPTER AT A GLANCE: The use of homecare therapeutics has had a significant impact on the overall management of cancer patients in the United States. Infusional chemotherapy, nutritional support, intravenous antibiotics, and pain management have each been applied for the cancer patient at home, both separately and in combination. An important aspect of homecare oncology is the use of palliative therapies at home for patients with terminal disease. Homecare can improve quality of life for cancer patients while preserving quality of care and reducing medical costs.

Introduction

During the last decade the practice of medicine has undergone many reforms, particularly in the economic arena. Cost containment measures have become a driving force in the evaluation and management of patients. This, in turn, has shifted the practice of medicine from the hospital to the ambulatory setting, and, most recently, the home.

Cancer is second only to heart disease as the leading cause of death in the United States. There are approximately 1.2 million new cases of cancer each year. The management of cancer patients constitutes a large portion of total healthcare expenditure. To decrease the cost of cancer care, many aspects have gradually moved from hospitals to outpatient centers. In a form of natural evolution, the next step has been to offer these services in the patient's home (1).

However, although the initial impetus for the use of homecare in oncology may have been economic, significant clinical benefits have been recognized. Homecare has an advantage over the hospital in that the home is a microbiologically simple environment and is less likely to expose an immune compromised patient to drug-resistant microorganisms. Most patients prefer to be at home rather than in the hospital for care, and thereby they experience an improvement in their quality of life with homecare.

Homecare oncology treatment may have advantages over outpatient infusion center therapy as well. Certain methods of chemotherapy administration, such as continuous-infusion therapy, are more suited to homecare than to outpatient infusion centers. Homecare also allows a physically or psychologically fragile individual to forgo the stress involved in traveling to the infusion center, waiting for laboratory work, and being confined in a treatment area.

The homecare option has been facilitated by technological advances and new chemotherapeutic agents, along with an increased awareness and participation of the caregivers. This chapter provides a review of the various components involved in the homecare of the cancer patient, including administration of chemotherapy, nutritional support, intravenous antibiotics, pain management, and palliative care.

Chemotherapeutic Agents

Chemotherapeutic agents can be utilized in either an adjunctive role, a palliative role, or a preoperative role. The primary goal of adjunctive therapy is either to increase the disease-free interval or to decrease the occurrence of relapsing disease. The goal of palliative therapy in patients with advanced disease is the prolongation of productive life. Lastly, preoperative chemotherapy is intended to decrease both the size and the extent of tumor prior to surgical excision.

Cancer can be defined as the replication and growth of abnormal cells. These cells reproduce, as do normal body cells, via the cell cycle (Fig. 17.1). During each phase of the cell cycle a different stage of cell replication occurs, such as DNA replication and RNA synthesis. Chemotherapeutic agents are capable of impairing cell division in cells with a high rate of replication. This results in the destruction of tumor cells, the reduction of tumor mass, or control of the growth of tumors.

Chemotherapeutic agents can be divided into two major categories: cell cycle specific and cell cycle nonspecific. The cell cycle–specific drugs are highly effective in cancers in which there are a large number of cells undergoing replication, such as hematologic malignancies. Cell cycle–nonspecific agents are effective in both cycling and resting stages and are most effective in the treatment of slower-growing, solid tumors.

In addition to the categories already mentioned, chemotherapeutic agents can be further classified according to their specific mechanism of action in cellular chemistry.

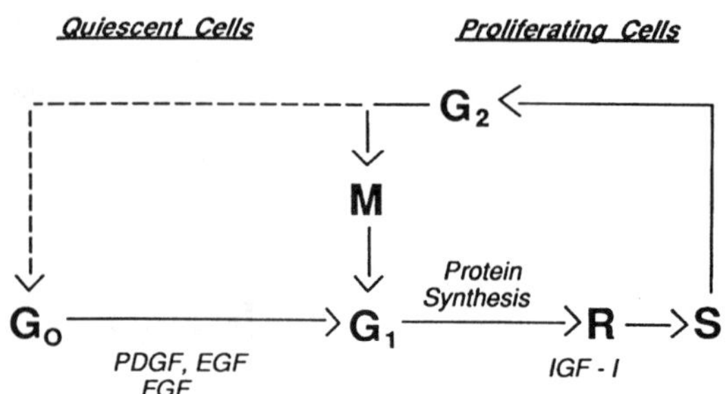

Figure 17.1. Growth factor requirements and temporal organization of the G_0 to G_1 transition and the cell cycle. For quiescent cells in G_0 to proliferate, they must first leave G_0 and enter G_1. For fibroblasts in culture, this transition is stimulated by growth factors such as platelet-derived growth factor (PDGF), epidermal growth factor (EGF), or fibroblast growth factor (FGF) and occupies an interval of 6–9 hr. From G_1, the cells require a rapid rate of protein synthesis and insulin-like growth factor-I (IGF-I) to pass the restriction (R) point and initiate DNA synthesis (S). The transition from G_1 to S also takes 6–9 hr, with the R point occurring in the last few hours. Once the cells begin to synthesize DNA, they no longer require exogenous factors to complete the S phase (8–12 hr), G_2 (2–4 hr), and mitosis (M; about 1 hr). If environmental conditions are permissive for proliferation, the daughter cells formed at M enter G_1 and the cell cycle. However, in the absence of positive environmental signals or in the presence of negative environmental signals, the cells return to G_0.

There are six major classes of agents:

1. Antimetabolites
2. Alkylating agents
3. Antitumor antibiotics
4. Plant alkaloids
5. Platinum-containing agents
6. Hormonal agents

With the exception of hormonal therapy, each of the agents acts to disrupt protein synthesis (2).

Antimetabolites, which act as fraudulent purines and pyrimidines, interfere in the formation of DNA. Examples of antimetabolites include folic acid antagonists such as methotrexate, purine antagonists such as mercaptopurine and thioguanine, and pyrimidine antagonists such as fluorouracil and cytarabine. These drugs are often utilized in the treatment of acute leukemias, choriocarcinoma, head and neck cancer, and cancers of the lungs and intestines. However because of their mechanism of action, they are toxic to normal body cells, causing bone marrow suppression and skin and gastrointestinal toxicity.

The alkylating agents act by forming reactive compounds that interfere with the conversion of DNA to RNA. The compounds they form join groups on the DNA that result in crosslinking of bases, abnormal pairing of bases, or breakage of DNA strands. They are used in combination therapies for the treatment of lymphomas, myelomas, and leukemias. Examples of the alkylating agents include nitrogen mustards, nitrosureas, and alkylsulfonates. This group of drugs and their toxicities are listed in Table 17.1.

The antitumor antibiotics intercalate between adjacent base pairs on the DNA structure, which results in an interruption of replication and transcription into RNA. They also cause disruption in the DNA strand itself and are capable of disrupting cellular replication.

Antitumor antibiotics can be divided into several classes. The anthracyclines (doxorubicin and daunorubicin) are cell cycle non-specific and are utilized in the treatment of breast, ovarian, testicular, and endometrial carcinomas as well as sarcomas and myelomas. These compounds are known to be cardiotoxic, a property that is often irreversible.

Bleomycin is a cell cycle–specific compound that is useful when used in combination with other chemotherapeutic agents for the treatment of cancers such as testicular and squamous cell carcinoma. Its adverse effects include pulmonary fibrosis, hyperkeratosis, fever, and anorexia. Mitomycin, which is activated by the cytochrome P-450 system, acts by crosslinking strands of DNA. This agent is extremely useful in combination therapy for the treatment of cervical carcinoma, as well as adenocarcinomas of the gastrointestinal system. However, mitomycin is known to cause severe myelosuppression, nephrotoxicity, and interstitial pneumonitis.

The plant alkaloids, which consist of the vinca alkaloids (vinblastine and vincristine) and the podophyllotoxins, cause arrest of the M phase in the cell cycle and hence inhibit cell division. They are useful in the treatment of lymphomas, Wilms' tumor, and choriocarcinoma. The most common toxicity seen is peripheral neuropathy; however, other noted side effects include alopecia, paralytic ileus, and bone marrow suppression.

Table 17.1. Alkylating Agents and Their Common Toxicities

Alkylating Agent	Toxicity
Nitrogen mustard	Nausea and vomiting
Cyclophosphamide	Nausea and vomiting
Chlorambucil	Nausea and vomiting
Busulfan	Adrenal insufficiency, pulmonary fibrosis, hyperpigmentation
Lomustine	Nausea and vomiting, leukopenia, thrombocytopenia
Carmustine	Nausea and vomiting, leukopenia, thrombocytopenia
Cisplatin	Nausea and vomiting, renal dysfunction, acoustic nerve dysfunction

Infusional Chemotherapy

Intravenous chemotherapy can be administered by intermittent or continuous infusion. Continuous infusion is advantageous for several reasons. It exposes cancer cells to the agent at all stages of the cell cycle, which increases efficacy. In addition, continuous infusion has been shown to produce fewer adverse reactions, which decreases morbidity and length of stay for hospitalized patients.

Outpatient, infusion center–based chemotherapy requires the patient to travel and be present in the center for each administration. Therefore, its use is more suited for intermittent rather than continuous infusions. From this perspective, homecare infusions are actually a closer approximation of hospital-based chemotherapy.

Table 17.2. Chemotherapeutic Agents Administered in the Home

Bleomycin
Doxorubicin
Etoposide
Fluorouracil
Methotrexate
Plicamycin
Vincristine

However, home chemotherapy can also serve as a reasonable alternative to intermittent infusion center therapy as well. This is particularly important to patients who are physically limited because of symptoms associated with advanced disease. The effort involved in traveling, waiting in the clinic, having laboratory studies done, being administered intravenous chemotherapy, and returning may be overwhelming. In these circumstances, home chemotherapy may be the only reasonable option for the patient.

Not all chemotherapeutic agents have been approved for home administration, however. Many agents have been excluded either because of the potential for adverse effects or for anaphylaxis. The agents depicted in Table 17.2, are generally considered safe for home administration (3).

Homecare Chemotherapy

Patient Selection

As with other aspects of intensive homecare, the process of homecare oncology begins with a careful evaluation of the patient's capacity to perform the medical functions expected (4). This subject is covered in many other areas within this book, particularly in Chapter 3.

The oncologist preparing a patient for homecare should undertake an evaluation to determine that both the patient and the therapy are appropriate for homecare (Table 17.3). The patient's medical condition should be stable and the home environment satisfactory. The patient and his or her caregivers should display responsibility, compliance, and knowledge of the therapeutic regimen (5). The home should be clean and contain ade-quate room for the storage of supplies. Refrigeration space is particularly important, since it will be needed for the storage of perishable items such as medications. The insurance and financial situation should be sufficient to ensure that the patient will receive the necessary nursing care and equipment.

The selection of patients for homecare administration of chemotherapy adds another layer to an already complex situation. Chemotherapy can be difficult to administer, even with experienced personnel. The homecare patient must be considered a novice, and extra preparation is necessary.

The patient should be accurately diagnosed and staged and should have an appropriate treatment plan. The patient's medical condition should be stable and without serious complications. It is also important that the patient be emotionally and psychologically stable.

The patient's first exposure to the chemotherapy should be given in a hospital or outpatient infusion center setting to monitor for adverse reactions. Secure venous access will be important for the successful continuation of intravenous therapy at home and should be in place prior to the beginning of homecare.

It is important to recognize that not all cancer patients are appropriate for homecare. Patients experiencing side effects or physical limitations secondary to chemotherapy, and those with advanced disease may not experience an improvement in quality of life on homecare (6). These patients may require more care than is available at home, particularly from the standpoint of psychosocial and emotional support. Inadequate preparation and anticipation of a patient's special needs in

Table 17.3. Criteria for Patient Selection

1. Physician approval
2. Appropriate medical and psychiatric condition
3. Satisfactory home environment and social support
4. Availability of a trainable caregiver
5. Insurance coverage and financial responsibility
6. Reasonable life expectancy of patient
7. Favorable assessment of drug toxicity and possible complications

this area can lead to failure of homecare and require rehospitalization of the patient.

The Homecare Team and Organization

Homecare is provided by a team of professionals—the physician, nursing staff, pharmacist, physical therapist, nutritionist, and laboratory staff—who work in conjunction with the family to care for the patient (6).

Organizations providing home chemotherapy must be able to demonstrate standards of care. Documented policies and procedures consistent with JCAHO standards should be in place. These include statements on patients' rights and responsibilities, patient care, safety management, infection control, homecare record, quality assurance management, and administration. Mechanisms for documentation of drug administration, nursing care plan, and nursing assessment should exist. Provision for safe disposal of excess antineoplastic agents and contaminated equipment should be made. Properly qualified personnel should be made available to ensure safe and effective treatments. For more information on the homecare organization please see Chapter 5. The homecare team is also covered in greater detail in Chapter 6.

An oncology nurse specialist certified to administer chemotherapy is also recommended. This is especially true if IV push methods are to be used. Nurses who administer intravenous chemotherapeutic drugs must be aware of their legal responsibilities to the patient, the physician, and their employing facility. Much of the nurses' time should be spent on educating the patient and family about cancer, its treatment, and the toxicity and side effects of chemotherapeutic drugs.

The pharmacy should also have personnel experienced in chemotherapeutics. In addition to proper techniques in mixing and handling of drugs, the services of a clinical pharmacy specialist is recommended. This includes review of the medication record and consultation with the case manager and physician. Other services include education, pharmacodynamics, drug and food interactions, and so forth.

Access to reliable, certified laboratory services is also required for adequate care of the home oncology patient. Dosage adjustments will often be guided by clinical laboratory reports. Laboratory results should be made available to both the nurse and the physician. "Panic values" should be immediately reported by telephone.

Patient/Environmental Hazards

The homecare nurse plays a critical role in patient safety at home. These nurses are trained to assess patients and provide appropriate care, including venipuncture and assessment of implanted catheters and access ports. However, those involved in the treatment of cancer patients must also be skilled in the handling and administration of chemotherapeutic agents as well as recognition of the adverse effects of these agents. In addition to the technical skills, the nursing staff is responsible for the education of the patient and family regarding disease, medications, expectations, and complications.

The handling of chemotherapeutic agents requires extreme caution. Nurses are advised never to prepare chemotherapeutic agents within the home. Doing so exposes the nurse, patient, and family to potential chemical hazards (7, 8). The administration of therapy should be performed in a well-ventilated setting without distractions. This will provide a safe environment and prevent accidental exposures. However, should an accident occur, the nursing staff should be well versed in the handling and disposal of these substances. Nurses should keep an emergency kit within the household in the event of a chemical spill. The contents of the spill kit are presented in Table 17.4.

Table 17.4. Contents of the Spill Kit

1. Latex gloves
2. Disposable gown
3. Chemical splash goggles
4. Respiratory mask
5. Sheets of absorbent material
6. Spill control pillows
7. Scoop and brush for glass fragments
8. Large plastic bags
9. Needle container
10. Toxic waste labels

Table 17.5. Vesicant Chemotherapeutic Agents

Amsacrine
Dactinomycin (actinomycin D)
Daunomycin
Doxorubicin (Adriamycin)
Mechlorethamine (nitrogen mustard)
Mitomycin
Vinblastine
Vincristine (Oncovin)

Moreover, it is essential that the nurses recognize complications associated with the intravenous access (9). The possible development of catheter sepsis or extravasation of the chemotherapeutic agent from the access site into the surrounding tissues must be watched for. The latter is particularly problematic, because if this occurs while using vesicant chemotherapeutic agents, damage to local tissues may result.

To avoid such complications, vesicant agents (Table 17.5) should be administered through a central venous access system. If extravasation has occurred, the nurse must immediately stop the infusion, clear the line, and administer an antidote. The physician should be notified in order to evaluate the patient for further treatment.

Homecare nurses must also be equipped to evaluate for and initiate treatment of anaphylaxis. The chemotherapeutic infusion must be stopped, the physician notified, and appropriate treatment initiated. The anaphylactic reaction should be documented and the patient observed for further symptoms. With the potential for both extravasation and anaphylaxis to occur, nurses should prepare an emergency kit equipped to treat these conditions.

Monitoring for Chemotherapy Toxicity

Homecare nurses must be able to recognize the side effects of chemotherapeutic agents (Table 17.6). They should anticipate these reactions and monitor for their development. As previously described, chemotherapeutic agents cause the destruction of rapidly dividing cells, which includes both normal and tumor cells. The most commonly affected areas are the gastrointestinal tract, the bone marrow, the hair follicles, and the skin.

The gastrointestinal system is extremely sensitive to chemotherapy. Adverse reactions in this system include nausea and vomiting, anorexia, diarrhea, and constipation. These vary, depending on the patient and the agent used. The effects of nausea and vomiting tend to occur within 2 to 6 hours of therapy and may persist up to 72 hours after treatment. Antiemetics have been useful in abating these symptoms, especially when administered prior to therapy.

Patients on chemotherapeutic regimens often experience a loss of appetite with concomitant weight loss. Some require appetite stimulants such as Megace or corticosteroids to reverse anorexia. In these patients, weight and nutritional status should be monitored carefully.

Both diarrhea and constipation are common in patients undergoing chemotherapy. Diarrhea, like nausea and vomiting, is usually experienced during the first 24 hours. It is essential to monitor the patient closely and treat with an antidiarrheal agent to prevent complications of electrolyte imbalance or dehydration. On the other hand, constipation tends to occur 5 to 8 days after treatment, especially with vincristine and vinblastine. If the patient has a history of constipation, treatment with stool softener and a high-fiber diet may be helpful.

Bone marrow suppression is a common risk of chemotherapy. It is the result of damage to the precursor or stem cells, which develop into erythrocytes, leukocytes, and platelets. Mature cells are unaffected, explaining the lag in laboratory test abnormalities. As the mature cells die, stem cells are unavailable to manufacture replacements. This results in anemia, leukopenia, and thrombocytopenia, leaving the patient susceptible to infection and bleeding.

The homecare team should monitor the patient carefully, especially 7 to 14 days after treatment, when the patient can be expected

Table 17.6. Drug Toxicity and Need for Monitoring

Agent	Toxicity	Monitoring
Cisplatin (Platinol)	Nausea; vomiting; nephrotoxicity; neuropathies; bone marrow suppression; hyperuricemia.	Check rate of infusion. Extravasation. Possible anaphylaxis. Adequate hydration.
Cyclophosphamide (Cytoxan)	Alopecia; interstitial pulmonary fibrosis; nausea; vomiting; hemorrhagic cystitis; bone marrow suppression.	Extravasation. Ambulation preferred to prevent accumulation of drug in bladder. Force fluids. Check rate of infusion.
Dacarbazine	Alopecia; nausea and vomiting; bone marrow suppression.	Discard if solution turns pink. Extravasation. Possible anaphylaxis. Check rate of infusion.
Dactinomycin (Cosmegen)	Alopecia; nausea and vomiting; gastrointestinal (GI) ulceration; bone marrow suppression.	Extravasation. Check rate of infusion. Pharyngitis; stomatitis; dysphagia; esophagitis; proctitis; diarrhea; hypocalcemia.
Doxorubicin (Adriamycin)	Alopecia; cardiotoxicity progressing to congestive heart failure; nausea and vomiting; GI ulceration; bone marrow suppression.	Check rate of infusion. Extravasation. Do not use aluminum-hubbed needles. Hyperpigmentation of nail beds. Local inflammation at injection site. Stomatitis, esophagitis. Red urine which is not hematuria; fever.
Etoposide (Vepesid)	Bone marrow suppression; nausea and vomiting; alopecia.	Extravasation; IV infusion to be slow; anorexia; hypotension; possible anaphylaxis.
Fluorouracil (5-FU)	Alopecia; nausea and vomiting; GI ulceration; bone marrow suppression.	Extravasation. Check rate of infusion. Do not refrigerate product; protect product from light. Skin hyperpigmentation; nail changes; stomatitis; diarrhea; headdache; blurred vision.
Interferon alfa-2B, recombinant (Intron-A)	Nausea and vomiting; tachycardia; mild thrombocytopenia; alopecia.	Patient to be well hydrated; diarrhea; taste alteration; weight loss; hypotension; hypertension; fever; flu-like symptoms; rash; pruritus; arthralgia.
Methotrexate	Alopecia; interstitial pneumonitis; nausea and vomiting; GI ulceration; hepatotoxicity; bone marrow suppression.	Extravasation. Check rate of infusion. Leucovorin rescue; or asparaginase recue prn; urticaria; photosensitivity; acne; stomatitis; diarrhea.
Mitomycin C (Mutamycin)	Alopecia; rate of pulmonary toxicity; dyspnea; nausea and vomiting; bone marrow suppression.	Extravasation; pruritus; anorexia; stomatitis; diarrhea; fever. Check rate of infusion.
Mitoxantrone (Novantrone)	Myelosupression; nausea and vomiting; tachycardia; electrocardiogram (ECG) changes.	Extravasation. Incompatible with heparin-containing solutions; rate of infusion; stomatitis; chest pain. Urine may turn bluish-green. Sclera may turn bluish.

Table 17.6—Continued

Agent	Toxicity	Monitoring
Vinblastine	Alopecia; nausea and vomiting; peripheral neuropathy; bone marrow suppression; ileus.	Extravasation; stomatitis; constipation; urinary retention; polyuria; loss of deep tendon reflexes; paresthesias.
Vincristine	Alopecia; pharyngitis; nausea and vomiting; ileus peripheral neuropathy.	Extravasation; anorexia; vertigo; stomatitis; constipation; diarrhea; mental depression; numbness; loss of deep tendon reflexes.

to be at a nadir. If the patient's laboratory data reveal leukopenia, anemia, or thrombocytopenia, the physician should be notified. Symptoms such as fevers, chills, bleeding, weakness, or fatigue should also be reported, as these may signal a dangerous developing condition.

A non–life-threatening complication of chemotherapy is alopecia, which usually occurs 2 to 3 weeks after the onset of treatment. Patients are often disheartened by this development and should be adequately prepared with the facts in advance. The homecare nurse may be a source of comfort and reassurance by emphasizing that alopecia will reverse after the completion of treatment .

Published Experience with Home Chemotherapy

With the advent of convenient venous access devices, ambulatory infusion pumps, and home chemotherapy infusions, homecare agencies and hospice programs have reported their experience with parenteral chemotherapy at home. However, many of these reports are in the form of abstracts presented at scientific meetings. The paucity of comprehensive studies in this area points to the need for greater emphasis on homecare research.

In 1975, The Visiting Nurse Association of Allegheny County, Pennsylvania (VNAC) (10) established a homecare oncology program that accepted both terminally ill patients who needed palliation and patients on maintenance chemotherapy. They reported safe home administration of methotrexate, fluorouracil, dacarbazine, doxorubicin, bleomycin, triethylenethiophosphoramide, vincristine, cyclophosphamide, and mithramycin. The drugs were administered singly or in combination, either as IV push or diluted in 50 to 100 mL of solution. Staff nurses administered the home infusional chemotherapy, while nurse-clinicians administered the IV push treatments.

Malone et al. (11) prospectively compared hospital-based chemotherapy with domiciliary chemotherapy in women receiving a cisplatin combination regimen for gynecologic cancers. The home therapy patients reported no extravasations or anaphylactic reactions. No patient required hospitalization for dehydration or for adverse reactions to the chemotherapy, and no patient wanted to return to the hospital environment. They preferred homecare because they had increased privacy and convenience as well as decreased anxiety.

High-dose chemotherapy was given at home by Rowland (12) using continuous infusion. Homecare was found to be a viable alternative to hospital treatment for solid tumors. Janson and Edberg (13) describe a homecare oncology working model. Their service has 12 homecare teams. Each consists of a doctor, nurses, a physiotherapist, and an occupational therapist. They are available to the patient 24 hours a day. The teams cooperate with oncology consultants located at three university hospitals. Because of the comprehensive nature of their service, they were better equipped to manage complex chemotherapy and homecare oncology.

Terzoli et al. (14) used a video-telephone system to monitor home chemotherapy between nursing visits. This increased patient contact and supervision without added personnel costs. Ophof et al. (15) reported improvement in quality of life for 102 patients treated with home chemotherapy. Vassilaros et al. (16) also reported improved quality of life in 175 cancer patients on homecare.

On the other hand, Bubela discovered difficulty in homecare patients receiving arterial pump chemotherapy infusion (17). Technical aspects of care (blood or air in the tubing, etc.), side effects, and psychological problems were observed. The mastery of the technical skills and the responsibility for the management of the treatment can be too much for some patients.

This may indicate that the more complex chemotherapeutic regimens are not yet appropriate for home use. However, the advent of programmable, multichannel drug delivery systems may alter this. For example, an Intelliject pump (Ivion Corp., Englewood, CO) can automatically administer several drugs in the home over a 4-day period. Lanning et al. (18) showed that such programmable, multichannel, pump-based therapy is accurate, reliable, and safe. It allowed precisely timed and sequenced IV chemotherapy in the home at 75% cost savings (from $920/day in-hospital to $225/day at home).

Home chemotherapy has particular advantages for children with cancer. It allows them to receive treatment without losing valuable educational and family time (19). Lange et al. (20) described a homecare program for administration of methotrexate by intermittent 24-hour infusion in children with acute lymphoblastic leukemia. The most common complication was subcutaneous infiltration of intravenous lines. No patients required antiemetic drugs.

Lange's group showed that homecare improved family satisfaction. Families could better plan their lives and prepare for when medicines were infused at home rather than in an outpatient center. The program saved 357 inpatient days while preventing exposure of the children to nosocomial infections.

The Sante-Service of Paris, France, one of the world's largest and most comprehensive homecare organizations, provides comprehensive support for homecare cancer patients (21). Their pediatric oncology institute treats approximately 150 solid tumor cases per year. Twenty percent receive treatment entirely at home (22). They report improved quality of life and reduced adverse reactions in this setting compared to the hospital. However, they also noted a tendency for parents to feel overly responsible and guilty regarding their child's illness.

Close (23) compared costs, medical outcome, and quality of life in 14 pediatric patients who received an identical course of chemotherapy in the hospital and at home. They reported that homecare reduced billed charges, out-of-pocket expenses, and lost income for parents. The patients' well-being, appetite, mood, and school work were significantly improved.

Nutritional Support

It is not uncommon for cancer patients to develop nutritional deficiencies during the course of their illness. In the most severe variety, these patients may develop overt protein-calorie malnutrition and require nutritional support.

Cancer patients can become malnourished for a variety of reasons, including the effects of the tumor as well as the side effects of cancer treatments. The tumor or metastasis may obstruct the alimentary tract at various points. This often involves the small and/or large bowel. If the omentum is seeded with metastasis, ascites may develop, which itself may produce a form of bowel obstruction.

The metabolic disturbances induced by the tumor, including futile cycling and cytokine release, may alter energy and protein utilization. In addition, factors responsible for the induction of anorexia and cachexia are suspected to be released by the tumor itself or by the body's immune response to tumor invasion.

Cancer treatments, including chemotherapy, radiation, and surgery can produce side effects that limit food intake. The entire process of eating can be affected at its various stages. Eating begins with a cerebral component, and cancer treatments can produce anorexia and an aversion to food. This may also be worsened by an induced alteration in the sense of taste or smell, which changes the perception of food. Some patients experience pain on chewing or swallowing due to oral or esophageal lesions induced by chemotherapy. Nausea and vomiting is often the result of chemotherapy-associated side effects. Lastly, malabsorption and diarrhea may be caused by radiation and/or surgery or by the development of an opportunistic infection.

Food safety is another important issue in the nutritional management of the cancer patient. This involves the avoidance of foods that may be contaminated and the careful handling and preparation of food to avoid secondary contamination. While these foods are usually safe for the average person, the immune-compromised patient may be harmed by the consumption of foods that are not sterile. These foods may be contaminated with significant pathogens, including *Salmonella* species, enteropathic *Escherichia coli,* and parasites such as *Cryptosporidium.* Infection with these organisms can cause a severe form of dysentery, which may require rehospitalization for fluid management.

The optimal management of the malnourished cancer patient remains controversial, especially with regard to total parenteral nutrition (TPN) (24). This is due to the lack of data demonstrating increased survival in cancer patients receiving TPN. Some studies have even shown a worsened outcome when TPN was administered poorly. Nonetheless, when viewed from the perspective of quality of life rather than length of survival, nutritional support appears to be of significant value (25). These modalities may include oral supplementation, tube feedings with enteral nutrition, or TPN (26). They have a long history in their application to homecare and can be successfully managed provided that the homecare team has sufficient experience in this area. For more information regarding nutritional support, please refer to Chapter 16.

Intravenous Antibiotics for the Cancer Patient at Home

Because of the immune-compromising effects of chemotherapy and radiation, cancer patients may develop fungal, viral, or bacter-

ial infections during the course of their illness. These are often associated with leukopenic episodes but may also be promoted by the presence of an indwelling catheter for venous access. In the past, these situations generally required hospitalization and triple-antibiotic therapy along with isolation. However, admission to the hospital exposes the patient to possible colonization with multiply resistant organisms. Therefore, it may be preferable to attempt to maintain the patients at home so long as they remain medically stable.

Otherwise stable patients with fever and leukopenia, and those with known infections, can be safely managed with intravenous antibiotics administered at home (27). The first doses of antibiotic therapy should generally be administered in a controlled environment, such as a physician's office or an outpatient clinic. This permits the monitoring of anaphylaxis or other adverse reaction. However, subsequent therapy can generally be continued at home under the supervision of a homecare nurse. Certainly, a home chemotherapy patient who is already well versed in intravenous techniques should be capable of adding intravenous antibiotics to his or her homecare regimen. More information on the subject of homecare antibiotics can be found in Chapter 12.

Pain Management

Another aspect of homecare oncology is aggressive pain management through the use of intravenous narcotics. These treatments are available through a system of patient-controlled analgesia (PCA), which makes use of a portable programmable pump that can be preset to administer appropriate therapy on a continuous basis. The patient is permitted a preselected amount of bolus therapy, which can be given within a range determined by the patient's physician. The programmable nature of the pump allows for the setting of a "lockout," which limits the dose of medication to a predetermined maximum. More information on the subject of pain management is available in Chapter 19.

Hospice and Palliative Care

Quality of Life

Care for the patient dying of cancer is another appropriate application for homecare. Issues related to quality of life and symptom control, particularly the control of cancer pain, must be addressed. Others symptoms, such as loss of appetite, dry mouth, thirst, nausea, vomiting, breathlessness, and depression also factor prominently and require attention.

Care in the home can enhance the patient's quality of life and is particularly appropriate for the final months of life. Recently, attention has focused on patient control as a mechanism of modifying the patient's pain response and suffering (28). Lewis has identified five types of control: processual control, contingency control, cognitive control, behavioral control, and existential control (29). The homecare or hospice nurse with training in this area can be of significant value to the patient with terminal cancer.

In addition to pain management, homecare technology can be used to support palliative aspects of homecare for patients with advanced cancer. For example, blood products (30, 31), IV fluids (32), and even dobutamine (33) have been applied in this situation. Roe (34) discussed the role of homecare for the control of suffering and the establishment of palliative care units.

Symptom Control

To meet the goal of providing patient comfort at home, control of troubling physical symptoms must be achieved, or at least attempted. Blum and Blum (35) have approached this problem from an organ system perspective, which provides a useful structure for review.

Mouth Care

Attention to mouth care has a significant impact on quality of life. In addition to brushing the teeth, oral hygiene may require cleansing mouthwashes such as those containing bicarbonate and peroxide. Xerostomia can be aided by the use of moistening therapy such as ice chips, glycerol lozenges, etc. Oral lesions due to fungal or viral infection can be treated with appropriate medications.

Nausea and Vomiting

After reversible causes such as drug reactions or tumor obstruction have been eliminated, symptomatic control with antiemetic agents such as prochlorperazine and metoclopramide may be useful. Recently, some patients have also observed a benefit in cannabis consumption.

Pulmonary Care

Respiratory symptoms may be related to reduced oxygenation (due to tumor mass effects, airway obstruction, plural effusions, and pneumonia) and recurrent aspiration. Low-flow oxygen can be easily applied in the home to provide comfort for the patient with advanced pulmonary disease. This reduces the sense of air hunger, which may be distressing to both the patient and the family.

If patients are aspirating oral secretions or food, the availability of a bedside suction unit may be very helpful.

Genitourinary Care

Urinary incontinence can be a major issue affecting quality of life. The loss of control experienced may be particularly distressing. Management includes increasing the frequency of voiding, using urinary drainage pads and, if needed, using urinary drainage catheters. Some patients may benefit from specific drug therapy such as Pyridium or Urecholine.

Skin Care

Special attention should be given to pressure relief, wound treatment, and avoidance of skin breakdown (36). Pruritus is another complaint that can be managed with topical emollients or systemic medications.

Ostomy and Bowel Care

If the patient has been discharged with an ostomy or if cutaneous fistulas require periodic drainage, appropriate arrangements must be made for ostomy care (37). The assistance of an enterostomal therapist can be extremely helpful to the patient or family.

Control of diarrhea and avoidance of constipation is another important aspect of homecare management. Alterations in the diet and the use of medication may be beneficial.

Conclusion

Health care reform and developing technology have shifted the management of cancer patients from the hospital to the home. This change has been facilitated by homecare organizations and the development of homecare teams. As a result, the responsibility of providing health care no longer rests solely on the healthcare establishment but includes the patient and family. In general, this has decreased the cost of care without sacrificing the quality of care. In some instances, homecare is actually superior to hospital or outpatient infusion center care because it eliminates the disadvantages associated with them. Many patients have been comforted by the ability to return home sooner. This, in turn, promotes an improvement in quality of life.

References

1. Haylock PJ. Home care for the person with cancer. Home Healthcare Nurse 1993;11:16–28.
2. Katzung BG, Trevor AJ. Pharmacology: Examination and Board Review, 3rd ed. East Norwalk, CT: Appleton & Lange, 1993:281–289.
3. Parker GG. Chemotherapy administration in the home. Home Healthcare Nurse 1992;10:30–36.
4. Maloney CH, Preston F. An overview of home care for patients with cancer. Cancer Nursing Perspectives 1992;19:75–79.
5. Matthews LE. Preparing your patient for home infusion. Nursing 1994;24:28.
6. Hinton J. Can home care maintain an acceptable quality of life for patients with terminal cancer and their relatives? Palliat Med 1994;8:183–196.
7. Michela NJ. High-tech home care infusion therapy. Geriatric Nursing 1995;16:249–250.
8. Granjy AE, Christie D, Tichy AM, Talashek ML. Chemotherapy. How safe for the caregiver? Home Healthcare Nurse 1993;11:51–58.
9. Danzig L, Short L, Collins K, Mahoney M, Sepe S, Bland L, Jarvis W. Bloodstream infections associated with a needleless intravenous infusion in patients receiving home infusion therapy. JAMA 1995;273:1862–1864.
10. DeMoss CJ. Giving intravenous chemotherapy at home. Am J Nurs 1980;80:2188–2189.
11. Malone J, Kavanagh J, Crosson K, Streckfuss B. Domiciliary chemotherapy for malignant disease. Eur J Gynaecol Oncol 1986;7:120–121.
12. Rowland CG. Home continuous infusion chemotherapy. Practitioner 1989;229:889–892.
13. Janson A, Edberg L. Consultant oncologist in cancer home care. In: Proceedings of the First World Congress on Home Care, Rome, Italy, 1989.
14. Terzoli E, Garufi C, Ranuzzi M, Saso U, Nistico C. Medical oncology and home care in Italy. Tumori 1993;79:30–33.
15. Ophof J, Leucht R, Frohmuller S, Dorsam J, Rouff G, Schlag P. Experiences in home care of cancer patients. Acta Oncol 1989;28:35–38.
16. Vassilaros S, Tsigouratos D, Halastani V, Tsitoura M. Cost-benefit ratio of home service in the treatment of terminal cancer patients. In: Proceedings of the First World Congress on Home Care, Rome, Italy, 1989.
17. Bubela N. Technical and psychological problems and concerns arising from the outpatient treatment of cancer with direct intra arterial infusion. Cancer Nurs 1981;4:305–309.
18. Lanning RM, Roemeling RV, Hrushesky WJ. Cost effective complex multi-drug infusional home chemotherapy. In: Proceedings of the First World Congress on Home Care, Rome, Italy, 1989.
19. Jayabose S, Escobedo V, Tugal O, Nahaczewski A, Donohue P, Fuentes V, Devereau G, Sunkara S. Home chemotherapy for children with cancer. Cancer 1992;69:574–579.
20. Lange BJ, Burroughs B, Meadows AT, Burkey E. Home care involving methotrexate infusions for children with acute lymphoblastic leukemia. J Pediatr 1988;112:492–495.
21. Goldberg J, Chigot B, Rodier S. An overview of the dietetic and nutritional support unit (DNSU): Sante-Service Ambulatory Health Care. In: Proceedings of the First World Congress on Home Care, Rome, Italy, 1989.
22. Pacquement H, Rosenblatt F, Renty MC, Quintana E, Zucker JM. Experience and questions about home care on children treated for cancer. In: Proceedings of the First World Congress on Home Care, Rome, Italy, 1989.
23. Close P, Burkey E, Kazak A, Danz P, Lange B. A prospective controlled evaluation of home chemotherapy for children with cancer. Pediatrics 1995;95:896–900.
24. Blackburn G. Round table discussion of nutritional support in the cancer patient. Nutrition 1990;6(Suppl):1s-16s.
25. Howard L, Ament M, Fleming CR, Shike M, Steiger E. Current use and clinical outcome of home parenteral and enteral nutrition therapies in the United States. Gastroenterology 1995;109:355–365.
26. Howard L. Home parenteral and enteral nutrition in cancer patients. Cancer 1993;72(Suppl 11):3531–3541.
27. Talcott JA, Whalen A, Clark J, Rieker PP, Finberg R. Home antibiotic therapy for low-risk cancer patients with fever and neutropenia: a pilot study of 30 patients based on a validated prediction rule. J Clin Oncol 1994;12:107–1014.

28. Houts PS, ed. American College of Physicians Home Care Guide for Cancer. Philadelphia: American College of Physicians, 1994.

29. Vallerand AH. Ferrell BR. Issues of control in patients with cancer pain. West J Nurs Res 1995;17:467–483.

30. Thompson HW, McKelvey J. Home blood transfusion therapy: a home health agency's 5-year experience [Letter]. Transfusion 1995;35:453.

31. Sciortino AD, Carlton DC, Axelrod A, Eng M, Zhukovsky DS, Vinciguerra V. The efficacy of administering blood transfusions at home to terminally ill cancer patients. J Palliat Care 1993;9:14–17.

32. Witteveen PO, vanBoxtel AJ, Nieuwland M, Neijt JP, Blijham GH. Feasibility of transferring medical-technological aid to the home situation for patients with cancer or a serious infection [published in Dutch]. Ned Tijdschr Geneeskd 1995;139:788–791.

33. Mercadante S, Simonetti MT. Dobutamine as palliative drug in home-care advanced cancer patients. Journal of Pain & Symptom Management 1994;9:480–483.

34. Roe DJ. Palliative care 2000—home care. J Palliat Care 1992;8:28–32.

35. Blum DS, Blum RH. Cancer care. In: Bernstein LH, Grieco AJ, Dete MK, eds. Primary Care in the Home. Philadelphia: JB Lippincott, 1987.

36. Agris J. Skin care. In: Bernstein LH, Grieco AJ, Dete MK, eds. Primary Care in the Home. Philadelphia: JB Lippincott, 1987.

37. Purcell EA, Gouge TH. Ostomy and bowel management. In: Bernstein LH, Grieco AJ, Dete K, eds. Primary Care in the Home. Philadelphia: JB Lippincott, 1987.

18

HOMECARE OF THE BONE MARROW TRANSPLANT PATIENT

Niculae Ciobanu

CHAPTER AT A GLANCE: High-dose chemotherapy with stem cell transplantation is frequently used for the treatment of different cancers. Treatment toxicity is higher in recipients of allogeneic transplants, as compared to autologous or syngeneic transplants, because of the occurrence of graft versus host disease (GVHD) and/or treatment of GVHD. Nevertheless, like other cancer patients, bone marrow transplant recipients prefer to be home as soon as possible. Despite early concerns, it has now been shown that homecare is a viable alternative for these patients. This chapter depicts the personal experience of the author in the development of homecare for the bone marrow transplant patient.

Intensive homecare of the bone marrow transplant patient requires assiduous management of the central venous catheter and strict adherence to protocol guidelines. When patients are home on parenteral nutrition, an overnight, 12- to 14-hour infusion is often utilized. Prophylactic administration of antibiotics to prevent opportunistic infections such as *Pneumocystis carinii* pneumonitis, cytomegalovirus, etc., is often necessary. Patients must be carefully monitored for the occurrence of chronic GVHD .

Introduction

A variety of cancers, including hematologic malignancies (acute and chronic myeloid and lymphoid leukemias, Hodgkin's disease and non-Hodgkin's lymphomas, multiple myeloma) and solid tumors (breast, ovarian, and testicular carcinomas and certain resectable primary brain tumors and melanomas) can be placed into long-term disease-free states with the use of high-dose chemotherapy/radiation therapy and stem cell support.

While the antineoplastic activity is due to the very intensive treatment administered, the survival of patients is ensured through the administration of viable stem cells. These repopulate the patient's bone marrow and regenerate hematopoiesis. In this way, the escalation of antineoplastic drugs and/or the dosage of radiation therapy becomes limited only by the extramedullary organ toxicity.

Chemotherapeutic doses 2 to 10 times higher than conventional doses of antineoplastic agents can be safely administered. Likewise, total body irradiation in excess of 1000 cGy can be delivered with acceptable toxicity.

According to the anatomical source of stem cells, transplants can be classified as being performed with bone marrow or peripheral blood stem cells (PBSC). The differences between these two categories are as follows:

1. The duration of severe pancytopenia after the high dose schedule—recipients of peripheral blood stem cells recover neutrophil and platelet counts in a shorter time (7 to 10 days earlier).
2. Peripheral blood stem cells have a lower rate of contamination with circulating malignant cells.

According to the donor source of stem cells, transplantation can be either (*a*) autologous, when the patient is his or her own donor; (*b*) allogeneic, when the donor is a different person, usually an HLA-matched sibling or, more recently, and HLA-matched unrelated donor, or (*c*) syngeneic, when the donor is an HLA-identical twin.

Autologous stem cell transplantation can be performed only if the patient's bone marrow is reasonably healthy—is uninvolved by malignancy or can be rendered as close to cancer-free status as medically possible. This may require several courses of conventional pretransplant chemotherapy or in vitro purging of the marrow. This form of stem cell support is used for the treatment of both hematologic malignancies and solid tumors. It has the advantages of immediate availability of stem cells (the patient), lack of graft versus host disease (GVHD), and lower mortality (only 2 to 4%), and as such can be performed up to ages 65–70. Its main disadvantage is felt when it is used for the treatment of hematologic malignancies, because under such circumstances the absence of GVHD is associated with the absence of beneficial graft-versus-leukemia effect.

Allogeneic stem cell transplantation requires the availability of an HLA-matched donor, is associated with a significant (20 to 70%) occurrence of acute or chronic GVHD, and carries a mortality of 20 to 30%. As such, the patient age is limited to less than 50–55 years. It may be used, however, for the treatment of bone marrow failure syndromes (e.g., aplastic anemia, severe combined immunodeficiency, myelodysplastic syndromes). Its advantage is precisely the occurrence of GVHD, with its associated anti-leukemia effect.

Nutrition

Pretransplant Nutritional Support

Malnutrition of patients prior to bone marrow or progenitor stem cell (PSC) transplantation may contribute to poorer outcome of the procedure, especially if previous chemotherapy and glucocorticoid therapy has been given. Recent hospitalization in the pretransplant period and psychological stress may amplify the problem. Steroids, integral components of numerous anticancer protocols (for acute lymphoblastic leukemia, Hodgkin's disease, non-Hodgkin's lymphomas) and antiemetic combinations, are well known to induce loss of muscle mass and protein stores. Underweight patients, with weight loss in comparison to their baseline, fare differently than patients with a low weight baseline. Objective impairment in ventilatory reserve and muscle strength was described in association with weight loss in excess of 15%, which in turn resulted in protein loss greater than 20% (1). Reduced serum protein levels and anthropomorphic measurements have not been associated with increased mortality (2).

However, a recent evaluation of patients undergoing marrow transplantation at Fred Hutchinson Cancer Center in Seattle, WA, disclosed significantly worse survival to 150 days after transplant for patients at 85–95% or less than 85% of ideal body weight, when compared to survival of patients at 95% to greater than 145% of ideal body weight (3). The observed effect was not explainable in terms of the composition of the lower weight categories in regard to other known or suspected risk factors (age, sex, race, diagnosis, transplant year, grade of acute GVHD, GVHD prophylaxis, or radiation dose received). Similar data were published regarding an increased morbidity and mortality in recipients of liver transplants who are malnourished at time of transplantation (4). While previous studies in patients with cancer have been equivocal as to the association of total parenteral nutrition (TPN) and nutritional rehabilitation (5, 6), others have suggested that even 1 week of TPN will improve wound healing in surgical patients (7). Obviously, in some patients, there will be no time to institute nutritional support before transplantation. In view of the Seattle data, however, intensive nutritional support at home should be strongly considered for those with a recent weight loss greater than 5%, if marrow or PSC transplantation is entertained.

Nutrition during Bone Marrow or PBSC Transplantation

Ideally, nutritional support should start prior to the transplant hospitalization. It should be maintained in the hospital and continue at home until full recovery occurs. There is an important role for nutritional support in the care of hospitalized transplant patients. The pretransplant conditioning regimen, be it high-dose chemotherapy or a combination of chemotherapy and total body irradiation, is responsible for significant nutritional problems that include nausea, vomiting, anorexia, diarrhea, malabsorption, and a negative nitrogen balance. All these problems may be aggravated by early or late posttransplant complications of GVHD and infection.

The rationale for nutritional support during marrow/PBSC transplantation is derived from the need to maintain a good caloric intake. There are data supporting the existence of increased nutritional requirements immediately after transplantation, especially since some of the complications may, in fact, simultaneously decrease the ability to eat and drink (8, 9). It is also important to remember that recovery of the immune function and to a certain degree of the hematopoietic functions is dependent on adequate nutrition (10).

Diminished Function of the Digestive System

Nausea and vomiting associated with high-dose chemotherapy and radiation therapy administration occurs in virtually all marrow transplant patients and may last for many weeks thereafter. The sedative effect of antiemetics may further impair any oral fluid and caloric intake. Oral mucositis may change the taste of food or, not infrequently, result in pain severe enough to require the use of narcotics. Diarrhea, a consequence of the mucositis that occurs in the gastrointestinal system, compounds the problem and may be prolonged by oral nonabsorbable antibiotics used for total gut decontamination. Viral or fungal esophagitis will invariably cause significant pain and further limit oral fluid intake.

Graft versus Host Disease

Degeneration of the intestinal mucosa results in watery or even bloody diarrhea, up to 5 to 10 liters per day. The clinical picture resembles ulcerative colitis or Crohn's disease. Significant protein loss may occur with associated hypoalbuminemia (11, 12). Jaundice and steatorrhea may appear in GVHD grades II-IV, due to small bile duct damage and cholestasis.

In-Hospital Nutritional Support

Transplant services mainly use two types of food services: sterile and neutropenic diets and low-microbial diets.

Sterile Diet

As its name implies, there are no bacteria or fungi in a sterile diet. Food preparation requires sophisticated separate facilities, including autoclaving, irradiation, or oven baking. Monitoring of bacterial growth is performed, and trays are made using laminar air flow. While this diet is less palatable, it is also more expensive and labor intensive (13).

Low-Microbial Diet

This diet is made of well-cooked foods, aimed at destruction of potential pathogens. Samples are cultured for microbial growth, and hygienic handling of foods is enforced. Separate kitchen facilities still may be needed, but there is a wider variation of meals (14).

It is unclear whether sterilizing the food has a more protective effect than simply lowering the bacterial content of the food. Several studies have shown a tendency to liberalize food service, at least in the United States (15).

Enteral Nutrition

As previously mentioned, oral food intake is rather scanty during transplant hospitalization, and fear of nausea and vomiting or fear of the unknown associated with the entire transplant treatment may further diminish the desire to eat. Gentle encouragement, counseling, and a varied menu may help increase the oral intake. Commercially available supplements like Sustacal and Ensure may be of help. Snacks, ice lollipops, and fortified drinks could bring extra energy and proteins as well (16). Overall, oral nutrition intake may be below 500 kcal per day. The main source of caloric support during hospitalization is still obtained via parenteral nutrition, once an assessment is made that the patient is unable or unwilling to eat and drink enough.

Parenteral Nutrition

With a better understanding of the role of stem cell transplantation, more patients are entering the high-dose treatment with good nutritional status (17). Even in this category of patients, in at least one study, prophylactic administration of TPN showed a modest improvement in survival, although it had no effect on the incidence of GVHD or the speed of engraftment (18). Under these conditions, the role of TPN is more to maintain rather than increase body cell mass.

Nutritional requirements are increased in the first month after transplantation, due to high-dose treatment, fever, and infection. When calculating TPN requirements, one has to consider both the basal and the stress energy requirements.

The Harris Benedict Basal Energy Expenditure (BEE) equation, which is used to determine the basal requirements, differentiates between males and females (16):

$$\textit{Males:}$$
$$66 + (13.7 \times ABW) + (5 \times Ht) - (6.8 \times age)$$

$$\textit{Females:}$$
$$665 + (9.6 \times ABW) + (1.7 \times Ht) - (4.7 \times age)$$

where ABW is the actual body weight (kg), Ht is the height (cm), and age is in years. The stress energy requirements will add an extra 70 to 90% following transplantation.

Home Nutritional Requirements: After Discharge

About 10 to 15% of patients undergoing bone marrow or stem cell transplantation may require home TPN following discharge. The reason for this need derives from the speed of discharge occurring nowadays with the use of growth factors, which allow a quick hematopoietic reconstitution, while recovery of the gut mucosa epithelium is not complete and the prolonged emetogenic effects of high-dose chemotherapy persist.

Home TPN should be administered on a cyclical basis 10 to 14 hours per day, with the understanding that conversion to oral nutrition should occur as soon as possible. This may take anywhere from 7 to 21 days. At home, under conditions of bed rest and light physical activity, one has to consider an extra 10 to 20% increase from BEE.

Protein Needs

Protein requirements are calculated at double the recommended daily allowance according to the following table (16):

Age	Ideal Body Weight (g/kg)
Adult	1.5
15–18 years	1.8
11–14 years	2.0
7–10 years	2.4
4–6 years	2.5–3.0
1–3 years	3.0

Fluid Needs

Notwithstanding the increased requirements due to fever and/or diarrhea, calculations are performed according to body surface area and/or weight.

For patients weighing more than 20 kg, a total of 1.5 L/m^2 is recommended. For those weighing less than 20 kg, the recommendation is 100 mL/kg for the first 10 kg plus 50 mL/kg per day for each kilogram between 10 and 20 kg (16).

Complications of TPN during and after Bone Marrow Transplantation

Infections

Administration of concentrated glucose solutions and usage of lines for administration of both TPN and other drugs, in addition to blood drawing, creates the opportunity for catheter-related sepsis. To diminish this risk, aseptic techniques have to be used at all times. It is also worth mentioning that needleless devices used for TPN seem to be associated with increased risk for bloodstream infections (19). The exact mechanism whereby the needleless device and TPN result in this increased risk is unknown. The suggested mechanism is compromised sterility of the luminal contents of the preslit injection caps, compared with the injection caps used with protected needles.

Fluid Overload

Fluid overload is less of a problem for patients with excellent heart and kidney function, but it may became an issue when impairment of either or both organs occurs after high-dose chemotherapy. Restriction of the sodium content of TPN and a higher concentration of dextrose may be entertained.

Fatty Liver Infiltration and Hyperglycemia

Administration of TPN solutions rich in glucose for long periods of time may induce hyperglycemia (requiring insulin administration) in the short term, and hepatomegaly with fatty liver in the longer term.

Enteral Nutrition

About 3 to 4 weeks following high-dose treatment, the appetite is significantly improved, but occasionally it may take several months for normalization of good oral food intake. Fortified drinks, snacks, and commercial supplements like Ensure or Sustacal may be used to replace or supplement meals. Food must be not only nutritious but also tempting.

Antimicrobial Prophylaxis

Catheter-Related Bacterial Infections and Catheter Care

Prophylaxis against catheter-related bacterial infections for patients undergoing either autologous or allogeneic transplantation could be considered once a central venous catheter of the Hickman or Quinton type is implanted, usually for stem cell collections. The rationale

for such prophylaxis is based on the increased risk for infection due to daily manipulations of the catheter during apheresis procedures. With a non-neutropenic patient, the most likely organisms to cause catheter-related bacteremia are *Staphylococcus* species, so oral dicloxacillin should be sufficient. Any confirmed line sepsis under these conditions should prompt intravenous antibiotic treatment. Vancomycin IV is probably the first choice, pending bacteriologic identification of the pathogen. Besides administration of antibiotics, good care of the catheter should be delivered, with dressings changed initially twice per week for the first 2 to 3 weeks and once per week subsequently. As to the need of anticoagulation for the maintenance of catheter patency, the best regimen to be used with large-bore Hickman or Quinton catheters is prophylactic heparin 5000 units IV to each port three times a week (20). When this intense heparin regimen is used, concurrent administration of oral Coumadin becomes unnecessary.

Prophylaxis of Pneumococcal Pneumonia

Graft versus host disease and its treatment with immunosuppressive agents delays the reconstitution of humoral and cellular immunity and creates favorable conditions for the development of bacterial infections, especially with *Streptococcus pneumoniae,* due to impaired reticuloendothelial function of the liver and spleen. Because pneumococcal vaccine administration was shown to be ineffective in bone marrow transplant recipients (21), oral penicillin administration is highly recommended, as 250 mg twice a day for as long as immunosuppressive therapy is given (22). It is important to be aware of the occurrence of penicillin-resistant pneumococci during prolonged penicillin prophylaxis (23). Because autologous transplant patients have a quicker reconstitution of their immune functions, routine antipneumococcal prophylaxis is not needed.

Prevention of Cytomegalovirus Infection

Cytomegalovirus (CMV) infection is one of the major causes of morbidity and mortality in allogeneic transplant patients. Therapy with ganciclovir and intravenous immunoglobulin have resulted in resolution of interstitial pneumonia in some instances (24, 25). Because the role of γ-globulin administration for prophylactic purposes is rather well established, the Eastern Cooperative Oncology Group (ECOG) recommends that all allogeneic transplantation patients who are CMV positive at transplant and those who receive a transplant from a CMV-positive donor should receive intravenous γ-globulin as prophylaxis (26).

Administration of Immunoglobulins

Immunoglobulins are given to allogeneic transplant recipients for two reasons: their known antimicrobial activity, most effective as antiviral prophylaxis, especially in CMV infections, and their potential immunomodulatory effect. While the latter usage did not result in any clear benefits, the former indication is well established. Besides their anti-CMV activity, immunoglobulins may exercise an overall antibacterial effect via enhancement of neutralization and opsonocytophagic function.

The ECOG recommendation is to administer intravenous immunoglobulins after allogeneic transplantation as CMV prophylaxis in seropositive patients and as a nonspecific antimicrobial prophylaxis in all patients, at a dose of 500 mg/kg given at least every 2 weeks for the first 3 months after transplantation (26).

When immunoglobulins are administered in the home setting, attention should be given to the speed of infusion because of known side effects (hypotension, malaise, facial flushing, etc.). The infusion is to be started slowly at 30 mL/hr for the first 30 minutes; the speed can be subsequently increased up to 75 mL/hr. Occasionally, premedication with Benadryl or Decadron may be needed.

Intravenous Ganciclovir

Following discharge from the hospital, some transplant centers will administer prophylactic ganciclovir to all CMV-seropositive recipients of allogeneic transplants. In a nonrandomized study, none of the 20 patients given ganciclovir developed infections, compared with 23% of matched historical controls with CMV pneumonia (27). The benefit was confirmed in two subsequent randomized, double-blind, placebo-controlled trials (27, 28). The survival benefit of the earlier trial could not be confirmed, however. Thus, a recommendation cannot be firmly made as to ganciclovir prophylaxis.

An acceptable schedule of administration for patients who are CMV positive is to administer ganciclovir intravenously, 5 mg/kg twice weekly from marrow engraftment to 100 days after bone marrow transplantation. The role of oral preparations of ganciclovir has not been established yet.

Prevention of *Pneumocystis carinii* Infection

With chemoprophylaxis, less than 10% of allogeneic transplants and almost none of the autologous transplants will develop *Pneumocystis carinii* interstitial pneumonia. Trimethoprim-sulfamethoxazole is very effective.

ECOG currently recommends one double-strength tablet orally twice daily two to three times per week, starting after engraftment and continuing for 3 to 6 months after transplant or, if chronic GVHD is present, for as long as immunosuppressive therapy is given. In patients allergic to trimethoprim-sulfamethoxazole or if severe cytopenia occurs, aerosolized pentamidine, 300 mg once a month can be used.

Prophylaxis of GVHD

The significant morbidity and mortality associated with acute and chronic GVHD justifies the need for prophylactic treatment of these conditions. There are two approaches to GVHD prophylaxis:

1. Treatment of the recipient with pharmacologic agents, primarily with cyclosporine, and
2. In vitro purging of donor T cells from the marrow.

Homecare of GVHD implies supervision of cyclosporine administration. In the absence of GVHD, cyclosporine is administered for 3 to 6 months, with gradual tapering according to a variety of schedules. Irrespective of the schedule of administration, it must be recognized that cyclosporine therapy may induce renal toxicity. Doses should be reduced if renal dysfunction appears according to the recommendation of the physician transplanter. There are no rigid guidelines for cyclosporine blood level monitoring.

Conclusions

Homecare of stem cell transplant patients is a challenging endeavor requiring an experienced nursing staff, excellent pharmacy support, an efficiently operating the laboratory, and ongoing consultation with the transplant physicians. Professional satisfaction of the home therapy team may be very rewarding, since a significant number of these very sick patients fully recover and are able to return to work and enjoy their lives.

References

1. Hill GL. Body composition research: implications for the practice of clinical nutrition. JPEN 1992;16: 197–218.
2. Dickson B, Barale KV. Section 2: Nutritional Assessment. In: Lensen P, Aker SN, eds. Nutritional Assessment and Management during Marrow Transplantation. A Resource Manual. Seattle: Murray, 1985:5–15.
3. Deeg HJ, Seidel K, Bruemmer B, Pepe MS, Appelbaum FR. Impact of patient weight on non-relapse mortality after marrow transplantation. Bone Marrow Transplant 1995;15:461–468.
4. Pikul J, Sharpe MD, Lowndes R, et al. Degree of preoperative malnutrition is predictive of postoperative morbidity and mortality in liver transplant recipients. Transplantation 1994;57:469–472.
5. Bozetti F, Ammatuna M, Migliavalla S, et al. Total parenteral nutrition prevents further nutritional deterioration in patients with cancer cachexia. Ann Surg 1987;205:138–143.
6. Chlebowski RT. Critical evaluation of the role of nutritional support with chemotherapy. Cancer 1985;55 (Suppl 1):268–272.
7. Deeg HJ, Klingeman HG, Phillips GL. A Guide to Bone Marrow Transplantation, 2nd ed. New York: Springer-Verlag, 1992.
8. Aker SN, Lenssen P, Darbinian, J, Cheney CL, Cunningham B. Nutritional assessment in the marrow transplant patient. Nutritional Support Services 1983;3(10):22–27.
9. Maxymiw WG, Wood RE. The role of dentistry in patients undergoing bone marrow transplantation. Br Dent J 1989;167:229–234.
10. Weisdorf S, Hofland C, Sharp HL, et al. Total parenteral nutrition in bone marrow transplantation: a clinical evaluation. J Pediatr Gastroenterol Nutr 1984;3:95–100.
11. Gavreau JM, Lenssen P, Cheney CL, Aker SN, Hutchinson ML, Barale KV. Nutritional management of patients with intestinal graft-versus-host disease. J Am Diet Assoc 1981;79:673–675.
12. Keenan AM. Nutritional support of the bone marrow transplant patient. Nurs Clin North Am 1989;24: 383–392.
13. Driegel L, Burstall CD. Bone marrow transplantation: dietician's experience and perspective. J Am Diet Assoc 1987;87:1387–1388.
14. Aker SN, Cheney CL. The use of sterile and low microbial diets in ultraisolation environments. J Parenter Enteral Nutr 1983;7:390–397.
15. Dezenhall A, Currie-Bartley K, Blackburn SA, De Lamerens S, Khan AR. Food and nutrition services in bone marrow transplant centres. J Am Diet Assoc 1987;87:1351–1352.
16. Souchon V. Nutrition during bone marrow transplantation. In: Treleaven J, Barrett J, eds. Bone Marrow Transplantation in Practice. New York: Churchill Livingstone, 1992:329–336.
17. Szeluga DJ, Stuart RK, Brookmeyer R, Utermohler V, Santos GW. Nutritional support of bone marrow transplant recipients: a prospective, randomized clinical trial comparing total parenteral nutrition to an enteral feeding program. Cancer Res 1987;47: 3309–3316.
18. Weisdorf SA, Lysne J, Wind D et al. Positive effect of prophylactic total parenteral nutrition on long-term outcome of bone marrow transplantation. Transplantation 1987;43:833–838.
19. Danzig LE, Short LJ, Collins K, et al. Bloodstream infections associated with a needleless intravenous infusion system in patients receiving home infusion therapy. JAMA 1995;273:1862–1864.
20. Kouides PA, Kaukeinen J, Heal J, Abboud CN and DiPersio JF. The potential benefit of mobilized peripheral blood stem cells (PBSC) in autologous bone marrow transplantation may be offset by the risks of PBSC harvesting with chemotherapy-CSF mobilization [Abstract]. Blood 1992;80(Suppl 1)10: 235a.
21. Winston DJ, Ho WG, Schiffman G, et al. Pneumococcal vaccination of recipients of bone marrow transplants. Arch Intern Med 1983;143:1735–1737.
22. Momin F, Chandrasekar PH. Antimicrobial prophylaxis in bone marrow transplantation. Ann Intern Med 1995;123:205–215.
23. D'Antonio D, Di Bartolomeo P, Iacone A, et al. Meningitis due to penicillin-resistant *Streptococcus pneumoniae* in patients with chronic graft-versus-host disease. Bone Marrow Transplant 1992;9: 299–300.
24. Reed EC, Bowden RN, Dandliker PS, Lilleby KE, Meyers JD. Treatment of cytomegalovirus pneumonia

with ganciclovir and intravenous cytomegalovirus immunoglobulin in bone marrow transplant patients. Ann Intern Med 1988;109:783–788.

25. Emanuel D, Cunningham I, Jules-Elysee K, et al. Cytomegalovirus pneumonia after bone marrow transplantation successfully treated with a combination of gancyclovir and high-dose intravenous immune globulin. Ann Intern Med 1988;109:777–782.

26. Rowe JM, Ciobanu N, Ascensao J, et al. Recommended guidelines for the management of autologous and allogeneic bone marrow transplantation. A report from the Eastern Cooperative Group (ECOG). Ann Intern Med 1994;120:143–158.

27. Atkinson K, Downs K, Golenia M, et al. Prophylactic use of gancyclovir in allogeneic bone marrow transplantation: absence of clinical cytomegalovirus infection. Br J Haematol 1991;79:57–62.

28. Goodrich JM, Bowden RA, Fisher L, Meyers JD. Gancyclovir prophylaxis to prevent cytomegalovirus disease after allogeneic marrow transplant. Ann Intern Med 1993;118:173–178.

29. Winston DJ, Ho WG, Bartoni K, et al. Gancyclovir prophylaxis of cytomegalovirus infection and disease in allogeneic bone marrow transplant recipients. Results of a placebo-controlled, double-blind trial. Ann Intern Med 1993;118:179–184.

19

OUTPATIENT MANAGEMENT OF CHRONIC PAIN

Jeffrey Askanazi[a,b]

CHAPTER AT A GLANCE: The management of chronic pain is an evolving field, with treatment options covering a wide spectrum. Homecare therapeutics plays a significant role in the management of chronic pain.This chapter reviews the background and classification of pain states. Neural pain mechanisms are covered in detail. Different types of procedural interventions, including stimulation therapies and implants, are discussed, with a special emphasis on their outpatient and homecare applications. New treatment options, such as lysis of epidural adhesions, are briefly reviewed.

Background

In evolutionary terms, pain can be considered as a protective reflex system warning an individual of hostile situations and tissue injury. Chronic pain, however, has lost its meaningful significance and is characteristically accompanied by several harmful and deleterious projections to other systems, e.g., the autonomic nervous system. In 1986, the International Association of the Study of Pain (IASP) defined pain as "an unpleasant sensory and emotional experience associated with actual or potential tissue damage, or described in terms of such damage" (1). In principle, pain is considered chronic if it has lasted more than 6 months.

Pain is cited as the main complaint in more than 20% of all visits made to practicing physicians. According to Bonica, approximately one-third of the American population suffers from obvious pain lasting more than 6 months at some point in their life span (2). Most pain disorders are nonmalignant in origin, with chronic low back pain characterizing the largest observed patient group in pain clinics around the world. Up to 70% of the population show evidence of degenerative joint changes by the end of their fifth decade. Among cancer patients, 40% have been reported to suffer remarkable pain before the appearance of metastases, and over 70% thereafter. Palliation of these symptoms is a fundamental component of improving quality of life.

The concept of multidisciplinary pain clinics, consisting of participants from various disciplines (anesthesiology, dentistry, neurology, physiotherapy, psychology, psychiatry, etc.), was generated during the 1950s and

---

[a]*Tuula Manner, Olli Kirvelä, and Paul L. Goldiner contributed to this chapter in the first edition.*
[b]*Our warm thanks are due to Dr. Edith Kepes, M.D., for her valuable suggestions and clinical advice during the preparation of this chapter.*

1960s by J.J. Bonica in Seattle. Thereafter, much work has been done to spread awareness of pain as a specific illness entity requiring specialized management. Pain clinics are now found all over the world as multidisciplinary groups of physicians work on difficult diagnostic and therapeutic pain problems. In addition to patient care, which is usually carried out on an outpatient basis, pain clinics frequently provide consultant and educational services. In general, the function of pain clinics is directed to diagnostic measures, the initial setting of the treatment, and technical procedures, whereas patient follow-up, including readjustment of dosage schedules, is usually carried out by practicing physicians. Homecare therapeutics—the provision of medical supplies and support services in the home—has permitted an expansion of multidisciplinary pain management. Furthermore, it allows for the practical application of these services to homebound, chronically ill patients. In this chapter we will try to provide insight into the basic principles and currently available facilities of pain management and their applicability to the homecare system.

Neural Pain Mechanisms

Pain is sensed by the unencapsulated nerve endings (nociceptors) of primary afferent neurons located in the dermis, mucosal membranes, muscles, tendons, and other tissues. The mechanisms by which different kinds of noxious stimuli (thermal, mechanical, electrical, and chemical) activate nociceptors are not fully understood, although they seem to involve the release and activation of chemical substances (e.g., bradykinin, histamine, serotonin, prostaglandins, and substance P). Sharp, well-localized pain is transmitted rapidly (at speeds of 12 to 30 m/s) by the myelinated, thick Aδ nerve fibers, whereas diffuse, blunt, and burning pain is conducted by the slow (0.5 to 2 m/s), thin, unmyelinated C fibers (3).

After entering the spinal cord via dorsal spinal roots, afferent pain impulses synapse in the substantia gelatinosa of the dorsal horn and, after crossing the midline, pass upward, contributing to the dorsal spinothalamic tract

with two divisions (neospinothalamic and paleospinothalamic). The neospinothalamic tract projects directly via thalamic and thalamocortical projections to the somatosensory cortex, the site of the discrimination and interpretation of pain. The paleospinothalamic tract runs from the thalamic nuclei diffusely to limbic and subcortical areas. In its course, the pain-conducting tract shows extensive convergence of sensory fibers and has diffuse projections to the limbic system (4). These interactions are probably mediators of autonomic and affective response to pain.

The neural mechanisms of pain suppression include the pathway projecting from the cerebral cortex via thalamic neurons to the dorsal horn of the spinal cord (5, 6). This serotonergic pathway has a moderate tonic inhibitory effect on spinal nociceptive inputs. The descending noradrenergic pathway mediates its inhibitory effects through α-adrenergic receptors. In contrast, substance P appears to be an excitatory transmitter or neuromodulator of the afferent neurons of the dorsal horn. The gate-control hypothesis, presented by Melzack and Wall in 1965, introduced the theory that the nociceptive excitability of afferent neurons can be inhibited by ongoing activity in other sensory afferents serving the same or adjacent spinal segments (7).

Prostaglandins (especially PGE_2, $PGF_{2\alpha}$, PGI_2, and thromboxane A_2) play a crucial role in inflammatory pain, primarily mediated by sensitization of the peripheral afferent fibers to other chemical mediators, which also induce vasodilation, increased vascular permeability, leukocyte migration, phagocytosis, and release of lysosomal enzymes (8, 9). The effect of nonsteroidal anti-inflammatory drugs is related to the inhibition of PG synthesis by reversible inactivation of the enzyme cyclooxygenase, which catalyzes the conversion of arachidonic acid to various PGs, thromboxanes, or prostacyclin (10).

At the level of the central nervous system (CNS), pain transmission is modulated by the function of endogenous opioid-acting peptides, "endorphins," with corresponding opioid receptors. Opioid analgesia is mediated through complex interactions of μ-, κ-, and δ-opioid receptors (11, 12). The antinociceptive action of endogenous opioid peptides is most probably not effective against acute, severe pain. These compounds are associated more with the experience of pain as well as concomitant fear and anxiety.

The distribution of opioid receptors in the spinal cord has been found to be as follows: μ-receptors, 40%; δ-receptors, 10%; and κ-receptors 50%. The endogenous opioid peptide metenkephalin is known to act as a transmitter of the inhibitory interneurons. The different narcotic analgesics used in clinical practice bind with varying affinities to the opioid receptors.

In addition to pain being an intractable and uncomfortable experience, it has to be considered detrimental due to its ability to stimulate the neuroendocrine stress response. This reaction stimulates the release of catabolic hormones and inhibits the release of anabolic hormones (for example, it stimulates the release of catecholamines and enhances the secretion of ACTH, prolactin, and growth hormone, which causes a metabolic shift of substrates from storage sites to circulation, etc.), resulting in additional organic stress for the patient (13, 14). Local release of adrenergic transmitters impairs the microcirculation in the traumatized tissue, producing ischemia. Ischemia further induces the release of chemical mediators of vasopermeability and tissue injury, which in turn enhance the secretion of catecholamines, thus continuing the vicious cycle.

Classification of Pain States

For practical purposes, chronic pain can be classified into three groups (Table 19.1): somatogenic, neurogenic, and psychogenic pain (1). Somatogenic pain is characterized by continuous nociceptive stimulation of peripheral afferent fibers, which is conducted via undamaged, intact nociceptors and nerve fibers. In neurogenic pain the nerve tissue itself has been injured at either the peripheral or the CNS level.

Typical examples of somatogenic pain include musculoskeletal, ischemic, and cancer pain. Impaired metabolism of nerve tissue, demyelination, or loss of nerve axons are characteristically seen in neuropathies. Reflex

sympathetic dystrophia is a complex clinical syndrome that occurs in peripheral nerves after trauma. A vicious cycle involving primary afferent neurons, postganglionic sympathetic neurons, and spinal cord interneurons maintains continuous local overactivity of sympathetic input with resultant vasoconstriction. At its final point this situation is called causalgia, and comprises muscle loss, osteoporosis, and trophic changes in the injured limb (15).

Phantom pain, associated with postamputation trauma, reflects central loss of normal sensory input because of the imbalance between thick proprioceptive and thin nociceptive fibers. From a clinical point of view, it is important to recognize that neurogenic pain responds poorly to centrally acting analgesic drugs. Pure psychogenic pain is rare, but psychic symptoms—such as depression, sleep disorders, vegetative disorders, or increased irritability—are commonly observed to be accompanied by chronic pain.

Table 19.1. Classification of Chronic Pain States

Somatogenic Pain
Musculoskeletal pain
   Osteoarthritis
   Lumbosacral back pain
   Posttraumatic pain
   Myofascial pain
Cancer pain
Visceral pain
   Chronic pancreatitis
   Ulcer
   Irritable colon
Ischemic pain
   Arteriosclerosis obliterans

Neurogenic Pain
Posttraumatic and postoperative neuralgia
Neuropathies
   Diabetic
   Toxic
   Other
Causalgia, reflex sympathetic dystrophy
Nerve entrapment
Facial neuralgia
Perineal neuralgia
Postamputation pain
Thalamic pain

Psychogenic Pain

Table 19.2. Main Methods Used in the Management of Chronic Pain

Medical Therapy
Nerve Blocks
Somatic nerve blocks
Regional nerve blocks
Autonomic nerve blocks
Spinal and epidural blocks
   Continuous administration
   Neurolytic blockades
Surgical neurolysis

Stimulation Therapy
Transcutaneous nerve stimulation
Acupuncture

Physiotherapy

Psychotherapy

Management of Chronic Pain

Owing to the complexity of the pain-mediating system, it is reasonable to prevent pain transmission at several levels, thus potentiating the effectiveness and decreasing the incidence and severity of side effects of the treatment. The available methods for treating chronic pain are summarized in Table 19.2. Most, if not all, of these techniques have an outpatient or homecare application. In addition, homecare plays a significant role in reducing anxiety and thereby helping to modulate the pain response.

Pharmacologic/Medical Treatment of Pain

Analgesic pharmaceutical agents are the most frequently used tools in the alleviation of somatogenic pain. The concept recommended by the World Health Organization (WHO) of steplike administration of analgesic agents has been widely applied to the management of chronic pain (Fig. 19.1). The choice of drug depends primarily on the intensity and quality of pain, although such matters as side effects or the facility of administration (e.g., oral versus parenteral) can also become important with long-lasting therapy. Regular, repeated administration with satisfactory doses is also of considerable importance for the pharma-

cologic effectiveness of drug therapy in pain patients.

Nonsteroidal anti-inflammatory drugs (NSAIDs) are useful in treating mild to moderate somatogenic pain, such as the degenerative syndromes, as well as the pain related to bone metastases (16). The mechanism of their analgesic action is purely peripheral, resulting from the inhibited synthesis of prostaglandins mediating the inflammatory reaction. The various NSAID preparations (e.g., 650 mg of acetylsalicylic acid, 400 mg of ibuprofen, or 50 mg of indomethacin) provide maximal analgesic effects that are essentially equal, and are comparable with 5 mg of morphine intramuscularly (17). Possible side effects are gastritis, disturbances in hemostatic functions, and central nervous system side effects (tinnitus). Paracetamol in large overdoses may potentially induce renal and hepatic toxicity (18).

If NSAIDs alone prove insufficient, a weak centrally acting analgesic may be added to the therapy. Dextropropoxyphene and codeine are frequently combined with NSAIDs in commercial preparations for this purpose.

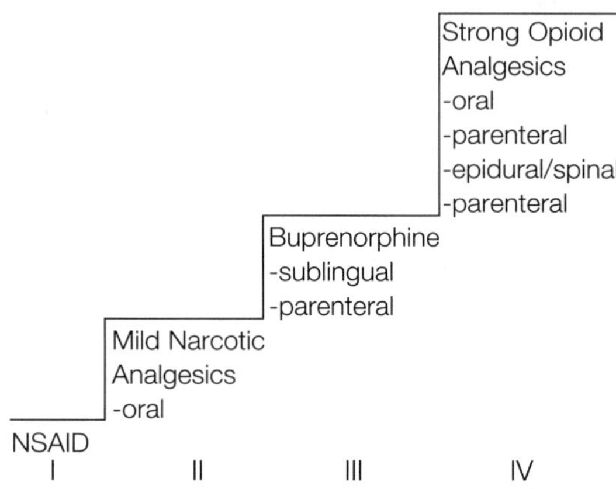

Figure 19.1.   A stepwise approach to the management of chronic pain, proposed by the World Health Organization, has been widely applied. The severity and intensity of pain guide the choice of drug therapy. Mild narcotics such as codeine are added to Step I (NSAID) therapy, progressing to mixed agonist-antagonists and the strong opiates.

If this level of pain management is insufficient, drugs such as buprenorphine can be added. Buprenorphine is a mixed agonist-antagonist analgesic with a long duration of action, moderate-to-strong analgesic activity, and a supposed lack of central side effects such as addiction and drug dependence (19). Sublingual administration of 0.4 to 0.8 mg of buprenorphine at 8-hour intervals provides adequate, continuing pain relief for the majority of patients with moderate pain. Unfortunately, buprenorphine typically induces nausea and psychotomimetic effects in about one-third of patients (20). Pentazocine, butorphanol, and nalbuphine are other agonist-antagonist narcotics with somewhat less analgesic activity and a shorter duration of action compared with buprenorphine (21).

With increasing intensity of pain, strong opiates are needed. However, the peroral administration route requires higher doses than the parenteral route by factors of two to five. This is due to the high degree of first-pass metabolism of these drugs. Morphine is a pure μ-agonist opiate with the classic opioid side effects (euphoria, nausea, urinary retention, constipation and, in large doses, respiratory depression) (22). Since the introduction of a slow-releasing tablet form of morphine sulfate (10- or 30-mg tablets, MS Contin), the usage of peroral opiate therapy has gained wide popularity among cancer patients, and by increasing the doses as needed, the great majority of cancer patients experience complete pain relief (23). Insufficient relief because of advancing tumor growth or opioid-resistant pain, nausea, itching, and urinary retention are the main reasons for the failure of peroral morphine treatment. The usefulness of methadone is limited because of its very long half-life (15 to 20 hours), which predisposes to accumulation with the danger of respiratory depression (24). Oxycodone is available in the United States as a parenteral formula only.

In addition to the analgesics, several adjuvant agents may be combined with the purpose of increasing the efficacy and tolerability of the treatment. Tricyclic antidepressants (amitriptyline, imipramine, and doxepin) have been shown to exert analgesic influences on chronic pain in addition to their antidepressive properties (25). This effect is most likely due to an increased activity in the descending, inhibitory serotonergic tracts. Antidepressants have been found to be beneficial in, for example, postherpetic neuralgia, diabetic neuropathies, chronic low back pain, chronic headache, and posttraumatic neuralgias. Anticonvulsant drugs (e.g., carbamazepine), which are chemically close to local anaesthetics, have been shown to be effective against burst-like pain syndromes like trigeminal neuralgia (26). Neuroleptics are commonly combined with the therapy due to their proposed additive potency on analgesics (levomepromazine) and, most importantly, due to their potent antiemetic effect (haloperidol, 4 to 8 mg/day). Benzodiazepines are widely used by pain patients because of their potent anxiolytic and, depending on the derivatives, sleep-inducing properties (27). In general, benzodiazepines can be considered safe drugs, but there is a certain risk of habituation, especially in association with long-term therapy. The suspected analgesic action of benzodiazepines is highly questionable.

Parenteral Administration

In the case of insufficient peroral dosage or the inability of the patient with severe chronic pain to take peroral medication, opiate analgesics can be administered in the home. This can be accomplished as a continuous parenteral infusion by the intravenous or subcutaneous route (28, 29). Subcutaneous continuous infusion offers ease of use and safety (less risk of infections). The intravenous route can provide higher levels of analgesia.

Sophisticated infusion pump devices, some of which allow the patient to repeatedly self-deliver minimal doses of an analgesic drug (patient-controlled analgesia [PCA]), have been developed using accurate programmable pumps and alarm systems. These systems are quite adaptable to the homecare setting. In addition, adjuvant medications (such as haloperidol) can be easily added to the same syringe with the analgesic solution.

Thus, the homecare patient can receive sophisticated pain management techniques in the comfort of familiar surroundings. This may reduce anxiety and further facilitate pain relief.

In general, all parenteral opioids are suitable for continuous infusions, but morphine or oxycodone are most often used in chronic pain patients (29). Home prescription of opiate analgesics is generally limited to the management of malignant diseases. However, in exceptional circumstances they may be used for carefully selected cases of excruciating nonmalignant pain, such as ischemic pain, spinal stenosis, or postherpetic neuralgia (30).

An opioid infusion can be started on an outpatient basis, with physician visits to adjust treatment. Alternatively, a homecare nurse may visit the patient at home and report the patient's condition to the doctor by telephone. Changes in the prescription can be ordered by the physician, with the nurse changing pump settings while in the patient's home. Common practice advocates starting morphine infusion for an opioid-naive patient with a dose of 1 mg/hr. If necessary, the dose can be increased once a day by 1 mg/hr until adequate pain relief is achieved. In pharmacologic investigations, the blood concentrations have been found to stabilize to a constant level 24 hours after a change in the subcutaneous infusion rate. If the patient has been on oral morphine medication, the equipotent parenteral daily dose can be estimated as one-third of the previous peroral dose. In hepatic or renal insufficiency, the metabolism or excretion of morphine metabolites may be reduced, and careful attention must be paid to the risk of overdosage and toxic opioid effects. With prolonged administration of opioids, the development of some degree of tolerance is inevitable. Regular follow-up and adjustment of the medication is therefore very important.

In comparison with repeated injections, the continuous administration regimen prevents both the peaks of opioid side effects (drowsiness, nausea, risk of respiratory depression) and the intermittent reversal of pain. Furthermore, the total daily dose of morphine can usually be reduced to a slightly lower level due to the stable administration rate.

Implantable Devices

A therapeutic alternative for traditional infusion therapy is the implantation of pain control devices. These include implantable morphine pumps and spinal cord stimulators. The former are reservoir systems that deliver a constant rate of morphine infusion. The reservoir can be refilled through a subcutaneous port on an intermittent basis. Spinal cord stimulators rely on the gate theory of pain. The principle is that gentle electrical stimulation of an affected nerve will blunt the sensation of pain. These devices generally have a life span of 2 to 3 years and can be externally programmed. They work best for extremity/radicular pain; a 60% success rate (success being defined as 50% or more pain relief) during the first 2 years can be expected.

For painful symptoms limited to the trunk, the success rate is lower. For this type of pain one can achieve better results with a morphine pump, a device that infuses morphine directly into the lower back. This allows the use of morphine in a localized area without the systemic effects. On the negative side, tolerance will occur, which mandates "drug holidays." Other compounds such as baclofen can be used for spasticity disorders.

Nerve Blocks

Nerve Blocks As Treatment for Chronic Pain

The generation of an action potential can be temporarily inhibited by local anesthetics, which bind to specific receptor sites of the nerve membrane (31). The blockage affects all modalities of a given nerve. Among the variety of local anesthetics, bupivacaine seems to be the most valuable for pain treatment, because of its prolonged duration of action and its preferable selectivity for sensory blockage at low concentrations (0.125 to 0.25%). Other agents commonly used for nerve blocks are lignocaine, mepivacaine, and etidocaine. For as-yet unknown reasons, local anesthetics, when used for nerve blocks in chronic pain—and particularly when used repeatedly—may provide analgesia far outlasting the predicted duration of action consistent with the pharmacologic properties of the agent.

Permanent ablation of nerve conduction can be achieved by chemical neurolytic agents, which induce local destruction of neural tissue at the place of injection. Neurolytic agents do not differentiate among various modalities of neural input, and interruption of nociperception thus may be accompanied by a block of motor function (32). Partial regeneration of nerve conduction occurs in several months. Neurolytic blocks are mostly used for the treatment of terminally ill patients with malignancies. A prognostic block using local anesthetics has to be performed before the neurolytic blockage to verify the extent and side effect profile of the block. Surgical dissection of pain-conducting pathways can be performed at several levels of the tract (rhizotomy, cordotomy, thalamotomy) (33). These operative procedures are very rarely indicated and require great caution because of the potential side effects and the severity of the treatment.

Somatic Nerve Blocks

Trigger points are well-localized, painful foci associated with inflammatory reactions of muscles (myalgia, myositis, myofascitis), joints, or connective tissues (fascitis, bursitis, myositis). It has been suggested that vasoactive substances, including noradrenalin, bradykinins, serotonin, and prostaglandins, play a role in the development of trigger points. Infiltration of local anaesthetic solution (5 to 10 mL of 0.25% bupivacaine) into the painful focus frequently provides significant pain relief for a duration greatly exceeding the pharmacologic action of the agent (34). Frozen shoulder syndrome and supras-capularis nerve entrapment are specific pain syndromes that react positively to the block of the suprascapular nerve at the scapular notch.

In the case of a posttraumatic peripheral neuroma, permanent pain relief can be obtained by injection of a minimal amount (0.1 to 0.5 mL) of a neurolytic chemical (6% phenol-glycerol or absolute alcohol) at the site of the palpable thickening of the nerve (35). As mentioned before, the response has to be tested by local anesthetics before the induction of a permanent, neurolytic blockage.

Sympathetic Nerve Blocks

The sympathetic nervous system is closely implicated in chronic pain, and a wide variety of pain states have been reported in the literature as responding to treatment with sympathetic blockages (36, 37). Despite some controversy concerning the indications and the efficacy of the treatment, visceral pains and ischemic symptoms in the extremities appear to respond positively to sympatholysis. The early use of sympathetic blockage for the treatment of acute herpes zoster may accelerate the healing process and prevent the development of the debilitating period of postherpetic neuralgia (38). Diagnostic sympathetic blockages are used to identify the patients with peripheral vascular insufficiency who will benefit from surgical sympathectomy.

A stellate ganglion block is commonly performed by the anterior paratracheal approach at the level of the transverse process of the sixth cervical vertebra in the vicinity of the cricoid cartilage (39). During the procedure, special care must be taken to avoid an intraarterial (arteria vertebralis) injection, which may cause toxic CNS effects. Clinical conditions that respond well to stellate ganglion block include circulatory insufficiency states like sympathetic dystrophia or causalgia, as well as acute herpes zoster and phantom limb pains of the upper extremities.

The celiac plexus is responsible for the autonomic innervation of the abdominal viscera. The plexus is located at the anterolateral position of the first lumbar vertebra (40). The percutaneous technique is somewhat difficult and is usually performed under x-ray or ultrasound control to verify the anatomic structures (41). Indications for celiac plexus block are pain due to pancreatic cancer and other severe visceral pains of the splanchnic region (42). Absolute alcohol is preferred for a permanent block. Possible complications of the procedure include hypotension, epidural or subarachnoidal injection, intravascular injection, pneumothorax, retroperitoneal hematoma, and visceral puncture. A more feasible alternative for the percutaneous technique is an abdominal, intraoperative puncture of the plexus in patients with inoperable cancer.

The lumbar sympathetic ganglia lie anterolaterally to the vertebral bodies of lumbar vertebrae L1–L4. Percutaneous injection is performed in a direction adjacent to the vertebral body of L2 (39). Circulatory disorders, phantom limb pain, and causalgias of the lower limbs, as well as pains in the urogenital region and renal colics, may benefit from this block. Effective blockage of the ganglia can be achieved with 20 mL of 0.25% bupivacaine. Somatic nerve puncture, intravascular or subarachnoidal injection, or renal tissue injury are possible complications of the procedure.

An alternative, easier approach to reduce the sympathetic activity of an extremity is the method of intravenous regional administration of guanethidine, which acts pharmacologically by displacing noradrenaline from the nerve endings (43). Performance of the block is relatively easy: after draining the superficial veins, a tourniquet is placed proximally on the limb with pressure 50 to 100 mm Hg above the patient's systolic pressure, and 15 to 20 mg of guanethidine is injected in a volume of 20 to 40 mL of physiological saline. Within 20 to 30 minutes, the guanethidine diffuses to neural tissue, and the tourniquet may be removed. While the pressure is being relieved, careful monitoring of blood pressure is required. The maximal response typically appears after repeating the block three to four times at 1-week intervals. Good results have been reported in the treatment of causalgias, sympathetic dystrophias, and posttraumatic pain syndromes (44).

Epidural and Spinal Administration of Analgesics

An intense and prolonged analgesia without motor blockage can be produced by epidural or spinal administration of analgesics. The degree of lipid solubility, ionization, and the affinity to opioid receptors are the major factors determining the analgesic efficacy, onset and duration of action, and safety of any given opioid (45). After epidural administration of a hydrophilic agent such as morphine, a rapid and extensive absorption occurs into the circulation with a plasma concentration-time profile comparable with that seen after intramuscular injection (46). However, a portion of the given dose apparently penetrates the dura, since the cerebrospinal fluid (CSF) concentrations of the drug considerably exceed the corresponding values in plasma. In the case of a more lipophilic agent (fentanyl and its derivatives), penetration into the CSF occurs rapidly with subsequent binding to the opioid receptors of the spinal cord and, hence, interruption of the transmission of pain signals segmentally at the spinal cord level (47). Absorption of lipophilic agents by epidural fat may decrease the amount available for crossing the dura. Intrathecal injection of a drug circumvents the diffusion barriers, and so considerably lower doses (commonly 2.5 to 5% of the corresponding parenteral dose) are needed.

Because of its hydrophilic nature and slow binding to spinal receptors, morphine is prone to rostral spread with CSF, which may lead to access into the medullary centers controlling respiration (46). The inherent danger of delayed respiratory depression, typically occurring 6 to 12 hours after morphine injection, is more likely to take place after bolus injections to opioid-naive patients (e.g., for treatment of postoperative pain) than in cancer patients accustomed to opioids (47). Advanced age, impaired respiratory function, and concomitant use of parenteral analgesics or other respiratory depressant drugs predispose to this serious complication. However, in a retrospective study of over 6000 patients receiving long-term opioids epidurally or intrathecally, a low incidence (0.25 to 0.4%) of respiratory depression was reported (48).

The side effect profile of epidural or spinal opioids is otherwise similar to that of systemic administration (nausea, vomiting, prorates, and urinary retention), but with slightly lower incidence. Only preservative-free preparations of analgesics (e.g., morphine hydrochloride) are suitable for epidural injections and especially for spinal injections, because of the risk of neurotoxicity and fibrosis induced by preservative agents.

With its strong analgesic potency and long duration of action (15 hours after 2 to 10 mg of morphine as an epidural bolus injection), morphine is still the most frequently used analgesic in epidural and spinal techniques, but good results have also been reported after administration of epidural fentanyl (0.1 mg lasting for 6 hours), meperidine (30 to 100 mg), buprenorphine (0.3 mg), nalbuphine, or diamorphine (49, 50). Local anaesthetics are often combined with the infusion solutions, and bupivacaine can be particularly recommended because of the bacteriostatic capacity of the pharmacologic solution.

A tendency to increase narcotic dosages over time is commonly seen in cancer patients, although tolerance may be difficult to distinguish from the progression of the disease or the prominence of a more opioid-resistant type of pain. Opioid infusion at a constant, slow rate appears to reduce the risk of tolerance. Several attempts have been made with alternative spinal agonists to decrease the tendency of receptor tolerance. In patients with advanced spinal morphine tolerance, intrathecally administered clonidine has been shown to produce analgesia (at a dose of 10 $\mu g/kg$) and to reduce the development of tolerance (at doses of 2 to 4 $\mu g/kg$) (51). The effect is apparently mediated through its α_2-agonist activity on spinal noradrenergic pain-suppressing pathways. Some authors have recommended clonidine to be routinely added to long-term epidural infusions of opioids (52). At the start of combination therapy, monitoring and control of blood pressure is of great importance due to the hypotensive action of clonidine in some patients.

When prolonged therapy with epidural or spinal opioids is required, intermittent injections increase the risk of infections. Special techniques with subcutaneously tunneled catheters and implanted injection ports or drug delivery systems are now available (53).

These catheters, in combination with small, portable infusion pumps, make the possibility of home continuous epidural narcotic administration feasible.

An overall complication rate of 15% has been reported with long-term delivery systems. These include mechanical problems such as catheter obstruction, leakage, and kinking; infectious complications (epidural abscess, sepsis, meningitis) are rare but require careful observation of patients, especially those with immunosuppressive or corticosteroid medication.

Alternative approaches to continuous opioid infusions in advanced cases of cancer pain of the visceral splanchnic and perianal region or the lower extremities are chemical neurolytic blockages (54). A fairly selective and long-lasting (up to 6 months) blockage of dorsal horn afferent pain fibers can be achieved by the injection of hyperbaric, 6% phenol-glycerine into the spinal space with subsequent careful positioning of the patient (55). Due to the possibility of concomitant blockage of ventral motor fibers, which may lead to the loss of bladder or bowel function, a prognostic block with a local anesthetic prior to the permanent neurolysis is necessary. Because of the difficulty of the technique, complications are seen in 1 to 15% of cases.

Epidural Injections of Steroids

Epidural steroid injections have been used to alleviate pain associated with acute herniated discs and related low back pain syndromes (56). By using the routine epidural space approach, 80 to 100 mg of methylprednisolone acetate or 25 to 50 mg of triamcinolone is injected into a mixture that also contains 4 to 5 mL of local anesthetic solution. A positive response may take several days to become apparent, and usually two to three injections over several days are needed for complete pain relief. Chronic low back pain syndromes appear to be resistant to anesthesiologic interventions (57).

Lysis of Epidural Adhesions

A neurolytic nerve block is done to remove adhesions in the epidural space of the back and neck. Adhesions can follow surgical procedures, resulting from either hemorrhaging into the epidural space or scar formation. The inflammatory response following injury can also cause adhesions.

Patients who have been unresponsive to epidural steroid injections and other therapies are candidates for this procedure. Definitive diagnosis is made with an epidurogram using injection of contrast media into the epidural space. Epidural scars or adhesions visualized are lysed with a Racz catheter. This catheter and the procedure were developed by Gabor B. Racz at Texas Tech University.

Seventy-two patients answered a questionnaire over the telephone. Improvement resulting from their having received this procedure was assessed by asking them to rate their improvement on a scale from 0 to 10 (0, no improvement; 5, noticeable improvement; 10, improved to normal). Nine patients were not included in the analysis because they were lost to follow-up (three patients), had additional problems (three patients), had new injuries (two patients), or did not want to answer the questionnaire (one patient). Overall, 90% of the men claimed an improvement by rating their improvement greater than 0 (average rating scores $\pm$ SEM were 6.6 $\pm$ 0.6 for men under 50, $n = 17$; 7.7 $\pm$ 0.8 for men over 50, $n = 10$). Eighty-five percent of the women also claimed improvement from the procedure (6.3 $\pm$ 0.8 for women under 50, $n = 16$; 6.3 $\pm$ 0.9 for women over 50, $n = 12$). Improvement was only temporary, lasting 1 month or less, in six of these patients. This procedure proved to be a viable therapeutic modality for a majority of patients that failed epidural steroid injections and had epidural adhesions on epidurogram.

Stimulation Therapies

The action of peripheral stimulation techniques is based on the theory of segmental pain inhibition, the gate-control theory (7). A concurrent activation of neurophysiologic (afferent input), humoral (endorphins), and psychic inhibitory mechanisms is apparently involved. Some evidence suggests that, in addition to its pain-relieving effect, transcutaneous nerve stimulation (TNS) may influence autonomic systems and suppress sympathetic overactivity (58). Acupuncture and TNS, the most frequently used stimulation therapies, are effective against myofascial and neurogenic pain. Chronic headache responds successfully to acupuncture, and in migraine acupuncture has been considered to be the treatment of first choice (59). Careful teaching of the patient is important for the effective use of the TNS apparatus. The more sophisticated surgical applications include spinal cord stimulation via epidurally placed catheters or electrical stimulation of thalamic nuclei associated with pain suppression (60). These techniques are used in specific cases of excruciating deafferentation or cancer pain.

In practice, the patient usually obtains a TNS device to be used at home, and careful teaching of the patient (by a physician or physical therapist) is therefore very important for the effective use of the TNS apparatus. Most recommendations include a minimum application trial of 20 minutes two to three times daily for adequate TNS therapy. However, a cumulative effect is most likely obtained with more frequent repetition of the treatment. The preferential application site for TNS electrodes is at the superior or contralateral segment next to the pain area. It should be emphasized that the pain stimulation may never be induced directly to the painful site but to the adjacent area with normal cutaneous sensation. Several anatomical locations, as well as variable frequencies and pulse widths, should be attempted before deciding that TNS is ineffective. The patient should also be informed about the time delay with the maximum pain relief by TNS. In most chronic pain states, TNS can be considered a favorable adjunct to other therapy due to its noninvasive nature and easy use at home.

Physiotherapy

Physical therapy, starting with simple motion, maintenance of muscle function, and physical activity, is a major part of the care of pain patients. Physiotherapeutics provide a great variety of treatments for pain patients, such as postural training, relaxation techniques, diadynamic pulses, galvanic stimulation techniques, etc. Muscle spasms can be effectively relaxed with massage or thermal therapies, which also facilitate the subsequent performance of muscular exercise. Biofeedback has been found to be successful in many patients with chronic headache refractory to previous treatments and relaxation therapies (61). Long-term results of studies performed on patients with back pain have not been as promising.

Psychological and Psychiatric Therapies

It is widely accepted that psychological variables exert a significant influence on the experience of pain. Psychological evaluation and interview should therefore be performed for every patient with chronic pain. The Minnesota Multiphasic Personality Inventory (MMPI) is a psychological instrument used widely in the assessment of personality factors contributing to the experience of chronic pain (62). When needed, individual cognitive strategies are used to manipulate the personal factors implicated in pain (anxiety, predictability, attention, sociocultural factors, etc.) (63). In chronic pain patients, group therapy has proved to be the most effective type of psychological support. Psychiatric consultants are important participants in the multidisciplinary pain clinic, and they are needed as well in their capacity as experts in the adjustment of psychoactive drugs.

Summary

During recent years, the different pharmacologic, physiologic, and psychological modalities of pain have received increasing attention, and important extrapolations have been made to the clinical management of pain. The importance of the attenuation and prevention of acute pain may become a matter of greater emphasis as our insight into the mechanisms mediating the suggested neural and biochemical learning effects of pain at the spinal level become more complete (64). It has been suggested that, in the future, the role of pain treatment may be directed more toward the prevention of chronic pain than to its management.

At present, successful pain relief can be provided for the majority of pain patients by combining different available methods of pain suppression. Medical treatment by peripherally active anti-inflammatory agents and centrally acting opioid analgesics is still the most widely used method, but neural blockages are becoming more popular due to their more limited mode of action on pain conducting tracts. Patients with complicated pain syndromes or severe pain should be referred to specialized pain clinics, but knowledge of the basic principles and the readiness to notice and treat pain are the duty of every physician, since effective pain treatment must be considered the right of every patient. New home techniques such as narcotic infusion and neural stimulation add considerably to the aggressive use of outpatient pain management.

References

1. Merskey H. Classification of chronic pain. Descriptions of chronic pain syndromes and definitions of pain terms. Pain 1986;Suppl 3:S1.
2. Bonica JJ. General considerations of chronic pain. In: Bonica JJ, ed. The Management of Chronic Pain. Philadelphia: Lea & Febiger, 1990:1883.
3. Raja SN, Meyer RA, Campbell JN. Peripheral mechanisms of somatic pain. Anesthesiology 1988;68:571.
4. Casey KL. Neural mechanisms of pain: an overview. Acta Anaesthesiol Scand 1982;74(Suppl):13.
5. Hole K, Berge O-G. Regulation of pain sensitivity in the central nervous system. Cephalalgia 1981;1:51.
6. Terenius L, Tamsen A. Endorphins and the modulation of acute pain. Acta Anaesthesiol Scand 1982;74 (Suppl):21.
7. Melzack R, Wall PD. Pain mechanisms: a new theory. Science 1965;150:971.
8. Hunskaar S, Hole K. The formalin test in mice: dissociation between inflammatory and non-inflammatory pain. Pain 1987;30:103.
9. Simon LS, Mills JA. Nonsteroidal antiinflammatory drugs. N Engl J Med 1980;302:1179.
10. Vane J. The evolution of non-steroidal anti-inflammatory drugs and their mechanisms of action. Drugs 1987;33:18.

11. Millan MJ. Multiple opioid system and pain. Pain 1986;27:303.
12. Pasternak GW. Multiple morphine and enkephalin receptors and the relief of pain. JAMA 1988;259:1362.
13. Kehlet H. Surgical stress: the role of pain and analgesia. Br J Anaesth 1989;63:189.
14. Kehlet H, Brandt MR, Rem J. Role of neurogenic stimuli in mediating the endocrine-metabolic response to surgery. J Parenter Nutr 1980;4:152.
15. Procacci P, Maresca M. Reflex sympathetic dystrophies and algodystrophies: historical and pathogenic considerations. Pain 1987;31:137.
16. Capetola RJ, Rosenthale ME, Dubinsky B, McGuire JL. Peripheral antalgesics: a review. J Clin Pharmacol 1983;23:545.
17. Helleberg L. Clinical pharmacokinetics of indomethacin. Clin Pharmacokinet 1981;6:245.
18. Mitchell JR. Acetaminophen toxicity. N Engl J Med 1988;319:1601.
19. Heel RC, Brogden RN, Speight TM, Avery GS. Buprenorphine. A review of its pharmacological properties and therapeutic efficacy. Drugs 1979;17:81.
20. Tigerstedt I, Tammisto T. Double-blind, multiple-dose comparison of buprenorphine and morphine in postoperative pain. Acta Anaesthesiol Scand 1980;24:462.
21. McQuay HJ. Opioids in chronic pain. Br J Anaesth 1989;63:213.
22. Sajwe J, Dahlstrojm B, Rane A. Morphine kinetics in cancer patients. Clin Pharmacol Ther 1981;30:629.
23. Hanks G, Truman J. Controlled release morphine sulphate tablets are effective in twice daily dosage in chronic cancer pain. In: Wilkes E, Levy J, eds. Advances in Morphine Therapy. London: Royal Society of Medicine, 1984:103.
24. Twycross RG. Relief of pain: strong narcotic analgesics. In: Saunders CM, ed. The Management of Terminal Malignant Disease. London: Edward Arnold, 1984:75.
25. Feinmann C. Pain relief and antidepressants' possible modes of action. Pain 1985;23:1.
26. Maciewicz R, Bouckoms A, Martin JB. Drug therapy of neuropathic pain. Clin J Pain 1985;1:39.
27. King SA, Strain JL. Benzodiazepines and chronic pain. Pain 1990;41:377.
28. Kerr IG, Sone M, DeAngelis C, Iscoe N, MacKenzie R, Scheuller T. Continuous narcotic infusion with patient-controlled analgesia for chronic cancer pain in outpatients. Ann Intern Med 1988;108:554.
29. Bruere E, Brennels C, MacDonald RN. Continuous SC infusion of narcotics for the treatment of cancer pain: an update. Cancer Treat Rep 1987;71:953.
30. Portenoy RK, Foley KM. Chronic use of opioid analgesics in non-malignant pain: Report of 38 cases. Pain 1986;25:171.
31. Strichartz GR. Neural physiology and local anesthetic action. In: Cousins MJ, Bridenbaugh PO, eds. Neural Blockage in Clinical Anesthesia and Management of Pain. Philadelphia: JB Lippincott, 1988:25.
32. Myers KM, Katz J. Neuropathy of neurolytic and semi-destructive agents. In: Cousins MJ, Bridenbaugh RO, eds. Neural Blockage, 2nd ed. Philadelphia: JB Lippincott, 1988:1031.
33. Gybels JM, Sweet WH. Neurosurgical treatment of persistent pain. Physiological and pathological mechanisms of human pain. Pain Headache 1989;11:1.
34. Fine PG, Milano R, Hare BD. The effects of myofascial trigger point injections are naloxone reversible. Pain 1988;32:15.
35. Kirvelaj O, Nieminen S. Treatment of painful neuromas with neurolytic blockade. Pain 1990;41:161.
36. Churcher MD, Ingall JRF. Sympathetic dependent pain. Pain Clin 1987;1:217.
37. Loh L, Nathan PW, Schott GD. Pain due to lesions of central nervous system removed by sympathetic block. Br Med J 1981;282:1026.
38. Milligan NS, Nash TP. Treatment of post-herpetic neuralgia. A review of 77 consecutive cases. Pain 1985;23:381.
39. Bonica JJ, Buckley FP. Regional analgesia with local anesthetics. In: Bonica JJ, ed. The Management of Pain. Philadelphia: Lea & Febiger, 1990:1883.
40. Moore DC, Bush WH, Burnett LL. Celiac plexus block: a roentgenographic, anatomic study of technique and spread of solution in patients and corpses. Anesth Analg 1981;60:369.
41. Kirvelä O, Svedstrojm E, Lundbom N. Ultrasonic guidance of lumbar sympathetic and coeliac plexus blockade: a new technique. Reg Anesth 1992:17:43–46.
42. Brown DL. Neurolytic celiac plexus: its place in your practice. Probl Anesth 1987;1:612.
43. Hannington-Kiff JG. Antisympathetic drugs in limbs. In: Wall PD, Melzack R, eds. Textbook of Pain. Edinburgh: Churchill Livingstone, 1984:566.
44. Loh L, Nathan PW, Schott GD, Wilson PG. Effects of regional guanethidine infusion in certain painful states. J Neurol Neurosurg Psychiatry 1980;43:446.
45. Moore RA, Bullingham RSJ, McQuay HJ, et al. Dural permeability to narcotics: in vitro determination and application to extradural administration. Br J Anaesth 1982;54:1117.
46. Nordberg G, Hedner T, Mellstrand T, Borg L. Pharmacokinetics of epidural morphine. Eur J Clin Pharmacol 1984;26:233.
47. Inturrisi CE. Management of cancer pain. Pharmacology and principles of management. Cancer 1989;63: 2308.
48. Rawal N, Arner S, Gustafsson LL, Allvin R. Present state of extradural and intrathecal opioid analgesia in Sweden. Br J Anaesth 1987;59:791.
49. Vainio A, Tigerstedt I. Opioid treatment for radiation cancer pain: oral administration vs. epidural techniques. Acta Anaesthesiol Scand 1988;32:179.
50. Morgan M. The rational use of intrathecal and extradural opioids. Br J Anaesth 1989;63:165.
51. Germain H, Neron A, Lomssy A. Analgesic effect of epidural clonidine. In: Dubne R, Gebhart GF, Bond MR, eds. Proceedings of the Vth World Congress on pain. Amsterdam: Elsevier, 1988:572.
52. Eisenach JC, Rauck RL, Buzzanell C, Lysak SZ. Epidural clonidine analgesia for intractable cancer pain: Phase I. Anesthesiology 1989;71:647.
53. Cherry DA. The use of opioids by implanted systems and self administration. Clin Anaesthesiol 1987;1:955.
54. Cousins MJ, Dwyer B, Gibb D. Chronic pain and neurolytic blockade. In: Cousins MJ, Bridenbaugh PO, eds. Neural Blockade in Clinical Anesthesia and Management of Pain. Philadelphia: JB Lippincott, 1988:1053.
55. Wood KM. The use of phenol as a neurolytic agent. A review. Pain 1978;5:205.
56. Dallas TL, Lin RL, Wu WH, Wolskee P. Epidural morphine and methylprednisolone for low-back pain. Anesthesiology 1987;67:408.
57. Fast A. Low back disorders: Conservative management. Arch Phys Med Rehabil 1988;69:880.
58. Ernst M, Gracely RH, Lee MHM. Influence of TENS on autonomic function. Acupunct Electrother Res 1987;12:259.

59. Richardson PH, Vincent CA. Acupuncture for the treatment of pain: a review of evaluative research. Pain 1986;24:15.
60. Budd K. Recent advances in the treatment of chronic pain. Br J Anaesth 1989;63:207.
61. Chapman SL. A review and clinical perspective on the use of EMG and thermal biofeedback for chronic headaches. Pain 1986;27:1.
62. Costello RM, Hulsey TL, Schoenfeld LS, Ramamurthy S. P-A-I-N: A four-cluster MMPI typology for chronic pain. Pain 1987;30:199.
63. Pilowsky I. Psychodynamic aspects of the pain experience. In: Sternbach RA, ed. The Psychology of Pain. New York: Raven Press, 1978:203.
64. Woolf CJ. Recent advances in the pathophysiology of acute pain. Br J Anaesth 1989;63:139.

20

Emergency Care in the Home

C. Gresham Bayne

CHAPTER AT A GLANCE: As medical care shifts out of the hospital and into the home, providers must struggle to meet regulatory requirements while solving the technical and logistical problems of delivering comprehensive physician services on an acute care basis. An innovative solution to this problem is the development of "high-tech" physician housecalls. This chapter provides an overview of the issues and solutions for providing such urgent care in the home setting. Providing these housecalls requires systems for dispatch, trained personnel, and modifications to equipment. Yet, despite its complexity, all of this is within the realm of practical application. The author describes his experience in establishing a comprehensive system for homecare emergency services.

Introduction

The national debate concerning cutbacks in Medicare/Medicaid funding in general, and homecare in particular, seldom addresses the unique opportunity provided by considering emergency housecalls as an alternative to high-cost emergency room treatments. The aging of the population, the continued scientific and medical advances that allow us to live longer despite disabilities, and the information revolution are all trends bringing the social pot to a boil over who is going to pay.

The argument usually reverberates around cost containment and questions about the cost effectiveness of homecare, defined as skilled nursing services provided under the remote telephonic direction of a physician. The logical progression of this service must include a reintroduction of the physician housecall. But how can one expect to provide the high level of care expected of a physician without the tools and technology we rely on? It is in the exploration of home-based solutions to this question that huge savings can be achieved while providing patients with what they most desire in the first place: staying home when they are ill.

The new paradigm of emergency housecalls fits the apparently competing political trends seeking cost containment while increasing access. In a 1994 report from the U.S. Department of Health and Human Services, Secretary Donna Shalala noted that 49.7 million (55.4%) visits to the emergency room in 1992 were nonurgent. This finding confirms an older study sponsored by the American Academy of Emergency Medicine, in which only 12.5% of 10,253 patients seen in 24 hospital emergency rooms needed immediate physician attention (1).

Although the elderly tend to use ambulances for nonurgent conditions, they are 1.7 times more likely to need ambulance transport than younger patients (2). Once they arrive in the emergency room, the elderly stay longer, receive more diagnostic tests, and incur higher average charges (3). About one-sixth of elderly emergency room patients arrive by ambulance, and between 10 and 30% of all emergency room patients are admitted to the hospital.

This chapter is intended to serve as an introduction to the innovative field of physician housecalls for urgent medical care. The discussion that follows represents the cumulative experience of over 40,000 housecalls made to patients with urgent medical needs supported by a physician/technician team in a specially equipped mobile "emergency room." It is worth noting here that the total charges for this type of service have generally been less than half the cost of an ambulance ride alone.

The Initial Call

Besides the obvious motivational problem of changing a trillion-dollar industry organized around physicians' office/hospital-based practice of medicine, significant functional barriers must be considered by the emergency housecall physician. Uncompensated travel time is increased by demographics, traffic patterns, and home security measures. There are difficulties in communicating with the physician on the road, prioritizing calls to treat the sickest patients first, and late cancellations. From a practical viewpoint, there are numerous impediments, beginning with the very basic ability of the patient to answer the door.

The liability of accepting the responsibility for acute housecalls cannot be taken lightly either. Patients do not know what an emergency is, and numerous articles have been written showing the lack of specificity for patient-perceived emergencies. However, some patient-perceived emergencies do require 911 responses, and a formal system of triage must exist to protect both the patient and the physician from an inappropriate delay in accessing the emergency medical system (EMS).

Once the question of the need for emergency response is addressed, efficiencies can

be built into the dispatching system. Placing patients in three categories (emergent, urgent, or same day) gives flexibility to the delivery system and allows both grouping of calls and meeting the realistic needs of sick patients. Emergent responses must be made within the hour, and urgent responses within 3 hours or with "next-in-line" attention. When calls are downgraded from patient-perceived emergency to same-day service, a 1-hour window is given, rather than a specific appointment time. This prevents patient dissatisfaction with the team coming either too early or too late.

The concept of triage is critical to the safe and efficient operation of an acute housecall system. Such a system could also be piggybacked on another program such as a managed-care gatekeeping system. However, one must be very cautious to account for the intense desires of a patient to stay at home, even when delays in care are liable to incur medical risks.

The best way to minimize such delays is to use an algorithm-based triage procedure, such as the military systems developed by both the U.S. Army and U.S. Navy, to prioritize patients coming to emergency rooms from outlying areas. Numerous commercial products ranging from computerized patient algorithms to interactive voice response systems to home software for member beneficiaries are now being explored by the managed-care industry. This is probably the most complex and poorly understood area in any acute medical model, including 911 systems nationwide.

Whatever system is used, there must be a recoverable logic specific to each chief complaint, and the interactive decision must be documented in the chart. For example, when I arrived at a 92-year-old woman's house for a routine housecall and found her dead in her chair (her daughter thought she was asleep), it was very reassuring to have the triage log documenting the daughter's request for a wound assessment of her pressure sores with the appointment scheduled 2 days earlier.

As in EMS services, communication with the providers is always a critical issue. The physician in the field is available both as a care provider and a final stop on the triage ladder. Without adequate two-way communication, the power of the physician's medical judgment is lost. Until geostationary wireless communication systems, such as Motorola's Iridium, are functional, the provider must choose between VHF, CB, UHF, and hybrid radios or the cellular telephone (with its more expensive services). Most radio systems now allow for scrambled channels to prevent eavesdropping and loss of patient privacy in often delicate home health communications. The type of communication decision is usually based on local geographic and cost-based factors.

Dispatch

Once a patient has called requesting acute medical services by a physician in the home, a triage priority is established by protocol, and dispatching considerations begin. There are three essential areas of discussion for dispatch: patient acuity, geography, and team preference. The patient's acuity level, as discussed above, will mandate certain patients to be seen out of order and may change during the day for various reasons. Urgent calls may be upgraded to emergent by an anxious spouse who can wait no longer. A home health nurse may visit unexpectedly and downgrade or remove the need for the physician visit. Unless an illness becomes extreme, patients are generally willing to await the physician housecall. However, the dispatching center must be attentive to the need for re-assessment when patients or caregivers call back repeatedly to request attention.

The geography of the area and local traffic patterns are then used to group calls as efficiently as possible. Since the majority of calls are downgraded to same-day service (analogous to the average 5-hour waiting times in our local emergency rooms), one has the luxury of planning the day around the traffic patterns, starting in a direction opposite to the afternoon rush hour patterns. Obviously, calls can be interrupted at any time by

patient care issues, but one generally adheres to this geographic concept. The experienced team quickly learns numerous "tricks of the trade" in getting the treatment team to the patient as efficiently as possible. Batching of calls, especially in congregate housing areas, is often impossible because of acute priorities, even after a formal triage decision has downgraded the patient's perception of urgency. Large complexes, use of elevators in high-rise apartments, steep driveways, and weather all play a role in making a home patient encounter time-efficient.

The recent change in federal reimbursement for ambulance transports will have a significant effect on the urgent housecall practice. As of January 1, 1995, Medicare and Medicaid will pay for ambulance transport only when "the patient's condition is such that other means of transportation would endanger the health of the patient" (4). This determination must be made at the time of transport, not when the patient calls for service, and payment by Medicare is not to be affected by any of the following factors:

- A particular physician does not have staff privileges in a hospital
- A more distant institution is better equipped
- A more distant institution is more convenient
- The nearer institution is in another state
- A particular insurance plan requires a specific hospital

Ambulances, therefore, are only paid when "the absence of immediate medical attention" could reasonably be expected to result in any of the following:

- Placing the patient's health in serious jeopardy,
- Serious impairment of bodily functions, or
- Serious dysfunction of any bodily organ or part.

Thus, patients are frequently transported to a hospital where their doctor does not have privileges and they have no health records.

The managed care patient is then transported again to their HMO hospital for reevaluation. Finally, the patient is liable for a governmental agency or managed-care utilization review committee to deny charges on the transport itself, not to mention the incurred emergency room charges. All of these induced inefficiencies can be avoided by employing the urgent care housecall, with the transport decision subordinated to the physician's evaluation, rather than the reverse.

The economic considerations to the patient have now become a reality. The Medicare beneficiary will be required to pick up the cost as more restrictive payment policies are invoked by both Medicare and managed-care payors. As of this writing, several states, such as California, have passed mandated payment laws requiring the HMO to pay for a reasonable "screening exam" in all cases of "patient-perceived" emergencies. Currently, Congress is considering a federal statute, sponsored by the American College of Emergency Physicians, to require full payment of the emergency room bill when a reasonable lay person perceives an emergency to exist at the time of arrival. Such legislation is far-reaching in its impact on patient and caregiver behavior evaluating the decision to seek hospital-based emergency care or an emergency housecall.

Site of Service

Triage encounters concentrate on the medical issues involved, whereas social and environmental influences often control the patient's agenda. The older the patient population, the more controlling these factors become. With 5% of Medicare beneficiaries dying each year and consuming 30% of the Medicare budget, access to acute care in the home could have significant economic advantages.

The average annual cost of a Medicare patient to the taxpayer is $1,924. This cost rises in the last year of life to $13,316. Physician housecalls can be seen as an alternative to expensive emergency medical systems. In the author's view, a considerable percentage of acutely ill Medicare patients could be voluntarily cared for at home.

A Harris poll done in 1993 indicated that 96% of Americans want to die at home; yet autopsy data show that only 4% do. Since Medicare patients account for 40% of all hospitalizations and a large percentage are admitted through the emergency room, the global financial effect of effecting patient choice at the point of hospital entry could be substantial.

Despite the obvious savings to be gleaned from a home-based delivery system of care, not every patient is a suitable candidate. Patients without telephones either cannot call for service or would be inappropriate to leave unattended. Patients who live alone must be cognitively intact enough to dial 911 if a subsequent emergency follows the housecall. The patient's emotional status must be stable enough to weigh the risks of staying home versus hospitalization, as well as awaiting a housecall rather than calling 911.

Spousal dynamics, including the difficulties of substance abuse, codependencies, and the enmeshed family syndrome, must be considered. The totally dependent patient must often be separated from the enmeshed caregiver to break the psychological ties that prevent reasonable decision-making. Agoraphobes must not be facilitated with repeated housecalls so as to allow them to fail in treatment plans designed to overcome their fear of going outside.

The physical dwelling plays a role in defining the appropriateness of an urgent housecall. We have a standing rule allowing the treatment team to cancel any call in which they feel unsafe, such as in a gangland area after dark. Certain areas of a city may be "off-limits" after dark, although medical personnel are usually treated with respect by even the hardest of criminals. Some housecalls uncover an unexpected problem; for example, the 650-lb patient who would not fit through the door, requiring the fire department to plan extrication by tearing down a wall of the house, as the treatment team began the resuscitation.

The delivery of acute care in the home also leads to a new core of technical knowledge, such as hanging intravenous bags on picture hooks in the wall, wearing headlamps to perform suturing, creative positioning with pillows to take x-rays in bedbound patients, and packaging equipment in efficient tackle boxes based on chief complaint or procedures rather than standard EMS stocking principles. A disposable Chux should be used in every case to take all trash out of the house, with a sharps disposal receptacle part of every doctor's bag. We have learned to treat all trash as hazardous in accordance with state laws, since separation of the trash is more trouble than it is worth. With all trash treated as hazardous materials, one does not have to worry about such situations as a grandchild getting hepatitis from a dirtied swab or gauze pad.

The Treatment Team

Acute care housecalls are significantly more labor-intensive than "black bag" housecalls. The latter involve the physician equipped with stethoscope, sphygmomanometer, ophthalmoscope/otoscope, and some limited medications. Acute care housecalls involve higher-level equipment, supplies, and therapeutics.The associated requirements of laboratory, x-ray, procedures, etc. often require a team of two professionals cross-trained in the various techniques involved. A two-person team provides increased security, a level of intrinsic quality control, an automatic "standby" for the patient's comfort, and more rapid assessment and treatment. The ideal would be a male/female team for obvious reasons, but staffing seldom permits that as a standard.

The old concept of physician team leadership is breaking down in managed care regions, and physician extenders or nurses are being used with or without a technical support person. Most states allow physician assistants or nurse practitioners a great deal of autonomy with telephone supervision by a physician, or even solo practitioner status for nurse practitioners. However, the current Medicare payment policies require direct, "in-the-building" supervision by a physician for both categories in urban areas. In designated Health Profes-

sions Shortage Areas, a physician assistant or nurse practitioner can practice with only telephonic supervision. In all rural areas, a nurse practitioner can practice with no direct supervision. The current presidential administration is attempting to broaden primary care access by expanding the autonomy of these physician-extenders, but at the time of this writing no real changes have been made.

Some programs, such as Doctors On Call in Brooklyn, New York, use off-duty policeman as drivers to support the physician on housecalls. This solves the security issue, but it does not permit a technician's input or facilitate female standby for pelvic examinations. A most difficult issue is the ethnicity of the treatment team, when the expectation of the patient may be different. Not only must one be sensitive with regard to the issue of discrimination, but one must also respect patients' right of privacy in their homes. We have made housecalls with physicians and technicians of all races, sexes, religions, and nationalities and have never received a complaint except for the inability of the physician to speak the language of the patient. The language problem has recently been aided by telephone company sevices that can provide rapid translation of virtually any language.

The two-person team, consisting of physician and technician, provides significant flexibility. The evolution of this team parallels that of physicians in the field with EMS programs, such as LifeFlight helicopters. Although the physician is the team leader, a unique and respected parity is established with the technician if portable services are carried with them. A technician trained as driver, laboratory technician, x-ray technician, ECG technician, and pharmacy technician can quickly determine the success or failure of a call. The hours of "windshield time" spent between calls leads to a personal bonding that I have not seen anywhere else in the practice of medicine.

In such a team approach, the physician quickly learns not only to do simple technical jobs, like the ECG, but also to trust the technician with surgical assisting, casting, or other procedures while the family is being counseled. A true blending of function not only characterizes the mature team, but allows for splitting the team when only technical services and a paramedic examination are anticipated. By using medics from the ambulance community, a technician can be trained to become the eyes and ears of the physician managing patients in his or her practice or referred by the managed care gatekeeper.

Radiology

It has never made me comfortable to make a black bag housecall on a patient with shortness of breath and order the portable chest x-ray from a independent carrier. Not only is there an administrative burden to connect the x-ray result back to the patient at a later time, often measured in days, but the x-ray will frequently require a face-to-face visit to explain unanticipated results. Thus, two housecalls separated by days result from the x-ray, unless a great deal of telephone communication is done with the patient, relatives, and often the payor.

The availability of stat portable x-rays is necessary for patients to be safely managed during emergency housecalls. Although many large cities have same-day services for portable x-ray in the home, getting the film or the radiological interpretation directly to the primary care physician, especially one making housecalls, is problematic. Several solutions to the dilemma exist.

First, the concept of teleradiology has been developing rapidly to the point where films can be taken, processed on site by an x-ray technician in a specialized vehicle, digitized, and sent by cellular modem to a radiologist for immediate reading. A remote, high-resolution monitor in the primary care physician's office could also receive a digitized copy of the film. This technique has long been in use to send CT scans to radiologists at home or in other sites for readings. The problem with sending a chest x-ray by digitizing camera is the much larger amount of information, approaching one gigabit, involved. Using portable x-rays of the chest, already limited in quality, a digitizing camera, transmission losses across cellular telephone lines, and in-

expensive office computer monitors will lead to a very limited quality of chest x-ray.

Another solution is taking the portable film immediately back to a hospital or central collecting point and having an on-duty physician read the actual film quickly. The transportation costs, stat professional fees involved, and loss of business taking each film back to the base station all remain uncompensated through current payor policies.

A third solution is to have the x-ray machine and developer in the same vehicle with the physician. With a technician to develop the film on site, the treating physician can look at it immediately and make therapeutic decisions. The efficiencies of this method are "one-stop shopping" with no subsequent visit or patient encounter required to change a plan of treatment, and the lower cost of operations of each film. The inefficiencies, however, concern the contingency costs of carrying the equipment on each housecall when the majority of housecalls do not require it.

Certain decisions must be made about the application of state and federal law when designing a portable x-ray system to support emergency care in the home. When the Health Care Financing Administration (HCFA) changed the basis of physician payment to a resource-based relative value scale (RBRVS) system, they removed the portable x-ray transport fees from allowable physician bills. This means that a physician must become a certified portable x-ray supplier, conforming to state laws and billing under a separate provider number.

One should decide whether all films, no films, or only selected films will be reviewed by a radiologist, since no state or federal regulations require it. The author's experience in literally thousands of portable x-rays taken on emergency housecalls has been that there is little use for the radiologist's reading days later, after the clinical decisions have been made.

It is apparent that the authors of Medicare reimbursement policy never anticipated the availability of new technologies providing these types of stat services in the home. Portable x-ray carriers are generally required to bill from their corporate address, rather than the customary site-of-service required for physicians. For instance, I have made housecalls in one carrier's area using a leased portable x-ray service based in another carrier's area. One could then reasonably expect to have to bill separate carriers for separate services made on a single housecall in the same day! When the physician's office is in a different state from the portable x-ray service, further billing problems ensue.

It is highly likely that conventional film-dependent radiology will become obsolete in 5 years. Using direct digitization of the exposure by x-ray excitation of single-pixel phosphors, a computer image can be created directly from the x-ray machine without processing of film. Under development is an even more exciting technology: the portable magnetic resonance imaging device. With a laptop computer, specialized software, and a catcher's mitt–sized electromagnet plugged into household current, one can image up to a depth of 8 cm in an uncontrolled environment. Without concerns about radiation, the continual imaging of the moving magnet seen on a portable computer could provide "home fluoroscopy" with an entirely new way of looking at pathology.

Finally, the reader should be aware of the general costs of conventional x-ray film techniques. A standard piece of x-ray film costs about $2.50, with some fifty cents of chemicals required to develop it. Since portable x-ray machines and tabletop developers cost about $10,000 together, the major expense consists of the amortization and employee time taking and developing the film. With physicians participating in taking stat films in the home, this labor cost can be the dominant economic reality defining a successful program.

Laboratory

The recent explosion in portable laboratory technologies makes emergency care in the home quite reasonable, even without on-site x-rays. A plethora of choices for testing equipment may be found in any medical electronics catalog. A decision must be made as to the minimum laboratory tests required for the physician to meet any foreseeable emergency. Beyond the disposition of the emergency lies the more complex rationale for comprehensive laboratory testing in the treatment of homebound patients.

Emergency rooms generally provide a limited number of stat laboratory tests. These values provide the clinician with the information they need for an acute treatment plan or disposition in the vast majority of cases. As the tabletop instrument industry rolled out a large number of innovative products, the government instituted a number of policy changes affecting the physician's ability to provide rapid, inexpensive laboratory tests to their patients. The largest change, besides a drastic reduction in reimbursement, occurred under the regulations known as the Clinical Laboratory Inspections Act (CLIA). Under this Act, the government now requires registration fees for ultimate certification and inspection of all physician laboratories that perform other than the most basic tests.

CLIA had a huge effect on the ability to provide emergency care in the home. The regulations were based on independent, volume laboratories and applied to physician office laboratories. But even office laboratories have a greater volume than a housecall physician could ever be expected to generate. Since one of the CLIA requirements is a set of control calibrations within 8 hours of the patient's test, the cost of registration and mandated control testing exceeds the possible Medicare revenues from the maximal volume of tests that could be done in a full-time housecall practice. The physician does not even have the right to avoid CLIA registration by not submitting a bill and giving the laboratory tests to the patient for free, since certification is tied to actual operations rather than reimbursement procedures!

The industry response to this dilemma has been a new technology using "electronic" controls that can be done at the time the patient's serum is being tested. At the time of this writing, the only point-of-service laboratory machine authorized for electronic controls is the iStat (iStat Corporation, Princeton, NJ) (Fig. 20.1). This unit allows the values listed in Table 20.1 to be measured from whole blood within 90 seconds of the arterial (or venous) sampling. A detailed cost analysis of this inexpensive machine and technician costs suggests a possible break-even with high utilization as expected in a full-time emergency housecall practice. Other technological developments include reagent-film polymers and rapid immunoassays that contain their own controls.

A number of tabletop machines can be custom-installed in a mobile unit, such as the Vitros DT60 (Johnson & Johnson, Rochester, NY), the Reflotron, the Vision, or the older Seralyzer. For such machines to be economically feasible using wet controls, the physician would have to develop a way to batch office laboratory tests for performance after hours.

A clear rationale exists for a more comprehensive laboratory capability, including cardiac enzymes and other important stat

Table 20.1. Laboratory Tests Available in 90 Seconds with a Hand-Held Instrument Using 100 μL Whole Blood or Plasma and a $12 per Panel Cartridge

Sodium
Potassium
Chloride
CO_2 (calculated)
Blood urea nitrogen
Glucose
Hemoglobin
Hematocrit
Po_2
Pco_2
pH

tests, under the managed care movement. A physician subcontracting with a managed care payor may now avoid the numerous federal anti-kickback regulations that impede the efficient delivery of innovations such as emergency care in the home. Under a flat per-housecall arrangement or a sub-capitated agreement, emergency housecalls can be performed with "lab-as-necessary" done in a CLIA-approved laboratory using free market negotiated rates. Such a structure removes the fee-for-service incentive to do more laboratory work under lucrative reimbursement policies while avoiding a rationing approach to laboratory work under the current Medicare reimbursement policy.

Cardiopulmonary Monitoring

There are numerous choices for inexpensive machines that perform electrocardiograms in a portable environment. Some also include an option for spirometry. Useful additional options include the ability to store many tracings in a database, an internal modem to transmit across the telephone for stat cardiology consultation, and computer reading of the tracing itself. These clinical decisions usually default to the experience of the physician delivering the care in the home.

Another extraordinary fact of life for the homecare physician is the federal policy of paying portable x-ray suppliers a transport fee

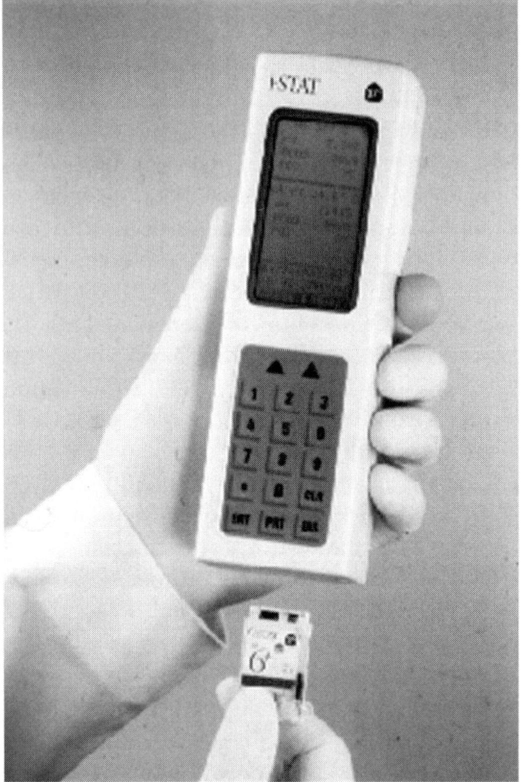

Figure 20.1. i-Stat, the only point-of-service laboratory machine authorized for electronic controls. (Courtesy of i-Stat Corporation, Princeton, New Jersey.)

for electrocardiograms. This transport fee usually equals or exceeds the global fee, which includes the technical and professional components. Thus, for a physician to be fully reimbursed for an ECG in the home, he or she must have a portable x-ray supplier's certification! Payor policies notwithstanding, portable electrocardiograms are perhaps the simplest technical service supporting physicians in the home.

As managed care policies become more widespread, the astute clinician will focus more and more on what is clinically important, rather than what is federally reimbursed. One of the least understood areas of emergency care is the selection of appropriate monitoring signals for the unstable patient. In the hospital, the use of invasive monitors with pressure lines such as central venous or pulmonary arterial catheters has had a long and controversial run. The high complication rates are now well known, and the iatrogenic problems of insertion can be life-threatening. Although central lines are often inserted at home, they are generally for long-term infusion, rather than monitoring. Unstable patients requiring intravascular monitoring are clearly more appropriate for treatment in the hospital.

That said, one might explore the data concerning noninvasive monitoring of more physiologic functions than blood pressure. A number of articles exists showing the correlation of clinical outcomes in critical patients to cardiac efficiency factors, such as the ratio of pre-ejection period (PEP) to left ventricular ejection time (LVET). The PEP is the time spent after electrical stimulation of the ventricle (determined by the onset of the QRS complex), and before the aortic valve opens (determined by simple phonocardiography). During this period the heart is maximally consuming oxygen but performing no useful work.

The LVET is the time between the opening and closing of the aortic valve determined by phonocardiography, during which the entire left heart cardiac output is performed. The ratio of the two factors represents the physiological state of the heart's performance and trends toward either improvement or de-

terioration long before pulse rate and blood pressure change. What is remarkable is the ease of measuring these parameters noninvasively, as well as the ease of measuring stroke volume and cardiac output through the principle of transthoracic impedance.

There are inexpensive, commercially available machines to monitor these important physiological variables and new techniques to monitor them over the telephone, which make the future home-base intensive care unit entirely plausible. What is missing is a cadre of physicians dedicated to understanding and implementing such monitors when the community standard is to admit unstable patients to the hospital and insert invasive hemodynamic lines.

Procedures

Once equipped with laboratory, x-ray, and appropriate monitoring such as portable oximetry, the physician can carry such supplies as are necessary to perform most procedures done in the home. A detailed list of equipage and an inventory restocking plan are mandatory to protect the physician from finding out a critical piece of equipment is missing in the middle of a procedure. One must be assured every time one performs a laceration repair in the home that one has the proper suture and sterile package of instruments before anesthetizing the skin. There is no central supply to call for backup, so duplicate gloves and kits must be stocked at all times. A classic example is a difficult Foley catheter insertion, when the physician contaminates the catheter on a bedsheet and asks the technician for another.

Procedures the author has performed in the home are listed in Table 20.2. This list only includes those performed on housecalls. It does not include lifesaving procedures performed in flight as a physician for LifeFlight at the University of California Medical Center. However, it was in performing such extraordinary procedures as an A-K amputation of the leg of an impaled workman, or the insertion of a chest tube in a man lying in a field

Table 20.2. List of Some Procedures Safely Done in the Home with Appropriate Equipment, Staffing, and Technology

Thoracentesis
Tube thoracostomy
Complex laceration repair
Stage IV decubiti débridement
Long-line insertion
Foley catheterization
Irrigation and drainage procedures
Casting and splinting of fractures
Shoulder and other reductions
Chemotherapy
Tracheostomy tube replacement
Ventilator management
Fecal disimpaction
Ear wax removel and irrigation
Foreign body removal, eye (Wood's light)

with 20 rib fractures after being run over by a car, that the concept of emergency care in the home originated. Most procedures are technically simple for the experienced physician. It is only convention that prevents us from changing the site of practice from the hospital to a home supported by technology waiting in a van parked outside.

In other words, if one has the equipment, the clinical skills, and the support of a trained technician, one can perform many procedures in the home. As the monitoring systems of the future are developed, other procedures will be done safely and efficiently in the patient's home. However, these will probably still require not only the requisite materials to do a procedure, but the x-ray, laboratory, and monitoring equipment required to handle any untoward complication of the procedure or illness itself. This comprehensive approach is generally beyond the capability of the private practitioner but has been developed by larger medical groups in at least four states.

Reimbursement

No treatise of clinical medicine today would be complete without an analysis of the policies toward reimbursement. It is generally accepted in this country that physicians do not make housecalls because it is not economically feasible. Perhaps a more detailed analysis can shed some light on the current state of policy and where the HCFA is likely to go.

Under RBRVS reform in 1991, a physician service was "scored" in a detailed financial model developed out of research in the Harvard School of Public Health. Some 5000 Clinical Procedural Terminology (CPT) codes were analyzed for the costs of the physician's cognitive work, practice, and insurance costs involved. Because so few housecalls were being made at the time of the study, the housecall CPT codes were never scored; yet, the five levels of service customarily used for Evaluation and Management (E&M) codes were arbitrarily reduced to three. Thus, there is no complex level of housecall service code nor is there a code for the briefest visit. Apparently, the reasoning was that patients requiring a complex level of evaluation should be seen in an institutional setting, and the transportation time for the briefest visit "upcoded" the cost to the next level.

The result of this action leaves a federal payment policy that is not only arbitrary and in violation of the Congressional intent of the Omnibus Budget Reconciliation Act (OBRA) of 1989 (which required the scoring of all physician services) but is one that compensates a physician more for a moderately complex patient seen in the office than for a highly complex patient seen in the home. It is little wonder that most physicians send an ambulance to take the patient to the emergency room rather than make an urgent housecall!

Another little-known attribute of the RVS system was the failure to time home visits, as was required of all other E&M coded services. Since home visits cannot be timed, Medicare carriers cannot calculate prolongation of service codes for difficult housecalls. They are based on a 30-minute period that begins 30 minutes after the scored time of the housecall. Likewise, Medicare carriers do not recognize emergency services in the home, critical care in the home, unusual travel, unusual caseloads endemic to the housecall physician who specializes in urgent care, or other modifiers without paper billing "by report." In other words, the federal government has designed physician reimbursement so that virtually any cost efficiencies for emergency care in the home are reimbursed below office rates for equivalent services. Medicare carriers can hide behind provisions for specialized reporting requirements to claim they may pay for services "as appropriate," but paper reporting is a costly and lengthy procedure.

For comparison of E&M services by physicians and nurses, one might look at the 1995 physician-allowed payment for a comprehensive home visit, established patient ($79), the allowed cost reimbursed for a routine home nursing visit ($89.93) and a home social work visit ($128.84). It is no surprise that every day 1 million nursing visits are made to the home, and only 300 physician housecalls nationwide.

Medicare carriers have variable policies concerning "bundling" of ancillary services in the home. Almost no costs for medical supplies are paid to physicians. In contradistinction, almost all medical supply costs, including routine bandages, are reimbursed to nurses using them. The Blue Cross/Blue Shield of Illinois Medicare Carrier bundles oximetry into the housecall fee for the physician, despite specific instructions in the Federal Register not to do so (5).

Emergency care, whether in the home or not, often requires that laboratory results be done and interpreted immediately. Not only are the laboratory fees paid the *same* when done stat for physicians, but the recent resumption of payment for transportation of specimen fees is restricted to main laboratories and specifically excludes physicians from such payment for carrying a laboratory to the patient or carrying the specimen back to the office for immediate results.

Section 1833(h)(2)(B)(i) of the Social Security Act allows "the Secretary to make adjustments or exceptions to the fee schedules to ensure adequate payment for emergency laboratory tests needed for the provision of bona fide emergency services." Despite years of meetings and notices to the Secretary and to officials of the Department of Health and Human Services and the HCFA, the author has been unable to stimulate any attempt to address this point.

Another inconsistency in federal reimbursement policy for homecare by physicians concerns the penalty paid by the physician for acute housecalls in non-residence settings. HCFA policy requires carriers to decrease the reimbursement for housecalls made to residential care facilities, the assumption being that batches of calls would be made on the same day. The effect of this policy is to reduce the opportunity for the most at-risk elderly population—those too infirm to live in their own homes—to receive an acute housecall. Emergency care in this setting is, by definition, an isolated event and receives reduced payment while incurring the greater contingency costs of fast response and higher levels of service.

In 1996, the HCFA began payment for care plan oversight. This code (99375) was for over 30 minutes of telephonic or face-to-face communication with other healthcare professionals, chiefly nurses, involved in the home treatment plan. Because of numerous restrictions and record keeping requirements, the projected Medicare expense of $310 million for the year was never realized. By September of 1995 they had only paid out $17 million for the service. It was, however, a significant step for HCFA to introduce and pay for a new code restricted to physician involvement in homecare.

In August of 1995, the HCFA requested public comments on a proposal to pay physicians for time spent in case management with the family, service representatives, and other nonprofessionals involved in the socioeconomic features of homecare. The American Academy of Home Care Physicians (AAHCP) submitted a unique proposal to consider using patients' disabilities as a qualifier and pay physicians a bundled capitated fee for all outpatient services monthly. HCFA requested further comment in December of 1995, and is considering a bundled fee for physicians undertaking Physician Case Management. When such a plan is implemented, the expert homecare physician will be rewarded for the cost efficiencies of avoiding ambulances and emergency rooms.

As this is being written, the Relative Value Scale Update Committee will hear in February 1996 a joint proposal for an approximately 60% increase in the physician payment for home visits. One can be cautiously optimistic not only for the legal and actuarial rationale developed, but for the impact of the sponsoring societies led by the AAHCP, the American Academy of Family Practice, the American Academy of Pediatrics, the American Geriatrics Society, the Podiatrists, and the American Nursing Association. Since home visit codes have been increased more than the RBRVS inflation rate for four consecutive years, such an additional increase will finally make home visits an economically worthwhile practice style.

Summary

Emergency care in the home is professionally rewarding, cost effective, and technologically supported. As the HCFA sorts out the reasonable and necessary aspects of these types of services; as home health agencies explore synergies with their medical directors armed with innovative new products; as managed care companies are forced to provide quality services by market competition and government oversight, we can expect new homecare-based solutions for the healthcare crisis in America.

References

1. Gifford MJ, Franaszek JB, Gibson G, et al. Emergency physicians' and patients' assessments: urgency of need for medical care. Ann Emerg Med 1980;9:502–505.
2. Gerson LW, Skvarch L. Emergency medical service utilization by the elderly. Ann Emerg Med 1982; 11:610–612.
3. Eliastam M. Elderly patients in the emergency department. Ann Emerg Med 1989;18:1222–1229.
4. Notice to physicians: ambulance transports. Medicare update. Los Angeles: Transamerica (Medicare Division). March 1995.
5. Federal Register, December 8, 1994;59(235):63426.

21

Intensive Homecare for the Pediatric Patient

Richard Lander and Michael M. Rothkopf

CHAPTER AT A GLANCE: Pediatric homecare has changed dramatically in recent years. Technological advances ranging from home phototherapy with fiberoptic-implanted blankets to cycled, overnight parenteral feeding via pediatric silastic catheters are examples of the breadth and scope of available services. Infusion therapies with antibiotics, chemotherapy, and chelation therapy keep children in school or at home and out of the hospital. The economic and psychosocial impacts on both the patient and the family are significant. This chapter provides an overview of the many applications employed in intensive pediatric homecare.

Introduction

Contrary to popular belief, pediatric homecare is not a new phenomenon. Years ago, babies were born at home. Sick children who could not afford to be cared for at home were placed in charitable hospitals. In the late 1800s, visiting nurses were the mainstay of homecare. In the 20th century, advances in surgery, anesthesia, and aseptic techniques brought the very sick patient back into the hospital. As these advances allowed children with critical problems to be cured, pediatric intensive care units were established.

The very definition of the term pediatric homecare changed with advancements in technology. Sixty years ago, homecare might have meant the quarantining of a home due to scarlet fever. Fifty years ago, it might have meant an intramuscular injection of Bicillin given by the pediatrician during a housecall

for a sore throat. Forty years ago, following the terrors of a polio epidemic, one might have seen an "iron lung" in someone's home. Today, homecare is seen as a replacement for intensive hospital-level services—continual mechanical respiratory support, intravenous antimicrobial therapy, or total parenteral nutrition (Table 21.1).

From the quarantining of a home to intensive homecare, pediatric homecare has come a long way. Pediatric homecare today is achieved by an interdisciplinary team that provides primary healthcare to the patient as well as support and education to the family. It coordinates and advocates all facets of the patient's health needs (1). This all-encompassing approach to homecare is beneficial not only to the physical well-being of the child but also to the psychosocial issues that confront the family (2).

Economics and the business of medicine have resulted in a formula that has promoted

"

Table 21.1. Pediatric Uses of Homecare

- Total parenteral nutrition
- IV antibiotics
- Chemotherapy
- IV γ-globulin
- Phototherapy
- Mechanical respiratory support
- Electrocardiographic monitoring
- Pain management
- IV fluid replacement
- Oxygen administration
- Renal dialysis
- Primary nursing care such as dressing changes or procurement of laboratory specimens
- Uterine activity monitoring

home healthcare. For reasons of cost containment, patients are being discharged more quickly than before, and some of them are going home while they are still "sick." Physicians are sometimes expected to discharge patients earlier than was previously thought beneficial.

At times, physicians are prodded by the prepaid health maintenance organizations (HMOs) based on financial rather than clinical criteria. These HMOs realize the tremendous cost savings of homecare. The physician must recognize his or her responsibility and make an appropriate decision on the use of homecare services.

For a variety of reasons, most pediatricians have avoided participation in homecare. Homecare was often not practical and fit poorly into the busy schedule of an active pediatrician. Training in the use of homecare services has been limited and was generally not included in the syllabus of medical school or residency programs. Furthermore, little attention was given to reimbursement for homecare in pediatrics.

Clinical procedural terminology (CPT) codes have recently been implemented to aid the physician in securing remuneration for homecare. CPT codes to report evaluation and management services at home for new patients are 99341, 99342, and 99343. The codes for established patients are 99351, 99352, and 99353. The length of time spent and the complexity of the issues will determine which code to use.

There are also two sections of coding under case management services. Where the physician is responsible for the direct care of patients and/or coordinating healthcare services or team conferences, codes 99361 or 99362 can be used. When telephone calls to the patient or for managing the case are required, codes 99371, 99372, or 99373 may be used (please refer to your Current Procedural Terminology references for a full explanation of these codes).

Pediatric training programs have slowly begun to incorporate homecare into their core curricula. Goldberg (3) and others (4, 5) have encouraged the development of pediatric training programs for home healthcare. Homecare can offer an area of practice expansion for the pediatrician. It can be professionally fulfilling because it involves interactions with numerous professionals and makes use of cutting-edge technologies.

Physicians in other disciplines, such as internal medicine and family practice, have already incorporated homecare into their practices. Who better to render home healthcare to infants and children than the pediatrician, who understands that an infant or child is not a physiologic "small adult"?

This chapter reviews the current status of intensive homecare from the perspective of the general pediatrician. More information on specific areas of homecare are available elsewhere in the book.

Psychosocial Concerns

Before moving on to other aspects of pediatric homecare, a brief discussion of the psychosocial implications of caring for a chronically ill child is warranted. There are many feelings that have to be dealt with by the family of a debilitated child or infant. These feelings are akin to the stages of grieving, outlined by Elisabeth Kübler-Ross in *On Death and Dying* (6). The parents experience a mourning for "the loss of . . . (their) wished-for perfect child, and accept and care for the real child who was born" (7).

Initially there is denial ("This can't be happening to me"). Anger follows, in which blame may be directed at the hospital, the doctor, a past trivial incident, or at themselves. Finally there is acceptance, and it is at this point that a firm commitment to the care that has already been initiated by the physician can be undertaken and continued by the family. This, however, is not the endpoint of the psychosocial implications of caring for a chronically ill or dependent child.

For every child with a chronic disability, there are other people in the family who are affected. These are the mother, the father, siblings, and other components of the extended family, who might be called on to aid in the care of the child. When there are other siblings included, a concerted effort must be realized so that these unaffected siblings do not feel neglected or abandoned.

In 1984, Haggerty (8) estimated that there were 1 million children in the United States with severe, chronic illness—and 10 million less severely affected children. This is approximately 10 to 20% of all American children. In 1992, Newacheck and Taylor (9) cited a higher prevalence of up to 35%. However, even if we use a conservative figure of 10 to 15 million index cases, an additional 20 to perhaps 55 million people may be affected secondarily. Therefore, the appropriate care of a chronically ill child has the potential to benefit a large circle of people in each case.

A particular challenge exists for parents with both healthy and chronically ill children. The mother of four children—twins with mucolipidosis IV, and two "normal" children—wrote of their family situation: "It's a fine line we walk to balance the needs of our regular children and our handicapped children. While we hate to split up our family, there are . . . times when it is necessary. I just hope it becomes easier for us to accept this without too much guilt and remorse" (10).

The parents also face the issue of lost wages due to the need to be present to care for their child. Sudden medical complications can force canceling of plans or work schedules (11). Two-income families may be reduced to one source of income because of the need for constant parental surveillance. Career changes may be needed to allow for greater availability of the parents at home. Other financial concerns also exist even if the patient has good health insurance coverage. There are out-of-pocket expenses that the insurance companies will not reimburse. These include items such as special clothing, over-the-counter medication, special furniture or bedroom adaptations, handicapped bathroom fittings, etc.

Another new phenomenon is the effect that having a chronically ill child at home can have on the grandparents, whose "golden age" may be diminished because they must help care for the disabled child. The presence of grandparents may benefit other family members because it allows both parents to work and/or gives time for the parents to cope with the "well" sibling(s). However, it may be a significant stressor for older family members, who are accustomed to slower-paced, less psychologically draining activities. Similarly, homecare siblings may experience a loss because of their responsibilities as caretakers or as a result of inadequate attention from the parents, who are focusing on the ill child (12).

The child's age at the onset of disease is a significant factor in determining the psychosocial impact of the illness or disability. The younger the child at onset, the more likely that he or she will, at some point, engage adaptive mechanisms to cope with the dysfunction in life (13). Studies have shown that the introduction of the disabling disease at key moments in the child's development can have a profound impact (14). This may be particularly true at such times as school entrance or adolescence, because these are stages at which there is a search for self-identity.

Children with chronic illnesses are often abused or neglected. Jaudes et al. (15) showed that 14% had been abandoned, 25% had been physically abused, and 65% had been neglected medically. Neglect was also seen physically in 9%, emotionally in 14%, and educationally in 8%. Life-threatening noncompliance was seen in 29%.

Another problem that affects these children is the multiplicity of their problems and their increased morbidity. Newacheck and Stoddard (16) demonstrated that ". . . the observed co-prevalence for the most common pairs of childhood chronic conditions ranged from one hundred forty percent to three hundred eighty percent above expected levels." Regardless of the reasons for the increase in morbidity, these children missed more school days and required more health services.

Because of the complex psychosocial issues, care of the chronically ill child is best accomplished by a team approach. In addition to the pediatrician, the multidisciplinary team should include a child psychiatrist, a psychologist, and/or a psychiatric social worker to meet the needs of the patient and family. The pediatrician, as the coordinator, must be aware of the potential problems and act on them appropriately. (17)

Physician Adaptation to Homecare

The physician-patient and physician-parent relationships also require special attention when dealing with homecare. The physician must not be lulled into a false sense that all is well with the child, simply because the family says so. Similarly, one must not assume that all is well with the family simply because of outward appearances. It is often important to families not to appear as failures to the physician. The family may have a perception that if the physician is happy with the progress being made, he or she will provide even better care. Our patient is the child and we must make certain that the family is doing what is expected of them to care for the patient.

The patient suffering a debilitating illness experiences a significant emotional impact. For a child, this can be equally true for a 6-week course of intravenous antibiotics for osteomyelitis, 6 months of total parenteral nutrition because of inflammatory bowel disease, or a lifetime dependence on mechanical ventilation. The pediatrician needs to be sensitive to the patient's fragile psyche, especially at the beginning of therapy.

The pediatrician must also address his or her own feelings. The vast majority of our training is hospital based and inpatient focused. Treating otitis media, sinusitis, or even pneumonia is something that is easily done in an outpatient setting. However, the pediatrician must make a transition from treating more serious conditions in the hospital to treating these conditions in the home. He or she must also learn to share some of the responsibility for patient care with the family.

The physician may struggle with care issues when determining whether to send a patient home or maintain that child in the hospital. As Lantos and Kohrman state (18), ". . . physician responsibility has at least two meanings: responsiveness to patient need, and responsibility for outcomes, good and bad." These two meanings often appear to be in conflict.

Is the physician keeping the child in the hospital because of his or her own reason; for example, reimbursement or unfamiliarity with homecare? Or is it because the family cannot cope with the responsibilities of caring for the child at home? Perhaps the physician does not have confidence in the home health-care company, or perhaps the homecare company chosen by the patient's insurance carrier is inappropriate. In the hospital, the primary care physician shares patient responsibility with the pediatric subspecialists who have been called in on consultation. In the home setting, the physician shares responsibility with the family, and it is the primary care pediatrician who receives the 2:00 AM emergency call, not the pediatric resident on call in the hospital.

Because of these challenges, intensive homecare must be addressed carefully by the pediatrician. Ongoing education is needed to ensure optimal use of the homecare team and system.

Perinatal Care

Home Uterine Activity Monitoring (HUAM)

Survival rates of premature infants and low–birth weight infants have improved dramatically. However, the very essence of prematurity can be partially prevented by home preterm monitoring. This generally includes the measurement of uterine activity along with an educational program to teach the expectant mother prudent steps to prevent premature delivery. Carlan et al. (19) demonstrated a benefit in a carefully selected group of women with preterm premature rupture of membranes. A report prepared by The U.S. Preventive Services Task Force on HUAM (20, 21) stated that the combination of HUAM and patient education can reduce the incidence of preterm births in women with risk factors for preterm labor. Prevention efforts include cessation of tobacco, alcohol, and drug usage, as well as improving prenatal care. Programs that focus on improving the mother's nutritional status and socioeconomic conditions may be beneficial.

Another modality of homecare to aid in the prevention of premature labor is the administration of pharmaceuticals that inhibit uterine contractions. Together with home uterine monitoring, this encompasses a field now known as home tocolytic therapy. Home tocolytic therapy is a multi-modality approach that includes home visits by homecare nurses (generally biweekly), daily home uterine monitoring, and single or combination drug therapy.

Among the more potent drugs that can be used as tocolytics are β agonists (particularly terbutaline sulfate), magnesium sulfate, prostaglandin synthetase inhibitors (i.e., indomethacin), and calcium channel blockers (22). No single agent has been totally effective, but the most commonly applied regimen includes intravenous or subcutaneous use of terbutaline; sometimes in conjunction with magnesium sulfate and antibiotics (the use of antibiotics is employed when there is premature rupture of membranes).

Improvement in clinical outcome has been shown by several studies but is not universal. Results include reduced incidence of preterm birth, increased birth weight, decreased neonatal morbidity, increased time in utero, decreased incidence of premature dilations, and decreased effacement and rupture of membranes.

Management of Hyperemesis Gravidarum

Episodic nausea and vomiting are common occurrences in early pregnancy. However, some pregnant women develop a syndrome of severe intractable vomiting that all but eliminates their ability to eat. This condition is referred to as hyperemesis gravidarum (HG). The etiology of HG is unclear but may involve increased levels of HCG or hypersensitivity of the sense of smell (23). It usually occurs in the first and second trimesters and rarely continues to term.

Management of patients is based on the severity of their condition. Mild to moderate cases can be managed with conservative measures such as eating small meals that are high in protein, eliminating iron from the perinatal vitamins, and using mild antiemetics.

Women with severe HG, presenting with weigh loss, dehydration, concentrated urine, and urinary ketones have traditionally been treated in the hospital. They are administered intravenous fluids, antiemetics, and total parenteral nutrition (TPN). However, it is now clear that most of these patients can be managed via homecare, particularly in conjunction with HUAM as detailed above.

A recent study by Naef et al. (24) compared homecare with hospital care for HG patients. They studied 50 women treated at home and 47 managed in the hospital. The patients were matched for gravidity, gestational age, and weight loss. The investigators found no significant difference in length of IV therapy, complications of therapy, or incidence of readmission between the hospital and the homecare groups. However, the difference in cost between the groups was statistically significant ($p<0.001$). The care for the home therapy group cost a mean of $708, while the hospital cost was a mean of $2701.

Apnea Monitoring

Apnea in infants is a significant clinical dilemma that may be the cause of sudden infant death syndrome (SIDS). It is defined as pathologic when the respiratory pause is greater than 20 seconds, is abrupt, or is associated with cyanosis, marked pallor, hypotonia, or bradycardia. Children who are born prematurely or who have graduated from the neonatal intensive care unit with chronic respiratory disease or upper-airway obstruction are at particularly high risk of developing apnea. Siblings of infants who died of SIDS are also considered at risk. When these children are discharged, a home apnea monitor (HAM) is generally indicated.

HAM units are noninvasive cardiorespiratory monitors. They utilize circuitry for measurement of transthoracic electrical impedance to recode respiratory effort. Some also use an abdominal strain gauge, impedance plethysmography, and a nasal thermistor. A simple ECG is also part of these systems. Alarm circuitry detects hypoventilation, apnea, bradycardia, and tachycardia with an audible signal.

Some new and more advanced HAM units include the capability of capturing and storing respiratory patterns surrounding apnea units for later analysis. In addition, the combination of standard HAM units with pulse oximetry offers the ability to confirm changes in oxygen saturation (25).

When a decision has been reached that an infant needs an apnea monitor, the parents and caretakers should be instructed in cardiopulmonary resuscitation. This training is frequently provided by the homecare companies but is also available at the Red Cross and most local hospitals.

The home monitoring of apnea introduces an important general issue in homecare: the transfer of responsibility from the medical professionals to the family. Professionals are fully aware of the potential consequences of improper compliance in medical care. When an apnea alarm is triggered in the Neonatal Intensive Care Unit, a nurse responds immediately. The nurse ascertains whether there is an equipment malfunction or if the alarm truly signaled a prolonged apneic attack. The infant is under constant surveillance by qualified staff. Although parents may be carefully instructed in the use of the equipment at home, their diligence in its use has been shown to vary significantly.

Through the use of apnea monitors equipped with electronic memories, Cordero et al. (26) demonstrated the unreliability of parental recall. In their study, 100% of the parents reported full-time use of the monitors, whereas the electronic memories in the monitors revealed that 70% of all infants went unmonitored for one night and 30% of all infants were unmonitored for three or more nights.

The rate of usage was also determined by the parents' perception of the risk of apnea at the time of hospital discharge. Parents who felt that their infants were at high risk monitored them an average of 18.5 hours a day, while those who perceived the risk of apnea to be low averaged 13.6 hours per day.

This study suggests that parents' perception of their responsibility for the care of their child at home can be modified by subjective factors. Parents must be diligent and fully compliant in following physician instructions for the care of their child. The physicians will deal with the complications that arise. However, the parents must live with the sequelae of those complications forever.

Home Phototherapy

Although it has been available for more than 20 years, home phototherapy has not been widely accepted by many pediatricians. Geographically, physicians in the Northeast have been reluctant to participate in the home treatment of hyperbilirubinemia (27). The reasons for this, as cited by Meropol et al. (28), include fears that parents would not comply with phototherapy itself or would not apply eyeshields, medicolegal concerns, lack of use by colleagues, and fears of overheating or dehydration.

In-hospital therapy of hyperbilirubinemia can interfere with breast feeding and disrupt family routines. The per diem cost of hospital phototherapy is significantly higher than that of home phototherapy. However, hyperbilirubinemia treatment with phototherapy requires careful monitoring because of possible adverse effects on body temperature and fluid balance. The Provisional Committee for Quality Improvement and Subcommittee on Hyperbilirubinemia (29) have recommended guidelines for monitoring the lamp position as well as fluid replacement. Parents can be taught to monitor the baby's temperature and to determine urine output. The homecare nurse obtains the necessary blood specimens at home and delivers them to the laboratory or pediatrician's office for processing.

The physician has several choices of ultraviolet (UV) lighting units to select from for use in phototherapy (30). The most simple of these is a bank of lamps with white and blue bulbs to deliver 8 to 10 μW/cm^2/nm in the blue-green region of the visible spectrum. Single-bulb units also exist. These "bili-lights" are usually positioned 15 to 20 cm from the infant. The infant should have eyepatches to limit retinal exposure to the UV light.

A popular alternative to standard "bili-lights" is the Wallaby unit. It is a "blanket" or fiberoptic panel in which the infant is wrapped. There is no need for eyepatches, and parents can better physically bond with their babies. No heat transfer occurs, and the risks of dehydration secondary to evaporation is diminished.

Another unit has the appearance of a suitcase. The bulbs are positioned close to the infant's body, which means that up to 20 μW/cm^2/nm can be delivered. A cloth separates the head from the bulbs, again obviating the need for eyepatches.

Cardiorespiratory Care

Home Oxygen Therapy

Over the past 20 to 30 years, survival rates for low birth weight for premature infants have increased. This increase in survival rates has resulted in a growing number of infants who are neurologically impaired, as well as infants needing tracheostomies. New, smaller tracheostomy tubes, along with skilled nursing care and appropriate suctioning machines, allow these infants and children to be cared for at home.

Low-flow oxygen therapy can easily be achieved in an outpatient setting. This is generally done through the use of either portable liquid oxygen or oxygen concentrators that remove nitrogen from ambient air. Most patients can be adequately managed using nasal

prongs that are comfortable and unobtrusive. In small children they can be taped down to the face for security.

Recently, home oxygen therapy has been offered in conjunction with pulse oximetry. This allows for the noninvasive measurement of oxygen saturation. Patients can be given parameters to monitor and a range of oxygen flow rates based on oxygen saturation. For example, it is not uncommon for infants to require 0.75 L of oxygen per minute when inactive but need 1 L/min when nursing.

The efficacy and reliability of home oxygenation has been established and the cost effectiveness demonstrated (31).

Cystic Fibrosis

Patients with cystic fibrosis (CF) have become heavy users of homecare services. Home management, beginning with postural draining and chest percussion, has provided CF patients with substantial benefits. Medical therapies ranging from home nebulizers for the delivery of bronchial dilator therapy to the use of home IV antibiotics for bronchitis or pneumonia have allowed many patients to stay at home despite exacerbation of their condition. In addition, greater attention has recently focused on the nutritional status and survival in the malnourished CF patient (32). This has resulted in the addition of home nutritional support to the management of CF.

Strandvik et al. (33) studied home intravenous treatment of patients with CF. They compared inpatient versus outpatient treatments and found that outpatient therapy was simpler and less time consuming. There were no differences between inpatients and outpatients with regard to weight gain, laboratory data, spirometry, and subjective findings, such as appetite or general well-being. This study also addressed the economic (significant cost savings at home versus in-hospital) and psychological (96% of the group opting for home therapy for the next IV antibiotic course) aspects of CF care. These patients had all but the first antibiotic dose given at home, and many had a combination of β-lactam and aminoglycoside therapy.

The mechanisms underlying interaction between nutritional status and pulmonary function are complex. Protein-calorie malnutrition decreases the strength of respiratory muscles, which results in diminished vital capacity, increased atelectasis, and retained secretions, as well as impairment of the pulmonary parenchyma (34, 35).

Shepherd et al. (36, 37) studied 12 patients before and after they received a 21-day course of parenteral nutrition in addition to conventional therapy. They found a favorable and persistent effect as measured by decreased number of respiratory infections, improved pulmonary function (forced vital capacity [FVC], forced expiratory volume in 1 second [FEV_1], and partial expiratory flow [PEF]), and chest x-ray.

Home parenteral nutrition (HPN) using a high percentage of fat emulsion may be particularly useful in CF patients (38, 39). This suggests that the high concentration of fatty acids in Intralipid may induce clinical benefit in CF via normalization of serum fatty acids (with concomitant effects on the metabolism of eicosanoids).

Electrocardiogram (ECG)

Transtelephonic electrocardiographic monitoring of infants and children is safe, reliable, and cost effective. These units are capable of either single or continuous monitoring. Units for single-time monitoring are activated by the patient or parent when symptoms occur. One electrode is placed under each arm, and once the unit is triggered, the electrocardiogram is recorded for 30 seconds. Telephone transmission is then performed by calling an automated terminal; the patient's home telephone is connected to the monitor, and the recording is transmitted.

Continuous monitoring can also be achieved by applying skin surface leads. One lead continuously feeds into a 70-second memory loop. Once this unit is activated, the 30 seconds previous to and the 40 seconds following activation are recorded.

Goldstein et al. (40) reported that 85% of pediatric patients with previously documented arrhythmias and 52% of pediatric patients with suspected but undocumented arrhythmias (62% overall) obtained transtelephonic recordings while experiencing symptoms.

Intravenous Therapy

Home intravenous therapy (HIT) is one of the most common modalities for pediatric intensive homecare. This includes a variety of therapies such as antibiotics, chemotherapy, analgesia, and TPN.

Antibiotics

Intravenous antibiotic therapy generally employs a stable antibiotic with a long half-life and has been used extensively (Table 21.2) for a variety of conditions. It has been shown to be a safe and effective means of discharging patients early and reducing therapeutic costs (41). However, there remains substantial opportunity for further development in this area of pediatric homecare (42).

Diseases such as osteomyelitis, septic arthritis, or severe cellulitis will have therapy initiated in the hospital. After cultures have properly identified the organism and its antibiotic susceptibility, peak and trough antibiotic levels can be utilized to determine proper dosage. Once started on therapy, the patient may be discharged to the home for a continuation of therapy.

Prior to discharge, it is imperative that the patient's insurance company be contacted to obtain authorization for the particular homecare company that the physician wishes to employ. Some insurance companies, particularly health maintenance organizations, will not

Table 21.2. Infections Treated by Home Antibiotic Therapy

Osteomyelitis
Pneumonia
Lyme disease
Septic arthritis
Severe cellulitis
Endocarditis
Pyelonephritis
Exacerbations of cystic fibrosis
AIDS

cover 100% of home healthcare costs if the home healthcare company is not their preferred provider.

Once the patient is home, the IV insertion site must be checked daily for signs of infection or infiltration. This is accomplished by a nurse from a home healthcare company or a nurse from the local or county Visiting Nurse Association. Obviously, for the pediatric age group, the nurse should be certified in pediatrics.

An infusion device is generally used that is programmed to deliver the antibiotic at a specific rate. Since the antibiotic is delivered premixed from the pharmacy, parents can be instructed on the instillation.

While frequent intermittent infusion antibiotic therapy is often not practical at home, other options exist. Ceftriaxone, which is a third-generation cephalosporin, can be given once or twice daily by IV push. Ceftriaxone has a long half-life and produces adequate blood levels. In order to monitor the course of home antibiotic therapy, an appropriate amount of blood can be drawn at home by the nurse and delivered to either the pediatrician's office, a hospital, or a private laboratory.

Stable patients may not require hospitalization for the initiation of intravenous antibiotic therapy. The initial treatment can be given in the pediatrician's office and the patient followed up at home. A patient with recalcitrant Lyme disease, an exacerbation of CF, or cellulitis can be discharged from the pediatrician's office to his or her home for treatment.

Some families will embrace the idea of treating their child at home rather than hospitalizing him or her. However, others can be more reticent. Parents can be fearful that tragedy will befall their child and want the traditional safety of a protected hospital environment. However, once a child has been treated at home, these same families become advocates for homecare and oppose returning to the hospital for further treatment.

For a more in-depth review of homecare antibiotics, see Chapter 12.

Chelation

Another use of home intravenous therapy is seen in the treatment of iron overload, which can occur from the treatment of sickle cell disease or β thalassemia major. Sickle cell disease is the most common genetic disease seen among African-Americans, with an incidence of 1:375. Cystic fibrosis, the most common genetic disorder in Caucasians, has an incidence of 1:1500.

Sickle cell disease can wreak havoc in one of two ways: vaso-occlusion, in which the vessels are obstructed from the abnormally shaped ("sickled") red blood cells, or hemolytic anemia, which leads to cell membrane damage. Wang et al. (43) reported that 10% of children with sickle cell disease will have neurological damage because of a stroke. Monthly blood transfusions can significantly lower the likelihood of a second recurrence. However, these transfusions are not without their risks. The probability of infectious or minor group incompatibility complications increases because of the recurrent nature of the treatment.

Another complication of frequent blood transfusion is hemosiderosis. This accumulation of excess iron occurs primarily in the heart and lungs and may increase morbidity and mortality (44). The treatment of choice is chelation, generally with deferoxamine mesylate (Desferal).

Normally, the body stores 3 to 4 g of iron. When the body has accumulated 15 to 20 g, symptoms of overload can occur. A unit of blood has 200 mg of iron. At two units a month, a child can accumulate 5 g of iron per year, resulting in iron overload in 3 to 4 years.

Iron chelation with deferoxamine binds 85 mg of iron to every gram of deferoxamine. Proper kidney functioning is imperative, since the kidneys are the primary route of deferoxamine excretion. Deferoxamine can be administered subcutaneously or intravenously, at a dose of 50 mg/kg over 12 hours. The intravenous administration of deferoxamine is more effective because higher doses can be used. Patient compliance is the keystone to success in chelation therapy. The disruptiveness of hospitalization and the pain inherent in the administration of deferoxamine all contribute to noncompliance.

Day et al. (45) demonstrated the effectiveness of the team approach in the treatment of iron overload with their five-step program.

Step 1 is an introduction to the program and is an educational process. Step 2 is a demonstration of technique in which the nurse is observed performing the infusion. The family is encouraged to rotate infusion sites monthly. Step 3 involves a nurse observing the family infusing. Older children are taught to help in the process. Step 4 is weekly monitoring of treatment, and step 5 is monthly surveillance.

Teenagers can take over the entire process by themselves, but parents are advised to monitor their teenagers. Adolescents with chronic illnesses have a tendency toward denial of their problem, or feel that they are omnipotent and no ill can befall them. In either scenario, the administration of their treatment suffers. Families are instructed to be alert for side effects. These can range from infusion site pain and swelling to an allergic reaction to the deferoxamine. The former can be managed by warm compresses and acetaminophen. The latter can be ameliorated with diphenhydramine for mild symptoms, such as pruritus and/or watery eyes. Subcutaneous epinephrine can be used for the more severe reactions such as laryngeal edema or acute bronchoconstriction.

Chemotherapy

Pediatric oncology has seen increasing survival rates as newer, more potent, and specific treatment regimens allow children to live longer and enjoy a higher quality of life than they could have anticipated in the past.

Home intravenous chemotherapy has been found to be less costly than hospital treatment, and families have incurred lower out-of-pocket expenses with home treatment. The patients were noted to have better appetites, had a perception that they felt better, and even performed better in their school work (46).

Wolfe (47) described an integrated service in which inpatient nurses rotated onto outpatient and homecare activities. This enabled patient and staff to experience a continuity of care in the management of pediatric cancer. Both staff members and patients report an increased satisfaction with this system.

Pain associated with the cancer and the palliation of terminal pediatric cancer patients is addressed later in the chapter in the section on analgesics.

Immunoglobulin Therapy

Intravenous immunoglobulin (IVIG) therapy is a widely accepted method of treating immunodeficient or autoimmune patients. The treatable diseases are listed in Table 21.3 (48).

Standard γ-globulin was first used in the 1940s as prophylaxis against hepatitis A and rubella. In 1952, Bruton successfully treated a boy with X-linked infantile hypogammaglobulinemia. These early treatments were with intramuscular injections. When standard γ-globulin was used intravenously, anaphylactoid reaction occurred due to aggregated proteins.

Intravenous immune globulins were used investigationally in the 1960s. These preparations did not have aggregated proteins. The two significant advantages of the intravenous route of administration over the intramuscular injection are (a) the quantity of IgG intravenously administrated is essentially unlimited, compared to a limit of 100 mg/kg when administrated intramuscularly, and (b) the total dose of intravenously administered IgG is immediately available.

Congenital immune deficiencies result from a partial to total lack of immunoglobulins, either quantitatively or functionally. Primary and secondary immune deficiencies demonstrate a decrease in one or more of the classes of immunoglobulins (IgG, IgA, IgE,

Table 21.3. Indications for IVIG

Congenital agammaglobulinemia
X-linked immunodeficiency
Post-transfusion purpura
Recurrent respiratory disease
Wiskott-Aldrich syndrome
Idiopathic thrombocytopenia purpura
Bone marrow transplantations
Severe infections in newborns and infants
Collagen vascular diseases (myasthenia gravis)
Ataxia-telangiectasia
Kawasaki syndrome
Chronic Epstein-Barr syndrome
Burns
AIDS

IgM, and IgD). The end result is the development of (or increased susceptibility to) bacterial, viral, or fungal infection.

Bielory (49) reviewed IVIG as the accepted standard in clinical practice for replacement therapy of patients with primary immunodeficiency, acute idiopathic thrombocytopenic purpura (ITP), and Kawasaki's syndrome (see also Chapter 14). Under investigation are the use of IVIG in the treatment of pediatric AIDS, infections in low–birth weight infants, rheumatoid arthritis, and myasthenia gravis.

It is important to note that when evaluating a child for immune deficiency, one should not accept a normal total serum IgG as proof that the child does not have an immune deficiency. IgG has four subclasses. IgG1 comprises 66% of the total IgG in serum, and IgG2 25%. IgG3 and IgG4 comprise the remainder. Since each subclass plays a specific role in immune response, a deficiency in any one class can result in repeated infections.

Home use of IVIG provides economic savings and less interruption of the patient's daily routine. However, patients must be prepared for side effects, which occur in up to 15% of all patients. Minor side effects include chills, fever, or headache. Severe side effects, such as anaphylaxis, should be prepared for in advance by providing patients with an anaphylaxis kit, to include at least diphenhydramine and epinephrine. Of particular note is that patients with IgA deficiency should be treated with an IVIG with the lowest concentration of IgA to minimize the risk of an IgE antibody response to IgA.

Nutritional Support

Intravenous total parenteral nutrition (TPN) is utilized by children with a wide array of problems. Gastrointestinal patients with short gut syndromes or malabsorption problems benefit from TPN. Some neurologically impaired children also require TPN. Pediatric oncology patients on multiple chemotherapy regimens need TPN to help maintain positive nitrogen balance.

Home TPN is generally employed as overnight therapy, allowing patients to sleep during infusion. Because it permits a patient who would otherwise require a long hospitalization to be discharged, it has a strong influence on reducing cost and improving quality of life (50). More detail on home TPN is found in Chapter 15.

However, not all home nutritional services need be delivered intravenously. Some of the previously mentioned patients can be fed at home through gastrostomies or jejunostomies using enteral infusion pumps (51). A gastrostomy button can be surgically implanted in the abdominal wall. This is then connected via an adapter to the infusion pump. Since the button is practically on the skin line, there is no need for any of the long tubes previously used in enteral feedings. The infusion pumps are programmed to deliver the amount of fluid needed over whatever time span is desired.

Analgesia

Pain is a frequently overlooked and undertreated problem in pediatrics. New methods of pain management have been devised that should be considered by the pediatrician.

However, the diagnosis of chronic pain in a child is difficult. The emotional immaturity and developing cognition of children influence their interpretation of pain (52). Definitive management relies on the use of rating scales (53), which can be applied even to young children. For example, the Oucher scale uses photographs of a face with different expressions of pain and can be used by young children. Older children can assess the intensity of their pain using poker chips, number rating scales such as pain thermometers, or visual analog scales. Children with chronic pain can use pain diaries to demonstrate the frequency and duration of their pain.

Similarly, management of pain in children relies on special tools. A multidisciplinary team with expertise in pharmacologic and nonpharmacologic methods can be particularly useful. Sensitivity to psychosocial and culture issues that can influence the response to pain is also important.

Chronic pain can be managed by a variety of methods, including medications, nerve blocks, acupuncture, and biofeedback. Drug therapy relies on a combination approach that includes nonsteroidal anti-inflammatory drugs (NSAIDs), mixed agonist/antagonist analgesics, and opioids. Severe pain often requires parenteral therapy. Morphine is often utilized as a first-line parenteral analgesic. Morphine sulfate can be administered as a continuous intravenous subcutaneous infusion whose dosage is adjusted based on the patient's symptoms. Other narcotics have also been utilized in pediatric pain management. For example, fentanyl is 100 times more potent than morphine (54). It can successfully induce analgesia without loss of consciousness. The usual dose is from 2 to 3 $\mu g/kg/hr$ IV. Fentanyl is also available in lozenge form, and because it is shaped like a lollypop (Fentanyl Oralet), there has been obvious acceptance by young patients. Infants receiving fentanyl for more than 7 days have to be weaned over a course of 10 to 20 days to prevent opiate withdrawal symptoms from occurring.

Meperidine has been used intermittently on an as-needed basis. The limitation of this is that someone must be available to draw up the medication and administer it. Because we are dealing with children or adolescents, the patient usually would not be unattended. However, this could be problematic in some cases.

Patient-controlled analgesia (PCA) is a viable alternative to intermittent IV pain control. Patients with chronic severe pain, such as some cancer patients, can self-administer their analgesia, usually morphine. (The usual starting dose for morphine is 0.015 mg/kg/hr). An infusion pump is preloaded with the medication and the patient activates the device at the time he or she experiences pain. An important safeguard is that the pump can be programmed to deliver a specified amount of medication over a predetermined amount of time, for a limited number of doses.

An indwelling epidural catheter can also be used to deliver a continuous infusion of pain medication. A physician must determine the rate and the duration of continuous therapy, dependent on the symptoms. Caudal infusions are used when therapy is limited to less than 72 hours. A lumbar catheter should be used if longer treatment is required.

Palliative care of the child dying of cancer may involve the use of methadone (55). Integration with a hospice program can be very useful for both patient and family (56). Bereavement and appropriate follow-up care can have a significant impact on surviving siblings and parents (57).

Equipment and IV Access

As there are many indications for intravenous therapy, so too there are many choices in the delivery of the intravenous therapy. Traditional IV catheters, while satisfactory for short-term therapy, require frequent replacement when long-term therapy is indicated. Catheters are available today that increase in size and soften when exposed to body fluid (e.g., the Landmark catheter). This allows a smaller-diameter catheter to be initially inserted. These catheters are available in different lengths.

Patients who require long-term therapy also have options for delivery of their intravenous therapy. A popular device in pediatrics is the peripherally inserted central catheter (PICC) line (58). This is a flexible Silastic catheter that is inserted with a butterfly-like device to the desired length. Hickman and Broviac catheters can also be used, but these need to be surgically implanted. Another alternative is the implantation of a subcutaneous reservoir in the chest, with a central line attachment. Delivery of therapy is accomplished by accessing the reservoir through the skin.

Insertion of any of these devices can be a painful procedure, particularly in pediatrics. To decrease the unpleasantness, the skin site can be prepared to decrease the degree of pain. In infants older than 1 month, EMLA cream (Astra USA, Inc.) can be used (59). This is a eutectic mixture of 2.5% lidocaine and 2.5% prilocaine. It is applied to the insertion site before the procedure for at least 60 minutes in children older than 5 years of age, and 30 minutes in children 1 month to 5 years of age. The site is then covered by an occlusive dressing. Side effects are local and transient, such as pruritus, erythema, or blanching of the skin.

EMLA is not approved for infants under 1 month of age because methemoglobin can be induced by prilocaine. Infants receiving sulfonamides, nitrites, and nitrates, which can also induce methemoglobin, cannot use EMLA. A recent study (60) has demonstrated the use of buffered 1% lidocaine intradermally to diminish pain in children 8 to 15 years old.

Another interesting development in pediatric homecare is the use of disposable devices (61). These are pressure-driven systems that provide a controlled infusion without an electric or mechanical pump. Because they are small and disposable, they have practical value in the management of the child who is attending school or who is away from home periodically. The entire infusion can be performed safely and the material disposed of without the child being restricted to the home.

Infections of the venous access system remains a major limitation of pediatric homecare. Pediatric infection rates of chronic in-

dwelling catheters appear to be higher than in adults (62, 63). Closer monitoring and more complete patient training may be needed to alleviate the situation.

Summary

Pediatric homecare has truly come full circle. From the 1880s with visiting nurses bathing babies and checking their weight at home, to the highly sophisticated technological respiratory, nutritional, and hematological supports of today, sick children can be safely cared for at home.

Further technological advances will permit greater application of intensive homecare for pediatrics. Specialized training of pediatric residents in homecare practice will expand utilization of these services.

References

1. Lessing D, Tatman MA. Paediatric home care in the 1990s. Arch Dis Child 1991;66(8):994.
2. Stein REK, Jessop DJ. Does pediatric home care make a difference for children with chronic illness? Findings from the Pediatric Ambulatory Care Treatment Study. Pediatrics 1984;73(6):845.
3. Goldberg AI, Gardner G, Gibson LE. Home care: the next frontier of pediatric practice. J Pediatr 1994; 125(5):686.
4. Wallgren-Pettersson C, Donner M, Holmberg C. Wasz-Hockert O. Interdisciplinary teaching of community pediatrics. J Med Educ 1982;16:290–295.
5. Steinkuller JS. Home visits by pediatric residents. A valuable educational tool. Am J Dis Child 1992; 146: 1064–1067.
6. Kübler-Ross E. On Death and Dying. New York: Macmillan, 1969.
7. Sabbeth B. Understanding the impact of chronic childhood illness on families. Pediatr Clin North Am 1984; 31:47.
8. Haggerty R. Foreword. Pediatr Clin North Am 1984; 31:1.
9. Newacheck P, Taylor W. Childhood chronic illness: prevalence, severity, and impact. Am J Public Health 1992;82:364.
10. R. Lander. Personal correspondence.
11. Schweitzer SO, Mitchell B, Landsverk J, Laparan L. The costs of a pediatric hospice program. Public Health Rep 1993;108(1):37.
12. Desguin BW, Holt IJ, McCarthy SM. Comprehensive care of the child with a chronic condition. Part 1. Understanding chronic conditions in childhood. Curr Probl Pediatr 1994;24:199.
13. Pless IB. Clinical assessment: physical and psychological function. Pediatr Clin North Am 1984;31:33.
14. Steinhauer PD, Mushin DN, Rate-Grant O. Psychological aspects of chronic illness. Pediatr Clin North Am 1974;21:825.
15. Jaudes P, Diamond L. Neglect of chronically ill children. Am J Dis Child 1986;140:655.
16. Newacheck PW, Stoddard JJ. Prevalence and impact of multiple childhood chronic illnesses. J Pediatr 1994; 124:40.
17. Desquin BW, Holt IJ, McCarthy SM. Comprehensive care of the child with a chronic condition. Part 1. Understanding chronic conditions in childhood. Curr Probl Pediatr 1994;Jul;24(6):199–218.
18. Lantos JD, Kohrman AF. Ethical aspects of pediatric home care. Pediatrics 1992;89(5):920.
19. Carlan SJ, O'Brien WF, Parsons MT, Lense JJ. Preterm premature rupture of membranes: a randomized study of home versus hospital management. Obstet Gynecol 1993;81(1):61.
20. U.S. Preventive Services Task Force. Policy statement. Home uterine activity monitoring for preterm labor. JAMA 1993;270(3):369.
21. U.S. Preventive Services Task Force. Review article. Home uterine activity monitoring for preterm labor. JAMA 1993;371(3):371.
22. Cowan M. Home care of the pregnant woman using terbutaline. MCN 1993;18:99.
23. Erick M. Hyperolfaction and hyperemesis gravidarum: what is the relationship? Nutr Rev 1995;53(10): 289–295.
24. Naef RW 3rd, Chauhan SP, Roach H, Roberts WE, et al. Treatment for hyperemesis gravidarum in the home: an alternative to hospitalization. J. Perinatol 1995;15(4) 289–292.
25. Ahmann E. Family impact of home apnea monitoring: an overview of research and its clinical implications. J Pediatr Nurs 1992;18(6)611–616.

26. Cordero L, Morehead S, Miller R. Parental compliance with home apnea monitoring. J Perinatol 1993;13(6): 448.
27. Rothkopf M, Lander R. Personal communication.
28. Meropol SB, Luberti AA, DeJong AR, Weiss JC. Home phototherapy: use and attitudes among community pediatricians. Pediatrics 1993;91:97.
29. American Academy of Pediatrics Provisional Committee for Quality Improvement and Subcommittee on Hyperbilirubinemia. Management of hyperbilirubinemia in the healthy term newborn. Pediatrics 1994; 94(4):420.
30. Schuman AJ. Homeward bound: The explosion in pediatric home care. Contemp Pediatr 1994:26.
31. Hudak BB, Allen MC, Hudak ML, et al. Home oxygen therapy for chronic lung disease in extremely low birth weight infants. Am J Dis Child 1989;143:357.
32. Kraemer R, Rudeberg A, Kadain B, et al. Relative underweight in cystic fibrosis and its prognostic value. Acta Paediatr Scand 1978;67:33.
33. Strandvid B, Hjelte L, Malmborg A-S, Widen B. Home intravenous antibiotic treatment of patients with cystic fibrosis. Acta Paediatr Scand 1992;81:340.
34. Rochester D. Malnutrition and the respiratory muscles. Clin Chest Med 1986;7:91–100.
35. Sahebjami H. Nutrition and pulmonary parenchyma. Clin Chest Med 1986;7:111–126.
36. Shepherd RW, Holt TL, Thomas BJ, et al. Nutritional rehabilitation in cystic fibrosis: controlled studies of effects on nutritional growth retardation, body protein turnover, and course of pulmonary disease. J Pediatr 1986;109:788–794.
37. Shepherd R, Cooksley WGE, Cooke WDD. Improved growth and clinical, nutritional and respiratory changes in response to nutritional therapy in cystic fibrosis. J Pediatr 1980;97:351–357.
38. Askanazi J, Rothkopf M, Rosenbaum SH, et al. Treatment of cystic fibrosis with long-term home total parenteral nutrition. Nutrition 1987;3:277–279.
39. Skeie B, Askanazi J, Rothkopf MM, et al. Improved exercise tolerance with long-term parenteral nutrition in cystic fibrosis. Crit Care Med 1987;15:960–962.
40. Goldstein MA, Hesslein P, Dunnigan A. Efficacy of transtelephonic electrocardiographic monitoring in pediatric patients. Am J Dis Child 1990;144:178.
41. Goldenberg RI, Poretz DM, Eron LF, et al. Intravenous antibiotic therapy in ambulatory pediatric patients. Pediatr Infect Dis 1984;3:514.
42. Tatman MA, Woodroffe C. Paediatric home care in the UK. Arch Dis Child 1993;69(6):677–680.
43. Wang WC, Kovnar EH, Tonkin IL, et al. High risk of recurrent stroke after discontinuance of five to twelve years of transfusion therapy in patients with sickle cell disease. J Pediatr 1991;118:377–382.
44. Cohen A. Management of iron overload in the pediatric patient. Hematol Oncol Clin North Am 1987;1:521.
45. Day S, Dancy R, Kelley K, Wang W. Iron overload? In sickle cell disease? MCN 1993;18:330.
46. Close P, Burkey E, Kazak A, Danz P, Lange B. A prospective, controlled evaluation of home chemotherapy for children with cancer. Pediatrics 1995;85(8):896–900.
47. Wolfe LC. A model system. Integration of services for cancer treatment. Cancer 1993;72(Suppl 11):3525–3530.
48. Minnefor AB, Oleske JM. IV immune globulin: efficacy and safety. Hosp Pract 1987;Oct:171.
49. Bielory L. Home health care: intravenous gamma globulin. N J Med 1992;89(1):56.
50. Howard L, Ament M, Fleming CR, et al. Current use and clinical outcome of home parenteral and enteral nutrition therapies in the United States. Gastroenterology 1995;109(2):355–365.
51. Orduna RM, Gimenez Martinez R, Valdivia Garvayo M, et al. Our experience with ambulatory enteral nutrition [Spanish]. Nutr Hosp 1995;10(5):268–271.
52. Stevens MM, Dalla Pozza L, Cavalletto B, et al. Pain and symptom control in paediatric palliative care. Cancer Surv 1994;21:211–231.
53. McGrath PA. Pain in the pediatric patient: practical aspects of assessment. Pediatr Ann 1995;24(3):126–133.
54. Holder KA, Patt RB. Taming the pain monster: pediatric postoperative pain management. Pediatr Ann 1995;24(3):164–168.
55. Martinson IM, Nixon S, Geis D, et al. Nursing care in childhood cancer. Methadone. Am J Nurs 1982;82(3):432–435.
56. Lauer ME, Mulhern RK, Hoffman RG, Camitta BM. Utilization of hospice/home care in pediatric oncology. A national survey. Cancer Nurs 1986;9(3):102–107.
57. Whittam EH. Terminal care of the dying child. Psychosocial implications of care. Cancer 1993;71(Suppl 10):3450–3462.
58. Stovroff MC, Totten M, Glick PL. PIC lines save money and hasten discharge in the care of children with ruptured appendicitis. J Pediatr Surg 1994;29(2):245–247.
59. Guttormsen AB, Nordahl SH, Olofsson J. Home application of EMLA cream prior to venipuncture. Is it feasible in pediatric ENT day care surgery? Int J Pediatr Otorhinolaryngol 1995;31(1):47–52.
60. Klein EJ, Shugerman RP, Leigh-Taylor K, et al. Buffered lidocaine: analgesia for intravenous line placement in children. Pediatrics 1995;95(5):709.
61. Rich DS. Evaluation of a disposable, elastomeric infusion device in the home environment. Am J Hosp Pharm 1992;49(7):1712–1716.
62. Rizzari C, Palamone G, Corbetta A, et al. Central venous catheter-related infections in pediatric hematology-oncology patients: role of home and hospital management. Pediatr Hematol Oncol 1992;9(2):115–123.
63. White MC, Ragland KE. Surveillance of intravenous catheter-related infections among home care clients. Am J Infect Control 1994;22(4):231–235.

22

PEDIATRIC HOME VENTILATORY SUPPORT

Michael M. Rothkopf and Allen I. Goldberg

CHAPTER AT A GLANCE: Home ventilatory support has been a spearhead for the field of pediatric intensive homecare. This chapter reviews the progress made thus far and outlines the criteria for successful management of children requiring long-term artificial ventilation at home. Technological, organizational, and financial issues are discussed in detail.

Introduction and Historical Perspective

Initial Homecare Experiences

Pediatric home healthcare represents a return to tradition. Historically, the customary site for providing care for illness or disability was in the home. Only children of families without economic means required institutional care; middle- and upper-class families converted bedrooms into sickrooms. Babies were delivered at home, relatively uncomplicated surgery was conducted in the home, and patients received care from physicians who made daily house calls (1).

Some families avoided entering institutions thanks to homecare services organized by religious orders and secular groups. A home nursing service was established in Boston as early as 1796. By the end of the 19th century, visiting nurse associations supported by philanthropy were the major source of homecare in the United States (1).

The modern hospital era began with the scientific advances of the late 19th and early 20th centuries. Asepsis, anesthesia, surgery, and medical technology accelerated further in response to necessity (World War I). This led to the possibility of safely conducting complicated antiseptic surgical procedures. Although the hospital became the site for treating seriously ill patients, most patients still remained at home with self- or family-provided care supplemented by privately funded visiting nurse associations. The experiences of the Second World War and the postwar era introduced new health concepts and practices and continued to stimulate community care (1).

During the middle and late 20th century, hospital care for pediatric patients evolved to permit treatment of complex conditions due to congenital defects and acquired illness. Because of modern advances in upper-airway management and artificial respiration with mechanical ventilators, it became possible to sustain infants and children after successful management of life-threatening medical and surgical conditions despite acute respiratory failure (2). These children were managed in pediatric multidisciplinary intensive care units such as Children's Hospital of Philadelphia (under the direction of Drs. Koop, Bachman, and Downes); Children's Memorial Hospital, Chicago (Drs. Allan and Seleny); and Kings County Hospital, Brooklyn (Dr. Torres).

These pioneering units renewed interest in pediatric homecare in the 1970s. As a result of successful acute care, an increasing number of infants and children remained in these ICUs with chronic conditions. They required prolonged support by a variety of life-sustaining medical technologies. Intensive homecare was considered an important option for these patients (3). Successful demonstrations of intensive homecare programs (4) were established in these centers, which defined the state of the art of homecare for long-term mechanical ventilation (5–7). From such locations, physicians were trained to understand homecare as an integral component of pediatric intensive or primary care (8).

In 1982, Surgeon General C. Everett Koop, himself a pioneer of homecare, increased public and professional awareness about community-based care for children (9). Special Projects of Regional and National Significance awarded in 1983 by the Division of Maternal and Child Health encouraged the development of models to evaluate outcomes (10). Public policy initiatives have recently been undertaken to define public policy for children who require high-technology homecare (11, 12).

The Polio Era

Pediatric intensive homecare began with respiratory care. This was made possible through modern advances in upper-airway management and mechanical ventilation. Although the origin of these techniques can be traced to ancient times (13), the modern era began with the poliomyelitis experiences of the mid-20th century. This prompted the modern use of the tracheostomy and the development of

the Engstrom positive-pressure ventilator, the prototype modern volume ventilator (14). Positive-pressure ventilation by tracheostomy reduced the mortality due to bulbar polio from 90 to 20% (15).

In the United States, the complex medical, social, and technological problems of polio patients were managed in regional centers of expertise under the auspices of the National Foundation for Infantile Paralysis—The March of Dimes (3). Regional centers provided an interdisciplinary approach to clinical care, integrated healthcare administration, and the coordination of basic and applied research. Although the discovery of polio prevention (the polio vaccine) was the major success of that period, it is important to note that management techniques developed in response to polio created a new standard of care. The centers also reintroduced home care, which resulted in financial savings and a greater degree of independence and self-sufficiency. The average hospital time was cut from more than a year to 7 months. The home care costs were one-tenth to one-fourth of hospital costs. (3)

The Critical Care Era

Pediatric ICUs continued to advance new techniques and technologies from a variety of disciplines. These included breakthroughs in nephrology, cardiology, gastroenterology, pulmonology, immunology, and infectious disease. Some of these techniques evolved into intensive homecare procedures such as home peritoneal dialysis and parenteral nutrition (16, 17), as discussed elsewhere in this book.

Medical Issues

Definition of Terminology and Concepts

It is important to define terminology and concepts for program development and operational purposes. This is especially true because community-based homecare (the wellness model) requires a different mindset than hospital-based intensive care (the medical model). These illustrative concepts apply to the homecare of infants and children who require long-term respiratory care.

Children should not be treated at home if they are experiencing *acute respiratory failure.* If acute respiratory failure is threatening or present, the child must be in the hospital, because his or her condition is unstable. Children suitable for home respiratory care generally have a more chronic condition. *Chronic respiratory failure* is defined as a life-*threatening* condition with a disorder in oxygenation and/or ventilation that has extended beyond 1 month. *Chronic respiratory insufficiency* is defined as a life-*affecting* and growth-affecting condition with a disorder in oxygenation and/or ventilation beyond 1 month.

One of the major requirements for intensive homecare is clinical stability. It is not possible to design, logistically operate, and finance a program that has frequent changes over a period of time. We define *medically stable* as a condition in which the level of technical support and clinical course have not varied for at least 1 month. On the other hand, we define a patient as *medically unstable* when he or she has a condition that requires one or more major diagnostic and/or therapeutic interventions during a month.

Children whose condition requires intensive respiratory care at home for chronic respiratory failure or insufficiency use life-supportive technology, which is defined as a *mechanical aid for breathing;* that is, any device, based on any principle, that gives augmentation (or replacement) to the natural efforts to breathe. These children are *chronically ventilator-dependent*, meaning that they require mechanical aid for breathing to improve oxygenation or ventilation for at least 4 hours per day for longer than 1 month.

The concept of optimal support describes the way in which we use the medical technology. *Optimal ventilation* is defined as the application of mechanical aids for breathing that tend to reproduce age-appropriate cardiopulmonary function to permit optimal growth and life.

Pediatric "Homecare-Specific" Conditions

The concepts presented for home respiratory care are generic and have universal application for all medical devices that have been adapted to pediatric intensive homecare. Other home techniques are available for infants and children with chronic, stable conditions. These illnesses, such as short bowel syndrome and chronic renal failure, can be considered homecare applicable or "homecare specific" and are discussed in other chapters of the book.

For appropriate indications, methodologies, and applications of any technology in the home, the prescriber must be aware of the uniqueness of the pediatric population. Adult techniques require significant modification. Certain approaches exist only in pediatric applications. For example, techniques of parenteral nutrition have been adapted to children (18) and consensus has been obtained about their use (19), whereas continuous ambulatory peritoneal dialysis (CAPD) began as a pediatric technique and was adapted for use with adults. Home apnea monitoring, bilirubin monitoring (20–22), and phototherapy at home are mainly pediatric approaches (23–25). These home therapies are discussed in Chapter 21.

Consensus panels have been helpful in defining the uses of pediatric intensive homecare. However, even consensus recommendations sometimes remain controversial (26). With more application of home technologies, new lessons and observations are reported that raise questions about their efficacy (27). Concerns about device safety have led to government and voluntary standards. Professional association consensus panels are active in establishing standards for activities such as apnea monitoring. Similar standards are now being developed by the U.S. Food and Drug Administration (FDA).

Controlled multicenter research is needed before it can be determined conclusively which are the appropriate conditions and technologies suitable for pediatric homecare. Taking these concerns into account, conditions suitable for pediatric respiratory homecare should be viewed with caution and attention to appropriate selective criteria, organizational design, and risk management (7).

Conditions Suitable for Home Respiratory Care

Chronic respiratory insufficiency can be caused by primary disorders of the respiratory system: upper airway, lower airway, or alveoli. Conditions due to upper-airway disorders usually result in lung soiling from inadequate upper-airway protective mechanisms. Examples include Pierre-Robin syndrome, Arnold-Chiari malformation, vocal cord paralysis, tracheomalacia (vascular ring), and tracheoesophageal fistula. Situations involving the lower airways include bronchopneumonia, aspiration syndrome, pulmonary hypoplasia, and chronic obstructive pulmonary disease. Chronic respiratory insufficiency due to alveolar disorders may be caused by infectious or chemical pneumonias, bronchopulmonary dysplasia, and alveolar or interstitial edema.

Chronic respiratory insufficiency may also be caused by the failure of one or several other organ systems. For example, it can be caused by conditions of the cardiovascular system such as a variety of congenital cardiac defects and acquired cardiac lesions. It may result from problems of the central nervous, neuromuscular, and/or skeletal systems. Examples of such diagnoses include myasthenia gravis, Werdnig-Hoffmann disease, infant botulism, congenital and childhood myotonias and hypotonias, muscular dystrophy, spinal cord injury, phrenic nerve paralysis, kyphoscoliosis, and thoracic wall deformity.

The classification of organ system insufficiency or failure depends on pathophysiology. Pathophysiological criteria determine (*a*) the nature of the condition, (*b*) how stable the condition is, and (*c*) whether or not the condition is suitable for homecare.

The defining criteria for chronic respiratory insufficiency due to cardiopulmonary disorders in infants and children are both clinical and physiological (Table 22.1). The criteria are slightly different for chronic respiratory insufficiency due to central nervous system, neuromuscular, and/or skeletal conditions (Table 22.2).

Understanding pathophysiology is a major part of the therapeutic process. It is the first step in rational clinical management and is essential in determining prognosis. Furthermore, it is a vital consideration for the design of the homecare program. The diagnostic criteria reflect expectations regarding cardiopulmonary function with consideration of the pathophysiology involved. The emphasis is on important "soft signs" that provide clinical evidence of organ system function adequate for normal growth and development.

Table 22.1. Criteria for Chronic Respiratory Insufficiency Due to Cardiopulmonary Disorders

Clinical
Decreased inspiratory breath sounds
Increased retractions; use of accessory muscles
Cyanosis in room air
Decreased level of normal activity, function (*Important*)
Poor weight gain (mass) (*Important*)
Physiological
$Paco_2$ greater than 45 mm Hg
Pao_2 less than 65 mm Hg in room air
O_2 saturation less than 93% in room air

Table 22.2. Criteria for Chronic Respiratory Insufficiency Due to Central Nervous System, Neuromuscular, and/or Skeletal Conditions

Clinical
Weak cough
Retained airway secretions
Increased use of accessory muscles
Incompetent swallowing
Weak or absent gag reflex
Decreased level of normal activity, function (*Important*)

Physiological
Vital capacity less than 15 mL/kg
Inspiratory force less than 20 cm H_2O
$Paco_2$ greater than 40 mm Hg
Pao_2 less than 70 mm Hg in room air
O_2 saturation less than 95% in room air

Growth and Developmental Factors

In pediatrics, consideration must be given to developmental anatomy and physiology as they affect expectations of organ system function. Understanding anatomical and physiological development will provide important insights into clinical management. For example, if one analyzes the generation of the tracheo-bronchial tree, one can see that there is a critical narrowing of the tree from the 16th branch level onward that is present from birth to 5 years of age (28). After 5 years of age, these critically narrow, small airways become larger. This initial anatomic manifestation has important clinical implications for small-airway obstructive phenomena during the first 5 years of life. If already small airways become further narrowed by intrinsic mechanisms (secretion retention, bronchospasm) or extrinsic means (peribronchial cuffing by interstitial fluid), a critical airway obstruction (increased airway resistance) will result. In addition, the anticipated increased dimension of smaller airways has prognostic implications for the potential of normal growth and development of the lung.

If the child is permitted optimal conditions, critically narrow distal airways will grow to a larger size. This normal developmental potential will dramatically improve the clinical status of the child. The growth in small-airway size is also paralleled by an increase in the number of alveoli during the first decade of life (29). Normally developed lung can functionally replace abnormal pulmonary parenchyma that results from congenital or acquired conditions. This may be the explanation for improvement in the mechanics of breathing (compliance and resistance) and increased functional residual reserve observed in long-term mechanically ventilated infants (30).

Clinical Management Principles

With the emphasis on pathophysiology, medical stability, growth and development, and wellness, the clinical management approach for pediatric intensive homecare is based on the concept of "optimal support" (Table 22.3). This implies that medical technology will be used not just to sustain life but to support function to the child's fullest potential.

Table 22.3. Criteria for Successful Pediatric Homecare

Medical stability
Optimal support
Family preparedness
Appropriate home equipment
Mechanism for repair and maintenance of
   medical equipment
Written operational plan
Written educational plan
Required funding available

The goals are to reduce the risk of frequent, intermittent, acute decompensation; to enhance functional reserve; and to create the best possible internal and external environment for growth and development.

For the pediatric patient with chronic respiratory failure or insufficiency, the goal of optimal support means a program of optimal ventilation, optimal pharmacy and nutrition, and optimal developmental stimulation. There is no exact prescription for this optimal care. Like a roadmap, it provides a destination, which can be met by a variety of routes.

Psychosocial Factors

Infants and children on prolonged mechanical ventilation experience a psychological impact as a result of living in an ICU for an extended period. In 1975, Goldberg began to address the management of the increasing number of such children at the Children's Hospital of Philadelphia. Programs were initiated with the psychological and developmental well-being of the child and family in mind (31, 32). After this program succeeded, the homecare option become necessary and obvious.

Developmental Stimulation, Rehabilitation, and Education

Every child has the potential for normal psychosocial development, even if it is interrupted by acute life-threatening conditions. To facilitate this development, the concept of "programming" a developmental agenda into each individual care plan has been devised.

The first steps in realizing the child's potential are to determine expected developmental outcomes, program means of accomplishment into a therapeutic plan, and document evaluative observations on a regular basis. Developmental stimulation, rehabilitation (habilitation), and educational responsibilities are given to an interdisciplinary primary team. This team should be under the direction of a designated leader and include various healthcare and educational professional disciplines. Nursing, respiratory care, physical therapy, occupational therapy, speech therapy, nutrition, child life therapy, and special education are commonly involved in the care of a child in the hospital. When the patient makes the transition from the institution to home, this care plan must be transferred to a community-based team of similar constituency.

Central Role of the Family

The family must become involved with decision making and providing care for the child as soon as possible. It is only by encouraging family participation that parents will develop and maintain essential emotional bonding to the child. Thus, "family-centered" programs are essential for successful long-term care. When families participate in difficult decisions and observe challenging clinical problems, they become emotionally invested and understand the outcomes. Parental participation leads to a greater commitment to the care of the child and often to the initiation by the family of determining options other than prolonged hospitalization (i.e., homecare).

Homecare requires that the family be motivated and understand what will be involved. This is not only necessary to ensure success, but it is "malpractice insurance" in what could become a medicolegal risk. With the occasional family that does not appear to follow through on expected involvement, a written "contract" must be drawn up with the family that mutually determines responsibilities and accountabilities (7).

Studies on the psychological impact of homecare on children have recognized the importance of the family-centered program (10, 12, 33, 34) on a positive outcome. Homecare programs have different approaches to the level of professional caregivers required in the home (5, 6, 35–40). Most families need flexibility with regard to such supplemental caregivers so that they can adapt their lifestyle (e.g., two jobs, shift-work schedules, lifestyle preferences, etc.), and allow for respite care (for psychological health). One alternative may be the utilization of nonprofessional personal attendants trained by the family (41–44).

Self-Help and Mutual Aid

Anthropological and sociological observations applied to children with special needs have determined the vital role of self-help and mutual aid (45). Few professionals have the experience, insight, and credibility to provide all the essential support that a family requires. However, professionals in partnership with self-help groups can make an important impact on meeting the psychosocial and needs of these children and their families (46).

Environmental Concerns

In Philadelphia and Chicago, special units were designed to provide optimal environments for the psychological and developmental well-being of the children (6, 31, 32, 47). This concern for a supportive environment extended to the home and community setting.

As homecare becomes an option, the homecare plan must consider factors important in the home that make possible the transfer of the child, delivery of equipment and supplies, and access for supplemental caregivers into the home (6, 7, 37). These factors include physical accessibility, storage, living space, and energy requirements. In addition, the plan must take into account emergency and supportive services from the community that will be required (6, 7, 37). The environment (home and community) must be appropriate and supportive.

Technological Issues

Home versus Hospital

Each infant or child who requires intensive homecare will need the flexibility of an individualized prescription of procedures, equipment, and supplies that will meet his or her unique situation. Many factors must be taken into consideration, including the basic pathophysiology, the amount of "free time" when the patient can function independently of technological support, the environment where the patient will be living, and the degree of human surveillance (trained family, professionals, alternative caregivers) that is available.

Patients will need some degree of technological surveillance (alarm systems) to alert others of equipment malfunction or change in clinical condition. Although most devices contain internal alarms, supplemental alarms that monitor physical parameters (e.g., pressure, volume) as well as physiological parameters (oximetry, end-tidal CO_2) may be desirable. However, no alarm system can replace a well-prepared, well-trained, alert, and concerned person. A well-designed homecare program with family input is the goal.

When a medically stable child on optimal support is sent home, it is possible to limit techniques designed for acute care in a hospital setting. Such practices and equipment are far too complicated, costly, and confusing for parents and caregivers to use at home. This equipment has been designed for maximum capability with a variety of options. The clinical situations of properly selected homecare candidates do not usually require such multiple selection options. Specific patient needs can best be met with innovative solutions and basic simple equipment that has been modified for homecare use. Working through creative problem solving also provides an investment and understanding of the solution that enables the homecare system to be appropriately used.

It is not necessary to recreate the medical model or an ICU in the home. For optimal wellness of the child and family, the less technology and technique reflect hospital practice, the more the living environment can encourage health. When complicated (expensive) equipment is prescribed, professional (expensive) care providers can justify control. To accomplish a family-centered program, techniques should be simple for parents and other family members to learn and teach. Furthermore, equipment should be durable and easy

to use, repair, and maintain. Due to limited space and the desire for mobility, it should be as small and lightweight as possible.

Pediatric patients and their families cannot be expected to be technical experts, although they must be trained and evaluated regarding their skill in using their equipment. It is essential that some designated experts be involved who are available for equipment surveillance and support in liaison with the distributors and/or manufacturers of homecare devices. Medical devices used in the home should be provided with mechanisms for emergency repair and routine maintenance service.

Standards

Unfortunately, past performance of home respiratory care devices has sometimes been disappointing. This is partially because homecare equipment was not designed for the requirements of smaller patients. Due to concern for safety, alternative (nonportable) devices had to be substituted or provided for backup purposes. In addition, backup technological surveillance (alarm systems) and additional caregivers were required, depending on the circumstances.

Equipment and supplies used in the home must be subject to basic safety standards of design and manufacture. As a result of concerns about the lack of device standards, consensus activities were conducted at the American Society for Testing and Materials (ASTM) (48). Devices used in the home and homecare practice regarding such devices must also meet certain basic requirements.

Several years ago, the American College of Chest Physicians suggested guidelines for home respiratory care equipment (49). More recently, consensus standards have been proposed (50), and the Joint Commission on Accreditation of Healthcare Organizations has made available an accreditation process (51).

Intensive homecare demands an individual approach to technology that is flexible and adaptable. Equipment in use must be well understood by all users and those who support its function. Since homecare devices may not always meet expectations, communication mechanisms must be in place to track performance and make the necessary adjustments.

Families require an integrated management system for surveillance and support of the equipment (52, 53).

Organizational Concerns

Pediatric intensive homecare requires a detailed organizational structure to facilitate communication among the various disciplines. However, the practical application of homecare for children with respiratory failure is frequently limited by inadequate communication (8). In other countries, regional programs serve large populations and are useful models for analysis of the organizational requirements (41, 54). Our challenge is to establish programs that fit the unique requirements of each locality and that permit the involvement of all required participants (55, 56).

Core Team/Extended Team

Most pediatric patients who require intensive homecare will have received acute critical care in a hospital setting. They will be known best to their primary caregivers, who should initiate plans for homecare as soon as their patients are medically stable. To enable continuity of care so important to the welfare of the child and family, the primary team members responsible for clinical management should join forces with a "core" team of homecare expert consultants during and after the discharge process (7).

The core team should include a physician, a nurse, related allied health professionals, and a social worker who will serve as resource persons to the primary care team members, parents, and representatives from hospital administration. Additional team members are integrated as appropriate to constitute the "extended team." This may consist of professionals from other disciplines involved with children (e.g, school officials, members of community boards and religious organizations).

Comprehensive Written Plan

Each infant or child requires a comprehensive written operational plan that outlines all components of the homecare program (5, 7).

These components reflect the input of members of the interdisciplinary professional team: medical, nursing, respiratory, physical/occupational therapy, child life therapy, speech/nutrition, etc. In addition, the plan should outline all anticipated emergency and elective procedures, with input from the appropriate community-based participants.

The plan should include documentation of an evaluation of the home and community environment with confirmed correspondence with the local emergency facilities (local hospital, emergency room), emergency services (fire, police, utility, highway departments), and required support services (nursing agency, durable medical equipment provider, funding authority). The plan outlines mechanisms for appropriate linkages to ensure that roles, relationships, and responsibilities are defined, coordination and communication are facilitated, and accountabilities are determined. The written plan serves as a legal document for risk management.

Written documentation is recommended for the training program as well. Objectives, methodology, and evaluation should be clearly defined. Most parents will have had several months of experience learning techniques in the ICU. However, some of the equipment and practices in the home are different, and when it is time to go home, education and training must be comprehensive.

For complicated cases, up to 2 full days of classroom education are required. This program is offered to the parents, family members, friends, and neighbors as well as the community-based home caregivers who must be oriented to the care of the child while still in the hospital. This is followed by extensive bedside training, observation, and evaluation using the same equipment setup that the child will have at home. Often, training will be continued and reinforced during the initial period at home.

Education and training of the family and home caregivers, including written documentation of evaluation, is an essential step for medicolegal purposes as well as to ensure that the future training of others by the parents will be as intended. Children receiving home ventilatory support should not be discharged until their families are prepared in this manner.

Individualized Approach

There are some basic practices and procedures that must be incorporated into any homecare program. Many patients may require similar services, and preset (modular) components of the program can be used for efficiency. These are reflected in the guidelines and evolving standards of community-based practice (49–53). However, since each individual patient and family is unique, it is important to permit flexibility and adaptability in each case. Furthermore, the comprehensive written operational and educational plans are legal documents, which can be considered the "homecare prescription."

Care Coordination and Management

Pediatric intensive homecare involves many participants and tasks that must be integrated and coordinated. The role of case coordinator must be a designated responsibility. For some families, it is appropriate and desirable for family members to fulfill this role. This is one component of the family-centered program (12). However, other families do not have the skills and do not want to learn or assume this responsibility. Under those circumstances, it is advisable to assign this role to a home-based caregiver with direct care responsibility who spends the majority of time with the child. This arrangement is preferable to a homecare agency supervisor based elsewhere in the community.

In addition to care coordination, case management must be assigned. A case manager must be capable of an overview of financial, administrative, and clinical aspects of the case. This individual should be accountable to all involved parties: the family, professionals, care providers, and reimbursement officials. Although this person may serve as an advocate for the family, credibility requires that he or she also determine what is medically necessary and appropriate within the requirements of acceptable quality, safety, and cost containment.

Quality and Risk Management

Each pediatric intensive homecare case must incorporate a mechanism to review and document compliance with preset indicators that ensure quality of services provided. There are many individuals and organizations providing these services. The discharging hospital and prescribing professionals are responsible to determine that the program arranged and the services provided meet their expectations. Written quality management procedures make certain that this responsibility is met and that it represents good risk management. Furthermore, documenting quality is also the means to evaluate outcomes and determine ways of modifying the program to ensure safety, improve quality, and reduce costs.

These concerns can be summarized as follows: A homecare program requires an individualized, written operational and educational plan with the input of a designated home discharge team of experts. The plan must define roles and responsibilities, determine mechanisms of care coordination and case management, and provide means for quality and risk management.

Financial Realities

Current Reimbursement Practice

Professionals, providers, and families must be assured that the necessary funding will be available to cover the cost of homecare. Homecare can offer significant cost savings in contrast to prolonged hospitalization (5, 43). However, the costs of homecare are beyond the means of most families, even if they are required to pay only a small percentage (spend-down, co-payment, deductible) of the total costs. Successful homecare requires 100% funding, which often requires a mix of both public and private sources. If such funding is not available, safety may be compromised and the economic burden on the family may be overwhelming.

There are also extra expenses to the family beyond the direct costs for healthcare. For example, the opportunity costs of lost work, extra charges for electric, utility, telephone services, and extra tax assessments on home improvement must also be considered.

Current reimbursement practice makes funding homecare a continuing challenge. On an individual case basis, reasonable people are usually able to establish a mutually acceptable arrangement for funding of homecare services. This is an interactive process among the service providers, payor(s), and family. However, difficulties arise when third party-payors determine that "a policy" is required. Since these cases are often unique, no existing policy applies. On the other hand, both public and private-sector officials are understandably concerned that new policies will potentially increase healthcare costs at a time when cost reduction is a major priority.

The development of a "managed-care" approach has been useful in determining what is appropriate and necessary for homecare. This works well when the professionals involved are knowledgeable experts, but it still becomes problematic when organizations refer to restrictive policies and procedures that limit flexibility, innovation, and "creative financing."

Funding Constraints

The current public funding policy for intensive homecare for children with special needs is determined by waivers to existing Medicaid policy. This approach began with a single case that required an exemption from policy. In 1981, President Reagan was made aware of the bureaucratic red tape preventing the cost saving and appropriate discharge of a child (Katie Beckett) who required intensive homecare services (57). The administration's public policy response to this event was to convene a special task force (58). This initiated a legislative process that established mechanisms for a series of waivers. These, in turn, require approval from the Health Care Financing Administration (59). It must be determined that homecare requires less public monies than alternative institutional care. This policy requires states to apply for waivers that are limited to a set number of cases. Only some states have applied. Waivers in operation have different provisions depending on the perspectives of the authors and approval authority. Furthermore, the emphasis has been on funding mechanisms rather than on innovative management approaches.

Quality Incentives

The future healthcare agenda calls for meeting the dual objectives of cost savings and quality care (60). This is possible with existing home healthcare providers. However, under current reimbursement policies, there is little incentive for innovation or flexibility. Most providers respond to funding constraints with justifiable concerns about inadequate reimbursement and cash flow limitations. If quality performance were designed into the reimbursement structure, and current fragmented delivery of services were coordinated by an integrated management system, operational efficiencies could result in improved services and cost savings. No current reimbursement approach is in place to encourage such management practices.

Family-Centered Managed Care

Families make a major investment in homecare. They also have important insights into operational improvements and cost savings that are not taken into consideration by funding authorities or professional managers. Families want to get the most out of their healthcare dollar and can contribute to efficient management of the homecare program.

The Homecare Era

The Present: Fragmented Health Care Delivery

From a historical perspective, we are experiencing a transition from the hospital era back to a homecare-based system of care for chronically ill children who require ventilatory support. Successful homecare has been demonstrated, and the benefits of the experiences have been recognized (10–12). Major efforts have been undertaken to increase public and professional awareness (49, 52, 53, 61–64). However, educational programs are not yet in place to help patients and families for their new roles and responsibilities. As a result, the intensive homecare option is still not universally accepted or understood.

Significant cost savings have been documented for pediatric intensive homecare (5, 35, 36). In the early 1980s, homecare with full professional caregivers up to 24 hours a day represented less than 30% of hospital ICU charges. However, such economies have been eroded by operational inefficiencies due to fragmentation of payment sources and providers of services. Services are not coordinated, and reimbursement is provided without rigorous cost accounting. Furthermore, homecare costs have risen due to "uncontrolled pricing" in a marketplace that is neither free nor regulated.

These considerations have increased the financial risk for payors and providers of homecare services. In addition, the lack of "a system" has resulted in less than complete satisfaction by all involved parties. Nonetheless, in a country known for both pluralism and individualism, there is understandable concern about the constraints a "system" would impose (56).

The Future: Integrated Health Management Systems

The most desirable scenario for the future of pediatric intensive homecare would include an integrated health management system. This system would be responsive to the needs of all beneficiaries and link all participants: payors, providers, and users. It should be a flexible, adaptable, and evolving system that can both meet the needs of individuals and maximize the utilization of available resources. Cooperation is the only approach to satisfy four mutually beneficial goals of homecare: safety in the home, medical necessity/appropriateness, quality of services, and cost containment.

References

1. Ginsberg E, Balensky W, Ostow M. Home care—its role in the changing health services market. Totowa, NJ: Rowman and Allanheld, 1984:6.
2. Downes JJ, Fulgencio T, Raphaely RC. Acute respiratory failure in infants and children. Pediatr Clin North Am 1972;19:423–445.
3. Faure EAM, Goldberg AI, eds. Proceedings of an International Symposium: What Ever Happened to the Polio Patient? Chicago: Northwestern University Press, 1982.
4. Goldberg AI, Kettrick R, Buzdygan D, Lis E, Schraeder B, Vaughn C. Home mechanical ventilation program for infants and children. Crit Care Med 1980;8:238.
5. Goldberg AI, Faure EAM, Vaughn CJ, Snarski R, Seleny FL. Home care for life supported persons: an approach to program development. Pediatrics 1984;104:785–795.
6. Kettrick RG, Donar ME. The ventilator dependent child: medical and social care. In: Critical Care—State of the Art, vol. IV(F). Fullerton, CA: Society of Critical Care Medicine, 1985:1–38.
7. Goldberg AI, Noah Z, Fleming M, Staniek L, Childs B, Frost L, Glynn W. Quality of care for children who require prolonged ventilation. Qual Rev Bull 1987;13:81–88.
8. Goldberg AI, Monahan CA. Home health care for children assisted by mechanical ventilation—the physician's perspective. J Pediatr 1989;114:378–383.
9. Report of the Surgeon General's Workshop. Children with handicaps and their families. Case example: the ventilator dependent child. Publication PHS-83-50194. Washington, DC: U.S. Department of Health and Human Services, 1983.
10. Aday LU, Wegener DH, Anderson RM, Aitken MJ. Home care for ventilator assisted children. Health Affairs 1989;8:137–147.
11. U.S. Congress, Office of Technology Assessment. Technology dependent children: hospital v. home care—a technical memorandum. Publication OTA-TM-H-38. Washington, DC: U.S. Government Printing Office, 1987.
12. U.S. Department of Health and Human Services. Report of the task force on technology dependent children, vols. 1 and 2. Publication HCFA 88-021271. Washington, DC: U.S. Government Printing Office, 1988.
13. Downes JJ, Goldberg AI. Airway management, mechanical ventilation, and cardiopulmonary resuscitation. In: Scarpelli EM, Auld PAM, Goldman HS, eds. Pulmonary Disease of the Fetus, Newborn, and Child. Philadelphia: Lea & Febiger, 1978:99–131.
14. Engstrom CG. Treatment of severe cases of respiratory paralysis by the Engstrom universal respirator. Br Med J 1954;2:666.
15. Kristensen HS, Neukirch F. Very long-term artificial ventilation (28 years). In: Rattenborg CC, Via-Reque E, eds. Clinical Use of Mechanical Ventilation. Chicago: Year Book, 1981:211.
16. Kohaut EC. Continuous ambulatory peritoneal dialysis: a preliminary experience. Am J Dis Child 1981;135:270.
17. Dudrick SJ, Wilmore DW, Vars HM, Rhodes JE. Long-term total parenteral nutrition with growth, development and positive nitrogen balance. Surgery 1968;64:134.
18. Luck SR. Nutrition and metabolism. In: Raffensperger JG, ed. Swenson's Pediatric Surgery, ed 5. East Norwalk, CT: Appleton & Lange, 1990:81–90.

19. Committee on Nutrition, American Academy of Pediatrics. Commentary on parenteral nutrition. Pediatrics 1983;71:547–552.

20. National Institutes of Health Consensus Development Conference on Infantile Apnea and Home Monitoring. Consensus statement. Pediatrics 1987;79:292–298.

21. Task Force on Prolonged Apnea, American Academy of Pediatrics. Prolonged infant apnea—1985. Pediatrics 1985;76:129–131.

22. Committee on Fetus and Newborn, American Academy of Pediatrics. Home phototherapy. Pediatrics 1985;76:136–137.

23. Von Lilien T, Salusky IB, Boechat I, Ettenger RB, Fine RN. Five years' experience with continuous ambulatory or continuous cycling peritoneal dialysis in children. J Pediatr 1987;111: 513–518.

24. Eggert LD, Pollary RA, Folland DS, Jung AL. Home phototherapy treatment of neonatal jaundice. Pediatrics 1985;76:579–584.

25. Slater L, Brewer MF. Home versus hospital phototherapy for term infants with hyperbilirubinemia: a comparative study. Pediatrics 1984;73:515–519.

26. Grabert BE. Home phototherapy recommendations questioned. Pediatrics 1985;78:373–374.

27. Weese-Mayer DE, Brouillette RT, Morrow AS, Conway LP, Klemka-Walden LM, Hunt CE. Assessing validity of infant monitor alarms with event recording. J Pediatr 1989;115:702–708.

28. Pang LM, Mellins RB. Neonatal cardiorespiratory physiology. Anesthesiology 1975;41:173.

29. Ream RS, Schreiner MS, Neff JD, et al. Volumetric capnography in children. Influence of growth on alveolar plateau slope. Anesthesiology 1995;82:64–73.

30. Morray JP, Fox WW, Kettrick RG, Downes JJ. Improvement in lung mechanics as a function of age in the infant with severe bronchopulmonary dysplasia. Pediatr Res 1982;16:290–294.

31. Schraeder BD. A creative approach to caring for the ventilator dependent child. Am J Matern Child Nurs 1979;4:165–170.

32. Schraelder BD, Donar ME. The child with chronic respiratory failure—a special challenge. Crit Care Nurs 1983;44:119.

33. Lis EF, Goldberg AI, Monahan CA, Murphy KE, Holm KJ. The Children's Home Health Network of Illinois— Pediatric home ventilation: a model of discharge and home care planning. [Grant MCH MC5173363.] Rockville, MD: U.S. Department of Health and Human Services, Division of Maternal and Child Health, 1987.

34. Aday LA, Aitken MJ. Pediatric home care—results of a national evaluation of programs for ventilator assisted children. [Grant PHS-MCJ-173363-03-0.] Rockville, MD: U.S. Department of Health and Human Services, Public Health Service, Division of Maternal and Child Health 1987.

35. Burr BH, Guyer B, Todres ID, Abraham B, Chiode T. Home care for children on respirators. N Engl J Med 1983;309:1319–1323.

36. Frates RC, Splaingard ML, Harrison GM. Outcome of home mechanical ventilation for children. J Pediatr 1985;106:850–856.

37. Johnson DL, Giovannoni RM, Driscoll SA, eds. Ventilator assisted patient care—planning for hospital discharge and home care. Rockville, MD: Aspen, 1986.

38. Schreiner MS, Donar ME, Kettrick RG. Pediatric home mechanical ventilation. Pediatr Clin North Am 1987;34:47–60.

39. Splaingard MC, Frates RC, Harrison GM, Carter RE, Jefferson LS. Home positive pressure ventilation— twenty years' experience. Chest 1983;84:376–382.

40. Hochstadt NJ, Yost DM, eds. The medically complex child: the transition to homecare. New York: Harwood Academic Publishers, 1991.

41. Goldberg AI, Faure EAM. Home care for life supported persons in France: the regional association. Rehabil Lit 1986;47:60–64, 103.

42. U.S. Congress, Office of Technology Assessment. Life sustaining technologies and the elderly. Publication OTA-BA-306. Washington, DC: U.S. Government Printing Office, 1987.

43. Goldberg AI. Home care for life-supported persons: the French system of quality control, technology assessment and cost containment. Public Health Rep 1989;104:329–335.

44. Goldberg AI, Alba AA, Oppenheimer EA, Roberts E. Caring for mechanically ventilated patients at home. Chest 1990;98:1543.

45. French GA. Self-help groups: More than a band-aid treatment? Chic Med Sch Q 1989;92:10–13.

46. Katz AH, Heddrick HL, Isenberg DH, Thompson LM, Goodrich T, Katscher AH, eds. Self-Help: Concepts and Applications. Philadelphia: The Charles Press, 1991.

47. McCarthy MF. A home discharge program for ventilator assisted children. J Pediatr Nurs 1986;12:331–335, 380.

48. American Society for Testing and Materials (ASTM), Committee F29.03.09. Philadelphia, PA.

49. O'Donohue WJ, Giovannoni AM, Goldberg AI, Keens TG, Make BJ, Plummer AL, Prentice WS. Long term mechanical ventilation: guidelines for management in the home and at alternative community sites. Chest 1986;90:1S–37S.

50. American Society for Testing and Materials (ASTM), Committee F31.01.02. Philadelphia, PA.

51. Joint Commission on Accreditation of Healthcare Organizations. Home Healthcare Standards. Chicago: Joint Commission on Accreditation of Healthcare Organizations, 1988.

52. American Association for Respiratory Care, U.S. Food and Drug Administration, and Health Resources Services Administration. Consensus Conference on Home Respiratory Care Equipment. Dallas: American Association for Respiratory Care, 1989.

53. Plummer AL, O'Donohue WJ, Petty TL. Consensus conference on problems in home mechanical ventilation. Am Rev Respir Dis 1989;140:555–560.

54. Goldberg AI, Faure EAM. Home care for life supported persons in England: the Responaut program. Chest 1984;86:910–914.

55. Goldberg AI. Home care for life supported persons—is a national approach the answer? Chest 1986;90:744–748.

56. Goldberg AI. Home care for life supported persons: the French system of quality control, technology assessment, and cost containment. Public Health Rep 1989;104:329–336.

57. "Girl Cited by Reagan Received Medicaid Under a Special Rule." New York Times. November 11, 1981.

58. HHS News. May 6, 1982.

59. Fox HB, Yosphe R. Technology Dependent Children's Access to Medicaid and Homecare Financing. Washington, DC: U.S. Congress, Office of Technology Assessment, 1986.

60. Arthur Anderson and Co., and The American College of Healthcare Executives. The future of healthcare: Changes and choices. Delphi Study, December 1986–May 1987.

61. Goldberg AI. Mechanical ventilation and respiratory care in the home in the 1990s: some personal observations. Respir Care 1990;35:247–259.
62. Webb-Waring Conference: Proceedings of the 1st International Conference on Home Mechanical Ventilation. March 3–4, 1988, Denver, CO.
63. JIVD Conference: 2nd International Conference on Home Mechanical Ventilation. January 26–27, 1989, Lyon, France.
64. GINI Conference: Fifth International Post-polio Conference. May 31–June 4, 1989, St. Louis, MO. St. Louis: Gazette International Networking Institute, 1989.

23

HOME MANAGEMENT FOR BLEEDING DISORDERS IN CHILDREN AND ADOLESCENTS

Eric J. Werner and Kim N. Stewart

CHAPTER AT A GLANCE: Many children suffer from congenital or acquired disorders of coagulation. Symptoms may range from minor epistaxis to life-threatening hemorrhage. In this chapter, we briefly review the hemostatic system and then describe clinical features and treatments for hemophilia, von Willebrand disease, and thrombocytopenia as examples of childhood bleeding disorders. The emphasis is on current methods of management—including new medications, self-infusion, prevention, and patient/family education—which have allowed the home to become the principal site of treatment.

Introduction

The management of most pediatric patients with hematologic disorders has centered around hospital-based tertiary care centers. Patient encounters have traditionally occurred within subspecialty clinics, emergency rooms, and inpatient facilities. In recent years, great progress has been made in the transition from incident-based care in a tertiary care environment to a preventive, homecare approach. In many ways, the homecare and comprehensive care systems developed for hemophilia have become models for the management of other chronic illnesses.

In this chapter we discuss childhood bleeding disorders that in years past would account for a sizable percentage of in-hospital and emergency room patients. We describe the newer approaches, such as family education, prevention, and home treatments, which have improved the quality of life for these patients. Most importantly, these techniques have allowed patients to take control of their own lives by providing the tools through which they can manage the majority of their own medical problems.

The hemostatic system is highly complex. It consists of both cellular components and plasma proteins; prohemostatic factors and natural anticoagulant and antiplatelet factors. A highly simplified schema of the prohemostatic system is shown in Figure 23.1. Many naturally occurring defects of this system have been recognized. As examples of bleeding disorders, in this chapter we discuss hemophilia, von Willebrand disease (vWD), and thrombocytopenia.

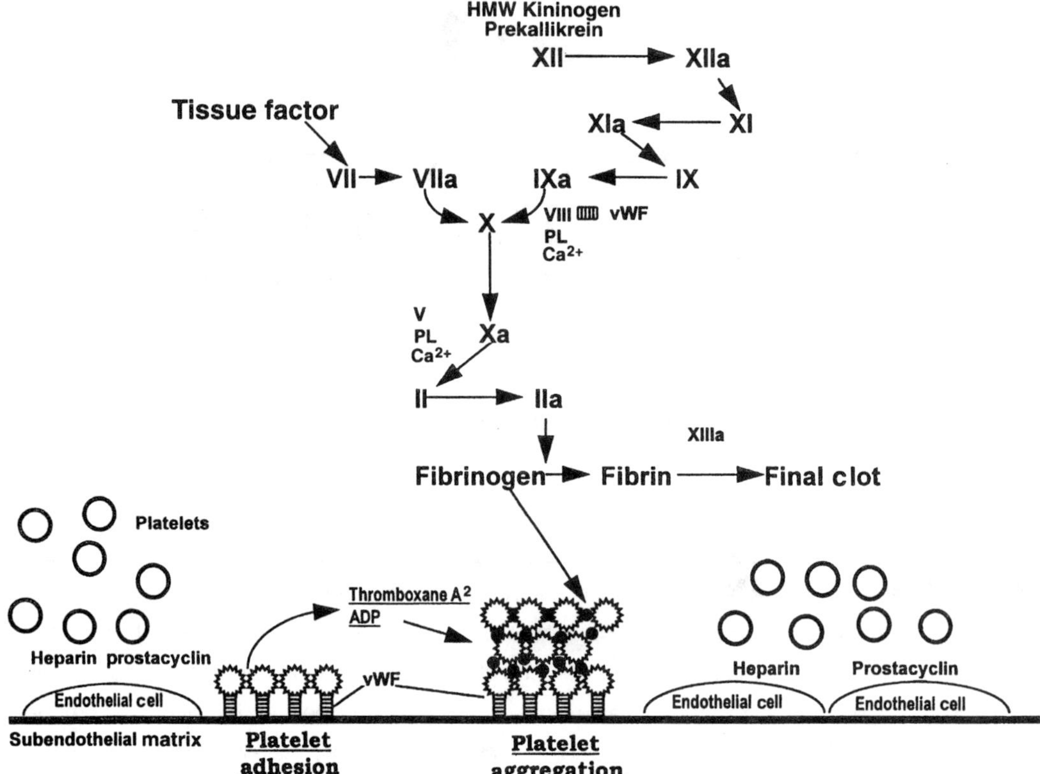

Figure 23.1.   The hemostatic system consists of cellular and plasma protein components. Platelets do not readily adhere to intact endothelial cells, in part due to the production of prostacyclin (PGI_2) by endothelial cells. Platelets adhere to exposed subendothelial matrix. Adhesion is facilitated by von Willebrand factor (vWF). Activated platelets release factors such as thromboxane and ADP, which stimulate platelet aggregation. Fibrinogen is the cofactor for platelet aggregation. The fibrin clot is formed through the interaction of a series of serine proteases that eventually lead to the production of thrombin (IIa), which stimulates the conversion of fibrinogen to fibrin. The fibrin strands are then covalently cross-linked by factor XIII. (Modified from Werner EJ. von Willebrand disease in children and adolescents. Pediatr Clin North Am 1996;43:683–707.)

Hemophilia

Factor VIII and factor IX deficiency account for most cases of hemophilia. Both are sex-linked recessive disorders. Factor VIII deficiency occurs in 1 in 10,000 births, while factor IX deficiency occurs in 1 in 40,000 (1).

The clinical severity of hemophilia is related to the patient's endogenous plasma factor level. By definition, the mean factor VIII and IX level of a normal population is 100 U/dL, and the normal range in adults is roughly 50 to 150 U/dL but will vary from laboratory to laboratory. Newborns and infants have lower levels of many of these factors, which rise gradu-

ally to adult levels during childhood (2). Individuals with severe hemophilia have plasma levels below 1 U/dL. Such people generally have frequent, significant bleeding episodes and spontaneous hemorrhages. In moderate hemophilia, the baseline level of the deficient factor is 1 to 5 U/dL. Such patients generally bleed following trauma; spontaneous hemorrhages are uncommon. Individuals with mild hemophilia (factor levels of 5 to 40 U/dL) have infrequent bleeding episodes, often fewer than one per year, and virtually always have a history of trauma or surgery inducing bleeding. Patients with mildly subnormal levels of factor VIII may in fact have vWD.

Treatment Options

The first goal of treatment for significant bleeding is to increase the plasma concentration of the deficient clotting factor. The target concentration to be achieved is determined by the location and severity of bleeding. There are now several options for use in hemophilia management. Desmopressin, a non-transfusional therapeutic agent, may cause a sufficient increase in plasma factor VIII levels to treat certain kinds of bleeding in patients with mild factor VIII deficiency (3). For the remaining factor VIII–deficient patients, factor VIII concentrates are the treatment of choice. The dosage of factor VIII is calculated by the assumption that 1 U/kg of factor VIII will increase the plasma concentration by 2 U/dL (4). The formula is thus

Amount of factor VIII to be infused =
[Concentration to be reached × Weight (kg)/2]

The half-life of infused factor VIII is estimated at 12 hours. Factor VIII concentrates are manufactured as lyophilized powders. They can be easily reconstituted within minutes and are then administered by intravenous infusion. Recombinant factor VIII concentrates, now commercially available, have a very low risk (if any) for transmission of human viruses (5, 6). Plasma-derived factor VIII concentrates available in the United States have been treated with various viral inactivation processes. These products have little risk for transmission of hepatitis B, hepatitis C, or HIV (7). Infusion of cryoprecipitate or fresh frozen plasma has been used in some settings (4). However, because the concentration of factor VIII in normal plasma averages 1 U/dL and the maximum amount of plasma one can infuse acutely is 15 mL/kg, normal plasma concentrations of factor VIII cannot be achieved with fresh frozen plasma. Cryoprecipitate has higher concentrations of factor VIII per milliliter and hence can be used to achieve normal factor VIII levels. However, neither fresh frozen plasma nor cryoprecipitate is currently available in a virally inactivated form. Because of the combination of safety and convenience, most physicians treating hemophilia prescribe either recombinant or virally inactivated plasma-derived factor VIII products for patients with factor VIII–deficiency hemophilia.

Factor concentrates are also available for factor IX–deficient patients. In recent years, highly purified factor IX concentrates have become available and are the optimal product for use. Prothrombin complex concentrates, which are less purified and contain other vitamin K–dependent clotting factors, were the mainstay of treatment for factor IX deficiency for many years. Prothrombin complex concentrates carry a risk of significant thrombosis, especially in patients receiving high concentrations or repeated doses of the product, who are taking anti-fibrinolytic agents, or who have co-existent liver disease. Recombinant factor IX is just entering clinical trials. Like the factor VIII products, factor IX concentrates are dispensed as lyophilized powders and are reconstituted with saline and administered intravenously in small volumes. The volume of distribution is greater for factor IX than for factor VIII, and the dosage of factor IX is calculated by the assumption that 1 U/kg of factor VIII will increase the plasma concentration by 1 to 1.5 U/dL (4, 8, 9). The formula is thus

Amount of factor IX to be infused =
Concentration to be reached × Weight (kg)

Clinical Manifestations

The bleeding manifestations of hemophilia may begin at birth. Roughly 30% of patients with severe hemophilia will have excessive bleeding following circumcision (10). Internal hemorrhage, including intracranial hemorrhage, may also occur in the neonate. After birth, there is a period of infrequent bleeding, often called the "honeymoon period," until the child becomes mobile. During the toddler years, the typical manifestations of hemophilia usually become apparent.

Hemarthrosis

The musculoskeletal system is the most common site of bleeding for patients with hemophilia. Joint bleeding (hemarthrosis) can occur in any joint but most frequently involves the ankles, knees, and elbows. Acute hemarthroses cause pain and limit joint mobility. In young children, joint bleeding presents as unexplained pain and decreased mobility of a joint. Older hemophilic individuals often recognize the onset of bleeding before such objective physical findings are apparent. Over time, recurrent hemarthroses damage the joint, resulting in hemophilic arthropathy, a condition with signs and symptoms similar to rheumatoid arthritis.

If a joint bleed is recognized and treated early, a single infusion calculated to bring the plasma levels between 30 and 60 U/dL will often resolve the problem. More advanced bleeding episodes require multiple infusions given at intervals of 12 to 24 hours. Temporary joint immobilization can help alleviate symptoms and prevent further joint damage; however, long-term immobilization may lead to further joint dysfunction. Prednisone, at a dose of 2 mg/kg/day for 5 days, may be used to decrease the inflammatory reaction to severe joint bleeding in patients for whom there is no medical contraindication to systemic corticosteroids.

Intracranial Hemorrhage

Intracranial hemorrhage is the most common cause of fatal hemorrhage in young people with hemophilia. Such events may be precipitated by trauma or may occur spontaneously. Because of the risk of intracranial hemorrhage, patients with hemophilia who have head trauma or severe headache should be carefully evaluated and empirically treated with coagulation factor calculated to bring the plasma level above 100 U/dL. A noncontrast CT scan is useful to identify an acute intracranial hemorrhage.

Oral Bleeding

Bleeding from the oral cavity can be problematic, especially for young children. Mouth bleeding may be the initial presenting symptom for infants with hemophilia. For patients with hemophilia treated with factor VIII concentrates, the ability to form clots is present only as long as sufficient plasma concentrations exist. Fibrinolytic enzymes, present in high concentrations in the mouth, rapidly degrade these clots, leading to prolonged oozing from injured sites. Severe anemia may result. Antifibrinolytic agents such as aminocaproic acid or tranexamic acid can inhibit this fibrinolytic process and can facilitate hemostasis in patients who have significant mouth bleeding or who are to undergo surgery in the oral cavity.

Intramuscular Bleeding

Intramuscular bleeding may occur in any muscle, is often quite painful, and can lead to fibrosis of the involved muscle. On occasion, intramuscular bleeding may be severe enough to cause compartmental syndrome. The treatment of intramuscular bleeding is similar to that of hemarthrosis; factor infusions are administered until the symptoms have resolved. Patients with signs of compartmental syndrome should have an orthopedic evaluation.

A particularly serious form of intramuscular hemorrhage occurs into the iliopsoas muscle. As the bleeding is retroperitoneal, the signs are more difficult to recognize. Usually the patient is most comfortable with the involved leg held in a flexed and inwardly rotated position. There can be substantial blood loss from bleeding of the iliopsoas muscle, hence early recognition is important.

Other

Physicians should have a high index of suspicion for bleeding when unexplained symptoms exist in a patient with hemophilia. Neck or retropharyngeal injuries can be life-threatening. Hematuria may occur without other cause, but patients should be evaluated for renal pathology before attributing hematuria solely to hemophilia. Infusion of coagulation factors, bed rest, and administration of corticosteroids have been recommended in the treatment of hematuria, but antifibrinolytic agents are contraindicated.

Complications of Hemophilia Treatment

Various blood products have been used to correct the plasma protein deficiency in patients with hemophilia. However, in recent years, complications of these treatments, especially viral infection and thrombosis, have been recognized. Recent advances in antihemophilic factor have reduced these risks enormously and improved the quality of life for affected individuals.

Viral Transmission

The recent epidemic of HIV and hepatitis C virus infection in patients with hemophilia has been among the greatest medical tragedies in history. Over half of the severe hemophilia patients treated with factor concentrates in the late 1970s and early 1980s have been infected with HIV (11, 12). The great majority of patients who were given either untreated or dry heat–treated antihemophilic factor have been infected with hepatitis C virus (13–15). Fortunately, current donor screening and viral inactivation processes are effective in preventing the transmission of these viruses (16). Furthermore, the availability of recombinant factor should virtually eliminate this risk. Nevertheless, there are many hemophilia patients with ongoing medical needs due to prior infection with these agents.

Inhibitors

Inhibitors are antibodies targeted against the deficient clotting factor in patients with hemophilia. Such inhibitors develop following exposure to this factor and interfere with its ability to promote hemostasis. Clinically significant inhibitors were thought to occur in 10 to 15% of severe factor VIII–deficient patients (17) but have recently been shown to be more common (5, 6, 18). Inhibitors are less common in those with factor IX deficiency or less severe factor VIII deficiency (19). Hemophilic patients with high titers of inhibitors do not bleed more often than those without inhibitors, but they do not respond to infusions of their deficient clotting factor. One alternative therapy for patients with high-titer inhibitors has been prothrombin complex concentrate (20). This product has some efficacy in treating bleeding complications for patients with inhibitors, but its effectiveness is limited and there is a risk for paradoxical thrombosis. A second alternative, highly purified porcine factor VIII, can initiate excellent hemostasis in factor VIII–deficient patients with high-titer inhibitors as long as that inhibitor does not cross-react with the porcine molecule (21). Complications may include allergic reactions and the eventual development of an anti–porcine factor VIII inhibitor. Some therefore reserve porcine factor VIII for the management of life-threatening bleeding episodes. In recent years, it has been shown that repetitive infusions of human factor VIII into factor VIII–deficient patients with high-titer inhibitors will often cause a decrease in the plasma level and the eventual disappearance of the inhibitor. Several protocols for initiation of this immune tolerance effect in factor VIII–deficient patients with high-titer inhibitors have been developed (19, 22).

Home Care for Hemophilia

Reasons for Home Care

There are many advantages to home therapy for patients with hemophilia. Most important is that prompt treatment of a bleeding episode decreases tissue damage to the injured site. Other important factors include fewer interruptions in school and job performance and improved quality of life. While there is some increased usage of coagulation factors, the overall long-term costs have been shown to be lower as a result of fewer emergency room visits, hospitalizations, and physician consultations (23).

Prior to initiating home training and treatment, several issues must be addressed. Antihemophilic factor is expensive. Some families have no health insurance coverage, while others may have policies that do not cover coagulation factors or necessary supplies. Case management may place restrictions on home care choices. The family must be made aware of their ultimate financial obligations prior to initiation of home therapy.

Safety to the family is an issue for two reasons. First, exposure to blood products carries the possibility of transmission of blood-borne disease. Second, in some communities the presence of intravenous equipment in the home may place some families in jeopardy. If the latter circumstance exists, it may be acceptable to keep antihemophilic supplies at a relative's safer residence.

Initiation and Maintenance of Hemophilia Home Infusion Therapy

Home therapy should begin if and when the family can identify appropriate times for blood factor infusion, can manage venous access or central venous catheter care, and can reconstitute and administer the blood factor. The child must be of sufficient maturity to allow the parent to perform the tasks necessary for treatment.

Home therapy of hemophilia should be supervised by the staff of a hemophilia treatment center (HTC). The center is composed of a team of healthcare providers dedicated to the goal of hemophilia health promotion. The core team members consist of a medical director, a nurse coordinator, a psychosocial professional, a program coordinator, a physical therapist, and a case manager. Extended team members include a dentist, a genetic counselor, an orthopedist, and an obstetrician/gynecologist. The center also has access to professionals with expertise in the areas of HIV and hepatitis care. Together they ensure that the child and all associated caregivers are kept abreast of current information regarding trends and developments related to hemophilia therapy. By close contact between HTC staff and patients—including home and school visits, comprehensive care clinic evaluations, coordination of ancillary needed services of physicians and consultants—hemophilia patient care improves. Furthermore, through data collection with other HTCs, new advances in hemophilia management are rapidly transmitted to affected individuals. The HTC staff must work together with the primary care provider, patient, and family for optimal medical care.

Several companies are in the business of providing antihemophilic factor and supplies to patients affected by hemophilia or related bleeding disorders. The homecare companies servicing the family's geographic area will each have their own benefits, services, and limitations, but in general most offer overnight delivery of antihemophilic factor, necessary supplies, and related medications to the home. Some also offer home nursing services. In some areas, HTCs also provide antihemophilic factor and supplies to patients. It is the family's and patient's right to choose their homecare company, supplies, and care provisions, but their payer coverage may vary. Information on the companies, products, and nursing services should be provided to families.

The nurse who teaches home infusion to a patient with hemophilia or his family must be competency qualified in the care of the pediatric patient with a bleeding disorder and have a proven foundation of care with regard to all aspects of infusion therapy, from accessing techniques to product care. The Joint Commission on Accreditation of Healthcare Organizations (JCAHO) Standards of Care now indicate that the RN must have his or her skills not only competency qualified, but also age-specific qualified. The nurse must accomplish the education in a language and at an educational level that is understood by all participants in the child's care. At times it may be necessary to enlist the services of an interpreter. When communication is necessary between hospital and home, the local telephone company's services may have to be used to set up a special language line. Cultural differences must also be taken into consideration; care delivery will vary from culture to culture.

The principal process of patient and family education should take place in the patient's home. The first few visits should consist mostly of education and demonstration. In most instances, the parent receives the infusion training. Eventually the child with hemophilia may express an interest in participating, whether it be simply gathering the necessary supplies or performing the infusion itself. Compliance is greater when the child becomes the active participant, as it gives him a sense of control over his body and disease that will exist for his lifetime.

The first few months of home therapy are often quite stressful for families. Not only must they make the decision of when to treat, but there is internal pressure to be successful; the anxiety of attempting to access an IV or central venous device on one's own child can be quite sizable. For patient safety, there must be quick access to a telephone. If the family is unable to have a telephone in their home, social service agencies are often able to make provisions for one. Additionally, the family must have backup technical services available in case they are unsuccessful in achieving venous access.

During the first visit, it may be necessary for the nurse to administer the therapy, with the family in close observation. It is helpful if the family can be provided with practice equipment such as a plastic practice arm for learning venipuncture, or a model central venous line or Port-A-Cath. Time to experiment with the equipment and solutions and positive reinforcement are imperative during this crucial learning period. One of the most important yet difficult concepts to grasp is the need for sterile technique. Additional time should be allocated for this teaching.

Patients and families must learn to check infusion products for expiration, identity, dosage, clarity, and broken seals. Outdated products must be discarded to eliminate the possibility of infusing incorrect product. Outdating of supplies is especially a problem for the child who only occasionally needs infusion treatment.

Instruction on signs and symptoms of infection and the need for medical attention to this matter must be understood, especially for children with central venous access devices. While allergic reactions to antihemophilic factor infusions are rare, symptoms should be understood by the family. The family should have an excellent understanding of how to gain immediate access to medical and home infusion company personnel.

The infusions performed, and the results and any complications of these treatments, need long-term monitoring. Patients receiving home therapy should be routinely evaluated in the HTC. A patient self-infusion log, which includes a record of any treatments, indications, effects, or complications, should be maintained by the patient and reviewed by the HTC. The patient should be investigated and, if possible, treated for complications of therapy such as viral infections or inhibitors. As stated earlier, the family may now also face the possibility of exposure to blood-borne pathogens. Occupational Safety and Health Administration (OSHA) guidelines must be understood and followed by all care participants.

Travel for Patients with Hemophilia Receiving Home Infusion Therapy

Through interaction with the supervising agency, families should have a plan to deal with emergencies, such as temporary loss of power, interruption of services, etc. When it is necessary for the patient to be seen in a local emergency room, the family should bring necessary supplies with them. Many facilities do not keep the appropriate infusion products in stock. There may also be financial and time incentives for the family to use their own antihemophilic supplies. A customized "emergency room letter" can be helpful for the patient as well as the medical care staff.

Travel outside the geographic coverage of the supervising agency requires added preparation. Ideally, the agency will be involved and will be able to provide the nearest appropriate medical facility with the pertinent information. Before their departure, the family should also be provided with the necessary telephone numbers to access medical care. The family should also understand how to pack their supplies for travel, ensuring that an adequate amount of antihemophilic factor is available to the child at all times. For instance, when traveling by automobile, supplies should not be kept in the trunk of the car, as an accident may prevent the trunk from opening. The supplies need to be stored in a crush-proof container labeled with a biohazard sticker and suitable identification to allow immediate recognition that medical supplies are stored inside.

Similarly, if traveling by boat or plane, the family should always keep several doses of antihemophilic factor and accompanying supplies close at hand. When it is necessary to prepare an infusion while in an airplane, less diluent may be required to reconstitute the factor. The family should check with their infusion company for such modifications.

Lastly, it is advisable for anyone traveling with intravenous medical supplies to have a letter of explanation from their physician, especially if they are venturing internationally.

New Approaches to Hemophilia Management

The availability of homecare, recombinant factor VIII, and immune tolerance treatments has led to a proactive approach to hemophilia care. While home management of acute bleeding problems has improved the quality of life for most patients with hemophilia, this bleeding still causes significant morbidity. Prophylactic therapy is now being tested. Scheduled infusions of antihemophilic factor (approximately three times a week for factor VIII and two times a week for factor IX) are timed to maintain measurable levels of the protein. Long-term follow-up of patients receiving prophylactic therapy in Sweden has documented dramatic decreases in the musculoskeletal complications of hemophilia (24). It has recently been recommended that prophylactic therapy be considered for young people with hemophilia in the United States.

von Willebrand Disease

von Willebrand disease (vWD) is the most common congenital bleeding disorder, with an estimated prevalence of approximately 1%. The clinical manifestations of vWD are typically less severe than those of hemophilia. von Willebrand disease occurs in several subtypes. A new classification system for vWD has recently been recommended (25). There are three major categories of vWD under this system.

In type 1 disease, subnormal levels of von Willebrand factor (vWF) exist in the plasma, but isolated vWF protein is normal in structure. This is by far the most common form of the disorder. Proving the presence of type 1 vWD can be difficult because vWF is an acute phase reactant (26); hence, levels often increase with various stresses. Repetitive testing is often necessary to document an abnormality.

Type 2 vWD is caused by a structurally abnormal vWF, and many subtypes exist. In type 2A vWD, the high–molecular weight form of vWF does not appear in the plasma. In type 2N vWD, the factor VIII molecule does not bind to vWF; these patients present with symptoms typical of mild hemophilia. In type 2B vWD, there is excessive adherence of vWF to platelets, which causes in vivo platelet agglutination and leaves inadequate amounts of intact vWF to promote normal hemostasis. Type 2M vWD encompasses other structural defects of vWF.

Type 3 vWD is the most severe form of the disorder. Individuals with type 3 vWD have no measurable circulating vWF, and hence factor VIII is essentially absent as well. Type 3 vWD is inherited in an autosomally recessive fashion and likely represents either a homozygous or doubly heterozygous state of another type of vWD.

Clinical Manifestations of von Willebrand Disease

von Willebrand disease typically presents with mucosal bleeding symptoms as opposed to the deep tissue bleeding associated with hemophilia. Epistaxis, menorrhagia, and easy bruising are common. Postoperative hemorrhage occurs, especially with surgeries that leave large amounts of denuded tissue such as tonsillectomy or extraction of secondary teeth. The clinical manifestations are extremely variable—some individuals are asymptomatic, while others have frequent bleeding problems. The bleeding manifestations of type 2 vWD are typically more severe than those of type 1 vWD. Type 3 vWD patients are the most significantly affected and have deep tissue bleeding similar to hemophilia as well as mucosal bleeding.

Treatment of von Willebrand Disease

Desmopressin, a synthetic analog of antidiuretic hormone, will cause a 1- to 5-fold increase in plasma vWF levels in most, but not all, patients with vWD (3). In patients previously proven to respond to the medication, desmopressin can be used to treat bleeding problems. Two preparations are available for this purpose. The intravenous preparation is administered at a dosage of 0.3 µg/kg in 50 mL of normal saline over 30 minutes. A new high-strength intranasal preparation, recently licensed in the United States, is given as one activation (150 µg) for children and two activations (300 µg) for adults (27). The older intranasal preparation, developed for patients with diabetes insipidus, has too low a potency to be useful for patients with bleeding disorders. Doses may be repeated at intervals of 12 to 24 hours for continued bleeding or for postoperative use (28, 29). While the intranasal preparation is the best alternative for home treatment, there is less experience with its use for postoperative patients.

When used appropriately, desmopressin has few side effects. Rapid intravenous administration can cause facial flushing and headache. The most serious complication of desmopressin reported is the occasional hyponatremic seizure (30, 31). Factors that predispose to this problem include a large intake of free water, use of general anesthesia, and extremes of patient age (28, 32).

Patients and their families should be educated regarding desmopressin, its risks, and its proper use. The patient's daily maintenance fluid requirement should be calculated and fluid intake should be restricted to that amount for 24 hours following use of desmopressin. Furthermore, patients and family should be educated regarding the salt content of various fluids. Patients receiving desmopressin should be evaluated for headache or persistent emesis.

Tachyphylaxis can be another problem with the use of desmopressin. Tachyphylaxis occurs when there is a diminishing plasma vWF response to subsequent doses of desmopressin. It is more likely to occur when doses are given more frequently than every 24 hours (29).

When patients with vWD who do not respond to desmopressin require treatment, plasma derivatives that contain high–molecular weight vWF may be administered. The dosage to be used is usually calculated on the basis of

factor VIII units. Although there is no FDA-licensed plasma product for the treatment of vWD, there is published experience with this approach. One option is cryoprecipitate, which contains high–molecular weight vWF. Because currently available cryoprecipitate units have not undergone any viral inactivation process, factor VIII products that contain multimeric vWF and that have also undergone viral inactivation are recommended. Only a few factor VIII products that contain von Willebrand factor are available in the United States.

Thrombocytopenia

Subnormal platelet counts may occur by several mechanisms. While the normal range for platelet counts is generally 150,000 to 400,000/µL, bleeding is seldom a problem if the platelet count exceeds 50,000 to 100,000/µL. The causes of thrombocytopenia are listed in Table 23.1.

Immune Thrombocytopenia

Patients with immune thrombocytopenia (ITP) may have surprisingly few bleeding problems, despite often severe thrombocytopenia. ITP in children tends to be a self-limited disorder (acute) in the vast majority, while in adults the chronic form predominates. Acute ITP resolves within 6 months of diagnosis, while chronic ITP persists beyond that time (33).

Table 23.1. Causes of Thrombocytopenia

Increased Platelet Destruction
Immune thrombocytopenic purpura
Hypersplenism
Sepsis
Disseminated intravascular coagulation
Thrombosis
Thrombotic thrombocytopenic
   purpura/hemolytic uremic syndrome
Decreased Platelet Production
Bone marrow failure syndromes
Bone marrow infiltration (malignancy,
   myelofibrosis, etc.)
Chemotherapy or other drugs
Congenital amegakaryocytic disorders

The management of ITP is controversial, especially in children. Treatments that increase the platelet count include corticosteroids, intravenous γ-globulin, splenectomy, and immunosuppressive medications. Most clinicians will manage children with acute ITP conservatively with preventive measures outlined below or will intervene with intravenous γ-globulin or corticosteroids. Recently, immune globulin directed at the D antigen of erythrocytes (anti-D) has been purified. Anti-D has a relatively slow effect in acute ITP (34). Even with chronic ITP, spontaneous resolution may occur. Anti-D, intravenous γ-globulin, and corticosteroids provide transient efficacy. Splenectomy will cause a remission for the majority of patients with chronic ITP, but should be reserved for those patients for whom it is truly necessary, especially in patients under 5 years of age, for whom the risk of sepsis is greatest (35).

Immunosuppressive medications are generally used for patients who have failed to resolve with splenectomy.

Chemotherapy-Induced Thrombocytopenia

Myelosuppressive chemotherapy, principally used in cancer treatment, is a common cause of severe thrombocytopenia. Mucosal bleeding symptoms occur in this population. Platelet transfusion are generally given to manage patients with symptomatic thrombocytopenia. Most clinicians transfuse platelet concentrates to maintain a platelet count above 5,000 to 20,000/μL (36). Cytokines that promote platelet production, such as thrombopoietin, may soon significantly decrease the risk of bleeding and the need for platelet transfusion in cancer patients.

General Treatments for Individuals with Bleeding Disorders

Preventive

Medications with known antiplatelet effects should be avoided (Table 23.2). Aspirin permanently impairs platelet cyclooxygenase and thus platelet function. Patients often use over-the-counter compounds unaware that they contain aspirin. Nonsteroidal anti-inflammatory agents also inhibit platelet function and are common ingredients of over-the-counter remedies. Glycerol guaiacolate, found in many cold treatments, can also inhibit platelet function. It is helpful to provide a bleeding disorder patient with a list of prescription and nonprescription medications to avoid.

In treating a patient with a bleeding disorder, the physician should emphasize the importance of accident prevention measures such as bicycle helmets, car seats, seat belts etc. For patients with mild vWD, excessive activity restrictions are probably unnecessary, but participation in sports with a high incidence of injuries may be unwise. The National

Table 23.2. Some Medications with Antiplatelet Effects

Over-the-Counter Medications
Aspirin
Salicylates
Nonsteroidal anti-inflammatory agents
Guaifenesin
Antihistamines
Ethanol
Antiplatelet agents
Dipyridamole
Ticlopidine
Antimicrobial Agents
High-dose penicillins
Cephalosporins
Nitrofurantoin
Hydroxychloroquine
Cardiovascular Medications
Propranolol
Furosemide
Calcium channel blockers
Quinidine
Other Medications
Caffeine
Tricyclic antidepressants
Phenothiazines
Valproate
Heparin
Prostacyclin
Aminocaproic acid
Ethanol

Hemophilia Foundation has published a booklet entitled *Hemophilia and Sports,* which outlines the relative risks of various athletic activities for patients with hemophilia.

Nontransfusional Therapies

Several home remedies can facilitate control of recurrent epistaxis. Use of a cool-air humidifier is advised. Local measures include application of pressure to the nares for 10 to 15 minutes, use of Neo-Synephrine spray, and/or intranasal application of porcine strips (37) with or without added microfibrillar collagen (Avitene) (38).

Oral contraceptives can be very useful for the patient with a bleeding disorder and menorrhagia. In vWD, birth control pills raise vWF levels and limit menstrual blood loss (39, 40). Other hormonal agents may be necessary for the patient with severe dysfunctional uterine bleeding. For documented responders, desmopressin may be used in conjunction with other therapies to manage menorrhagia.

As noted in the section on hemophilia, bleeding frequently follows oral surgery or mouth injuries in patients with disorders of hemostasis. An antifibrinolytic agent should be used either before oral surgery or following trauma with bleeding in the oral cavity. ϵ-Aminocaproic acid (Amicar) can be ingested orally. The usual loading dose is 200 mg/kg followed by 100 mg/kg every 6 hours. The syrup (250 mg/mL) is more convenient than the 500-mg tablets for most individuals. Nausea may occur. Cyclokapron is an alternative and can also be ingested orally, but a 4.8% mouthwash of this medication is generally well tolerated (41). As it should be swished for 2 minutes every 6 hours, patients must be old enough to understand and comply with its proper use. Antifibrinolytic agents are continued for at least 5 days.

Anemia can promote bleeding, especially in individuals with underlying hemostatic disorders. Patients who have anemia secondary to blood loss should take ferrous sulfate at a dosage of 3 to 6 mg/kg/day and should continue the medication at this dosage for 2 to 3 months after resolution of the anemia. Supplemental doses of ferrous sulfate (1 to 2 mg/kg/day) should be used by patients at risk for iron deficiency. Erythropoietin has had a significant impact on the incidence of anemia in patients with renal failure and is now being tried in other populations with impaired red cell production.

Synopsis

The home is increasingly becoming the site for management of most pediatric patients with bleeding disorders. Hemostatic defects such as hemophilia, von Willebrand disease, and thrombocytopenia may each produce significant clinical problems for affected patients. Management includes nontransfusional therapies in many instances. For patients with severe coagulopathies such as hemophilia, home intravenous infusion of antihemophilic factor, administered by the patient or the parent, is standard therapy. The treatments may also be related to significant complications. The patient and family must receive adequate training and support for optimal outcome. Preventive approaches should be stressed. Coordination of the care provided by the primary care practitioner, the hematologist, the bleeding disorder nurse coordinator, the home supply company, and the patient and family is necessary.

References

1. Miller CH. Genetics of hemophilia and von Willebrand's disease. In: Hilgartner M, Pochedly C, eds. Hemophilia in the Child and Adult. 3rd ed. New York: Raven Press, 1989:297–345.
2. Andrew M, Schmidt B. Hemorrhagic and thrombotic complications in children. In: Colman RW, Hirsh J, Marder VJ, Salzman EW, eds. Hemostasis and Thrombosis. Basic Principles and Clinical Practice. 3rd ed. Philadelphia: JB Lippincott, 1994: 989–1022.
3. Mannucci PM, Cattaneo M. Desmopressin: a nontransfusional treatment of hemophilia and von Willebrand disease. Haemostasis 1992;22:276–280.
4. Hilgartner M. Factor replacement therapy. In: Hilgartner M, Pochedly C, eds. Hemophilia in the Child and Adult. New York: Raven Press, 1989:1–26.

5. Lusher J, Arkin S, Abildgaard C, Schwartz R. Recombinant factor VIII for the treatment of previously untreated patients with hemophilia A. N Engl J Med 1993;328:453–459.

6. Bray GL, Gomperts ED, Courtier S, et al. A multicenter study of recombinant factor VIII (Recombinate): safety, efficacy and inhibitor risk in previously untreated patients with hemophilia A. Blood 1994;83: 2428–2435.

7. Julius C, Westphal RG. The safety of blood components and derivatives. Clin Hematol Oncol North Am 1992;7:1057–1078.

8. Furie B, Limentani S, Rosenfield C. A practical guide to the evaluation and treatment of hemophilia. Blood 1994;84:3–9.

9. Brettler DB, Levine PH. Clinical manifestations and therapy of inherited coagulation factor defects. In: Colman RW, Hirsh J, Marder VJ, Salzman EW, eds. Hemostasis and Thrombosis. Basic Principles and Clinical Practice. 3rd ed. Philadelphia: JB Lippincott, 1994: 169–183.

10. Montgomery R, Scott J. Hemostasis: diseases of the fluid phase. In: Nathan D, Oski F, eds. Hematology of Infancy and Childhood. 4th ed. Philadelphia: WB Saunders, 1993:1605–1650.

11. Goeddert JJ, Kessler CK, Aledort LE. A prospective study of HIV-1 infection and the development of AIDS in persons with hemophilia. N Engl J Med 1989; 321:1141–1148.

12. Phillips A. The epidemiology of HIV disease in men with haemophilia in the UK. Hemophilia 1995;1(Suppl):6–7.

13. Blanchette VS, Vorstman E, Shore A, et al. Hepatitis C infection in children with hemophilia A and B. Blood 1991;78:285–289.

14. Brettler DB, Alter HJ, Dienstag JL, Forsberg AD, Levine PH. Prevalence of hepatitis C virus antibody in a cohort of hemophilia patients. Blood 1990;76:254–256.

15. Tibbs C, Williams R. Hepatitis C and hemophilia: a report of a meeting held at the Royal Free Hospital. London, 12 December, 1994. Haemophilia 1995;1: 207–209.

16. Schimpf K, Mannucci PM, Kreutz W, et al. Absence of hepatitis after treatment with a pasteurized factor VIII concentrate in patients with hemophilia and no previous transfusions. N Engl J Med 1987;316:918–922.

17. Bloom A. The treatment of FVIII inhibitors. Thromb Haemost 1987;58:447–471.

18. Ehrenforth S, Kreuz W, Scharrer I, Linde R, Funk M, Gungor T. Incidence of development of factor VIII and factor IX inhibitors in haemophiliacs. Lancet 1992; 339:594–598.

19. Hay CRM. Factor VIII inhibitors. Haemophilia 1995;1 (Suppl):14–21.

20. Lusher JM. Use of prothrombin complex concentrates in management of bleeding in hemophiliacs with inhibitors—benefits and limitations. Semin Hematol 1994;31(Suppl 4):49–52.

21. Brettler DB, Forsberg AD, Levine PH, et al. The use of porcine factor VIII concentrate (Hyate:C) in the treatment of patients with inhibitor antibodies to factor VIII. A multicenter US experience. Arch Intern Med 1989; 149:1381–1385.

22. Nilsson IM. Immune tolerance. Semin Hematol 1994;31(Suppl 4):44–48.

23. Aledort LM, Branch I. The cost of care for hemophiliacs. In: Hilgartner MW, Pochedly C, eds. Hemophilia in the Child and Adult. 3rd ed. New York: Raven Press, 1991:137–147.

24. Nilsson I. Experience with prophylaxis in Sweden. Semin Hematol 1993;30:16–19.

25. Sadler JE. A revised classification of von Willebrand disease. For the Subcommittee on von Willebrand Factor of the Scientific and Standardization Committee of the International Society on Thrombosis and Haemostasis. Thromb Haemost 1994;71:520–525.

26. Pottinger BE, Read RC, Paleolog EM, Higgins PG, Pearson JD. von Willebrand factor is an acute phase reactant in man. Thromb Res 1989;53:387–394.

27. Rose EH, Aledort LM. Nasal spray desmopressin (DDAVP) for mild hemophilia A and von Willebrand disease. Ann Intern Med 1991;114:563–568.

28. Lusher JM. Response to 1-deamino-8-D-arginine vasopressin in von Willebrand disease. Hemostasis 1994; 24:276–284.

29. Aledort LM. Treatment of von Willebrand's disease. Mayo Clin Proc 1991;66:841–846.

30. Shepherd LL, Hutchinson RJ, Worden EK, Koopmann CF, Coran A. Hyponatremia and seizures after intravenous administration of desmopressin acetate for surgical hemostasis. J Pediatr 1989;114:470–472.

31. Smith TJ, Gill JC, Ambruso DR, Hathaway WE. Hyponatremia and seizures in young children given DDAVP. Am J Hematol 1989;31:199–202.

32. Logan LJ. Treatment of von Willebrand's disease. Hematol Oncol Clin North Am 1992;6:1079–1094.

33. Buchanan GR. Overview of ITP treatment modalities in children. Blut 1989;59:96–104.

34. Blanchette V, Imbach P, Andrew M, et al. Randomised trial of intravenous immunoglobulin G, intravenous anti-D and oral prednisone in childhood acute immune thrombocytopenic purpura. Lancet 1994;344:703–707.

35. Beardsley DS. Platelet abnormalities in infancy and childhood. In: Nathan DG, Oski FA, eds. Hematology of Infancy and Childhood. 4th ed. Philadelphia: WB Saunders, 1993:1561–1604.

36. Warkentin TE, Kelton JG. Management of thrombocytopenia. In: Colman RW, Hirsh J, Marder VJ, Salzman EW, eds. Hemostasis and Thrombosis. Basic Principles and Clinical Practice. 3rd ed. Philadelphia: JB Lippincott, 1994:469–488.

37. Heywood BB, David RB, Yonkers AJ. Treatment of epistaxis with porcine stripped packing. Trans Am Acad Ophthalmol Otolaryngol 1976;82:255–260.

38. Smith P. von Willebrand's disease: pathophysiology, diagnosis and treatment. In: Hilgartner MW, Pochedly C, eds. Hemophilia in the Child and Adult. New York: Raven Press, 1989:275–295.

39. Alperin JB. Estrogens and surgery in women with von Willebrand's disease. Am J Med 1982;73:367–371.

40. David JL, Gaspard UJ, Gillain D, Raskinet R, Lepot MR. Hemostasis profiles in women taking low-dose oral contraceptives. Am J Obstet Gynecol 1990;163: 420–423.

41. Sindet-Pedersen S, Ramstrom G, Bernvil S, Blomback M. Hemostatic effect of tranexamic acid mouthwash in anti-coagulant treated patients undergoing oral surgery. N Engl J Med 1989;320:840–843.

24

AMBULATORY MANAGEMENT OF CARDIAC ARRHYTHMIAS

Kevin J. Ferrick

CHAPTER AT A GLANCE: Over the last 10 years, many diagnostic and interventional cardiovascular techniques that formerly required a hospitalized setting are being performed on an ambulatory basis. Improved microprocessor technology has allowed for the development of miniaturized recording devices with sophisticated computational ability, resulting in the ability to detect, quantitate, and in the case of implantable defibrillators, initiate therapy for a variety of complex arrhythmias. These techniques have facilitated the outpatient diagnosis and management of a broad spectrum of cardiac rhythm disturbances. The advent of radiofrequency techniques has fostered an era in which patients can be cured of disabling arrhythmias, often in an ambulatory setting. Sophisticated arrhythmia recognition algorithms are now routinely utilized to recognize and treat lethal ventricular arrhythmias as they occur, limiting the need for lengthy hospitalizations for arrhythmia management in many patients.

Introduction

The recognition and treatment of complex cardiac arrhythmias has evolved significantly over the last 15 years. Coupled with the rapid evolution of electrophysiologic testing, advances in microprocessor technology have enhanced our ability to detect cardiac rhythm disturbances. At the same time, improved understanding of the mechanisms of cardiac arrhythmias has enhanced our ability to treat formerly refractory rhythm disturbances. Concomitantly, spiraling healthcare costs have prompted a greater emphasis on the outpatient diagnosis and treatment of disorders that in the past have been evaluated on an inpatient basis. Although the detection and management of cardiac arrhythmias has historically been performed in a hospital setting, an emerging outpatient arrhythmia service is developing. This chapter presents a profile of the present state of cardiac rhythm analysis and therapy, with an emphasis on the modalities that can be utilized in an ambulatory or homecare setting.

Arrhythmia Detection

A number of techniques have evolved to detect cardiac arrhythmias on an ambulatory basis (Table 24.1). These devices, in effect, provide initial documentation of the nature and frequency of a patient's spontaneous arrhythmia.

"

Table 24.1. Ambulatory Arrhythmia Detection

24-Hour ambulatory recording (Holter monitor)
Real-time recording
Transtelephonic monitoring
Continuous-loop recording
Signal-averaged electrocardiography
Heart rate variability
T-wave alternans

Although many of these devices can provide similar information, each has its own distinct advantages, and an understanding of the features of each device can be of significant use in the management of cardiac rhythm disturbances.

24-Hour Ambulatory Recordings

The primary advantage of hospitalization for arrhythmia evaluation is continuity of observation. Cardiac arrhythmias are often transient and infrequent events that can require long periods of monitoring for detection. Because of the limited duration of recording, 12-lead electrocardiography lacks the sensitivity to detect all but the most frequent events. The development of 24-hour ambulatory electrocardiography (ECG) recorders, the so-called "Holter monitor," greatly enhanced the sensitivity of ECG recording for detecting infrequent events. First described in 1961 (1), the early Holter monitors utilized cumbersome reel-to-reel tape recorders of limited frequency response, which made the interpretation of ST segment shifts difficult. Arrhythmia analysis was qualitative, using manually operated scanners that detected ectopic beats based primarily on their degree of prematurity. The ability to obtain quantitative counts was therefore highly dependent on operator skill, and the counts were often, upon review, found to be inaccurate. Currently available devices utilize compact cassette or solid-state recorders that are capable of multi-lead recordings with an enhanced frequency response (2–4). Improved fidelity has contributed to the ability to perform quantitative analysis of ST segment shifts, which have been found to correlate with periods of myocardial ischemia (5–9).

Additional timing channels assist in the analysis of pacemaker function, which has become progressively more complex, as evidenced by the now common use of dual-chamber and rate-responsive devices (10–14). Current Holter analysis systems are complex, computer-based devices that are capable of highly accurate recognition of both supraventricular and ventricular arrhythmias, as well as atrioventricular block. Arrhythmia recognition algorithms now incorporate a variety of techniques, including templating, area determination, superimposition, and fast Fourier transforms. These are microprocessor controlled, but in the most accurate and sophisticated units they require technician overview and verification. Appropriate user interaction has been demonstrated to enhance detection accuracy (15). The most sophisticated units are now capable of performing adjunctive functions of ST segment analysis, heart rate variability determination (which has been correlated to mortality), and late potential detection. The development of accurate timing channels to minimize variation in cassette tape speed has allowed for the development of algorithms to determine heart rate variability. The human heartbeat is not metronomically regular, and variations in the interval between successive QRS complexes is normally seen. The degree of heart rate variability (or period, as it is changes in the interbeat interval that is quantitated) has been attributed to alterations in sympathetic and parasympathetic autonomic input. Diminished heart rate variability has been associated with increased mortality in patients surviving myocardial infarction, in those exhibiting congestive heart failure, and in patients with diabetic neuropathy. Quantitation of heart period variability can be expressed using either time domain or frequency domain parameters. Close correlations exist between measurements in the time and frequency domains and are related to fluctuations in sympathetic or parasympathetic tone. Using specially designed recorders, some scanners are capable of analyzing ambulatory blood pressure data.

Real-Time Recorders

These solid-state recorders were initially introduced with an emphasis on ST segment analysis and were capable of triggering an alarm when significant ST segment depression was noted (16, 17). Although they were able to perform arrhythmia recognition, full disclosure of all recorded waveforms was not possible with the early devices. Therefore, only a limited sample of "significant arrhythmias" could be reviewed for accuracy. Through the use of data compression, newer units are now capable of providing more complete waveform review. However, the fidelity of recorded data is still limited. Quantitative review and correction is thereby compromised such that the conventional Holter monitor appears to provide greater flexibility and accuracy for detailed arrhythmia analysis.

Transtelephonic Recorders

These devices are portable, patient-activated units that are designed to transmit a single-lead rhythm strip via telephone to a central monitoring station (18–20). Most units are capable of recording 30 to 90 seconds of data for each of up to three separate episodes. The major advantage of such devices is that they allow the recording of relatively infrequent events because they are not overshadowed by the large amount of information in a 24- to 48-hour recording. The use of these devices is limited to patients who are aware of their arrhythmia and can tolerate the hemodynamic sequelae of their arrhythmia long enough to activate the device. These devices are not suitable for very brief events, as it usually takes 30 to 60 seconds to locate and activate the recorder, even under the best of circumstances.

A modification of the basic transtelephonic monitor is the continuous-loop recorder, which is worn by a patient using a modified two-lead system. The device continuously records using a 30-second to 5-minute recording loop. Upon a signal from the patient, the device "freezes" the preceding 30 to 90 seconds of recording while recording "online" for an additional programmed period.

The onset of a symptomatic arrhythmia can thus be recorded, and even extremely brief events can be documented due to the continuous nature of the recording.

The use of memory-loop recorders is also limited to symptomatic events, and the units themselves are inconvenient to use for long periods of time, as they require continuous attachment. Battery consumption is significant with these devices, and an average 9-volt battery lasts approximately 48 hours. Several commercial services provide 24-hour transtelephonic arrhythmia surveillance using these units, and they have been shown to be useful in the follow-up of patients with a history of sustained ventricular tachycardia or implantation of a pacemaker or automatic implantable cardioverter defibrillator (AICD) (20, 21). Recently, several manufacturers have introduced even smaller, more convenient units that approach the size of a credit card. One manufacturer has introduced an event recorder as part of a functioning wristwatch, which allows for acquisition of up to 30 seconds of ECG data by merely pressing one's finger against a brass electrode plate built into the watch casing. While the electrocardiograms recorded using this wristwatch system are not as artifact-free as those obtained from systems utilizing a dedicated, disposable electrode, the convenience of use and the ability to record even brief symptoms in real time represent significant advantages over older units.

Signal-Averaged Electrocardiography

This technique utilizes high-gain amplification and repetitive waveform averaging to reduce random noise levels and thereby enhance the detection of high-frequency signals in the terminal portion of the QRS complex (Fig. 24.1). These signals have been termed "late potentials," and their recording is enhanced through the use of special filtering that assists in the recording of signals of microvolt amplitude. Late potentials are believed to represent delayed conduction in abnormal myocardium and are often considered

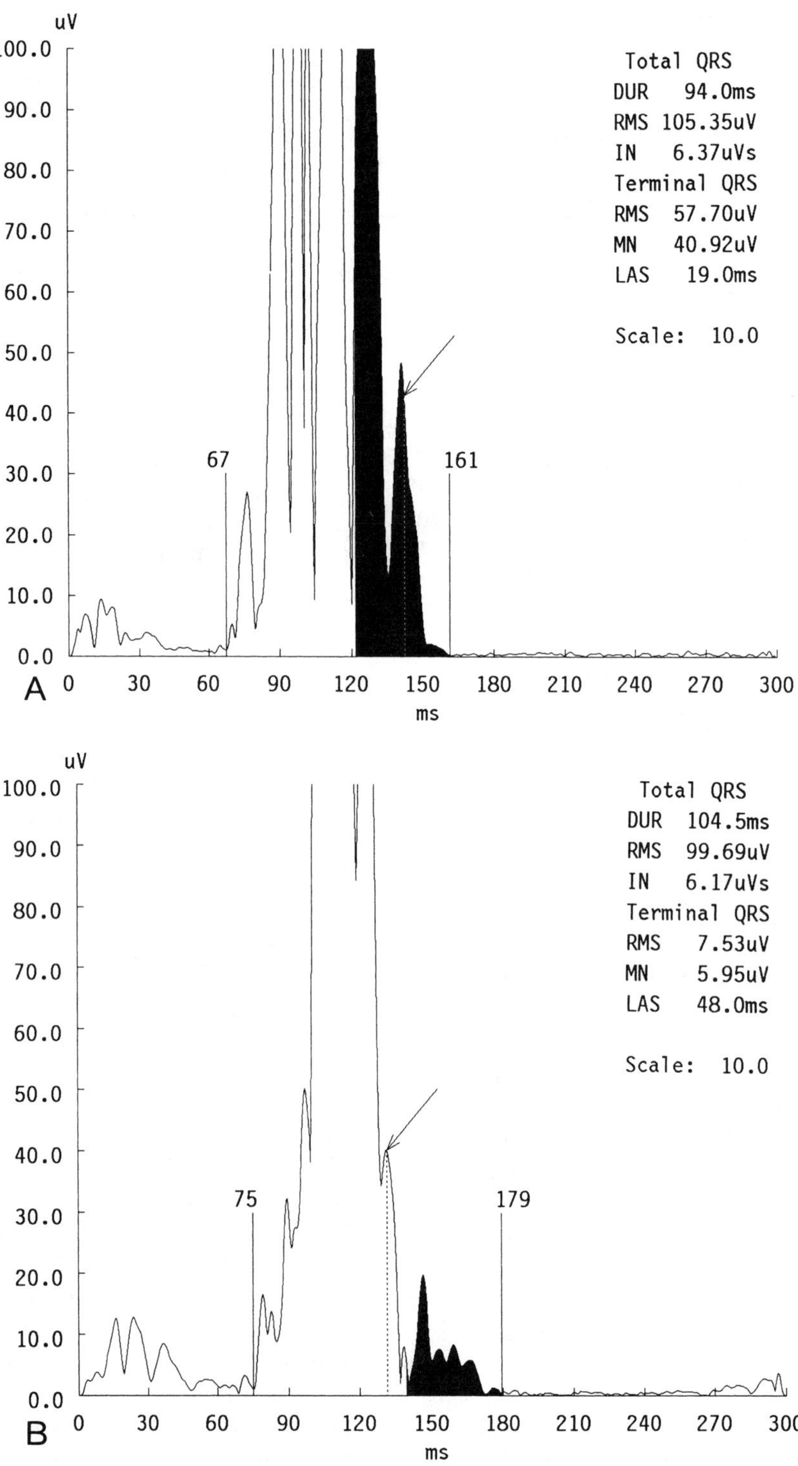

Figure 24.1. Signal-averaged electrocardiograms with time-domain analysis. **A,** Normal signal-averaged electrocardiogram from a patient with isolated ventricular ectopy. RMS_{40}, LAS_{40}, and QRS duration are all within normal limits. **B,** Abnormal signal-averaged electrocardiogram from a patient with a history of myocardial infarction and sustained ventricular tachycardia. RMS_{40} and LAS_{40} are abnormal.

the electrocardiographic manifestation of an arrhythmogenic substrate (22).

Although this technique was first used to record His bundle depolarizations as early as 1973 (23), more recent attention has focused on the terminal QRS complex. Whereas qualitative analysis was originally used, more recent quantitative analysis has focused on two different approaches. Time-domain analysis, as described by Denes et al., involves measuring the amplitude and duration of the terminal summed QRS complex according to predetermined criteria (Table 24.2) (24). An alternative analysis approach using a computer-facilitated mathematical transformation has been advocated by Cain and Lindsay (25–27). Known as fast Fourier transform analysis (FFTA), this approach calculates a spectral plot determined by the proportion of specific frequency ranges constituting the terminal QRS complex. This approach has been advocated as being less dependent on filtering than time-domain analysis. Both techniques have been demonstrated to yield reproducible results (22).

Although the criteria used to define the presence of late potentials has not been standardized, it has been suggested that late potentials are more common in patients with coronary artery disease and are present in 80 to 90% of patients with coronary artery disease and a history of sustained ventricular tachycardia (22, 26, 27). Conversely, only 3% of normal individuals have late potentials (22). The frequency of late potentials in patients with congestive cardiomyopathy and a history of sustained ventricular tachycardia has been reported to be 45%, and the overall sensitivity

Table 24.2. Signal Averaging—Time Domain Analysis

RMS_{40}	Root mean square of the high-frequency signals in the terminal 40 msec of the summed QRS complex
LAS_{40}	Duration of the high-frequency signals of the terminal summed QRS complex less than 40 μV in amplitude
QRS duration	Total duration in msec of the summed QRS complex

and specificity of signal averaging in identifying patients with ventricular arrhythmias has been reported to be in the range of 70 to 80%. Signal-averaged electrocardiography in concert with left ventriculography has been shown to be of powerful predictive accuracy in identifying high-risk patients with recent myocardial infarction (28, 29). Signal-averaging techniques have recently been applied with the analysis of microvolt-level variations in T-wave amplitude. Available microprocessor analysis can now quantitate the degree of T-wave alternans using frequency-domain analysis. Abnormalities in T-wave alternans power spectra have been correlated with increased risk of sudden death as well as the inducibility of sustained ventricular tachycardia by electrophysiologic techniques in high-risk patients.

Arrhythmia Analysis

Analysis of cardiac rhythm disturbances may require provocative maneuvers beyond simply waiting for spontaneous events to occur. Several of these procedures are applicable to the ambulatory setting (Table 24.3).

Single-Catheter Electrophysiologic Study

The analysis of complex cardiac arrhythmias has evolved significantly since the introduction of His bundle electrocardiography as a clinical tool by Damato in 1969 (30). Multiple-catheter studies are now routinely used both to elucidate the mechanism and to guide therapy for a variety of supraventricular and ventricular arrhythmias (31–35). Traditionally, these studies have been performed on an inpatient basis to allow for cardiac rhythm surveillance after initial evaluation, as well as between serial studies. However, limited electrophysiologic studies can be performed on an ambulatory basis in patients with hemodynamically well-tolerated arrhythmias or to screen patients with potentially lethal arrhythmias. These patients can then be admitted for additional evaluation if the study demonstrates them to be at risk for lethal arrhythmias. Single-catheter studies

Table 24.3. Ambulatory Arrhythmia Analysis

Single-catheter electrophysiologic study
Transesophageal recording and stimulation
Noninvasive programmed electrical stimulation
Exercise testing
Tilt-table test

make use of a percutaneously inserted multipole catheter from either the median basilic or the femoral vein. This catheter can be used to provide data regarding basic conduction intervals, parameters of sinus and AV node function, as well as atrial and ventricular vulnerability to sustained arrhythmias. The information obtained is comparable to that of a more formal "complete" study.

Fisher et al. have described a technique of low right atrial pacing using a standard multipole pacing catheter, which allows for recording of a His bundle potential (36). Parameters of His-Purkinje conduction and their response to pharmacologic maneuvers can thus be determined in patients felt to be at risk for high-degree atrioventricular block.

Using a single-catheter study in patients with Wolff-Parkinson-White syndrome, the effective refractory period of the accessory pathway can be determined and its response to procainamide administration assessed. In addition, a patient's vulnerability to atrial fibrillation as well as the hemodynamic response to this arrhythmia can be quantitatively determined. Risk stratification of patients with asymptomatic or minimally symptomatic Wolff-Parkinson-White syndrome can thereby be performed on an ambulatory basis. Wolff-Parkinson-White patients with documented paroxysmal supraventricular tachycardia, syncope, or other symptoms suggestive of hemodynamically unstable cardiac rhythms, as well as those considering surgical ablation of the accessory pathway, should undergo more complete electrophysiologic study. As this requires the placing of multiple catheters from several central venous sites, detailed electrophysiologic study should be performed subsequently on an inpatient basis (33–35). With the advent of radiofrequency ablative techniques, even more complex diagnostic and interventional studies are being performed virtually on an outpatient basis. A patient with paroxysmal supraventricular tachycardia (PSVT) can undergo a diagnostic study whereby the mechanism of the supraventricular tachycardia can be determined and, using a localized application of radiofrequency energy, the region of abnormality can be cauterized. Initially these techniques involved postprocedure observation in a hospital setting for several days. Recently, procedures such as AV node modification and ablation of right atrial tachycardias have been performed as "same-day" procedures, with patients being discharged after a relatively limited period of observation. Similarly, pacemaker replacement is routinely performed without overnight hospitalization. There may come a time when initial pacemaker implantation is done on an outpatient basis, at least for patients who are not pacemaker dependent.

Transesophageal Recording

Positioning a bipolar catheter in the esophagus at the level of the atrium allows for the recording of a discrete atrial electrogram (37–39). Determining the relationship, if any, between atrial and ventricular depolarizations is often critical to determining the nature of a sustained tachycardia. Therefore, transesophageal electrograms can be an important adjunct in arrhythmia interpretation. Although an appropriate electrode can be fashioned by placing a 4 Fr bipolar temporary pacing catheter inside a standard nasogastric tube, specially designed pill electrodes consisting of a thin bipolar wire encased in a gel capsule have been manufactured (40). The pill electrode can then be swallowed and positioned at the appropriate level using centimeter markings on the pacing wires, as well as by using the amplitude of the recorded atrial electrogram. A specially designed external stimulator capable of rectangular impulses of long duration and high amplitude can be used for atrial pacing. Atrial pacing can be used to effectively terminate supraventricular arrhythmias such as atrial flutter and atrioventricular reciprocating tachycardia (37, 39).

As with single-catheter electrophysiologic studies, transesophageal pacing can be used to determine the conduction properties of accessory pathways as well as to induce atrial fibrillation to assess the minimum preexcited RR interval in patients with Wolff-Parkinson-White syndrome. Transesophageal pacing is a benign procedure without significant morbidity, although the energy required for atrial capture can be associated with a sense of epigastric distress commonly described as "heartburn."

Noninvasive Programmed Electrical Stimulation

A number of currently available permanent pacemakers are capable of performing electrophysiologic studies noninvasively (Table 24.4) (41–45). The Medtronics Spectrax pacemaker, an otherwise conventional VVI (ventricle paced and sensed; response inhibited) pacemaker, is capable of ventricular burst pacing to rates up to 400 beats/min using a hand-held external activator. This device is approximately the size of a package of cigarettes and can be used either to initiate or to terminate sustained arrhythmias. A special programmer for the device is capable of complete programmed stimulation using up to three premature stimuli. Other devices, such as the Pacesetters Synchrony and the Cordis Gemini, are DDD (atrium/ventricle paced and sensed; response to sensing triggered and inhibited) pacemakers capable of be-

ing placed in DDT (atrium/ventricle paced and sensed; response triggered) or VVT (ventricle paced and sensed; response triggered) mode with short ventricular refractory periods. Thus programmed, these pacemakers can be triggered by low-amplitude chest wall stimulation using a programmable stimulator or external pacemaker. Noninvasive programmed stimulation can be performed using this technique, which can be useful in assessing either short-term or long-term drug efficacy in patients with sustained atrial and ventricular arrhythmias. Arrhythmias recurring spontaneously despite antiarrhythmic therapy can be effectively terminated using this technique if the arrhythmia is hemodynamically tolerated long enough to allow presentation to an emergency room or physician's office.

However, termination of sustained ventricular arrhythmias by this technique can occasionally result in acceleration of the ventricular tachycardia rate or degeneration into ventricular fibrillation. Obviously, either one can result in the need for emergency direct-current cardioversion (44, 45). This concern has limited the use of antitachycardia pacing algorithms in an automatic mode without automatic defibrillator backup. The risk of ventricular tachycardia acceleration can be limited, but not eliminated, by appropriate patient selection. Specifically, before permanent pacemaker implantation, the efficacy of pacing modalities to terminate ventricular tachycardia should be tested in the electrophysiology laboratory on multiple occasions over the course of several days. Ventricular tachycardia exhibiting slower rates is often more amenable to termination by pacing techniques, and the risk of ventricular tachycardia acceleration appears to be minimized in this setting (41, 44). Occasionally, underdrive pacing using single ventricular capture can terminate ventricular tachycardia. This modality is associated with a very low incidence of acceleration.

Table 24.4. Pacemakers Capable of Noninvasive Programmed Stimulation

Model	Manufacturer
Spectrax	Medtronic
Symbios	Medtronic
Thera	Medtronic
Versatrax	Medtronic
Gemini	Cordis
Omni-Orthocor	Cordis
Prism	Cordis
Cosmos	Intermedics
Paragon	Pacesetters
Synchrony	Pacesetters
Vigor	CPI

Exercise Testing

Symptom-limited exercise testing can be a useful adjunct in arrhythmia analysis. Although exacerbation of ventricular arrhythmias has not been shown to predict the presence of underlying coronary artery disease, exercise-induced ventricular tachycardia has been well described and may involve multiple electrophysiologic mechanisms, including reentry, enhanced automaticity, and triggered automaticity (46).

Grayboys et al. have described the use of exercise testing in concert with 24-hour ambulatory electrocardiographic recording to guide antiarrhythmic therapy in patients with a history of ventricular tachycardia or cardiac arrest (47). In this study, patients in whom antiarrhythmic therapy successfully suppressed ventricular tachycardia (Lown grade IVB ectopy) at rest and with exercise exhibited improved survival compared with those in whom antiarrhythmic therapy failed to suppress ventricular tachycardia.

Exercise testing can also be used to noninvasively estimate the effective refractory period of accessory pathways in patients with Wolff-Parkinson-White syndrome. Patients in whom evidence of preexcitation is abolished either with exercise or after procainamide administration generally have longer effective refractory periods than those in whom electrocardiographic evidence of preexcitation persists. Patients with short effective refractory periods appear to be at increased risk for hemodynamically unstable rhythms, including (potentially) ventricular fibrillation. Symptomatic individuals with Wolff-Parkinson-White syndrome in whom evidence of preexcitation persists throughout exercise should be referred for complete invasive electrophysiologic evaluation.

Tilt-Table Testing

Patients with syncope or symptoms suggestive of vasomotor instability can be evaluated through the use of a "standing" or tilt-table test. Although the specific protocols utilized for these studies vary among institutions, hypotension and/or symptomatic bradycardia can be provoked in selected individuals by placing them at inclines varying from 45° to 90° over a duration of 15 to 30 minutes (48–50). The use of agents such as edrophonium (Tensilon) or

isoproterenol enhances the diagnostic yield of tilt-table testing by evoking a cholinergic or barrow receptor response. Transdermal scopolamine has been shown to be effective in ameliorating symptoms in patients with a positive tilt-table test (50).

Ambulatory Antiarrhythmic Therapy

Initiation of antiarrhythmic therapy in patients with potentially lethal (nonsustained ventricular tachycardia and decreased ejection fraction) or demonstrably lethal (sustained ventricular tachycardia/ventricular fibrillation) arrhythmias has classically been performed in an inpatient setting under telemetric monitoring (31, 32, 34, 35, 47). The rationale behind this conservatism has been the knowledge that antiarrhythmic agents can, under certain circumstances, actually exacerbate arrhythmias. This concept of arrhythmogenesis or "proarrhythmia" is not new. William Withering, in his 1785 manuscript describing the use of digitalis in the treatment of congestive heart failure, noted several clinical vignettes that suggest an awareness of the potential of digitalis for proarrhythmia (51). The association linking the malignant ventricular arrhythmia torsades des pointes with quinidine administration was first described by Selzer more than 30 years ago (52). Subsequently, proarrhythmia as assessed by both invasive and noninvasive techniques has become a major concern of contemporary cardiology. Definitions by which to judge proarrhythmia by Holter monitoring have been suggested by Velebit and Morganroth (Table 24.5) (53, 54). Using these definitions, conventional antiarrhythmic agents have been shown to exacerbate arrhythmias in 5 to 15% of patients. Proarrhythmia can vary from merely an increase in the frequency of detected ventricular ectopy to the first appearance of sustained ventricular tachycardia or torsades des pointes. Although the clinical significance of increased ectopy frequency has not been established, the adverse effect on survival of sustained ventricular arrhyth-

Table 24.5. Definitions of Proarrhythmia

Velebit et al. (53)
I.   Fourfold increase in hourly VPD[a] frequency
II.   Tenfold increase in the hourly frequency of repetitive forms
III. First occurrence of sustained VT (>60 sec)

Morganroth and Horowitz (54)
I.   Presence of a new ventricular tachyarrhythmia not related to other factors
II.   Change in a previously documented ventricular arrhythmia:
    A.   Increased frequency of VPD

Mean Hourly VPD Frequency at Baseline	Increase Required for Proarrhythmia
1–50	10×
51–100	5×
101–300	4×
>301	3×

    B.   Marked increase in rate of VT
    C.   Change in type of ventricular tachyarrhythmia, such as nonsustained VT to sustained VT, sustained VT to torsades des pointes, or VT to ventricular fibrillation
    D.   Marked change in ease of termination of ventricular tachyarrhythmia

[a] VPD, Ventricular premature depolarization.

mias is clear. Proarrhythmia appears to occur most frequently in patients with poor ventricular function and a history of sustained arrhythmias (55). The Cardiac Arrhythmia Suppression Trial (CAST) has demonstrated that lethal proarrhythmia—once believed to occur soon after the initiation of antiarrhythmic therapy—can be a late phenomenon, at least in postinfarction patients (56).

In general, clinical parameters have not been shown to be useful in predicting proarrhythmia. However, patients with a history of sustained ventricular tachycardia in the setting of diminished left ventricular function have been shown by Podrid to be at highest risk for proarrhythmia (55). It is unclear at this time whether or not arrhythmia exacerbation by one drug predicts arrhythmia exacerbation by others. Podrid did not identify a "crossover" risk of proarrhythmia. However, in a study of 40 episodes of drug-induced ventricular fibrillation, Zipes reported a 16% crossover risk of ventricular fibrillation in patients treated with class Ia antiarrhythmic agents (57). Of note, QT prolongation did not predict the occurrence of proarrhythmia in this study. Unlike the CAST study, proarrhythmia appeared to be an early event, occurring after a median of 3 days of drug therapy.

Concern over lethal proarrhythmia effectively limits the potential initiation of antiarrhythmic therapy on an ambulatory basis. The incidence of proarrhythmia in patients without manifest structural heart disease is small. However, Morganroth has reported that in addition to structural heart disease, atrial fibrillation and hypokalemia are independent risks for proarrhythmia in patients treated with quinidine (58). When these risk factors were avoided, serious proarrhythmia was not seen in 370 patients treated with quinidine on an outpatient basis. There is also a general consensus that agents such as mexiletine, tocainide, and β-blockers have a relatively small potential for proarrhythmia. However, this has not been studied in either randomized or controlled clinical trials.

On the basis of this information, ambulatory initiation of antiarrhythmic therapy in selected patients may be appropriate. Several unconventional modes of antiarrhythmic therapy may be considered for ambulatory antiarrhythmic therapy.

Cocktail Therapy

Patients with hemodynamically well-tolerated supraventricular tachycardia that occurs infrequently may be suitable for intermittent therapy aimed at terminating episodic sustained arrhythmia rather than event suppression. Agents such as verapamil, propranolol, and procainamide have been shown to be effective in acutely terminating a variety of supraventricular arrhythmias and can be used on an "as-needed" basis to terminate episodic tachycardia in patients who have been shown to be at low risk for proarrhythmia. This approach is most useful when the sustained arrhythmia occurs without associated hemodynamic compromise and where the side effect profile of long-term "suppressant" therapy outweighs the benefit of continuous arrhythmia suppression. Patients who fail to respond to "cocktail" therapy administered orally may be managed on an outpatient basis with ultrashort-acting intravenous agents such as esmolol or adenosine in addition to the more conventional agents verapamil or procainamide. While these agents are most often administered in an emergency room or office setting, this concept could be expanded in selected circumstances to include a homecare setting. The agent could be administered by a nurse using transtelephonic monitoring, if it has been previously shown to be effective and well tolerated.

Lidocaine Pen

A variant of cocktail therapy is the so-called lidocaine pen, which is a device approximately the size of a ballpoint pen that can be used to self-administer subcutaneous or intramuscular lidocaine. The use of this device has been advocated for prophylaxis of perimyocardial infarction arrhythmia. It has also been shown to be effective in terminating ventricular tachycardia in patients who have previously been shown to be lidocaine responsive at the time of electrophysiologic testing (59, 60). The potential role of this type of device with other antiarrhythmic agents remains to be determined.

Home Defibrillation

Families of patients identified as being at high risk for sustained ventricular arrhythmias (sudden death survivors, high-risk postinfarction patients, hypertrophic cardiomyopathy patients with nonsustained ventricular tachycardia) are often trained in basic life support. Additional adjunctive support can be offered to certain patients in the form of home defibrillators (61). Application of these devices can permit arrhythmia identification and automatic defibrillation if predetermined criteria are met. A variation of this is a device being marketed in Europe. This unit transmits the patient's electrocardiogram transtelephonically to a central monitoring station and can, after physician verification, enable a defibrillating discharge (62). Although such devices are demonstrably effective in terminating sustained arrhythmias, it is perhaps understandable that patient and family compliance with them has been limited. Difficult to transport, such devices tend to limit a patient's mobility and are ineffective when an individual is alone or asleep. Despite these limitations, home defibrillation can be of use in selected high-risk patients who are not candidates for automatic antitachycardia devices.

Antitachycardia Devices (ATDs)

Currently available pacemakers are capable of automated arrhythmia detection and therapy (63–65). With advances in microprocessor technology, even conventional pacemakers are capable of auxiliary functions such as determining pacing thresholds and lead impedance. More sophisticated units are capable of tracking how frequently the device is called upon to sense or pace. Some are capable of tabulating both atrial and ventricular ectopic activity, in effect duplicating the function of a 24-hour ambulatory ECG recording (14). The efficacy of antiarrhythmic drug therapy can thereby be assessed on a long-term basis with the use of such devices. Recording of intracavitary electrograms from the permanently implanted leads can be accomplished by telemetry link between certain pacemakers and their programmers. This can be of use in diagnosing the nature of both spontaneous and pacemaker-mediated arrhythmias. Differentiation of supraventricular from ventricular arrhythmias can be facilitated using this technique.

As noted previously, appropriately timed pacing is often effective in terminating sustained arrhythmias. While this can be utilized effectively to perform noninvasive programmed electrical stimulation (NIPS) to guide the selection of effective antiarrhythmic therapy, the same techniques can be used to automatically identify and terminate sustained tachycardia. Specially designed pacemakers can utilize a variety of programmable arrhythmia detection algorithms (Table 24.6) to recognize abnormal rhythms. Once activated, these devices use programmable tachycardia termination algorithms in an attempt to interrupt sustained arrhythmias (Table 24.7). A termination hierarchy can be established to activate the most effective sequence first, with automatic switching to backup sequences if the first series proves to be ineffective. The pacing sequences can be programmed to scan electrical diastole in an attempt to identify the tachycardia termination zone, which can vary with fluctuations in sympathetic and parasympathetic tone (45, 63–65).

The current automatic antitachycardia pacemakers appear to have the greatest applicability in the management of supraventricular arrhythmias. This is due in part to the fact that supraventricular arrhythmias are generally tolerated well enough from a hemo-dynamic perspective to allow the time for a pacemaker to identify the proper pacing sequence to effect arrhythmia termination. The hemodynamic significance of tachycardia acceleration, a common problem with these devices, is minimized if the arrhythmia being terminated is supraventricular.

In one series of 23 patients in whom 573 episodes of ventricular tachycardia were evaluated (41), 89% of episodes were terminated by bursts of ventricular pacing; ventricular tachycardia was accelerated in only 4% of episodes. Unfortunately, 43% of patients exhibited at least one episode of tachycardia acceleration.

The advent of the automatic implantable cardioverter-defibrillator (AICD) allows for protection from this occurrence. Originally described by Mirowski in 1980 (66), this device is currently able to identify ventricular tachyarrhythmias by programmable rate and morphology criteria. In response to a detected episode, the device delivers a cardioverting/defibrillating shock of 2 to 30 joules in an attempt to restore sinus rhythm.

Entirely a reactive device, the AICD has been shown to improve survival in patients with a history of sustained ventricular arrhythmia or aborted sudden cardiac death (67). The early-generation AICDs were not capable of automatic antitachycardia pacing, and a variety of adverse pacemaker-AICD interactions—including oversensing, undersensing, and inappropriate shock delivery—were initially described when both units were implanted in the same patient (68–70). Present-generation devices are capable of sophisticated antitachycardia pacing as well as bradycardia support, in addition to their primary function of rendering high-output shocks for defibrillation. Over the last several years, the development of transvenous lead systems in concert with tiered therapy devices has facilitated the management of patients with drug-refractory ventricular tachycardia and patients who have been resuscitated from out-of-hospital cardiac arrest. These devices are also capable of complete noninvasive programmed stimulation, which simplifies the testing and postimplant programming of these

Table 24.6. Arrhythmia Recognition Algorithms

1. High rate
2. Sustained high rate
3. Abrupt onset
4. Rate stability
5. Combinations of above

Table 24.7. Arrhythmia Termination Algorithms

1. Single extra stimuli
2. Bursts
3. Decremental bursts
4. Scanning
5. Bursts plus extra stimuli
6. Other

units. More recently, implantable cardioverter-defibrillators (ICDs) have become smaller in size and weight, approaching 125 g and 70 cc. These smaller units have been implanted with success in the pectoral region, obviating the need, in many patients, for tunneling the ICD lead under the skin to an abdominal location. These units are now primarily implanted in the cardiac catheterization laboratory and can be implanted using conscious sedation, obviating the need for an operating room and general anesthesia. These tiered therapy devices are often successful in terminating the majority of episodes of ventricular tachycardia, with shock therapy being reserved for more unstable rhythms or rhythms refractory to antitachycardia pacing. Optimal reprogramming of these devices can be performed on an outpatient basis. Many individuals with these more sophisticated units require concomitant pharmacologic therapy to slow the ventricular tachycardia rate to allow its termination by antitachycardia pacing techniques. Under current development are plans for the introduction of an atrial defibrillator, which would allow for automated shock therapy for paroxysmal atrial fibrillation. Because of the need for lower output (on the order of 1 to 3 joules), these units will be smaller and more like present-generation pacemakers in size.

References

1. Holter NJ. A new method for heart studies. Continuous electrocardiography of active subjects over long periods is now practical. Science 1961;134:1214–1220.
2. Zeldis SM, Levine BJ, Michelson EL, Morganroth J. Cardiovascular complaints. Correlation with cardiac arrhythmias on 24-hour electrocardiographic monitoring. Chest 1980;78:456–462.
3. Kennedy HL, Chandra V, Sayther KL, Caralis DG. Effectiveness of increasing hours of continuous ambulatory electrocardiography in detecting maximal ventricular ectopy. Continuous 48-hour study of patients with coronary heart disease and normal subjects. Am J Cardiol 1978;42:925–930.
4. Sheffield TL, Berson A, Bragg-Remschel D, et al. Recommendations for standards of instrumentation and practice in the use of ambulatory electrocardiography. Circulation 1985;71:626a-636a.
5. Schang SJ Jr, Pepine CJ. Transient asymptomatic ST segment depression during daily activity. Am J Cardiol 1977;39:396–402.
6. Tzivoni D, Benhorin J, Gavish A, Stern S. Holter recording during treadmill testing in assessing myocardial ischemic changes. Am J Cardiol 1985;55:1200–1203.
7. Bragg-Remschel DA, Anderson CA, Winkle RA. Frequency response characteristics of ambulatory ECG monitoring systems and their implications for ST segment analysis. Am Heart J 1982;103:20–31.
8. Imperi GA, Lambert CR, Hill JA, Pepine CJ. Ambulatory ECG (Holter) monitoring in management of acute myocardial ischemia. Cardiovasc Clin 1988;18:5–22.
9. Kunkes SH, Pichard AD, Smith H, et al. Silent ST segment deviations and extent of coronary artery disease. Am Heart J 1980;100:813–820.
10. Barold SS. The DDI mode of cardiac pacing. PACE 1987;10:480–484.
11. Parsonnet V, Furman S, Smyth NPD, et al. Optimal resources for implantable cardiac pacemakers. Pacemaker study group. Circulation 1983;68:226a-244a.
12. Humen DP, Kostuk WJ, Klein GJ. Activity sensing, rate responsive pacing: improvements in myocardial performance with exercise. PACE 1985;8:52–59.
13. Webb SC, Lewis LM, Morris-Thurgood JA, et al. Respiratory dependent pacing: a dual response from a single sensor. PACE 1988;11:730–735.
14. Furman S, Hayes SL, Holmes DR Jr. A Practice of Cardiac Pacing. Mount Kisco, NY: Futura Publishing, 1989.
15. Anonymous. Ambulatory ECG monitors. Health Devices 1989;18:295–321.
16. Barry J, Campbell S, Nabel E, et al. Ambulatory monitoring of digitized electrocardiogram for detection and early warning of transient ischemia. Am J Cardiol 1987;60:483–488.
17. Jamal S, Mitra-Duncan L, Kiely D, et al. Validation of a real time electrocardiographic monitor for the detection of myocardial ischemia secondary to coronary artery disease. Am J Cardiol 1987;60:525–527.
18. Hasin Y, David D, Rogel S. Diagnostic and therapeutic assessment by telephone electrocardiographic monitoring of ambulatory patients. Br Med J 1976;2:609–611.
19. Judson P, Holmes DR, Baker WP. Evaluation of outpatient arrhythmias utilizing transtelephonic monitoring. Am Heart J 1979;97:759–761.
20. David D, Michelson EL. Transtelephonic electrocardiographic monitoring for the detection and treatment of cardiac arrhythmias. Cardiovasc Clin 1988;18:73–82.
21. Hasin Y, David D, Rogel S. Transtelephonic adjustment of antiarrhythmic therapy in ambulatory patients. Cardiology 1978;63:243–247.
22. Hall PA, Atwood JE, Myers J, Froelicher VF. The signal averaged surface electrocardiogram and the identification of late potentials. Prog Cardiovasc Dis 1989;31:295–317.
23. Berbari EJ, Lazzara R, Samet P, Scherlag BJ. Non-invasive technique for detection of electrical activity during the PR segment. Circulation 1973;48:1005–1013.
24. Denes P, Santarelli P, Hauser RG, et al. Quantitative analysis of the high frequency components of the terminal portion of the body surface QRS in normal subjects and in patients with ventricular tachycardia. Circulation 1983;67:1129–1138.
25. Cain ME, Ambos HD, Witkowski FX, Sobel BE. Fast Fourier transform analysis of signal averaged electrocar-

diograms for identification of patients prone to sustained ventricular tachycardia. Circulation 1984;69:711–720.

26. Cain ME, Ambos HD, Markham J, et al. Quantification of differences in frequency content of signal averaged electrocardiograms in patients with compared to those without sustained ventricular tachycardia. Am J Cardiol 1985;55:1500–1505.

27. Lindsay BD, Ambos HD, Schechtman KB, Cain ME. Improved selection of patients for programmed ventricular stimulation by frequency analysis of signal averaged electrocardiograms. Circulation 1986;73:675–683.

28. Kuchar DL, Thorburn CW, Sammel NL. Late potential detected after myocardial infarction: natural history and prognostic significance. Circulation 1986;74:1280–1289.

29. Kanovsky MS, Falcone RA, Dresden CA, et al. Identification of patients with ventricular tachycardia after myocardial infarction; signal averaged electrocardiogram, Holter monitoring, and cardiac catheterization. Circulation 1984;70:264–270.

30. Damato AN, Lau SH, Helfant RH, et al. Study of atrioventricular conduction in man using electrode catheter recordings of His bundle activity. Circulation 1969; 39:287–296.

31. Fisher JD, Cohen HL, Mehra R, et al. Cardiac pacing and pacemakers II. Serial electrophysiologic-pharmacologic testing for control of recurrent tachyarrhythmias. Am Heart J 1977;93: 658–668.

32. Horowitz LH, Josephson ME, Farshidi A, et al. Recurrent sustained ventricular tachycardia. 3. Role of the electrophysiologic study selection of antiarrhythmic regimens. Circulation 1978;58: 986–997.

33. Josephson ME, Seides SF. Clinical Cardiac Electrophysiology. Techniques and Interpretations. Philadelphia: Lea & Febiger, 1979.

34. Prystowsky EN. Electrophysiologic-electropharmacologic testing in patients with ventricular arrhythmias. PACE 1988;11:225–251.

35. Skale BT, Miles WM, Heger JJ, et al. Survivors of cardiac arrest: prevention of recurrence as predicted by electrophysiologic testing or electrocardiographic monitoring. Am J Cardiol 1986;57:113–119.

36. Fisher JDF. Pull-out His bundle/electrophysiologic studies using leads previously inserted via the subclavian vein. PACE 1985;8:671–677.

37. Gallagher JJ, Smith WM, Kasell J, et al. Use of the esophageal lead in the diagnosis of mechanisms of reciprocating supraventricular tachycardia. PACE 1980; 3:440–451.

38. Copeland GD, Tullis IF, Brody DA. Clinical evaluation of a new esophageal electrode, with particular reference to the bipolar esophageal electrogram. Part I. Normal sinus mechanism. Am Heart J 1959;57:862–873.

39. Benson DW Jr. Transesophageal electrocardiography and cardiac pacing: state of the art. Circulation 1987;75: III86–III90.

40. Arzbaecher R. A pill electrode for the study of cardiac arrhythmia. Med Instrum 1978;12:277–280.

41. Fisher JD, Kim SG, Furman S, et al. Role of implantable pacemakers in control of recurrent ventricular tachycardia. Am J Cardiol 1982;49:194–206.

42. Fletcher R, Cohen A, DelNegro A. Noninvasive electrophysiologic studies using implanted pacemakers. In: Barold S, ed. Modern Cardiac Pacing. Mount Kisco, NY: Futura Publishing, 1985:421–428.

43. Fletcher R, Keimel J, Larca L, et al. Noninvasive serial electrophysiologic testing using an implanted pacemaker to track chest wall stimuli. PACE 1981;4:A11-A17.

44. Fisher JD, Mehra R, Furman S. Termination of ventricular tachycardia with bursts of ventricular pacing. Am J Cardiol 1978;41:94–102.

45. Friehling TD, Marinchak RA, Kowey PR. Role of permanent pacemakers in pharmacologic therapy of patients with reentrant tachyarrhythmias. PACE 1988; 11:83–92.

46. Sung RJ, Huycke EC, Lai WT, et al. Clinical and electrophysiologic mechanisms of exercise-induced ventricular tachyarrhythmias. PACE 1988;11: 1347–1357.

47. Grayboys TB, Lown B, Podrid PJ, DeSilva RA. Long-term survival of patients with malignant ventricular arrhythmia treated with antiarrhythmic drugs. Am J Cardiol 1982;50: 437–443.

48. Allen SC, Taylor CL, Hall VE. A study of orthostatic insufficiency by the tilt board method. Am J Physiol 1945;143:11–17.

49. Kenny RA, Ingram A, Bayliss J, Sutton R. Head up tilt: a useful test for investigating unexplained syncope. Lancet 1986;1:1352–1354.

50. Milstein S, Reyes WJ, Benditt DG. Upright body tilt for evaluation of patients with recurrent, unexplained syncope. PACE 1989;12:117–124.

51. Withering W. An Account of the Foxglove and Some of Its Medical Uses with Practical Remarks on Dropsy and Other Diseases. Birmingham, England: M. Sweeney, 1785.

52. Selzer A, Wray HW. Quinidine syncope: Paroxysmal ventricular fibrillation occurring during treatment of chronic atrial arrhythmias. Circulation 1964;30: 17–26.

53. Velebit V, Podrid P, Lown B, et al. Aggravation and provocation of ventricular arrhythmias by antiarrhythmic drugs. Circulation 1982;65:886–894.

54. Morganroth J, Horowitz LN. Flecainide: its proarrhythmic effect and expected changes on the surface electrocardiogram. Am J Cardiol 1984;58:89A-94A.

55. Podrid PJ, Lampert S, Graboys TB, et al. Aggravation of arrhythmia by antiarrhythmic drugs—incidence and predictors. Am J Cardiol 1987;59:38E-44E.

56. The Cardiac Arrhythmia Suppression Trial Investigators. Preliminary report: effect of encainide and flecainide on mortality in a randomized trial of arrhythmia suppression after myocardial infarction. N Engl J Med 1989;321:406–412.

57. Zipes DP. Proarrhythmic effects of antiarrhythmic drugs. Am J Cardiol 1987;59:26E-31E.

58. Morganroth J. Risk factors for the development of proarrhythmic events. Am J Cardiol 1987;59:32E-37E.

59. Chadda KD, Barry MF, Bodenheimer MM. Efficacy of out-of-hospital self-injectable intramuscular lidocaine in patients with ventricular tachycardia. PACE 1987;10:988.

60. Capone RJ, Visco J, Curwen E. The effect of early prehospital transtelephonic coronary intervention on morbidity and mortality: experience with 284 post-myocardial infarction patients in a pilot program. Am Heart J 1984;107:1153–1160.

61. Chadda KD, Miller K, Kammerer RJ, Bodenheimer MM. External countershock by family members of victims of out-of-hospital sudden death. PACE 1987;10: 975.

62. Dalzell GWN, Cunningham SR, Pouzina S. Transtelephonic synchronized cardioversion. PACE 1987; 10:975.

63. Reddy CP, Todd EP, Kuo CS, DeMaria AN. Treatment of ventricular tachycardia using an automatic

scanning extrastimulus pacemaker. J Am Coll Cardiol 1984;3:225–230.

64. Palakurthy PR, Slater D. Automatic implantable scanning/burst pacemakers for recurrent tachyarrhythmias. PACE 1988;11:185–192.

65. Davies DW, Butrous GS, Spurrell RA, Camm AJ. Pacing techniques in the prophylaxis of junctional re-entry tachycardia. PACE 1987;10:519–532.

66. Mirowski M, Reid PR, Mower MM, et al. Termination of malignant ventricular arrhythmias with an implanted automatic defibrillator in human beings. N Engl J Med 1980;303:322–324.

67. Echt DS, Armstrong K, Schmidt P, et al. Clinical experience, complications and survival in 70 patients with the automatic implantable cardioverter/defibrillator. Circulation 1985;71:289–296.

68. Cohen AI, Wish MH, Fletcher RD. The use and interaction of permanent pacemakers and the automatic implantable cardioverter/defibrillator. PACE 1988;11:704–711.

69. Kim SG, Furman S, Waspe LE, et al. Unipolar pacer artifacts induced failure of an automatic implantable cardioverter/defibrillator to detect ventricular fibrillation. Am J Cardiol 1986;57:880–881.

70. Kim SG, Furman S, Matos JA, et al. Automatic implantable cardioverter/defibrillator: inadvertent discharges during permanent pacemaker magnet tests. PACE 1987;10:579–582.

25

OUTPATIENT MANAGEMENT OF SEVERE CONGESTIVE HEART FAILURE

Stuart D. Katz, Mark H. Goldberger, Nuala Ronan, and Christine Lawrence[a]

CHAPTER AT A GLANCE: This chapter reviews the evaluation and treatment of patients with severe congestive heart failure. The therapeutic options are detailed and an illustrative case report is presented. Criteria for identifying patients likely to benefit from home intravenous positive inotropic therapy, and guidelines for the use of home intravenous positive inotropic therapy, are outlined.

Introduction

Congestive heart failure (CHF) is an increasingly common cardiovascular disorder in the United States, with an estimated prevalence of more than 2 million cases and more than 400,000 new cases diagnosed each year (1, 2). Heart failure was listed as the primary discharge diagnosis in almost 600,000 hospitalizations in 1985, and it accounted for almost 4 million outpatient office visits (3). Healthcare costs related to the diagnosis of congestive heart failure are conservatively estimated to exceed $10 billion annually. Despite recent advances in the treatment of CHF, the prognosis associated with this diagnosis remains grim, with an estimated 5-year mortality of 50% (2, 4). Approximately one-half of the deaths related to CHF are sudden; that is, occurring within 1 hour of the onset of unstable symptoms (1). The remaining patients die of progressive ventricular failure and are often subject to repeated, prolonged hospitalizations. In an era when concerns over rising healthcare costs are gaining wide public recognition and managed care and diagnosis-related groups (DRGs) are limiting hospital revenues, the concept of outpatient management of severe CHF has financial appeal that has acquired the support of some major private insurance carriers (5). The pathophysiology and conventional treatment of CHF are the subjects of recent reviews (6–8). Accordingly, this chapter is limited to considerations directly pertinent to the intensive homecare of patients with advanced heart failure.

Identification of Candidates for Intensive Homecare

Recognition of the clinical signs and symptoms of advanced heart failure is necessary to identify patients most likely to benefit from home

---

[a]*Marie Galvao contributed to this chapter in the first edition.*

Table 25.1. Clinical Conditions That May Precipitate Acute Congestive Heart Failure

Infection (viral or bacterial)
Anemia (hemoglobin < 10 mg/dL)
Myocardial ischemia
Arrhythmias
Thyrotoxicosis
Noncompliance with medical regimen
Noncompliance with dietary sodium restriction
Adverse drug effects
    Negative inotropic agents
        β-blocking agents
        Calcium channel antagonists
        Antiarrhythmic agents
    Nonsteroidal anti-inflammatory agents

intensive therapy. When evaluating an episode of decompensated CHF in a previously stable patient, the presence of underlying precipitating factors must be considered before the clinical deterioration can be attributed to the natural progression of the disease. Common conditions associated with worsening heart failure are listed in Table 25.1. Most of these factors will be readily apparent from the initial history, physical examination, and laboratory data. Identification of precipitating factors is important, because many patients will improve dramatically once the underlying cause of decompensation has been corrected. Medical and

Table 25.2. Clinical Characteristics of High-Risk Patients with Advanced Heart Failure

Absence of precipitating factors
More than three hospital admissions within the
   last 6 months
Duration of CHF symptoms >2 years
Left ventricular ejection fraction <20%
Systolic blood pressure <90 mm Hg
Resting heart rate >100
Evidence of cachexia and malnutrition
BUN >50 mg/dL or serum creatinine >2.2
   mg/dL
Serum sodium <132 mEq/L
Marked jugular venous distention
Clinical findings of pulmonary hypertension
   (loud P_2, tricuspid regurgitation, RV heave)
Ascites or severe edema above the knees

dietary noncompliance are common causes of decompensated heart failure. Patients should be questioned carefully about medical and dietary compliance, as a more intensive management approach may be costly, ineffective, and perhaps even dangerous in these patients.

The absence of identifiable precipitating factors, along with other clinical features listed in Table 25.2, identify high-risk patients most likely to benefit from intensive home-care after discharge from the acute hospitalization. Early identification of these high-risk patients will lead to more aggressive management in the hospital and facilitate discharge planning to shorten the length of the hospital stay. A therapeutic approach to patients with advanced heart failure is presented below. The discharge planning should include pre-discharge placement of long-term intravenous access devices, psychosocial evaluation to determine whether homecare is appropriate and feasible, and arrangement of specialized home-based nursing support.

CASE REPORT

History and Physical Examination

A.G., a 74-year-old man, was referred to our institution for management of severe heart failure. He had a history of coronary artery disease dating back 15 years, at which time he sustained a myocardial infarction. The patient underwent coronary artery bypass grafting after a second small heart attack 8 years ago. Postoperative ejection fraction was 35%. The patient first presented with clinical congestive heart failure 5 years ago and had a favorable response to medical therapy. For 2 years, he reported slowly progressive exercise intolerance despite a medical regimen that included digoxin, furosemide, and captopril. He had been admitted to the hospital with decompensated congestive heart failure twice in the last 6 months despite good compliance with his medical regimen and low-sodium diet. Left ventricular ejection fraction, determined by radionuclide angiography during his most recent hospitalization, had decreased to 18%.

Over the 4 weeks since his last discharge from the hospital, the patient had been largely house bound, with complaints of severe dyspnea with minimal exertion, anorexia, and sleep disturbance. Over the last 48 hours, symptoms had progressed to dyspnea at rest. No precipitating causes of worsening heart failure listed in Table 25.1 were present. The patient was rehospitalized by his physician and transferred to our institution.

Upon physical examination, the patient appeared fatigued and chronically ill and was noted to have bitemporal wasting. Blood pressure was 90/60; resting heart rate was 100 beats/min. Respiratory rate was 24 breaths per minute. There was jugular venous distention present at 90° with large V waves consistent with the presence of tricuspid regurgitation. Lungs were clear to auscultation with decreased breath sounds throughout all lung fields. On cardiac examination, the point of maximum impulse (PMI) was laterally displaced to the anterior axillary line. There was a soft S_1, a loud P_2 and a harsh systolic murmur consistent with mitral regurgitation. The abdomen was slightly distended, and the liver was noted to be palpable but nontender at the right costal margin. The extremities were somewhat cool to touch and there was a trace amount of pretibial edema. The laboratory evaluation was notable for a serum sodium of 134 mEq/L, a BUN of 55 mg/dL, and a serum creatinine of 1.7 mg/dL.

Therapy for Advanced Congestive Heart Failure

The therapy discussed in this review is appropriate for a patient population with chronic dilated cardiomyopathy and advanced CHF without evidence of active myocardial ischemia, primary valvular heart disease, or other systemic illness.

Patients with advanced heart failure will most often present with clinical evidence of increased plasma volume (pulmonary congestion and edema), systemic hypoperfusion or "low cardiac output syndrome" (borderline hypotension, prerenal azotemia, fatigue), and

more rarely frank cardiogenic shock (symptomatic arterial hypotension with clinical signs of vital organ hypoperfusion). The primary therapeutic goals in these patients are to relieve congestive symptoms and maintain adequate perfusion to vital organs. These goals are achieved through the combined use of sodium restriction, fluid restriction (if serum sodium is below 128 mEq/L), diuretics, vasodilating agents, and positive inotropic agents. A general algorithmic clinical approach for evaluation and treatment of patients with severe heart failure is presented in Figure 25.1 and discussed below.

Diuretics

Diuretics relieve congestive signs by enhancing renal sodium excretion and reducing total-body sodium and water overload. Furosemide, the most commonly used diuretic agent for patients with advanced heart failure, is a loop diuretic that inhibits the ATP-dependent sodium-potassium-chloride cotransport pump in the ascending loop of Henle (9). Since bioavailability after oral dosing is delayed in patients with decompensated CHF (10), an intravenous route of administration is preferred. Doses range from 20 to 160 mg once or twice daily as required to induce a negative fluid balance of 1 to 3 L daily until clinical signs and symptoms of congestion have resolved (absence of jugular venous distention and edema) or pulmonary capillary wedge pressure is less than 20 mm Hg. Daily weight measurements are the simplest method for assessment of diuretic efficacy. Symptomatic patients with edema should lose 1 to 2 kg daily when administered an effective diuretic dose.

Bumetanide is another loop diuretic that is approximately 40 times more potent than furosemide on a milligram basis. Doses range from 0.5 to 5 mg once or twice daily. In contrast to furosemide, bumetanide does not rely entirely on renal tubular secretion for its diuretic action. This theoretical advantage of bumetanide may be clinically important in some patients who do not respond to high doses of intravenous furosemide (11).

Torsemide is a recently introduced loop diuretic that offers greater oral bioavailability

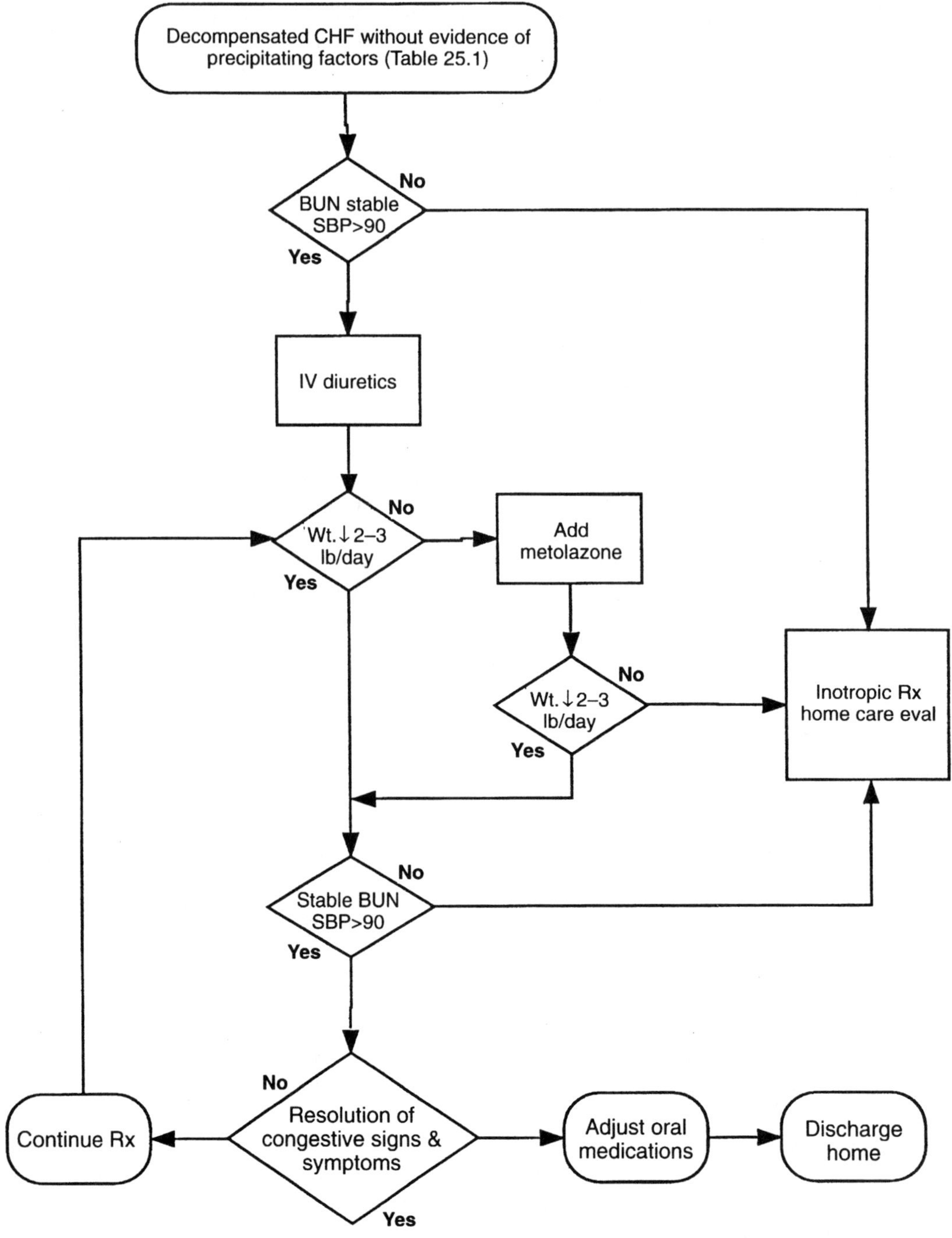

Figure 25.1. Algorithm for initial medical management of patients with decompensated congestive heart failure. Diamond-shaped boxes indicate clinical decision points. Rectangles with square or rounded edges indicate therapeutic options. This algorithm is meant to provide a general guide to therapy; individual treatment plans must be tailored to the patient's needs. This general approach may be appropriate for many patients with the high-risk clinical characteristics listed in Table 25.2. Determination of clinical stability during treatment can be assessed as indicated by following systolic blood pressure and BUN. In addition, appearance of any of the high-risk characteristics listed in Table 25.2 during diuretic therapy is an indication to consider right heart catheterization and addition of positive inotropic therapy. Therapy must be tailored for each patient in a manner that is appropriate for the overall clinical setting.

than furosemide and is approximately twice as potent as furosemide on a milligram basis. Doses range from 20 to 100 mg once or twice daily. The increased oral bioavailability of torsemide may be of particular importance in patients with severe right-sided congestion (12). Controlled trials in patients with advanced liver disease with ascites, and anecdotal experience in patients with severe right-sided congestive heart failure indicate that torsemide may be a more effective oral diuretic agent than furosemide in these clinical settings.

For patients with persistent edema unresponsive to high doses of loop diuretics, the combination of metolazone and a loop diuretic is a synergistic agent in promoting renal sodium excretion through combined inhibition of sodium reabsorption at the proximal and distal tubules and the ascending loop of Henle (13, 14). This combination must be used with caution, however, since metolazone has a long half-life (24 to 36 hours), and prolonged marked diuresis may occur with resultant hypokalemia, hyponatremia, hypovolemia, and hypotension. Metolazone may often be used once or twice weekly in combination with daily loop diuretics. Since the clinical response to metolazone is highly variable, serum electrolytes should be monitored on a daily basis at the initiation of therapy, and potassium supplements should be adjusted accordingly. For patients with recurrent congestion despite high doses of combination oral diuretic therapy, home intravenous diuretics may be considered.

During intravenous diuretic therapy, serum electrolytes must be followed daily and potassium supplements adjusted to maintain serum potassium concentrations of 4.2 to 5.0 mEq/L. Serum magnesium levels do not accurately reflect intracellular magnesium stores (15). Moreover, low serum magnesium levels do not appear to be linked to increased risk of sudden death in patients with advanced heart failure (16). Controlled clinical trials are needed to determine whether the routine long-term use of oral magnesium supplements is beneficial for patients with CHF. In patients requiring large amounts of potassium supplements, in those with low serum magnesium levels, or in patients with clinically significant ventricular arrhythmias, em-

piric oral magnesium supplementation may be considered. The addition of potassium-sparing diuretics, particularly spironolactone (25 to 50 mg twice daily), may also be considered in patients with persistent hypokalemia or hypomagnesemia despite the use of oral potassium and/or magnesium supplements. The combination of spironolactone with angiotensin-converting enzyme (ACE) inhibitors must be used with caution, as life-threatening hyperkalemia may result.

Diuretic therapy is often associated with reduction in renal blood flow and glomerular filtration rate and consequent prerenal azotemia. Increasing prerenal azotemia is not a contraindication to continued diuretic therapy in a patient with persistent signs or symptoms of biventricular congestion. Severe prerenal azotemia indicates greater severity of the underlying heart failure (reduced renal perfusion) and/or coexisting intrinsic renal disease and is a clinical indicator of high-risk patients most likely to benefit from home intensive care.

In diuretic-resistant patients, right heart catheterization should be performed to optimize myocardial loading conditions and determine the need for concomitant positive inotropic support. Low-dose dopamine (1 to 2 μg/kg/min) is a useful adjunctive therapy that increases renal blood flow (17) and promotes sodium excretion through dopaminergic receptor–mediated vasodilation in the renal vasculature (18, 19). Long-term home therapy with low-dose intravenous dopamine may be considered in patients with edema refractory to treatment with high-dose intravenous diuretics. Oral levodopa therapy has also been reported to improve clinical status in patients with advanced heart failure despite a high incidence of gastrointestinal side effects (20).

Vasodilators

In the last decade, ACE inhibitors have been shown to improve functional capacity and reduce mortality in patients with moderate to severe left ventricular systolic dysfunction, with or without concomitant clinical congestive heart failure (21, 22). As the principal benefits of ACE inhibition are long-term improvements in exercise tolerance and survival,

ACE inhibition therapy should generally not be initiated in a decompensated patient until the patient has been clinically stabilized. In patients receiving long-term treatment with ACE inhibitors, therapy may be continued in patients with decompensated heart failure in the absence of arterial hypotension and deterioration of renal function. As with other vasodilating agents, ACE inhibitors should not be initiated in the setting of intravascular volume depletion to avoid side effects of systemic hypotension and azotemia. Diuretics may be reduced or discontinued 1 to 3 days prior to initiation of an ACE inhibitor in patients without clinical signs of congestion, in order to minimize the risk of hypotension.

For patients with baseline hypotension (systolic blood pressure less than 90 mmHg), ACE inhibition therapy should be interrupted until cardiac status has been optimized with the use of positive inotropic agents. However, low systolic arterial pressure is not an absolute contraindication to therapy with ACE inhibitors if clinical signs of organ hypoperfusion are not evident. Small, asymptomatic increases in serum creatinine (0.2 to 0.5 mg/dL) in response to initiation of an ACE inhibitor are to be expected and are not a contraindication to continued therapy. Despite increased serum creatinine, ACE inhibitors increase renal blood flow in patients with CHF (23).

In patients with progressive symptoms despite chronic ACE inhibition therapy, the addition of a second class of vasodilating agents may be considered in the absence of symptomatic hypotension. Organic nitrates mediate vasodilation through activation of soluble guanylate cyclase in vascular smooth muscle (24). Although nitrates are often considered to be primarily venodilating agents, generalized systemic vasodilation occurs with high doses (25). For acute management of decompensated CHF, intravenous nitroglycerin may be rapidly titrated to lower pulmonary capillary wedge pressure and systemic arterial pressure to desired levels. Nitroglycerin acutely reduces mitral regurgitation volume and increases forward cardiac output in this subset of patients (26). Unfortunately, rapid development of tolerance during continuous nitrate infusions is frequently observed (27). For long-term use, isosorbide dinitrate in daily dosage of 160 to 240 mg has been shown to improve exercise capacity in patients with CHF (28). To avoid tolerance, three daily doses may be given at 4-hour intervals either during the day or at night, whenever congestive symptoms are most troublesome (29). Longer-acting isosorbide mononitrate preparations with once- or twice-daily dosing regimens have been shown to prevent the development of tolerance in patients with coronary artery disease and angina but have not been studied in patients with congestive heart failure.

Positive Inotropic Agents

In patients with advanced congestive heart failure, the use of vasodilating agents is often limited by clinically evident tissue hypoperfusion. Clinical manifestations of tissue hypoperfusion include systolic blood pressure below 90 mm Hg, lightheadedness or lethargy, extreme fatigue, cool extremities, oliguria, anorexia, abdominal distress, and prerenal azotemia. Although the safety and efficacy of long-term positive inotropic support as a treatment for patients with advanced congestive heart failure has not been fully documented, clinical practicalities dictate that some patients require such support to maintain adequate perfusion to vital organs. Three classes of positive inotropic agents are currently available for clinical use: digitalis glycosides, synthetic catecholamines, and specific phosphodiesterase inhibitors.

The positive inotropic effects of digitalis glycosides are attenuated in failing myocardium (30). Nonetheless, digoxin has been demonstrated to exert modest beneficial acute hemodynamic effects and improve exercise capacity in patients with severe CHF (31, 32). The risks of digitalis toxicity can be minimized by carefully adjusting the dose in relation to the level of renal function and closely following serum drug levels. Recent controlled clinical trials support the use of digoxin in patients with severe congestive heart failure (33).

Due to its unique pharmacologic and hemodynamic profiles, dobutamine has emerged as the most useful synthetic catecholamine for management of decompensated CHF. By virtue of its agonist activity on β_1, β_2, and α_2 receptors, dobutamine primarily increases cardiac output with relatively small changes in heart rate and systemic arterial pressure (34). The dose must be individually titrated based on hemodynamic criteria, as the hemodynamic response is dependent on baseline hemodynamic function and is highly variable (35). An initial dosage of 2.5 μg/kg/min is recommended, with subsequent upward titrations of 2.5 μg/kg/min at 30- to 60-minute intervals. The effects of therapy may be determined either clinically or by invasive hemodynamic monitoring. Clinical indicators of a beneficial response include an increase in arterial blood pressure, increase in urine output, and subjective improvement in clinical status (decreased fatigue and dyspnea). During hemodynamic monitoring, an increase in cardiac index of 30 to 50% (or cardiac index greater than 2.5 L/min/m^2) without associated excessive tachycardia (more than 20% over baseline heart rate or more than 120 beats/min), or a clinically significant increase in ventricular arrhythmias is desirable. The recommended maximal dosage is 15 μg/kg/min. Although dobutamine increases myocardial oxygen consumption in association with increased inotropy, this metabolic effect is often mitigated by concomitant decreases in myocardial systolic wall stress and does not often induce clinically detected myocardial ischemia as long as excess tachycardia is avoided (36, 37). If clinical signs or symptoms of myocardial ischemia are evident, the addition of nitroglycerin in conjunction with dobutamine or changing to a positive inotropic agent with intrinsic vasodilation properties, such as milrinone, should be considered.

Ideally, dobutamine is utilized to provide temporary inotropic support while reversible causes of decompensation are treated and ventricular loading conditions are optimized by adjusting doses of diuretics and vasodilators. Unfortunately, some patients demonstrate a rapid clinical deterioration when dobutamine therapy is withdrawn, which can be reversed by re-initiation of dobutamine at the previous dosage. These patients have been termed "dobutamine dependent." This term must be used with caution, as no precise definition or reliable physiologic parameters are available for objective determination of dobutamine dependency. In our institution, over 30% of patients referred for dobutamine dependency are eventually weaned from dobutamine following aggressive medical management and a very slow tapering schedule of a 1 μg/kg/min decrease in dosage every 24 hours as tolerated (38). Similarly, Stevenson and colleagues have reported that, following a period of intensive medical management, many severely ill patients receiving inotropic support referred for urgent cardiac transplantation could be successfully weaned from intravenous agents and discharged on an oral medical regimen (39). Patients who are unable to discontinue dobutamine therapy in spite of all efforts have a very poor prognosis and constitute a group of patients who may benefit from home intensive care.

Leier and colleagues were first to report that a short-term (72 hours) infusion of dobutamine was associated with a sustained (1 week) clinical improvement in 68% of patients studied with severe CHF (40). In a subsequent open-label trial, the same investigators reported that following a single 72-hour infusion of dobutamine, clinical improvement was evident for longer than 4 weeks in the majority of the patients studied and persisted for up to 10 months in some patients (41). These clinical findings were confirmed by Liang and colleagues, who used a high dosage of dobutamine (25 μg/ kg/min) in a 4-week placebo-controlled trial (42).

The physiological mechanisms by which a short-term dobutamine infusion induces a sustained clinical response are poorly understood. Changes in left ventricular function are not consistently present after dobutamine therapy and, in any case, are not directly related to changes in exercise capacity (43, 44). Studies examining right ventricular endomyocardial biopsy specimens offer evidence that dobutamine may improve subendocardial myocellular energetics (45, 46). Dobutamine also affects the peripheral circulation. Renal blood flow is increased but skeletal muscle blood does not acutely increase (47). Finally, intermittent dobutamine infusion may induce some of the physiologic changes in cardiac and skeletal muscle blood flow and metabolism associated with exercise (43, 48, 49). Intermittent 30-minute infusions of dobutamine have been shown to induce hemodynamic and metabolic effects in patients with congestive heart failure that resemble those seen in response to physical training (50).

Hemodynamic tolerance during dobutamine infusions lasting longer than 72 hours has been reported (51) and is presumably related to decreased β_1-adrenoceptor density (downregulation) or uncoupling of β_1 receptors from their postreceptor cellular effector mechanisms in the myocardium. However, many patients may be maintained on constant infusions of dobutamine for longer than 72 hours without deterioration in hemodynamic or clinical status. Lack of tolerance may be related to dobutamine's agonist activity on myocardial β_2 and α_2 receptors, which are not downregulated in failing myocardium and which may mediate positive inotropic effects in this setting (52).

Several investigators have conducted open-label trials of intermittent and/or continuous outpatient dobutamine infusions (Table 25.3) (53–60). The results of these trials are difficult to interpret because the study populations are small (fewer than 30 patients) and were generally conducted at a single center. Moreover, most of the trials were conducted without a control group, and objective endpoints of clinical improvement were not reported. Many of these studies were performed before angiotensin-converting enzyme inhibitors were in general use, and in some studies, patients with coronary artery disease were excluded. Doses of dobutamine, hemodynamic endpoints, clinical characteristics of the study populations, concomitant medications, and criteria for the use of dobutamine are vastly different among published studies.

Overall, dobutamine therapy was associated with clinical improvement in these studies. Mortality was high in many of the studies, a finding that is expected in a population with severe CHF (21, 61). Of note, a placebo-controlled trial was stopped prematurely when 15 of 20 deaths in the trial occurred in patients either randomized to or blindly crossed over to dobutamine therapy (60). In this report, although exercise time improved significantly following administration of dobutamine when compared with a placebo, the subjective clinical improvement in the placebo and active treatment groups was similar. In a more recent small, placebo-controlled clinical trial, dobutamine (7.5 to 10 µg/kg/min) infused at 72-hour intervals over 4 weeks was well tolerated and was associated with increased exercise capacity when compared with placebo (58). In an uncontrolled trial in patients awaiting cardiac transplantation, home dobutamine therapy was well tolerated and was associated with clinical improvement in functional capacity (59). Despite aggressive use of antiarrhythmic agents in this study, mortality was high (24%).

The sustained clinical improvement during dobutamine therapy observed in open-label trials may be partially related to correction of the underlying cause of decompensation, close medical follow-up, and improved patient compliance, in addition to the direct pharmacological actions of dobutamine. Nonetheless, based on limited data available from published trials, outpatient dobutamine infusion appears to be effective in the treatment of selected patients with advanced congestive heart failure. Since the risks of long-term dobutamine therapy are uncertain, this therapy should be reserved as a last resort when all other therapeutic options have failed.

The third pharmacologic class of positive inotropic agents is composed of the specific type III phosphodiesterase inhibitors. These agents exhibit both positive inotropic and direct-acting vasodilatory properties mediated by increases in intracellular cyclic AMP (62). Although phosphodiesterase inhibitors have acute hemodynamic effects that are similar to that of dobutamine (63), these agents differ from dobutamine in several important aspects.

Table 25.3. Clinical Trials of Outpatient Dobutamine Infusions

Study (Reference No.)	No. of Patients	Age (yr)	LVEF (%)	NYHA Class	ACE Inhibitors	DBA Dose	DBA Schedule	Outcome
Applefeld et al., 1983 (53)	3	51	13–26	IV	None	1.5–8	48 hr/week	3/3 improved functional class; no mortality at 6 months
Hodgson et al., 1984 (54)	1	19	17	IV	None	6	48 hr/week	Class III at 11 weeks; transplanted at 11 weeks
Krell et al., 1986 (55)	13	62	10–22	III-IV	54%	7.5	48 hr/week	54% improved functional class; 77% mortality at 26 weeks
Applefeld et al., 1987 (56)	21	55	7–30	III-IV	38%	7.1	48 hr/week in 11; continuous in 8	86% improved functional class; 95% mortality at 8.1 months
Miller et al., 1990 (57)	11	54	N/A	IV	All	5	2–6 days/week in 5; continuous in 6	64% improved functional class; 64% eventually weaned of dobutamine; 36% mortality at 29 months
Miller et al., 1991 (59)	25	48	N/A	IV	All	5	80% continuous; 20% intermittent	Improved functional class with dobutamine; 64% transplanted; 24% mortality at 4.5 months
Erlemeier et al., 1992 (58)	20	57	N/A	IV	All	7.5–10	24 hr Q 3 days	Only 1 month follow-up; improved functional class with dobutamine; 10% mortality

Milrinone and amrinone are the two phosphodiesterase inhibitors currently approved for intravenous use. Although milrinone and amrinone produce similar hemodynamic effects, milrinone is the preferred drug of this class because the half-life of milrinone is shorter (2 hours) than that of amrinone (6 to 8 hours), and milrinone has a better side effect profile than amrinone (64). Milrinone is initiated with a bolus dose of 50 μg/kg (administered over 10 to 15 minutes) and an initial infusion rate of 0.5 μg/kg/min. The dose may be adjusted upward at increments of 0.25 μg/kg/min (with concomitant additional bolus doses) to a maximum dose of 1.0 μg/kg/min. Clinical and hemodynamic endpoints of therapy are the same as those for dobutamine. Since milrinone is excreted renally, the dose should be adjusted in patients with elevated serum creatinine.

In contrast to dobutamine, milrinone and amrinone are direct-acting vasodilators as well as positive inotropic agents (65). Due to their combined positive inotropic and vasodilatory actions, neither milrinone nor amrinone increases myocardial oxygen consumption (66). Thus, milrinone may be of particular benefit in patients in whom active myocardial ischemia is suspected to be contributing to the episode of decompensated heart failure. The direct-acting vasodilatory effects of milrinone may also be of benefit in patients with extremely high baseline pulmonary and/or systemic vascular resistance. Despite these direct vasodilatory properties, significant hypotension complicating a careful titration is unusual. In addition, since the action of milrinone is not dependent on adrenergic receptors, hemodynamic tolerance has not been observed (67).

Although the oral form of amrinone was never approved for clinical use because of a high incidence of adverse side effects in a large clinical trial, long-term amrinone infusions, including home infusions, have been reported to be well tolerated (68). However, a controlled trial of long-term therapy with oral milrinone versus placebo demonstrated increased mortality in patients with severe heart failure treated with oral milrinone (69). In contrast, an investigational oral phosphodiesterase inhibitor, enoximone, was associated with improved survival in dobutamine-dependent patients with advanced heart failure (38). Until further information is available, milrinone is recommended only for short-term inotropic support in patients with heart failure.

CASE REPORT CONTINUED

History and physical examination at the time of admission were consistent with biventricular congestive heart failure and a low cardiac output syndrome. Medications at the time of admission included digoxin 0.25 mg daily, furosemide 160 mg daily, and captopril 25 mg TID. The patient was initially treated with intravenous furosemide 160 mg daily. The patient lost several pounds over the first 48 hours of hospitalization but reported no symptomatic improvement. During diuretic therapy, arterial blood pressure decreased to 80/60 mm Hg and the serum creatinine increased to 2.3 mg/dL. During a previous hospitalization for decompensated heart failure, the patient had received dobutamine with right heart catheter monitoring. In response to a dose of 5 μg/kg/min, cardiac index increased from 1.9 to 2.5 mL/min/m^2. Since the patient was deteriorating during diuretic therapy, dobutamine was once again initiated at a dose of 5 μg/kg/min. The patient reported a dramatic relief of dyspnea within 3 hours of the start of therapy.

After 72 hours of dobutamine therapy, blood pressure and creatinine had returned to baseline values. While receiving dobutamine therapy, the patient was able to ambulate in the hallways of the hospital without difficulty. On the fourth day of dobutamine therapy, the dose was lowered to 3 μg/kg/min. Thirty minutes later the patient appeared ashen and was complaining of dyspnea at rest. The dyspnea resolved after increasing dobutamine back to the previous dosage. Another attempt at withdrawing dobutamine therapy was made the next day with similar consequences. Physical examination and laboratory values were otherwise without change.

Investigational Drugs and Devices

For patients with advanced heart failure who are not responding to conventional therapy as discussed above, alternative empiric treatments, including investigational drugs and/or devices, should be considered prior to enrollment into a home dobutamine therapy program. Oral inotropic agents that increase contractility by mechanisms other than phosphodiesterase inhibition are under investigation (70). Other classes of cardiovascular drugs, including β-receptor blocking agents and calcium channel antagonists, appear to be promising in early trials (71). Although it is difficult to implement in severely ill patients, physical training in cardiac rehabilitation programs has been demonstrated to improve exercise capacity and function class in patients with heart failure (72). In lieu of a structured monitored rehabilitation program, all patients should be encouraged to walk as far as their condition allows once or twice daily. Isometric exercise should be avoided. Finally, early clinical investigations with an implantable left ventricular assist device indicate that long-term mechanical support for the failing heart may be a future alternative for patients failing medical therapy (73).

Intensive Homecare of Advanced Heart Failure

For patients with recurrent admissions for decompensated heart failure without obvious precipitating causes, home intensive care is an alternative to repeated hospitalizations (Figure 25.2). Intensive homecare of patients with severe CHF differs from hospital care only by virtue of a change in locale and personnel administering the daily care rather than any substantive change in the principles of management outlined in the previous discussion. Successful home management depends on the proper selection of a compliant patient with good insight into the disease process; a supportive family; reliable home nurses, nurse's aides, therapists, and technicians; and, lastly, good communication between all involved parties and the physician directing care. Clinical considerations for entry into a home dobutamine therapy program are listed in Table 25.4. Guidelines for nursing care plans in the homecare of heart failure patients receiving dobutamine therapy are the subject of recent reviews (74, 75).

Extensive patient education is the essential component of successful homecare therapy (76, 77). Patient education should begin in the hospital setting and continue when the patient is discharged home. Counseling and instruction on a variety of issues—including diet, exercise, medication, and stress reduction—must be provided to the patients and their families on an ongoing basis. Written materials (preferably in the patient's native language) should be given to patients and discussed during outpatient visits and in the homecare setting. For patients who have limited reading ability or language barriers, teaching can be initiated and reinforced with frequent verbal sessions. Patients and their families should be encouraged to be active participants in their plan of care.

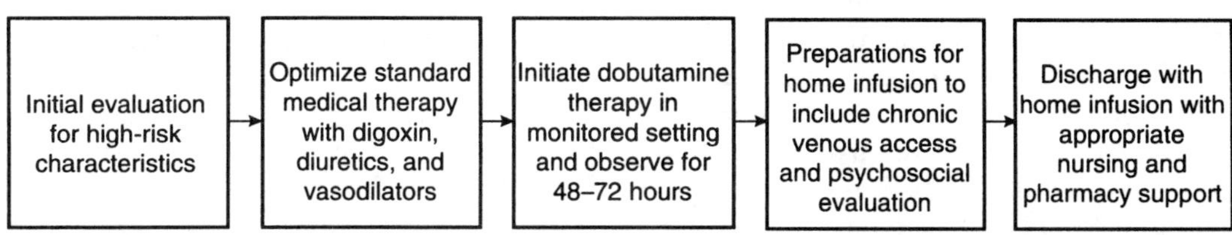

Figure 25.2.   Algorithm for evaluation and treatment of patients with severe heart failure. This general approach is applicable to many patients with the high-risk clinical characteristics listed in Table 25.2. Early discharge planning in these patients will shorten the hospital stay and facilitate the transition to home-based care.

Table 25.4. Clinical Considerations for Entry into a Home Dobutamine Therapy Program

1. Prior to initiation of therapy
    Consider alternative or investigational therapy
- Addition of a second vasodilating agent
- Oral levodopa
- Heart transplantation
- Investigational drugs or devices

    Review psychosocial profile
- Good cognitive function (able to operate pump)
- Adequate insight into disease (able to understand risk/benefit ratio)
- Receptive to educational efforts
- Family support (24-hour companion)
- Outpatient insurance coverage
- Determination of resuscitation status (DNR)

2. Upon initiation of therapy
    Establish chronic central venous access (Hickman, Groshong, or PICC catheter)
    Initiate dobutamine treatment in monitored setting
    Monitor at least 48 hours in hospital to assess for rapid development of tolerance
    Use lowest dose possible to achieve desired clinical effect
    Home nursing and pharmacy support (24-hour availability)
- Patient and family education
- Monitor clinically daily
- Home scale for daily weights
- Monitor serum chemistries 3 to 5 times weekly
- Physician visits as needed

    Careful adjustments in background therapy as needed

To enhance patient compliance, medical regimens should be kept as simple as possible. Patients should understand the purpose for each of their medicines and the importance of compliance with the prescribed regimen. The cost of medications should be discussed, since the cost of prescription drugs is often not covered by insurance and may be an impediment to adequate compliance.

Assiduous management of fluid and electrolyte balance is an extremely important component of successful intensive home-based heart failure treatment. Strict adherence to a 1- or 2-g sodium diet and fluid restriction (if hyponatremia is present) is essential. Extensive education is needed to help patients comply with severe sodium restriction. Accurate daily weights are essential. Many highly motivated patients can also keep a daily log of their intake and output. A weight increase of more than 3 to 5 lb over a 1-week period should be reported to a health care provider.

Based on daily weights, diuretic dosage (either oral or parenteral) and potassium supplementation may be adjusted up or down on a sliding-scale basis (78). The desired "dry" weight may need to be reassessed every few weeks, as most patients with severe CHF exhibit progressive cachexia (79, 80). Serum electrolytes, blood urea nitrogen, and serum creatinine must be monitored at least twice weekly. Drugs that are excreted primarily by the kidney, notably digoxin and most angiotensin-converting enzyme inhibitors, must be continually adjusted for variations in renal function.

Home oxygen therapy may be useful in selected patients. Although hypoxemia is unusual for patients with CHF without evidence of overt pulmonary edema or intrinsic lung disease, sleep apnea and Cheyne-Stokes breathing pattern are common and may merit the use of nocturnal low-flow oxygen supplements (81).

For patients requiring outpatient parenteral positive inotropic and/or diuretic therapy, chronic central venous access with a Hickman catheter has the lowest complication rate (82). Alternative chronic central venous access options include Groshong catheters and peripherally inserted central catheters (PICCs) (83, 84). A double-lumen catheter is often useful to facilitate blood sampling and combination intravenous drug therapy. Proper training of the patient and family is necessary to avoid infectious complications and recurrent hospitalizations. For many patients receiving continuous dobutamine infusions, functional capacity is quite limited, and a standard volumetric pump mounted on a mobile pole with long tubing will allow enough mobility for a bed-to-chair existence. For patients with greater mobility, portable pumps that fit in a shoulder sling are available (85). Portable pumps are preferred over pole-mounted pumps for most patients, as smaller pumps increase ease of ambulating and facilitate the performance of routine activities of daily living (86).

Initiation of intensive homecare therapy is often limited by the availability of adequate social supports and outpatient insurance coverage. The cost of a home infusion pump, drugs, and nursing support is substantially less than the cost of hospital-based care, but is still too high for most patients without adequate insurance. Our own recent clinical experience highlights the difficulties in finding ideal patients for intensive homecare. As a specialized, tertiary referral heart failure center, our institution admits nearly 500 patients annually for acute management of severe heart failure. Over the last year, 40 patients were considered possible candidates for home dobutamine therapy, but only nine patients had adequate insurance coverage. Of these nine patients with end-stage heart failure, three died before hospital discharge, three died within 6 months of discharge, one patient died after 12 months, one patient had dobutamine discontinued after a Groshong catheter infection, and one patient remains ambulatory after 3 months of home therapy.

For patients with severe CHF despite therapy with digoxin, diuretics, and vasodilating agents, prognosis is very poor. These issues must be discussed with the patient, and

his or her wishes regarding resuscitative efforts must be defined clearly. This is especially important with regard to outpatient dobutamine therapy, which—although effective in relieving symptoms—may actually increase mortality. Nonetheless, home dobutamine and intravenous diuretic therapy is an increasingly available option that will improve quality of life for many patients with advanced congestive heart failure.

CASE REPORT CONTINUED

After the second attempt to withdraw dobutamine had failed, arrangements were made to administer continuous dobutamine therapy at home. A Groshong catheter was placed under local anesthesia, and the patient and his wife were instructed in the use of a portable infusion pump. The risks and benefits of home dobutamine therapy, as well as resuscitation status, were discussed. The patient expressed relief to be able to continue dobutamine therapy at home, and, accepting the severe nature of his disease, agreed that a DNR code status was appropriate. The patient was discharged home with continuous dobutamine infusion at a dose of 5 μg/kg/min in addition to his oral medications. While receiving dobutamine at home, the patient remained ambulatory and was able to perform most activities of daily living, including light household chores and shopping. Nursing visits were conducted in the home three times weekly, and physician visits were conducted at the office once monthly. His clinical course was marked by a slow deterioration in functional status over the next 12 months. Episodes of worsening dyspnea and fatigue occurred at 2- to 3-month intervals and were invariably associated with hypotension and worsening azotemia. Each episode of worsening heart failure improved with incremental increases in the dobutamine dose. Eventually, metolazone was added to the diuretic regimen for worsening fluid retention. After 12 months of dobutamine therapy his dose had reached 10 μg/kg/min. The patient died of complications of pneumonia and worsening congestive heart failure after 12 months of dobutamine therapy.

COMMENTARY ON CASE REPORT: *This patient had many typical features of patients who are suitable candidates for dobutamine therapy at home. Continuous dobutamine infusion was associated with a dramatic improvement in the patient's quality of life. Although the patient demonstrated slowly progressive tolerance to the effects of dobutamine during the course of therapy, his condition did not require recurrent hospitalization for over a year. It is important to note that not all patients will experience such a dramatic improvement in functional capacity during dobutamine infusion. Response to dobutamine therapy should be assessed on an inpatient basis, and plans for outpatient dobutamine therapy should be reserved for those patients with the greatest improvement in functional capacity. Dobutamine therapy may also be used in conjunction with cardiac rehabilitation to improve functional capacity in patients with advanced heart failure and severe deconditioning.*

Summary

- Patients with severe congestive heart failure who are at high risk for recurrent hospital admissions can usually be identified from routine data collected in the initial history and physical examination.
- Patients with clinical risk factors for recurrent hospital admissions for heart failure should be identified early to ensure adequate time for arrangement of homecare.
- Conventional therapy for severe congestive heart failure includes high-dose diuretics, digoxin, angiotensin-converting enzyme inhibitors, and possibly additional vasodilators, if blood pressure allows.
- Home therapy with dobutamine, milrinone, and/or intravenous diuretics should be considered when an aggressive oral medical regimen has failed and the patient demonstrates an improvement in functional class in response to inpatient intravenous positive inotropic support.

References

1. Smith WF. Epidemiology of congestive heart failure. Am J Cardiol 1985;55:3A-8A.
2. Garg R, Packer M, Pitt B, Yusuf S. Heart failure in the 1990s: evolution of a major public health problem in cardiovascular medicine. J Am Coll Cardiol 1993;22 (Suppl A):3A-5A.
3. Gillum RF. Heart failure in the United States 1970–1985. Am Heart J 1987;113:1043–1045.
4. Kannel WB, Plehn JF, Copples LA. Cardiac failure and sudden death in the Framingham study. Am Heart J 1988;115:869–875.
5. Reinhardt UE. Future trends in the economics of medical practice and care. Am J Cardiol 1985;56:50C-59C.
6. Mancini DM, LeJemtel TH, Factor S, Sonnenblick EH. Central and peripheral components of cardiac failure. Am J Med 1986;80(Suppl 2B):2–13.
7. Packer M. Pathophysiology of chronic heart failure [Review]. Lancet 1992;340(8811):88–92.
8. Packer M. Treatment of chronic heart failure [see comments] [Review]. Lancet 1992;340(8811):92–95.
9. Puschett JB. Clinical pharmacological implications in diuretic selection. Am J Cardiol 1986;57(Suppl): 6A-13A.
10. Vasko MR, Brown-Cartwright D, Knochel JP, Nixon JV, Brater DC. Furosemide absorption altered in decompensated congestive heart failure. Ann Intern Med 1985;102:314–318.
11. Feig PV. Cellular mechanism of action of loop diuretics: implications for drug effectiveness and adverse effects. Am J Cardiol 1986;57(Suppl):14A-19A.
12. Dunn CJ, Fitton A, Brogden RN. Torasemide: an update of its pharmacological properties and therapeutic efficacy. Drugs 1995;49:121–142.
13. Friedland JS, Ledingham JGG. Oral metolazone plus furosemide for home therapy in patients with refractory heart failure. Lancet 1989;1:727–728.
14. Ghose RR, Gupta SK. Synergistic action of metolazone with loop diuretics. Br Med J 1981;282:1432–1433.
15. Ralston MA, Murnane MR, Kelley RE, Atschuld RA, Unverferth DV, Leier CV. Magnesium content of serum, circulating mononuclear cells, skeletal muscle and myocardium in congestive heart failure. Circulation 1989;80:573–580.
16. Eichhorn EJ, Tandon PK, DiBianco R, Timmis GC, Fenster PE, Shannon J, et al. Clinical and prognostic significance of serum magnesium concentration in patients with severe chronic congestive heart failure: the PROMISE Study. J Am Coll Cardiol 1993;21(3): 634–640.
17. Maskin CS, Ocken S, Chadwick B, LeJemtel TH. Comparative systemic and renal effects of dopamine and angiotensin converting inhibition with enalaprilat in heart failure. Circulation 1985;72:364–369.
18. Goldberg LI, McDonald RH, Zimmerman AM. Sodium diuresis produced by dopamine in patients with congestive heart failure. N Engl J Med 1963; 269:1060–1064.
19. Goldberg LI. Cardiovascular and renal actions of dopamine: potential clinical application. Pharmacol Rev 1972;24:1–29.

20. Rajfer SI, Rossen JD, Nemanich JW, Douglas FL, Davis F, Osinski J. Sustained hemodynamic improvement during long-term therapy with levodopa in heart failure: role of plasma catecholamines. J Am Coll Cardiol 1987;10(6):1286–1293.

21. The CONSENSUS Trial Study Group. Effects of enalapril on mortality in severe congestive heart failure. N Engl J Med 1987;316:1429–1435.

22. The SOLVD Investigators. Effect of enalapril on survival in patients with reduced left ventricular ejection fractions and congestive heart failure. N Engl J Med 1991;325:293–302.

23. LeJemtel TH, Maskin CS, Mancini D, Sinoway L, Feld H, Chadwick B. Systemic and regional hemodynamic effects of captopril administered alone and concomitantly in patients with heart failure. Circulation 1985;72:364–369.

24. Abrams J. Pharmacology of nitroglycerin and long-acting nitrates. Am J Cardiol 1985;56:12A-18A.

25. Imhof PR, Ott B, Frankhauser P, Chu LC, Hodler J. Difference in nitroglycerin dose response in venous and arterial beds. Eur J Clin Pharmacol 1980;18:455–460.

26. Keren G, Katz S, Strom J, Sonnenblick EH, LeJemtel TH. Dynamic mitral regurgitation. An important determinant of the hemodynamic response to load alterations and inotropic therapy in severe heart failure. Circulation 1989;80(2):306–313.

27. Packer M, Lee WH, Kessler PD, Gottlieb SS, Medina N, Yushak M. Prevention and reversal of nitrate tolerance in patients with congestive heart failure. N Engl J Med 1987;317:799–804.

28. Franciosa JA, Goldsmith SR, Cohn JN. Contrasting immediate and long-term effects of isosorbide dinitrate on exercise capacity in congestive heart failure. Am J Med 1980;69:559–566.

29. Parker JO, Fung H-L, Ruggirello D, Stone JA. Tolerance to isosorbide dinitrate: rate of development and reversal. Circulation 1983;68:1074–1080.

30. Spann JFJ, Buccino RA, Sonnenblick EH, Braumwald E. Contractile state of cardiac muscle obtained from cats with experimentally produced ventricular hypertrophy and heart failure. Circ Res 1967;21:341–354.

31. Gheorghiade M, St. Clair J, St. Clair C, Beller GA. Hemodynamic effects of intravenous digoxin in patients with severe heart failure initially treated with diuretics and vasodilators. J Am Coll Cardiol 1987;9:849–857.

32. Lee DC-S, Johnson RA, Bingham JB, et al. Heart failure in outpatients: a randomized trial of digoxin versus placebo. N Engl J Med 1983;308:363–368.

33. Packer M, Gheorghiade M, Young JB, Costantini PJ, Adams KF, Cody RJ, et al. Withdrawal of digoxin from patients with chronic heart failure treated with angiotensin-converting-enzyme inhibitors. RADIANCE Study [see comments]. N Engl J Med 1993;329(1):1–7.

34. Sonnenblick EH, Frishman WH, LeJemtel TH. Dobutamine: a new synthetic cardioactive sympathetic amine. N Engl J Med 1979;300:17–22.

35. LeJemtel TH, Keren G, Reis D, et al. The role of novel inotropic agents in the treatment of heart failure. J Cardiovasc Pharmacol 1986;8(Suppl 9):S47-S54.

36. Kupper W, Waller D, Hanrath P, et al. Hemodynamic and cardiac metabolic effects of inotropic stimulation with dobutamine in patients with coronary artery disease. Eur Heart J 1982;3:29–34.

37. Pozen RG, DiBianco R, Katz RJ, Bortz R, Meyerburg RJ, Fletcher RD. Myocardial metabolic and hemodynamic effects of dobutamine in heart failure complicating coronary artery disease. Circulation 1981;63:1279–1285.

38. Jondeau G, Dubourg O, Delorme G, Arnal JF, Chikli F, Kamoun L, et al. Oral enoximone as a substitute for intravenous catecholamine support in end-stage congestive heart failure. Eur Heart J 1994;15(2):242–246.

39. Stevenson LW, Dracup KA, Tillisch JH. Efficacy of medical therapy tailored for severe congestive heart failure in patients transferred for urgent cardiac transplantation. Am J Cardiol 1989;63:461–464.

40. Leier CV, Webel J, Bush CA. The cardiovascular effects of the continuous infusion of dobutamine in patients with severe cardiac failure. Circulation 1977;56(3):468–472.

41. Unverferth DV, Magorien RD, Lewis RP, Leier CV. Long-term benefit of dobutamine in patients with congestive cardiomyopathy. Am Heart J 1980;100(5):622–630.

42. Liang CS, Sherman LG, Doherty JU, Wellington K, Lee VW, Hood WB. Sustained improvement of cardiac function in patients with congestive heart failure after short-term infusion of dobutamine. Circulation 1984;69:113–119.

43. Leier CV, Huss P, Lewis RP, Unverferth DV. Drug-induced conditioning in congestive heart failure. Circulation 1982;65(7):1382–1387.

44. Maskin CS, Forman R, Sonnenblick EH, Frishman WH, LeJemtel TH. Failure of dobutamine to increase exercise capacity despite hemodynamic improvement in severe chronic heart failure. Am J Cardiol 1983;51(1):177–182.

45. Unverferth DV, Leier CV, Magorien RD, Croskery R, Svirbely JR, Kolibash AJ, et al. Improvement of human myocardial mitochondria after dobutamine: a quantitative ultrastructural study. J Pharmacol Exp Ther 1980;215(2):527–532.

46. Unverferth DV, Magorien RD, Altschuld R, Kolibash AJ, Lewis RP, Leier CV. The hemodynamic and metabolic advantages gained by a three-day infusion of dobutamine in patients with congestive cardiomyopathy. Am Heart J 1983;106(1 Pt 1):29–34.

47. Leier CV, Heban PT, Huss P, Bush CA, Lewis RP. Comparative systemic and regional hemodynamic effects of dopamine and dobutamine in patients with cardiomyopathic heart failure. Circulation 1978;58:466–475.

48. Liang CS, Tuttle RR, Hood WB, Gavras H. Conditioning effects of chronic infusions of dobutamine. Comparison with exercise training. J Clin Invest 1979;64:613–619.

49. Sullivan MJ, Binkley PF, Unverferth DV, Ren JH, Boudoulas H, Bashore TM, et al. Prevention of bedrest-induced physical deconditioning by daily dobutamine infusions. Implications for drug-induced physical conditioning. J Clin Invest 1985;76(4):1632–1642.

50. Adamopoulos S, Piepoli M, Qiang F, Pissimissis E, Davies M, Bernardi L, et al. Effects of pulsed beta-stimulant therapy on beta-adrenoceptors and chronotropic responsiveness in chronic heart failure. Lancet 1995;345:344–349.

51. Unverferth DA, Blanford M, Kates RE, Leier CV. Tolerance to dobutamine after a 72 hour continuous infusion. Am J Med 1980;69(2):262–266.

52. Hayes JS, Bowling N, Pollack GD. Effects of β-receptor down regulation on the cardiovascular responses to the stereoisomers of dobutamine. J Pharmacol Exp Ther 1985;235:58–65.

53. Applefeld MM, Newman KA, Grove WR, Sutton FJ, Roffman DS, Reed WP, et al. Intermittent, continuous outpatient dobutamine infusion in the management of congestive heart failure. Am J Cardiology 1983;51(3): 455–458.

54. Hodgson JM, Aja M, Sorkin RP. Intermittent ambulatory dobutamine infusions for patients awaiting cardiac transplantation. Am J Cardiol 1984;53:375–376.

55. Krell MJ, Kline EM, Bates ER, Hodgson JM, Dilworth LR, Laufer N, et al. Intermittent, ambulatory dobutamine infusions in patients with severe congestive heart failure. Am Heart J 1986;112(4):787–791.

56. Applefeld MM, Newman KA, Sutton FJ, Reed WP, Roffman DS, Talesnick BS, et al. Outpatient dobutamine and dopamine infusions in the management of chronic heart failure: clinical experience in 21 patients. Am Heart J 1987;114(3):589–595.

57. Miller LW, Merkle EJ, Herrmann V. Outpatient dobutamine for end-stage congestive heart failure. Crit Care Med 1990;18(1 Pt 2):s30–33.

58. Erlemeier HH, Kupper W, Bleifeld W. Intermittent infusion of dobutamine in the therapy of severe congestive heart failure—long-term effects and lack of tolerance. Cardiovasc Drugs Ther 1992;6(4):391–398.

59. Miller LW, Merkle EJ, Jennison SH. Outpatient use of dobutamine to support patients awaiting heart transplantation. J Heart Lung Transplant 1994;13(4): 126–129.

60. Dies F, Krell MJ, Whitlaw P, et al. Intermittent dobutamine in ambulatory patients with chronic cardiac failure. Circulation 1986;74(Suppl II):II-38.

61. Cohn JN, Archibald DG, Ziesche S, Franciosa JA, Harston WE, Tristani FE, et al. Effect of vasodilator therapy on mortality in chronic congestive heart failure. N Engl J Med 1986;314:1547–1552.

62. Endoh M, Yamashita S, Taira N. Positive inotropic effect of amrinone in relation to cyclic nucleotide metabolism in canine ventricular muscle. J Pharmacol Exp Ther 1982;221:775–783.

63. Biddle TL, Benotti JR, Creager MA, Faxon DP, Firth BG, Fitzpatrick PG, et al. Comparison of intravenous milrinone and dobutamine for congestive heart failure secondary to either ischemic or dilated cardiomyopathy. Am J Cardiol 1987;59(15):1345–1350.

64. Baim DS, McDowell AV, Cherniles J, Monrad ES, Parker JA, Edelson J, et al. Evaluation of a new bipyridine inotropic agent—milrinone—in patients with severe congestive heart failure. N Engl J Med 1983;309(13):748–756.

65. Cody RJ, Muller FB, Kubo SH, Rutman H, Leonard D. Identification of the direct vasodilator effect of milrinone with an isolated limb preparation in patients with chronic congestive heart failure. Circulation 1986; 73(1):124–129.

66. Monrad ES, Baim DS, Smith HS, Lanoue A, Brauwald E, Grossman W. Effects of milrinone on coronary hemodynamics and myocardial energetics in patients with congestive heart failure. Circulation 1985;71(5): 972–979.

67. Maskin CS, Forman R, Klein NA, Sonnenblick EH, LeJemtel TH. Long-term amrinone therapy in patients with severe heart failure: drug-dependent hemodynamic benefits despite progression of disease. Am J Med 1982;72(1):113–118.

68. Maskin CS. Intermittent parenteral inotropic therapy in patients with chronic heart failure: concept and clinical results. Heart Failure 1986;2:117–127.

69. Packer M, Carver JR, Rodeheffer RJ, Ivanhoe RJ, DiBianco R, Zeldis SM, et al. Effect of oral milrinone on mortality in severe chronic heart failure. The PROMISE Study Research Group [see comments]. N Engl J Med 1991;325(21):1468–1475.

70. Katz SD, Kubo SH, Jessup M, Brozena S, Troha JM, Wahl J, et al. A multicenter, randomized, double-blind placebo-controlled trial of pimobendan, a new cardiotonic and vasodilator agent, in patients with severe congestive heart failure. Am Heart J 1992;123:95–103.

71. Fowler MB. Beta-blockers in heart failure: potential of carvedilol [Review]. J Hum Hypertens 1993;7(Suppl 1):562–567.

72. Coats AJS, Adamopoulos S, Radaelli A, McCance A, Meyer TE, Bernardi L, et al. Controlled trial of physical training in chronic heart failure. Exercise performance, hemodynamics, ventilation, and autonomic function. Circulation 1992;85:2119–2131.

73. McCarthy PM. HeartMate implantable left ventricular assist device: bridge to transplantation and future applications [Review]. Ann Thorac Surg 1995;59(Suppl 2):S46-S51.

74. Coffin MR. Dobutamine infusion for the treatment of congestive heart failure in the home care setting. J Intravenous Nursing 1994;17(3):145–150.

75. Sherman A. Critical care management of the heart failure patient in the home [Review]. Critical Care Nursing Quarterly 1995;18(1):77–87.

76. Dracup K, Baker DW, Dunbar SB, Dacey RA, Brooks NH, Johnson JC, et al. Management of heart failure. II. Counseling, education, and lifestyle modifications. JAMA 1994;272(18):1442–1446.

77. Hagenhoff BD, Feutz C, Conn VS, Sagehorn KK, Moranville HM. Patient education needs as reported by congestive heart failure patients and their nurses. J Adv Nursing 1994;19(4):685–690.

78. Hattersley AT, Langley S, Thompson JR, Blackwood RA. Home intravenous diuretic therapy for patients with refractory heart failure. Lancet 1989;1:446.

79. Levine B, Kalman J, Mayer L, Fillit HM, Packer M. Elevated circulating levels of tumor necrosis factor in severe chronic heart failure. N Engl J Med 1990;323: 236–241.

80. Quinn T, Askanazi J. Nutrition and cardiac disease. Crit Care Clin 1987;3:167–184.

81. Hanly PJ, Millar TW, Steljes DG, Baert R, Frais MA, Kryger MH. Respiration and abnormal sleep in patients with congestive heart failure. Chest 1989;96: 480–488.

82. Hickman RO, Buckner CD, Cliff RA, Sanders JE, Stewart P, Thomas ED. A modified right atrial catheter for access to the venous system in transplant recipients. Surg Gynecol Obstet 1979;148:871–875.

83. Graham DR, Keldermans MM, Klemm LW, Semenza NJ, Shafer ML. Infectious complications among patients receiving home intravenous therapy with peripheral, central, or peripherally placed central venous catheters. Am J Med 1991;91:3B.

84. Lam S, Scannell R, Roessler D, Smith MA. Peripherally inserted central catheters in an acute-care hospital. Arch Intern Med 1994;154(16):1833–1837.

85. Bernstein LH, Brink SJ, Homza S, Stewart IE. Portable medicine pumps in primary care. Patient Care 1993; 27:91–115.

86. Koeppen MA, Caspers SM. Problems identified wit home infusion pumps. J Intravenous Nursing 1994;17:151–156.

26

HOME POSITIVE-PRESSURE VENTILATORY SUPPORT FOR RESPIRATORY FAILURE DUE TO PULMONARY DISEASE

William D. Marino[a]

CHAPTER AT A GLANCE: This chapter reviews the evolution of home-based positive-pressure mechanical ventilation for respiratory failure due to lung disease. Modes of interface between ventilator and patient (tracheostomy, mouth masks, full-face masks, nasal masks, and the Pneumobelt) are described and evaluated with regard to their specific utility. Noninvasive positive-pressure ventilation (NIPPV), its utility in acute and chronic hypercapnic respiratory failure, the probable mechanisms of benefit from NIPPV, and specific aspects of its application are reviewed in detail.

Introduction

Since the introduction in the late 1950s of positive-pressure ventilators, it has been clear that a subpopulation of patients requiring mechanical ventilation for acute respiratory failure are unable to regain the capacity for long-term independent ventilation. This may be the result of the severity of the acute lung injury (e.g., Paraquat lung) or of chronic conditions such as neuromuscular disease or chronic lung disease. In patients with restrictive or obstructive lung disease, an acute exacerbating condition such as infection or left ventricular failure may result in total dependence on assisted ventilation.

As these patients have increased in number, strategies for meeting their special needs have been adopted. Chronic respiratory care institutions, such as New York's Goldwater and Bird S. Coler Hospitals, quickly became (and remain) filled with respirator-dependent patients. The only hope these patients had for living outside of an institution was the provision of full-time home mechanical ventilation via permanent tracheostomy. This technique was used sporadically, as documented in several case reports (1–4).

Stemming from the success of such infrequent home ventilator use and the concurrent success of negative-pressure intermittent ventilation at home (5–8), studies began in the 1970s on the use of intermittent positive-pressure ventilatory support via fenestrated tracheostomy tubes (Fig. 26.1) (6, 9, 10). This was done primarily in patients who were not

---

[a]*Vladimir Kvetan contributed to this chapter in the first edition.*

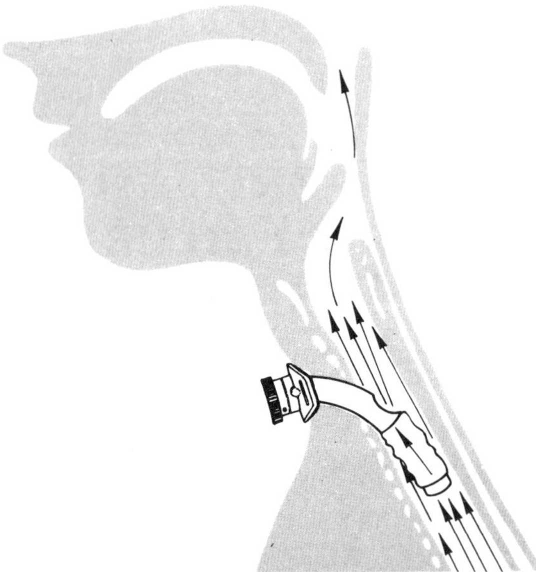

Figure 26.1.   Fenestrated tracheostomy tube in situ, showing laryngeal airflow with plug in place. When plug is removed, airflow occurs through this tube. (Courtesy of the Shiley Company, Irvine, CA.)

constantly ventilator-dependent but were in borderline chronic respiratory failure. It seemed that patients responded to this therapy, as they did to intermittent negative pressure ventilation, on the basis of an improvement in respiratory bellows function. This appears to be partially due to the effect of intermittent rest of an otherwise fatigued muscle system.

In addition to intermittent ventilation, methods of noninvasive positive pressure respiratory support began to be reported. One of these was the Pneumobelt, which intermittently compressed the abdomen, driving the diaphragm upward. This provides a mechanically supported expiratory phase during use of the Pneumobelt (11). The second appliance was the lipseal mouthpiece, which consisted of a mouthpiece bite block with a surrounding cup-like structure that held the lips firmly against the mouthpiece. This provided a relatively airtight seal when fastened by a strap around the back of the head (Fig. 26.2).

However, these forms of ventilation were incapable of providing much of the work of breathing. The Pneumobelt provided only expiratory support, and the lipseal did not provide an adequate seal for high inspiratory pressures. Thus, both devices found their major utility in the treatment of chronic respiratory failure due to neuromuscular diseases, in which the work of breathing is essentially normal (12–15).

In the late 1970s and early 1980s, therapeutic strategies employing intermittent mechanical ventilation with both positive-pressure and negative-pressure ventilators were developed for the treatment of chronic respiratory failure. A second mode of disease-specific, appliance-meditated home respiratory therapy was also shown to be effective. This was the use of continuous positive airway pressure (CPAP) applied by mask to either the nose alone or to the nose and mouth for the treatment of obstructive sleep apnea (OSA) (16–18). This form of therapy was shown to significantly reduce the incidence of sleep apnea syndrome due to upper-airway obstruction without a requirement for tracheostomy or other invasive measure. The mechanism of action of CPAP in OSA seems to be a pneumatic "splinting" of the otherwise collapsible upper airway (Fig. 26.3) (17).

The development of this therapy has had two major areas of significance. One is in the treatment of OSA at home without the need for resorting to surgical intervention. The sec-

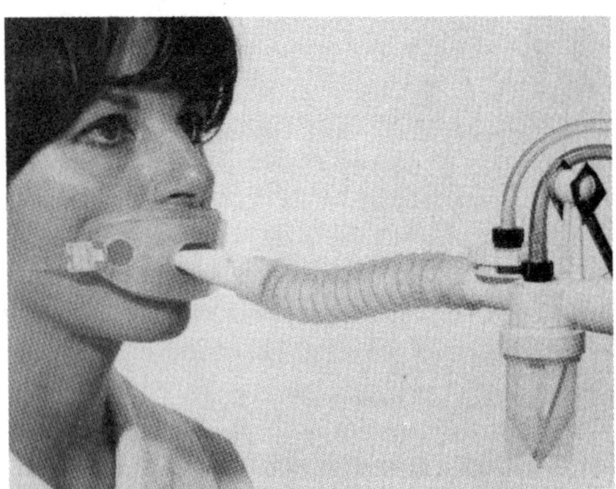

Figure 26.2.   Bennett lipseal mouthpiece adjusted to provide oral positive-pressure ventilation. (Courtesy of the Puritan-Bennett Company, Carlsbad, CA.)

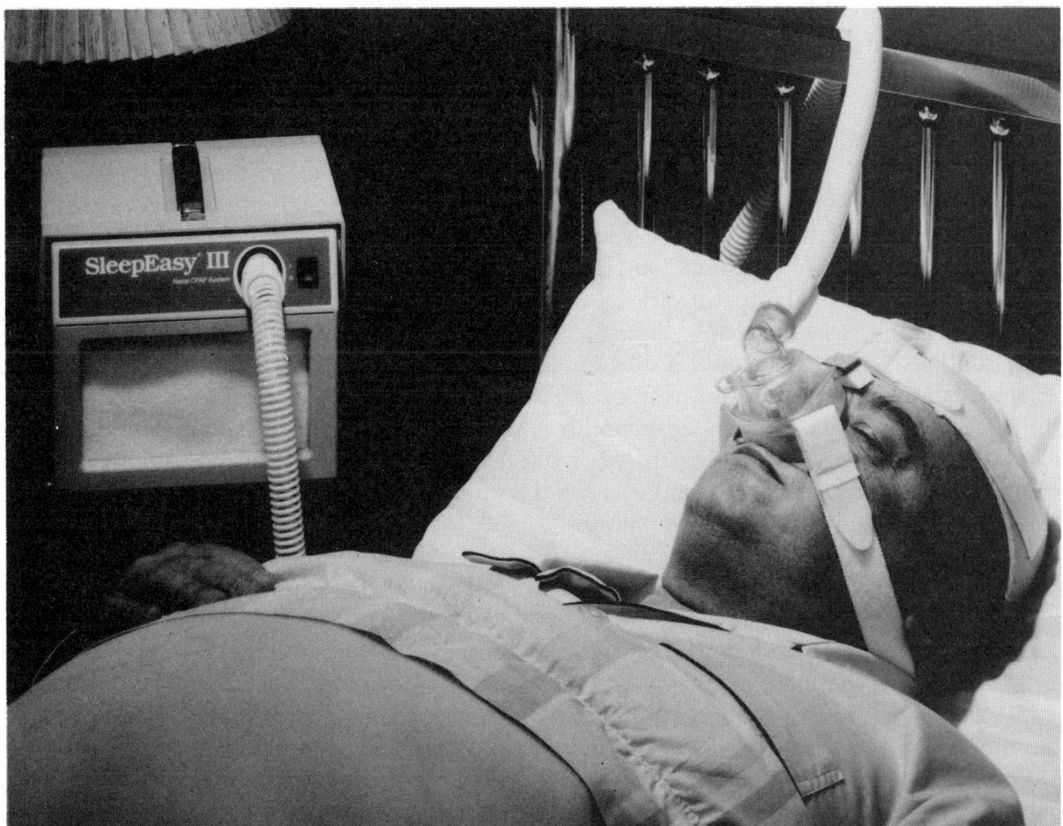

Figure 26.3.   Nasal CPAP mask in situ, in this case for the provision of nocturnal nasal CPAP. (Courtesy of Respironics Inc., Murrysville, PA.)

ond is in the impetus for the development of more effective and comfortable masks to apply positive pressure to the upper airway, either through the nose or through both the nose and the mouth.

The availability of nasal and full-face masks that achieve a seal capable of containing substantial (15 to 25 cm H_2O) positive airway pressure has led to a number of studies examining their utility as a mode of delivering volume-cycled or pressure-cycled positive-pressure ventilation. This was applied first to patients with neuromuscular diseases (13, 19–21) and more recently to patients with respiratory failure, both acute and chronic, due to lung disease (22, 23). Studies of such therapy have shown results similar to those reported in earlier studies employing either tracheostomy-delivered positive-pressure ventilation or negative-pressure ventilation (6, 10, 24). These results include improvements in respiratory muscle function, blood gases, and functional status (13, 19–21, 25–27).

The use of CPAP masks for the application of positive-pressure ventilation has been described as effective in many disease states (13, 19–23, 25–27). These masks are more comfortable than the lipseal mask (13) and are capable of relatively easy self-application, unlike negative-pressure body ventilators (27). However, problems remain with this system, including pressure effects on the face such as nasal bridge skin necrosis (26), the development of nasal congestion (26), and the feeling that some patients have of being shut in and claustrophobic (28). Some of these problems have been successfully addressed by the use of custom-made nasal masks with concurrent use of a chin strap to prevent opening of the mouth (26) and by the development of new full-face masks that avoid pressure points by use of a gasket surrounding the face (22, 23).

The availability of constantly improving means of noninvasive home-based positive-pressure ventilatory support will complement the ongoing utility of home-based negative-pressure ventilation for patients suffering from chronic respiratory failure of various etiologies. Nonetheless, these forms of mechanical ventilation seem to be useful for different subsets of patients with chronic respiratory failure (27). Their concurrent availability should therefore make the treatment of chronic respiratory failure with home-based intermittent mechanical ventilation feasible for a larger group of patients with respiratory insufficiency than has ever been possible. The convenience of mask positive-pressure mechanical ventilation can reduce the need for negative-pressure ventilatory support.

Three major groups of patients benefit from the use of equipment providing positive pressure to the upper airway. First are the patients who are dependent on constant mechanical ventilation. They are best treated with volume-cycled mechanical ventilation via tracheostomy. The second group of patients have obstructive sleep apnea, which can be noninvasively treated with continuous positive airway pressure applied with a tightly sealing mask to either the nose or the full face. The last group consists of patients who suffer from chronic ventilatory insufficiency with hypercapnia. These patients have been shown to benefit from intermittent use of various forms of mechanical ventilatory assistance probably due, at least in part, to resting of the respiratory muscles.

Specific Modalities

Tracheostomy

Tracheostomy has been the definitive method for the application of long-term positive-pressure ventilation essentially since the introduction of this type of respiratory support. In the setting of long-term mechanical ventilation it minimizes tracheal mucosal trauma, eliminates laryngeal trauma, provides a positionally secure airway, and permits highly effective tracheal suctioning (1–4). In addition, chronic tracheostomy has historically been the definitive treatment for obstructive sleep apnea (29). It bypasses the hypopharynx, which is the site of obstruction in this disease (30). In this way, tracheostomy is a highly effective therapy (29). Finally, tracheostomy has been used in the application of intermittent mechanical ventilation, with time off the ventilator spent using the natural airway by the virtue of the use of fenestrated tracheostomy tubes (Fig. 26.1) (6, 10).

As noted in Figure 26.1, the fenestrated tracheostomy tube consists of an outer cannula, which remains fixed in the tracheostomy track. It features a pneumatic tracheal seal cuff at its distal end and a hole (fenestra) on its upper surface positioned to fall within the tracheal lumen. When this outer cannula is plugged and the cuff is deflated, there is relatively little to obstruct airflow through the trachea, and air exchange occurs via the normal translaryngeal route. However, if the tube is unplugged, the cuff is inflated, and the nonperforated inner cannula is inserted, then gas exchange via the mouth is impossible. Positive-pressure ventilation can then be applied to the orifice of the tracheostomy tube. Using this system, a large number of patients requiring intermittent mechanical ventilation have been allowed normal speech during their time off the ventilator.

The second device for providing intermittent mechanical ventilation via tracheostomy is the tracheostomy button (Fig. 26.4) (31). This is a short tube or rod of the same diameter as the tracheostomy tube. The essence of this device is the removal of the entire tracheostomy tube and its replacement with the button, which serves to preserve the tracheostomy track. When the patient returns to mechanical ventilation, the button is removed and is replaced with a standard tracheostomy tube.

Tracheostomy for application of positive-pressure ventilation to the upper airway, for

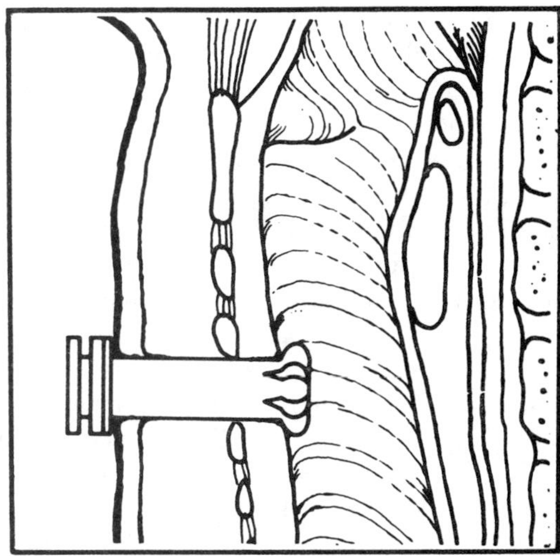

Figure 26.4. Olympic trach button in situ for the preservation of tracheostomy stoma. (Courtesy of Olympic Medical Corp., Seattle, WA.)

protection of the upper airway, and for bypassing the upper airway is highly effective and safe (1–3, 6, 10, 29). However, it is invasive. Although it is irreplaceable in patients with clear respirator dependence, those with disease processes permitting some degree of daily activity often object to such disfigurement.

In addition to problems with patient acceptance, there are certain technical difficulties associated with fenestrated tracheostomy tubes. Foremost among these is the fact that fenestrated tracheostomy tubes are mass-produced. Although the manufacturers will move the fenestra a bit along the tube in an effort at customization, the tube itself is of standard dimensions. Reference to Figure 26.1 will make it clear that if, for example, the pretracheal tissues are thick (for instance, in very obese individuals), or if any other factors make the stoma track unusually long, the fenestra will no longer be within the tracheal lumen and the plugged outer cannula will cause a substantial occlusion of the upper airway. Marsupialization of the tracheal stoma, defatting of the neck, and sometimes partial thyroidectomy may ameliorate this problem to some extent. However, there are some patients (in particular the very obese) who simply cannot suc-

cessfully utilize the tracheostomy tube fenestration feature.

Another problem with tracheostomy is the fact that tracheostomy tubes need to be replaced intermittently. Some patients do this for themselves, but those who cannot or will not need the ready availability of a person who can perform this for them.

Finally, a subpopulation of the patients given mechanical ventilation via a tracheostomy tube, either intermittently or continuously, will develop some softening and distention of the trachea in the area of the sealing cuff. This can result in progressively poorer air seals and sometimes bleeding. It is best treated by prevention using minimal effective cuff pressures of less than 20 mm Hg. Once this complication occurs, there is relatively little than can be done other than trying alternative tubes to find one that will maintain an effective seal.

Thus, tracheostomy can effectively and safely treat all three groups of patients who receive long-term treatment at home with positive-pressure devices. It is, in fact, the gold standard against whose efficacy all alternative forms of positive-pressure therapy have been evaluated. Despite its safety and efficacy, however, tracheostomy has a number of significant technical and aesthetic problems, and this has given impetus to the development of therapeutic alternatives that avoid invasion, disfigurement, or the obligatory use of indwelling hardware in the bodies of patients.

Lipseal

Mouthpiece ventilation has been shown to be practical during waking hours when the patient can consciously maintain the mouthpiece air seal (12–14). However, during sleep the relaxation of mouth and lip muscles often results in the loss of seal and inadequate ventilatory support. The Bennett lipseal is a cup-like device (Fig. 26.2) that holds the mouthpiece and lips in secure apposition. Using this, patients with neuromuscular disease who possess little or no functional respiratory musculature have been provided with adequate long-term continuous positive-pressure ventilation (12–14).

The mouthpiece-lipseal combination with a noseclip is quite easy to use and has been shown to be effective (12–14), primarily in the setting of neuromuscular disease. This predilection is largely related to the limitation of pressure that can be contained by this lipseal system. As only relatively low pressures may be applied to this system (generally 10 to 15 cm H_2O at most), its use is generally limited to diseases characterized by relatively normal airway resistance and respiratory system compliance. In addition, failure to clear saliva or even vomitus with the mouthpiece in place, especially during sleep, may be uncomfortable and dangerous. These problems tend to occur during the early application of the lipseal system. In the long term, the use of mouthpiece ventilation can cause bite deformities (13, 19).

Pneumobelt

The Pneumobelt is a 2- to 3-L bladder with a belt that holds it in immediate apposition to the abdominal muscles. Cyclic inflation of this bladder by a positive-pressure ventilator causes assisted exhalation, while inhalation takes place by gravity-assisted downward motion of the abdominal contents and diaphragm during the passive cycle of the respirator (11).

This device is very easy to use and requires no manipulation of the upper airway. However, it is incapable of assisting ventilation in the presence of an abnormal chest or lungs. By its nature, it decreases functional residual capacity. Nonetheless, the Pneumobelt has been useful in providing long-term ventilatory assistance in selected patients with respiratory failure secondary to Duchenne's muscular dystrophy and Charcot-Marie-Tooth disease (6, 20).

Nocturnal CPAP

In OSA, inadequate respiratory center output reaches the muscles of the upper airway during inspiration. This results in a passive collapse of the flaccid walls of the hypopharynx when inspiration causes intrapharyngeal pressure to be lower than the surrounding atmos-

pheric pressure (29, 30). Initial therapies for this included tracheostomy (discussed earlier) and pharmacotherapy, the latter having been proven ineffective for severe cases (32, 33).

In the early 1980s, investigators in Europe, the United States, and Australia began examining the possibility of providing a "pneumatic splint" to hold the upper airways open during inspiration, regardless of the adequacy of upper-airway muscle tone (16–18). This was done by providing CPAP, which helps to hold the hypopharynx open. CPAP was applied in these studies in one of four ways. First, it could be provided with a tightly fitting bombardier mask that applies CPAP to both the mouth and nose (Fig. 26.5). Second, it could be applied to the nose with a tightly fitting nasal mask that covered only the nose (Fig. 26.3). Third, it could be applied to the nose by a modified tightly fitting nasal cannula. Finally, most recently, a large-volume full-face mask has been produced whose seal is a circumferential facial gasket.

All of these appliances have been shown to provide improvements in apnea frequencies, sleep oxygenation, blood gases, cor pulmonale, and symptoms of lethargy in a large proportion of the patients treated (16–18, 34). Each has idiosyncratic problems associated with it. Custom-made nares cannulas are often perceived as uncomfortable (28), require frequent revision and replacement (13), and are not readily available in many areas. Bom-

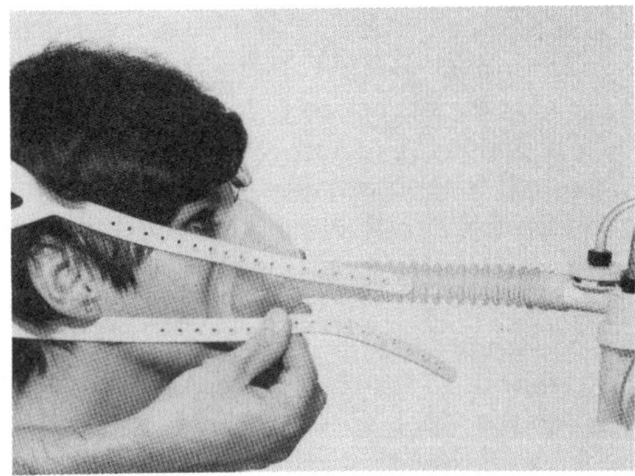

Figure 26.5. Full-face bombardier mask in situ with harness for provision of IPPB. (Courtesy of the Puritan-Bennett Company, Carlsbad, CA.)

bardier masks are relatively uncomfortable and often fail to achieve a good seal in thin patients due to lack of adequate buccal tissue to achieve mask-cheek apposition. These masks share with nasal masks a propensity for nasal bridge skin erosion (26, 35) but have an additional problem of full-face coverage of both nose and mouth. This can be dangerous in the event of vomiting, which can occur as a result of aerophagia (35).

As noted above, the nasal mask, which is currently the most widely used of these appliances, can cause erosion in the skin of the nasal bridge (26). However, it is safer than the bombardier mask in terms of aspiration since it does not occlude the mouth. By virtue of this it must be noted that some patients experience air leakage at the mouth during such therapy (26, 28). This can be easily reversed by the application of an elastic strap supporting (but not tightly binding) the chin. With this addition, effective CPAP is achieved while protecting against aspiration. The problem of nasal bridge erosion has most recently been addressed by the production of custom-fitted nasal masks that redistribute the seal pressure, eliminating "pressure points" (26).

Lastly, the large-volume full-face mask eliminates buccal, mouth, and other air leaks. It provides a large enough volume to minimize the danger of aspiration of vomitus and eliminates pressure points, thus improving comfort. This too has been shown to be effective in improving sleep ventilation (34).

Noninvasive Positive-Pressure Ventilation

Considerable progress was made in the late 1970s and early 1980s with the management of chronic respiratory failure and its acute exacerbation by intermittent mechanical ventilation. This was initially provided with negative-pressure ventilators (5–8, 36) and subsequently with positive-pressure ventilation via fenestrated tracheostomy tubes (6, 9, 10).

The negative-pressure ventilator, in the form of either the cuirass or the tank ("Iron Lung") respirator, has a long history in the management of respiratory failure (37–40).

This form of mechanical ventilation is quite effective in managing hypercapnia, but its use is attended by certain difficulties, including gastroesophageal reflux and the development of substantial hyperinflation with auto-PEEP (39). In addition, negative-pressure ventilation causes relative patient helplessness (especially in the tank-type respirator). It is also labor intensive, requiring dedicated personnel immediately in attendance to the mechanically ventilated patient. On the other hand, tracheostomy, the other early means of providing chronic intermittent ventilatory support, is invasive and unacceptable to many patients.

Therefore, the development of snug-fitting full-face and nasal masks and the documentation of their usefulness in providing mechanical ventilation to patients with neuromuscular diseases (12, 19, 20) was much appreciated. The utility of positive-pressure ventilation applied via such masks (noninvasive positive-pressure ventilation [NIPPV]) in the setting of acute and chronic respiratory failure was first evaluated in the late 1980s (35, 41, 42). Several series (25, 43–48) have subsequently demonstrated success in improving both clinical status and blood gases without the use of tracheostomy or intubation in patients with respiratory failure due to lung disease.

One cooperative study (49) reported no benefit from noninvasive ventilation in the acute setting. However, there are significant problems related to patient selection and control in this study. Another series (50) reported no success and a substantial increase in the nursing workload associated with such therapy in the acute setting. No other group has reported such an increase in nursing work. At our institution we have conducted extensive interviewing of nursing personnel. We conclude that the nursing staff do not consider NIPPV a significant influence on the workload of the nurse caring for a patient with an acute exacerbation of COPD.

More recently, randomized controlled studies of prospective design (51, 52) have shown substantial success in improving the acute outcome of respiratory failure using noninvasive mechanical ventilation. Some reports describe long-term intermittent mechanical ventilation following acute mechanical ventilation in the treatment of acute exacerbations of COPD. This may improve functional status and reduce the frequency of subsequent hospital admissions in selected patients (42, 44).

It is well to note that, although there is unanimity in the literature regarding the efficacy of intermittent NIPPV in improving the patient with restrictive lung disease, controversy exists regarding the efficacy of chronic intermittent ventilatory support of the patient with COPD and chronic respiratory failure. Although significant improvements have been reported in several series and controlled studies (6, 10, 42, 44, 53–57), others have not found such improvement (58–60).

This apparent discrepancy in study findings is disconcerting. However, on review of the original publications, it becomes clear that those studies in which no benefit was found from intermittent mechanical ventilation included substantial numbers of patients without significant gas exchange derangement during waking hours. The pressure of hypercapnia not only defines a critical level of respiratory muscle dysfunction but can also contribute to it. Therefore, it is intuitive that only patients with hypercapnia would be expected to respond significantly to intermittent mechanical ventilatory support. In this light, the routine use of mechanical ventilation on patients with lung disease who did not exhibit significant and consistent hypercapnia would be inappropriate.

The Mechanism of Clinical Improvement in Response to NIPPV

The mechanism of the benefit derived from NIPPV in respiratory failure due to lung disease is multifactorial. A major component is probably related to resting and strengthening the respiratory muscles, and permitting improved bulk gas exchange during periods of independent ventilation. A number of studies have provided electromyographic and physiologic data demonstrating resting of the respiratory muscles during the use of NIPPV (61–64). These results are similar to those found with the acute utilization of negative-pressure ventilation in patients with hypercapnic respiratory failure (24, 36).

A second factor in the benefit derived from NIPPV in respiratory failure due to lung disease is the improvement in bulk gas exchange achieved during NIPPV. On the most basic level, increased total ventilation allows improved oxygenation with much less concern for the potential development of severe hypercapnia. However, it must be noted that hyperinflation may occur during any positive-pressure mechanical ventilation in the COPD patient (65, 66). This may increase the ratio of deadspace volume to tidal volume (V_{DS}/V_T), offsetting the gas exchange improvement achieved.

By allowing other treatments (steroids, theophylline, antibiotics) to act without the need for intubation, NIPPV can play a major role in the management of respiratory failure due to pulmonary disease. Further, improved gas exchange can benefit diaphragmatic contractility either by decreasing the P_{CO_2} (67) or by increasing arterial oxygenation (68–70). Some investigators have suggested that NIPPV during sleep (specifically, applied during the night) may exert its beneficial effect by virtue of improvements in the disordered nocturnal ventilation of patients with respiratory failure (44). However, in our institution, patients choose to utilize NIPPV at various times during the day or night according to their preference and convenience, and all appear to benefit to the same extent.

It is not clear to what extent the concentration on nocturnal ventilation can contribute to optimization of an NIPPV regimen for respiratory failure due to lung disease. If there is a significant component of obstructive sleep apnea (OSA), the patient will be subject to repetitive inspiratory upper-airway obstruction. Such obstruction causes impaired bulk gas exchange and increases in the inspiratory workload. In this setting, any positive pressure applied to the upper airway may improve ventilation (16, 71). CPAP alone has been applied to patients with acute respiratory failure due to COPD in levels of 5 to 10 cm H_2O with some apparent benefit in clinical status and blood gas tensions. This may not be related to OSA but rather to auto-PEEP, alterations in respiratory muscle activity pattern, or effects on airway patency (72, 73).

The third possible effect of NIPPV on hypercapnic respiratory failure in COPD is a resetting of the constitutive drive level of the respiratory center, and possibly of chemoreceptor sensitivity (25, 74–76). In the face of a fatiguing workload for the maintenance of normal ventilation, the respiratory center may decrease its constitutive activity, thus avoiding the imposition of a fatiguing workload on the respiratory muscles. This is done at the expense of carbon dioxide retention, and this is sometimes referred to as central fatigue (59, 70, 77). Evidence for such a progressive desensitization of the respiratory center and decreased constitutive respiratory drive (due perhaps to progressive bicarbonate retention and metabolic alkalosis) exists in the sleep apnea literature (78). There are studies with both negative pressure (79) and positive pressure (80) that report changes in nocturnal ventilation caused by intermittent ventilatory assistance, independent of changes in muscle function. However, it is not clear that the controls for muscle function and measurement of constitutive respiratory drive in these studies are adequate to demonstrate a change in respiratory center activity without a change in muscle function.

Thus, NIPPV in acute respiratory failure of COPD can function first by stabilizing the hypoventilating patient. Following this, its salutary effects on respiratory muscle function and respiratory drive can improve lung and airway function as well as independent ventilation itself.

Operational Aspects of Noninvasive Ventilation in Respiratory Failure

Application of NIPPV in the treatment of respiratory failure due to pulmonary disease involves several unique components. First is the choice of ventilators. Any ventilator capable of assist control or pressure-support ventilation can be employed in this application. Although

assist control (A/C) and pressure-support ventilation (PSV) have both been shown to be effective in delivering NIPPV (35, 41, 42, 47, 51, 52, 81–83), PSV allows for much greater patient-ventilator synchrony (53) and is thus much more comfortable for the alert patient on chronic ventilatory support. With regard to this, the most cost-effective and convenient machine for home use at this time is the BIPAP pressure support system by Respironics, Inc.

The second operational issue in the application of NIPPV in the acute setting is the choice of interface between the machine and the patient. Three mask designs have been shown to be useful in the acute provision of NIPPV. The masks used initially in this setting were the so-called "bombardier" full-face masks (Vital Signs, Inc., Totowa, NJ) typified by the Downs CPAP mask (35). This type of mask is very effective, as it provides both mouth and nose coverage, but its use is beset by problems with pressure at the nasal bridge, air leaks in the area of the cheeks, and rather uncomfortable retention harness arrangements. In addition, this type of tightly fitting mask has a small volume and covers both mouth and nose, thus providing a certain risk of aspiration in the event of vomiting.

More recent studies have evaluated the use of nasal masks (nostril prongs as well as nose-covering masks) as mechanical ventilation interfaces (41, 42, 51). These masks, developed during the 1980s for the treatment of obstructive sleep apnea, have no buccal leak and no increased risk of aspiration. They are relatively comfortable and allow for free speech during mechanical ventilation. However, the problem of pressure points remains and there is an additional difficulty of severe air leakage when the mouth opens, which occurs often during sleep. This problem has been addressed with various strategies, including chin straps and changes in ventilator settings (44, 63). Although these strategies are often successful, a number of patients continue to have difficulty with leaks, at least occasionally. Most recently, a third mask type has been evaluated in the provision of chronic (22) and acute (23) mechanical ventilatory support. This is a full-face mask, similar in shape to a fencing mask, with a soft gasket around its entire perimeter. This creates a seal around the perimeter of the face during positive mask pressure. This mask obviates the previously noted difficulties of discomfort, pressure points, mouth leaks, and focal perimeter leaks. Although it covers the entire face, its volume is large enough to minimize the risk of aspiration in the event of vomiting. This mask is currently in the prototype stage but may soon be available on a limited production basis from Respironics, Inc.

The third practical issue is the actual application protocol for the use of NIPPV in the treatment of respiratory failure due to lung disease. Essentially all studies have employed an initial evaluation trial in which one or more physiologic parameters were evaluated for acute changes, presumably reflecting a beneficial effect of mechanical ventilation. In our institution, we evaluate the response to mechanical ventilation for 6 to 10 hours initially, while measuring respiratory rate, heart rate, and arterial carbon dioxide tension. A reduction in respiratory rate or heart rate is used to indicate that an effective level of ventilatory support has been achieved, after which blood gases are measured in order to document an improvement in alveolar ventilation.

After initial evaluation, all studies report the use of daily intermittent periods of mechanical ventilation of durations varying from 8 to 20 hours, provided in short (2 to 3 hours), long (8 to 10 hours), or both short and long (2 to 3 hours in the morning and afternoon, then overnight) treatment periods. Mechanical ventilation is then removed progressively until only 6 to 8 hours per day remain, usually during the night. This is prescribed as the chronic daily regimen. No study has clearly addressed the issue of further removal of mechanical ventilatory support. This may be because the majority of patients in whom this is an appropriate acute treatment prove to be reasonable candidates for long-term management of chronic hypercapnic respiratory failure with intermittent mechanical ventilation (42).

Finally, one must address the issue of patient selection. It seems that any patient with clearly demonstrable chronic (not episodic) hypercapnia due to a pulmonary disease causing an increased respiratory workload should be evaluated for long-term home-based noninvasive positive-pressure ventilatory support. Issues of patient symptomatology, lifestyles, goals, and preference will largely define the utility of intermittent NIPPV for a given patient. For example, a special case for early institution of such ventilatory support is in the cystic fibrosis patient awaiting lung transplantation. Intubation or tracheostomy would eliminate such a patient from the transplant lists. In this setting, NIPPV may thus allow survival without intubation until transplantation is possible (84).

CASE REPORT

A number of the points alluded to above are illustrated by the example of a typical patient who presented with severe hypercapnic respiratory failure as the end result of severe long-standing type A COPD.

A 53-year-old white female heavy smoker with a history of mitral stenosis was admitted for theophylline intoxication. She had a history of progressive dyspnea on exertion for 3 years, chronic atrial fibrillation, and admissions for hypercapnic respiratory failure.

On admission, her physical examination was remarkable for jugular venous distention, peripheral edema, rales at the base of the right lung, a I/IV mitral stenosis murmur, and a right ventricular third heart sound. The abdomen revealed a pulsatile liver and paradoxical abdominal motion on respiration. The chest radiograph showed cardiomegaly and a small right pleural effusion. The ECG disclosed atrial fibrillation with a rightward axis deviation. Arterial blood gases on 2 L nasal cannula oxygen supplementation were pH, 7.44; P_{CO_2}, 79; P_{O_2}, 57. Spirometry revealed a severe combined obstructive and restrictive ventilatory defect with emphysematous change.

The patient was continued on her usual medications (theophylline and albuterol) and was begun on pressure-support ventilation with a 22-cm support pressure via the BIPAP (Respironics, Inc.) device. The patient's respiratory rate immediately fell from about 30 to 20, with resolution of the paradoxical abdominal motion noted previously. The initial period of mechanical ventilation was continued for 10 hours overnight, after which the patient was allowed rest during breakfast. She was then provided with 2 hours of mechanical ventilation in the morning, allowed off the ventilator during midday, received another 2 hours during the afternoon, and had a rest during dinner and evening. By 10:00 PM, the ABGs on independent ventilation utilizing 2 liters of oxygen delivered by nasal cannula were pH, 7.48; Pco_2, 63; Po_2, 86.

The same regimen was continued daily, and by the seventh day of hospitalization the independent Pco_2 was 59 with a Po_2 of 70. She was discharged on her previous medications and overnight mechanical ventilation daily. Ten months later at follow-up she was ambulatory with ABGs on room air of pH, 7.48; Pco_2, 45; Po_2, 49; and on 2 L/min of oxygen via nasal cannula pH, 7.48; Pco_2, 43; Po_2, 79. Her previously noticed signs of cor pulmonale, including edema, were resolved without any need for diuresis. She continues to use pressure-support ventilation via the BIPAP machine daily.

Summary

Various forms of positive-pressure respiratory assistance suitable for use in the home are currently available. One therapy (CPAP) is specific for obstructive sleep apnea but may have utility in other disease processes. The other appliances and strategies discussed here address the application of positive-pressure mechanical ventilation in the treatment of chronic respiratory failure. They can be utilized in patients whose respiratory insufficiency is due either to chest disease or to neuromuscular disease.

These conditions may require either full-time or intermittent use of mechanical ventilation, depending on the degree of impairment. Many patients with a full-time requirement for mechanical ventilation are served best with tracheostomy, which is relatively comfortable and permits independent use of mouth and nose as well as improved pulmonary toilette. However, an increasing number of patients can be managed via the lipseal mouthpiece and CPAP masks. Patients with less impairment who can be managed with intermittent ventilatory support have utilized fenestrated tracheostomy tubes, full-face CPAP masks, mouthpiece with lipseal, and nasal CPAP masks.

All these devices and strategies are relatively easy to apply and should be usable by any physician or therapist familiar with standard respiratory equipment (Table 26.1). Each has advantages and disadvantages and each is best suited to a specific subgroup of patients. Patients benefiting from these mechanical ventilatory strategies are not always identical to those benefiting from negative-pressure mechanical ventilation. Thus, these different modalities are seen to be complementary rather than competitive. This is encouraging because it means that the addition of positive-pressure ventilatory support strategies to the home ventilator armamentarium should broaden the group of patients who can benefit from this form of therapy.

Unfortunately, home positive-pressure ventilation is a cost- and labor-intensive form of therapy (Table 26.2). It requires considerable monitoring by the physician. Additional equipment and reasonably trained personnel are needed to help the patient with equipment at home. The possibility of this role being filled by a family member or caregiver is important to consider. Many home health

Table 26.1. Equipment Needed for Home Positive-Pressure Ventilatory Care[a]

1. Ventilator
2. Cascade humidifier
3. Suction pump
4. Sidearm nebulizer
5. Oxygen source
6. Suction catheters; and
   a. CPAP mask, or
   b. Tracheostomy tubes and tracheostomy care supplies

[a]In addition to the equipment listed, professional visits by physicians, respiratory therapists, and sometimes nurses are required

Table 26.2. Daily Charges for Maintenance of Ventilator-Dependent Patients with Medicare and Private Insurance Coverages*[a]*

	Private	*Medicare*
Home	$146.00 ($53,000/yr)	$44.00 ($16,000/yr)
SNF	$330.00	$165.00
Acute hospital	$1,000.00	$500.00

[a]The above figures are averages over 1 year of 12 patients receiving ventilatory support at home, 16 patients receiving ventilatory support in the setting of a skilled nursing facility (SNF), and 16 patients receiving ventilatory support in the acute hospital setting. (Ventilatory support cost analysis provided courtesy of Mr. August DelGiacco, R.P.T., 6010 NW 61st St., Parkland, FL 33067.)

agencies will not, for reasons of liability, provide a paid assistant whose duties include responsibility for the operation of mechanical ventilatory equipment. The requirement for help at home has denied a number of patients the potential benefits of home ventilatory assistance.

In conclusion, devices and strategies for providing home-based positive-pressure ventilatory assistance are currently available. The systems have been shown to be safe and efficacious, providing improvement in physiologic parameters, quality of life, and survival in appropriately treated patients. The use of such therapy, however, is limited at this time by its labor-intensive nature. Of concern is the possibility of further limitation in the near future based on fiscal and administrative difficulties. Guidelines are needed to more clearly define the appropriate patients and therapies chosen for home positive-pressure ventilation.

References

1. Fisher AD. Poliomyelitis: late respiratory complications and management. Orthopedics 1985;8:891–894.
2. Splaingard ML, Frates RC Jr, Harrison GM, Carter RE, Jefferson LS. Home positive pressure ventilation: twenty years' experience. Chest 1983;84:376–382.
3. Robert D, Gerard M, Leger P, Blank P, Holzapfel L, Salamond J, et al. Long term IPPV at home of patients with end stage respiratory insufficiency. Chest 1982;82:258–259.
4. Peters SG, Viggiano RW. Home mechanical ventilation. Mayo Clin Proc 1988;63:1208–1213.
5. Garay SM, Turino GM, Goldring RM. Sustained reversal of chronic hypercapnea in patients with alveolar hypoventilation syndromes. Am J Med 1981;70: 269–274.
6. Marino WD, Braun NMT. Reversal of the clinical sequelae of respiratory muscle fatigue by intermittent mechanical ventilation. Am Rev Respir Dis 1982;125:85S.
7. Weirs PWJ, LeCoultre R, Dallinga OT, Van Dijl W, Meinesz AF, Sluiter HJ. Cuirass respirator treatment of chronic respiratory failure in scoliotic patients. Thorax 1977;32:2221–228.
8. Zibrak J, Hill N, Federman E, Kwan S, O'Donnell C. Evaluation of long term negative pressure ventilation in patients with severe chronic obstructive pulmonary disease. Am Rev Respir Dis 1988;138:1515–1518.
9. Braun NMT. Intermittent mechanical ventilation. Clin Chest Med 1988;9(1):153–162.
10. Braun NMT, Marino WD. Effect of daily intermittent rest of respiratory muscles in patients with severe chronic airflow limitation (CAL). Chest 1984;855–59.
11. Adamoon JP, Lewis L, Stein JD. Applications of abdominal pressure for artificial respiration. JAMA 1959;169:1613–1617.
12. Bach JR, Alba AS, Bohatiuk G, Saporito L, Lee M. Mouth intermittent positive pressure ventilation in the management of post-polio respiratory insufficiency. Chest 1987;91:859–864.
13. Bach JR, Alba A, Mosher R, Delaubier A. Intermittent positive pressure ventilation via nasal access in the management of respiratory insufficiency. Chest 1987;92:168–170.
14. Bach JR, O'Brien J, Krotenberg R, Alba A. Management of end stage respiratory failure in Duchenne muscular dystrophy. Muscle Nerve 1987;10:177–182.
15. Yang GFW, Alba A, Lee M. Respiratory rehabilitation in severe restrictive lung disease secondary to tuberculosis. Arch Phys Med Rehabil 1984;65:556–558.
16. Sanders M. Nasal CPAP Effect on Patters of Sleep Apnea. Chest 1984;86:839–844.
17. Strohl KP, Redline S. Nasal CPAP Therapy, Upper Airway Muscle Activation and Obstructive Sleep Apnea. Am Rev Respir Dis 1986;134:555–558.
18. Sullivan CE, Issa FG, Berthon-Jones M, Eves L. Reversal of obstructive sleep apnea by continuous positive airway pressure applied through the nares. Lancet 1981;1:862–865.
19. Ellis EK, Bye PTP, Bruderer JW, Sullivan CE. Treatment of respiratory failure during sleep in patients with neuromuscular disease. Positive pressure ventilation through a nose mask. Am Rev Respir Dis 1987;135:148–152.
20. Kerby G, Mayer L, Pingleton S. Nocturnal positive pressure ventilation via nasal mask. Am Rev Respir Dis 1987;135:738–740.
21. Segal D. Noninvasive nasal mask assisted ventilation in respiratory failure of Duchenne muscular dystrophy. Chest 1988;93:1298–1300.

22. Criner G, Travdine J, Brennan K, Kreimer D. Efficacy of a new full face mask for non-invasive positive pressure ventilation. Chest 1994;106:1109–1113.

23. Marino W. The efficacy and comfort of mask positive pressure ventilation via a unique full face mask. Chest 1994;106:159S.

24. Marino W. The acute effects of negative pressure mechanical ventilation on patients with chronic respiratory insufficiency. Am Rev Respir Dis 1986;133:A167.

25. Ellis E, Grusten R, Chen S, Bye P, Sullivan C. Non-invasive ventilatory support during sleep improves respiratory failure in Kyphoscoliosis. Chest 1988;94:811–815.

26. Gay P, Viggiano R, Edell E, Staats B. Treatment of complications from intermittent nasal ventilation (INV) for neuromuscular disease (NMD) and hypercarbic respiratory failure (HRF). Chest 1989;96:174S.

27. Marino W. The utility of chronic positive pressure ventilation via the nasal CPAP mask in patients with chronic respiratory failure due to COPD. Chest 1989;96:298S.

28. Marino W. Unpublished observations.

29. Guilleminault C, Eldridge FL, Tilkian A. Simmons FB, Dement WC. Sleep apnea syndrome due to upper airway obstruction. A review of 25 cases. Arch Intern Med 1977;137:296–300.

30. Hudgel DW, Chapman KR, Faulks C, Hendriks C. Changes in inspiratory muscle electrical activity and upper airways resistance during periodic breathing induced by hypoxia during sleep. Am Rev Respir Dis 1987;135:899–906.

31. Long J, West G. Evaluation of the Olympic Trach-Button as a precursor to tracheostomy tube removal. Respir Care 1980;25:1242–1243.

32. Bonora M, St. John WM, Bledsoe TA. Differential elevation by protriptyline and depression by diazepam of upper airway respiratory motor activity. Am Rev Respir Dis 1985;131:41–45.

33. Orr WC, Imes NK, Martin RJ. Progesterone therapy in obese patients with sleep apnea. Arch Intern Med 1979;139:109–111.

34. Sanders M, Kern N, Stiller R, Strollo P, Martin T, Atwood C. CPAP therapy via oronasal mask for obstructive sleep apnea. Chest 1994;106:774–779.

35. Meduri GU, Conoscenti CC, Menashe P, Nair S. Non-invasive face mask ventilation in patients with acute respiratory failure. Chest 1989;95:865–870.

36. Rochester D, Braun M, Laine S. Diaphragmatic energy expenditure in chronic respiratory failure: the effect of assisted ventilation with body ventilators. Am J Med 1977;63:223–232.

37. Corrado A, DePaola E, Messori A, Bruscoli G, Hutini S. The effect of intermittent negative pressure ventilation and long term therapy for patients with COPD: a four year study. Chest 1994;105:95–99.

38. Gigliotti F, Spinelli A, Duranti K, Gorin M, Goti P, Scano G. Four weeks negative pressure ventilation improves respiration function in severe hypercapnic COPD patients. Chest 1994;105:87–94.

39. Marino W, Pitchumoni CS. Reversal of negative pressure ventilation induced lower esophageal sphincter (LES) dysfunction with metoclopramide. Am J Gastroenterol 1992;87:190–194.

40. Plum F, Lukas DS. An evaluation of the Cuirass Respirator in acute poliomyelitis with respiratory insufficiency. Am J Med Sci 1951;221:417–424.

41. Brochard L, Isabey D, Piquet J, Amoro P, Munchero T, Messachi A, Brun-Buisson C, Ramos A, Lemoire F, Harp A. Reversal of acute exacerbation of chronic obstructive lung disease by inspiratory assistance with a face mask. N Engl J Med 1990;323:1523–1530.

42. Marino W. Intermittent volume cycled mechanical ventilation via nasal mask in patients with respiratory failure due to COPD. Chest 1991;99:681–684.

43. Carroll N, Branthwaite MA. Control of nocturnal hypoventilation by nasal intermittent positive pressure ventilation. Thorax 1988;43:349–353.

44. Gay P, Patel A, Viggiano R, Hubmayr R. Nocturnal nasal ventilation for treatment of patients with hypercapnic respiratory failure. Mayo Clin Proc 1991;66:695–703.

45. Goldstein R, DeRosie J, Avendaro M, Dulmage T. Influence of non-invasive positive pressure ventilation on inspiratory muscles. Chest 1991;99:408–415.

46. Leger P, Jennequin J, Gerard M, Robert D. Home positive pressure ventilation via nasal mask for patients with neuro muscular weakness or restrictive lung of chest wall deformities. Respiratory Care 1989;34:73–77.

47. Meduri G, Abu-Shila N, Fox R, Jones C, Leeper K, Wunderlink B. Non-invasive mechanical ventilation in patients with hypercapnic respiratory failure. Chest 1991;100:445–454.

48. Waldorn E. Nocturnal nasal intermittent positive pressure ventilation with bi-level positive airway pressure (BiPAP) in respiratory failure. Chest 1992;101:516–521.

49. Foglio C, Vitaca M, Quadri A, Scalvani S, Marangoni S, Ambrosino N. Acute exacerbation in severe COPD patients. Treatment using positive pressure ventilation by nasal mask. Chest 1992;101:1533–1538.

50. Chevrolet J, Jolliet P, Abajo B, Toussi A, Louis M. Nasal positive pressure ventilation in patients with acute respiratory failure. Difficult and time consuming procedure for nurses. Chest 1991;100:775–782.

51. Bott V, Carroll M, Conway J, Keilty S, Ward E, Brown A, Paul E, Elliot M, Godfrey K, Wezicka J, Moxham J. Randomized controlled trial of nasal ventilation in acute ventilatory failure due to chronic obstructive airways disease. Lancet 1993;342:1555–1557 .

52. Vitaca M, Rubini F. Foglio K, Scalvani S, Nava S, Ambrosino N. Non-invasive modalities of positive pressure ventilation improve the outcome of acute exacerbations in COLD patients. Intensive Care Med 1993;19:450–455.

53. Ambrosino N, Montagna T, Nava S, Negri A, Brega S, Fracchia C, et al Short term effect of intermittent negative pressure in COPD patients with respiratory failure. Eur Respir J 1990;3:502–508.

54. Elliot M, Carroll M, Wedzicka J, Branthwaite M. Nasal positive pressure ventilation can be used successfully at home to control nocturnal hypoventilation in COPD. Am Rev Respir Dis 1990;141:A322.

55. Elliot M, Mulvey D, Moxham J, Green M, Branthwaite M. Domiciliary nocturnal nasal intermittent positive pressure ventilation in COPD: mechanisms underlying changes in arterial blood gas tensions. Eur Respir J 1991;4:1044–1052.

56. Gutierrez M, Beroiza T, Contreras G, Diaz O, Cruz E, Moreno R, et al. Weekly cuirass ventilation improves blood gasses and inspiratory muscle strength in patients with chronic air flow limitation and hypercarbia. Am Rev Respir Dis 1988;138:617–623.

57. Scano G, Gigliotti F, Duranti R, Spinaldi A, Gorin M, Shiavina M. Changes in ventilatory muscle function with negative pressure ventilation in patients with severe COPD. Chest 1990;97:322–327.

58. Celli B, Lee H, Criner G, Bermudez M, Passulo J, Gilmartin M, et al. Controlled trial of external negative pressure ventilation in patients with severe air flow obstruction. Am Rev Respir Dis 1989;140:1251–1256.

59. Shapiro SN, Ernst P, Gray Donald K, Martin JG, Wood-Dauphinier S, Beaupne A, et al. Effect of negative pressure ventilation in severe chronic obstructive pulmonary disease. Lancet 1992;340:1425–1429.

60. Strumpf D, Millman R, Carlisle C, Gratham C, Ryan S, Erickson A, et al. Nocturnal positive pressure ventilation via nasal mask in patients with severe chronic obstructive pulmonary disease. Am Rev Respir Dis 1991;144:1234–1239.

61. Ambrosino N, Nava S, Bertone P, Fraccia C, Rempulle C. Physiologic evaluation of pressure support ventilation by nasal mask in patients with stable COPD. Chest 1992;101:385–391.

62. Belman M. SooHoo G, Kuei J. Shadmehr R. Efficacy of Positive vs. Negative pressure ventilation in unloading the respiratory muscles. Chest 1990;98:850–856.

63. Carrey Z, Gottfried S, Levy R. Ventilatory muscle support in respiratory failure with nasal positive pressure ventilation. Chest 1990;97:150–158.

64. Nava S, Ambrosino N, Rubini F, Fracchia C, Rempulle C, Torri G, Calderini E. Effect of nasal pressure support ventilation and external PEEP on diaphragmatic activity in patients with severe stable COPD. Chest 1993;103:143–150.

65. Gay PC, Rodante JR and Hubmayr RJ. The effects of positive end expiratory pressure on isovolume flow and dynamic hyperinflation in patients receiving mechanical ventilation. Am Rev Respir Dis 1989;139:621–626.

66. Kimball W, Leith D and Robins A. Dynamic hyperinflation and ventilator dependence in chronic obstructive pulmonary disease. Am Rev Respir Dis 1982;126:991–995.

67. Juan G, Calverly P, Talamo C, Schnader J, Rousses C. Effect of carbon dioxide on diaphragmatic function in human beings. N Engl J Med 1984;310:874–879.

68. Goldstein R, DeRosie J, Avendaro M, Dulmage T. Influence of non-invasive positive pressure ventilation on inspiratory muscles. Chest 1991;99:408–415.

69. Jardim J, Farkas G, Prefaut C, Thomas D, Macklem P, Roussos C. The failing inspiratory muscles under normoxic and hypoxic conditions. Am Rev Respir Dis 1981;124:274–279.

70. Roussos C, Macklem P. The respiratory muscles. N Engl J Med 1982;307:786–797.

71. Shivaram V, Cash M, Beal A. Nasal continuous positive airway pressure in decompensated hypercapnic respiratory failure as a complication of sleep apnea. Chest 1993;104:770–774.

72. De Lucas P, Tarancon C, Puente L, Rodriguez C, Tatay E, Monturial J. Nasal Continuous positive airways pressure in patients with COPD in acute respiratory failure: a study of the immediate effects. Chest 1993;104:1694–1697.

73. Miro A, Shivaram V, Mertig I. Continuous positive airways pressure in COPD patients in acute hypercapnic respiratory failure. Chest 1993;103:266–268.

74. Ellis E, McCauley V, Mellis C, Sullivan C. Treatment of alveolar hypoventilation in a six-year-old girl with intermittent positive pressure ventilation through a nose mask. Am Rev Respir Dis 1987;136:188–191.

75. Roussos C. Function and fatigue of respiratory muscles. Chest 1985;88:124S-132S.

76. Strumpf D, Millman R, Hill N. The Management of chronic hypoventilation. Chest 1990;98:474–480.

77. NHBLI Workshop Summary. Respiratory Muscle Fatigue. Report of the Respiratory Muscle Fatigue Workshop Group. Am Rev Respir Dis 1990;142:474–480.

78. Berthon-Jones M, Sullivan C. Time course of change of the ventilatory response to CO_2 with long term CPAP therapy for obstructive sleep apnea. Am Rev Respir Dis 1987;135:144–147.

79. Goldstein R, Molotiu N, Skrastins R, Long S, deRosie J, Canteras M, Popkin J, Rutherford R, Phillipson E. Reversal of sleep induced hypoventilation and chronic respiratory failure by nocturnal negative pressure ventilation in patients with restrictive ventilatory impairment. Am Rev Respir Dis 1987;135:1049–1055.

80. Hill N, Eveloff S, Carlisle C, Goff S. Efficacy of nocturnal nasal ventilation in patients with restrictive thoracic disease. Am Rev Respir Dis 1992;145:365–371.

81. Benhemou D, Girault C, Faire C, Portier F, Muir J. Nasal mask ventilation in acute respiratory failure. Experience in elderly patients. Chest 1992;102:912–917.

82. Fernandez R, Blanch L, Valles J, Bargorrt F, Artigas A. Pressure support ventilation via face mask in acute respiratory failure in hypercapnic COPD patients. Intensive Care Med 1993;19:456–461.

83. Pennoch B, Kaplan P, Carter B, Sabanya J, Magoven J. Pressure support ventilation with a simplified ventilatory support system administered with a nasal mask in patients with respiratory failure. Chest 1991;100:1371–1376.

84. Piper A, Parker S, Torzillo P, Sullivan C, Bye P. Nocturnal nasal IPPV stabilizes patients with cystic fibrosis and hypercapnic respiratory failure. Chest 1992;102:846–850.

27

HOME MANAGEMENT OF PATIENTS WITH ADVANCED NEUROMUSCULAR DISEASES

John R. Bach and Michael M. Rothkopf

CHAPTER AT A GLANCE: Effective strategies for ventilatory support have been developed for patients with advanced neuromuscular diseases. These approaches were first utilized in hospitals and chronic ventilatory units but can be successfully transferred to home. This chapter describes the available options in detail. The authors present a comprehensive review of the literature and homecare experience.

Introduction

Respiratory failure from complications of paralytic restrictive pulmonary syndromes is the most common cause of death in patients with high-level traumatic tetraplegia, severe myopathies, idiopathic kyphoscoliosis, and anterior horn cell disorders. Duchenne muscular dystrophy alone has an incidence of 1 in 3000 to 3500 males, and 85 to 90% of mortality is due to respiratory complications (1). The lives of many patients with neuromuscular ventilatory insufficiency can be prolonged by both tracheostomy and noninvasive methods of respiratory support (2–9). Noninvasive methods are preferred for patients with neuromuscular disease, since these methods avoid the complications associated with tracheostomy (10).

Global alveolar hypoventilation (GAH) can result from any neuromuscular or skeletal disorder that causes respiratory muscle dysfunction. It usually leads to episodes of acute respiratory failure, which require endotracheal intubation for positive-pressure ventilation and airway suctioning. When ventilator weaning fails, the patient often must undergo tracheostomy. Ultimately, discharge back to the community is only possible with support services needed to maintain a ventilator user with an indwelling tracheostomy tube. For most patients with paralytic and neuromuscular conditions, however, episodes of acute respiratory failure and hospitalization may be avoidable.

To maximize benefit from physical medicine and general rehabilitation interventions, individuals must have the ability to learn and to follow directions. They must also have adequate bulbar muscle function to use equipment and techniques that can optimize respiratory and general physical functioning. Such conditions are listed in Table 27.1. However, some patients whose bulbar muscle weakness precludes safe use of noninvasive inspiratory aids may still benefit from mechanical cough assistance methods.

Technical advances in transportation, computers, environmental control systems, and augmentative communication, along with the recent proliferation of home healthcare agencies that provide portable ventilators and

Table 27.1. Common Neuromusculoskeletal Conditions Leading to Global Alveolar Hypoventilation and Amenable to Physical Medicine Intervention

Myopathies
Muscular dystrophies
   Dystrophinopathies—Duchenne and Becker dystrophies
   Other muscular dystrophies—limb-girdle, Emery-Dreifuss, facioscapulohumeral, congenital, childhood
     autosomal recessive, and myotonic dystrophy
Non-Duchenne myopathies
   Congenital and metabolic myopathies like acid maltase deficiency
   Inflammatory myopathies such as polymyositis diseases of the myoneural junction such as
     myasthenia gravis, mixed connective tissue disease
   Myopathies of systemic disease such as carcinomatous myopathy, cachexia/anorexia nervosa,
     medication associated

Neurological disorders
Spinal muscular atrophies
Motor neuron diseases
Poliomyelitis
Neuropathies
   Hereditary sensory motor neuropathies including familial hypertrophic interstitial polyneuropathy
   Phrenic neuropathies—associated with cardiac hypothermia, surgical or other trauma, radiation,
     phrenic electrostimulation, familial heredity, paraneoplastic or infectious etiology, and lupus
     erythematosus
   Guillain-Barré syndrome
Multiple sclerosis
Disorders of supraspinal tone such as Friedreich's ataxia
Myelopathies of rheumatoid, infectious, spondylitic, vascular, traumatic, or idiopathic etiology
Tetraplegia associated with pancuronium bromide, botulism

Sleep disordered breathing/central hypoventilation
Obesity hypoventilation, congenital, familial dysautonomia, diabetic microangiopathy

Skeletal pathology
Kyphoscoliosis, osteogenesis imperfecta, rigid spine syndrome

After lung resection

Chronic obstructive pulmonary disease

other durable medical equipment with 24-hour on-call service to the patient, have made home ventilatory therapy both feasible and economical. These advances permit many ventilator-assisted neuromuscular patients to be managed safely, less expensively, and with better quality of life in the community. This chapter explores various noninvasive options for providing total respiratory support in the home setting.

Statement of the Problem

Disorders can be divided into those with sudden and those with insidious development of ventilatory failure. Conditions such as acute poliomyelitis (11, 12) and traumatic high-level spinal cord injury (2, 3) (traumatic tetraplegia) are examples of the former. In these conditions, ventilatory failure can not only occur suddenly but can be permanent.

For most patients, ventilatory failure occurs insidiously. To avoid respiratory muscle fatigue, patients with weakened or otherwise severely dysfunctional respiratory muscles breathe with increasingly shallow breaths. This results in chronic hypercapnia, retention of bicarbonate to offset the elevated CO_2 tensions, and resulting depression of ventilatory drive sensitivity to hypoxia and hypercapnia. With the resetting of respiratory chemotaxic centers associated with GAH, cor pulmonale develops. Concomitant expiratory muscle weakness exacerbates the problem by impairing coughing. These conditions progress until the patient develops acute respiratory failure or a cardiopulmonary arrest due to some combination of CO_2 narcosis and airway congestion.

Some patients who initially experience sudden ventilatory failure and then recover ventilatory function may develop late, insidious chronic ventilatory insufficiency (5, 13). Individuals with certain degenerative central nervous system conditions who have relapsing or intermittently exacerbating episodes of ventilatory failure can also benefit from physical medicine respiratory interventions (4). Except for individuals with isolated phrenic neuropathies, virtually all patients with GAH also have skeletal and at times cardiac muscle dysfunction that may require treatment (14).

Management of Ventilatory Failure

The Invasive Modes

IPPV via Endotracheal or Tracheostomy Tube

Although used for the delivery of surgical anaesthesia since 1869 and popular for the tracheal suctioning of patients supported by body ventilators in the late 1940s, tracheostomy for intermittent positive-pressure ventilation (IPPV) was not used for assisting ventilation until the Copenhagen polio epidemic of 1952, when an insufficient quantity of body ventilators was available (15). Body ventilators necessitated recumbency on the part of the user, while tracheostomy IPPV permitted the patient wheelchair mobility. For this reason, it became the conventional method of ventilatory support after 1952.

Tracheostomy and IPPV are associated with numerous complications (3, 16–18). Death from accidental disconnection is not uncommon despite the use of alarms (7, 19). Long-term complications relate to pathogenic bacterial colonization (20), bronchial mucus plugging, loss of the ability to generate adequate thoracoabdominal pressures for coughing or assisted coughing, and failure to enter the left main stem bronchus during routine suctioning (21). In addition, granulation tissue may accumulate and tracheal wall damage can lead to tracheal stenosis in 17 to 65% of patients (22).

Trachiectasis and tracheal perforation can also result from tracheostomy, as can subcutaneous and mediastinal emphysema. Mucus plugs that are adherent to the tracheostomy tube wall or cuff may also be impossible to clear and can occlude a bronchus, causing sudden respiratory distress. Other complications include hemorrhage, tracheoesophageal fistula (23), painful hemorrhagic tube changes, and psychosocial impairment. The presence of a tracheostomy tube stimulates bronchial secretions, necessitating regular bronchial suctioning and routine stomal care as well as regular changing of the tube and ventilator tubing itself. Supplemental humidification must be provided and attended to daily.

An indwelling tube impairs swallowing and speech. Swallowing difficulties result from restriction of upward laryngeal movement and rotation by the anchoring of the trachea to the strap muscles and skin of the neck. This results in reduced glottic closure and increased laryngeal penetration, thus increasing the chances of aspiration. Interference with relaxation of the cricopharyngeal sphincter (24), compression of the esophagus, and changes in intratracheal pressure can add to the problem (25). Tube-induced airway edema, wheezing, and bronchospasm can also occur.

In many states the tracheostomy is considered an open wound. This prohibits the individual from community living without the 24-hour care of family members or nursing care for tracheal suctioning. Some schools and places of employment also prohibit patients with "open wounds." There is also considerable expense associated with the use of disposable suction catheters, tracheostomy tubes, stomal care, and the employment of healthcare personnel when family members are unavailable 24 hours a day (26).

Electrophrenic Respiration

Electrophrenic respiration (EPR) is an option for the ventilatory assistance of traumatic tetraplegics with intact diaphragm and phrenic nerve function. Other criteria include no ventilator-free breathing ability, an inability to turn the neck sufficiently, or inadequate bulbar muscle function to grab a mouthpiece for IPPV. It may also be useful for some small children with traumatic tetraplegia who cannot cooperate with the use of noninvasive methods of ventilatory support (27).

The technique works by transmission of a radio wave signal by an antenna placed on the skin to an implanted receiver. The signal is converted to electrical impulses, which are carried to electrodes in contact with the phrenic nerves.

The advantage of EPR is that the impulse transmitter is small and lighter than a ventilator. Disadvantages include the operative risk of infection or trauma to the phrenic nerve, which is easily damaged. The in-hospital training period is 6 to 16 weeks but not infrequently longer. Total expenses amount to a minimum of $300,000 but are often greater. Unilateral pacing causes paradoxical diaphragmatic movement and often suboptimal ventilation. EPR may also increase microatelectasis. There is inability to routinely modify tidal volumes, so in situations calling for increased inspiratory volumes the patient must resort to a manual resuscitator or ventilator. Voice quality is poorer than for patients using an intermittent abdominal pressure ventilator (IAPV), and increasing voice volume is not possible. In addition, despite the expense, most of the time phrenic pacing is ineffective or inadequate for total ventilatory support (28).

Patients are also subject to the potential complications that accompany the maintenance of a tracheostomy. A tracheostomy must usually be maintained because of the upper-airway collapse that occurs during sleep while using EPR and because of episodic operational failure (29). This is particularly dangerous because of the lack of internal alarms and the inability to use glossopharyngeal breathing (GPB) effectively in the presence of a tracheostomy. Infection can occur during pacer

placement and with long-term use. Neuromuscular fatigue can also lead to irreparable phrenic nerve and diaphragm damage (29–31).

When EPR is not adequate, the tracheostomy tube must be left unplugged even though this may make verbal communication ineffective. One-way valves applied to the tube to improve communication are not always tolerated. There is not yet sufficient experience with newer protocols that encourage bilateral pacing, quadripolar electrode systems, and supplemental intercostal muscle pacing to determine whether EPR can be more effective without the associated deterioration of the phrenic nerve and diaphragm (32).

The Noninvasive Methods

Noninvasive methods of ventilatory assistance or support include body ventilators and direct noninvasive positive airway pressure techniques (noninvasive IPPV). Because of their relative simplicity, safety, effectiveness, and low cost, the noninvasive IPPV techniques have supplanted the use of negative-pressure body ventilators as the methods of choice for long-term ventilatory support for up to 24 hours a day. Negative-pressure body ventilators are still occasionally useful to facilitate stomal closure during the transition from tracheostomy IPPV to noninvasive IPPV, and they are being used by some patients with chronic obstructive pulmonary disease. Noninvasive IPPV methods are ideal, however, for home management of the adolescent or adult with chronic paralytic/restrictive respiratory insufficiency.

Direct positive airway pressure methods include IPPV delivered via the mouth, nose, or mouth and nose via oral-nasal interfaces. The portable ventilators used for these techniques are ideal for home use and can also be used for intermittent abdominal pressure ventilation.

Intermittent Abdominal Pressure Ventilator

The IAPV (Fig. 27.1) is a body ventilator that consists of an inflatable rubber bladder in a cloth abdominal corset. The bladder, which is fit over the abdomen, is intermittently inflated by a positive-pressure ventilator. The

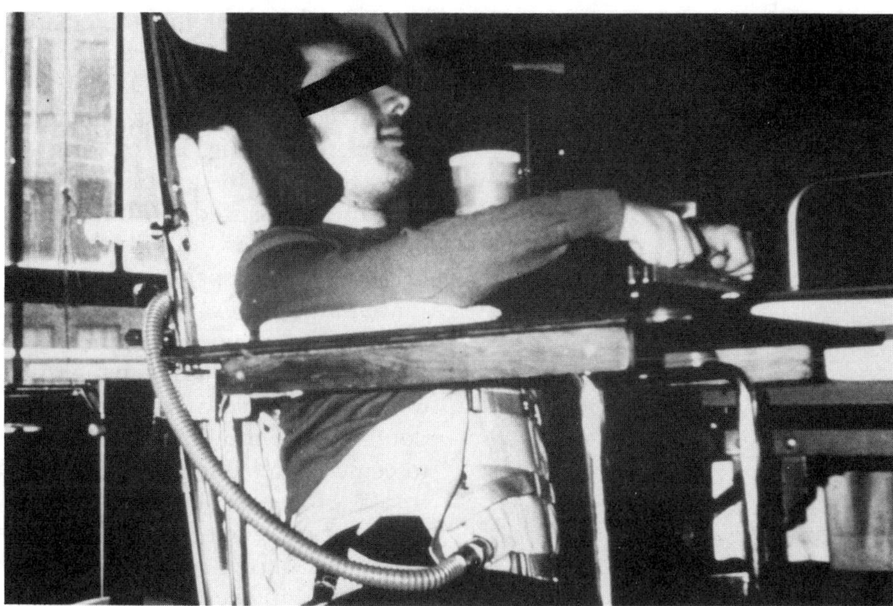

Figure 27.1. Traumatic tetraplegic patient with no ventilator-free breathing ability except with the use of glossopharyngeal breathing who was converted from tracheostomy to nocturnal mouthpiece ventilation and daytime use of the intermittent abdominal pressure ventilator (pictured here: ventilator manufactured by Lifecare International Inc, Lafayette, CO).

action of the inflated bladder moves the abdominal contents against the diaphragm, thus forcing exhalation. Deflation of the bladder allows passive inspiration, to which the patient can then add if he or she has residual inspiratory muscle function. The IAPV generally augments tidal volumes by 350 to 500 mL, but we have achieved volumes exceeding 1200 mL for a patient with no measurable vital capacity (VC). Because the passive downward excursion of the diaphragm relies on gravitational forces, the patient must sit at an angle of 30° or greater, with the optimal angle being about 75° from horizontal (33).

The IAPV has been used for decades by many patients with little or no measurable VC (5, 34). When combined with GPB, the IAPV virtually normalizes the rhythm and volume of speech. However, it is not effective in the presence of scoliosis or extremes of body weight.

The Noninvasive Intermittent Positive Airway Pressure Methods

Small, portable (22 to 38 lb), volume-triggered positive-pressure ventilators (Lifecare Inc., Lafayette, CO; Aequitron Medical Inc., Minneapolis, MN) are convenient for placement at bedside or on a wheelchair ventilator tray. Air is delivered to the patient through the mouth (2, 3, 5, 34), nose (19, 35, 36), or mouth and nose (37, 38) via appropriate patient-ventilator interfaces. In all three methods the air can be delivered to the patient via custom interfaces for enhanced comfort and efficacy (8, 38).

MOUTHPIECE IPPV. Mouthpiece IPPV is ventilatory support via a mouthpiece (Fig. 27.2). Mouthpiece IPPV is as effective as tracheostomy IPPV for the patient with functional oropharyngeal muscles and has been used by many patients with little or no measurable VC for long-term 24-hour ventilatory support (2, 5, 34). It is also ideal for use in combination with other forms of noninvasive aids.

For daytime use, the mouthpiece is either kept in the mouth or is more commonly fixed onto motorized wheelchair controls adjacent to the mouth for insufflation as needed (34). The mouthpiece has the advantage of

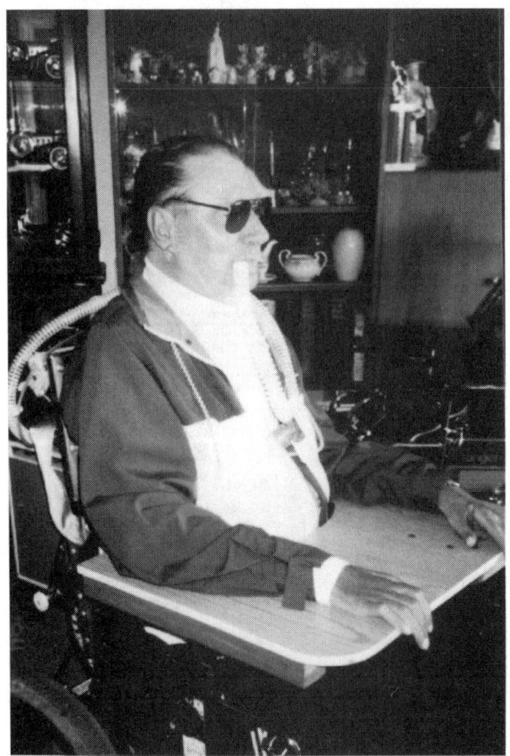

Figure 27.2. Post-polio ventilator user with no ventilator-free breathing ability using mouthpiece intermittent positive-pressure ventilation.

being simple, inexpensive, and commercially available. It is used predominantly for daytime IPPV. The mouthpiece may be flexed to enhance retention and comfort.

In 1964, Alba et al. (39) discovered that mouthpiece IPPV could be used safely during sleep by patients with little or no measurable VC. With use during sleep, however, transient severe oxyhemoglobin desaturation and hypercapnia can occur unless the mouthpiece is securely retained and insufflation leakage is minimized by using a Bennett lip seal (Puritan-Bennett Inc., Boulder, CO) (Fig. 27.3). System pressures of 30 to 40 cm H_2O can be maintained with this system.

Since mouthpiece IPPV can safely and effectively ventilate patients both day and night and can be an effective alternative to tracheostomy IPPV, it can be used for the transition to noninvasive aids in general and can also be used in weaning patients from tracheostomy IPPV. The tracheostomy tube can

be plugged and the mouthpiece placed adjacent to the patient for use as the patient becomes short of breath. Oximetry monitoring during conversion to mouthpiece IPPV is helpful, reassuring, and a form of biofeedback. Early on, the patient may need to have each breath assisted. With time and successful weaning he or she will take fewer assisted breaths until independent of ventilator use.

Disadvantages of long-term IPPV by mouthpiece include the appearance of orthodontic deformity in some patients and allergy to the plastic. Early on, aerophagia with abdominal distention may occur. Patients tend to cease complaining of aerophagia after the first few weeks of mouthpiece IPPV. Although it may continue to occur on occasion, it has not caused us to discontinue mouthpiece IPPV in over 150 patients who use the technique for nocturnal ventilatory support (40). Supplemental humidification is necessary for mouthpiece IPPV users during sleep.

NASAL IPPV. In 1981, Delaubier, Rideau, and Bach first used nasal IPPV as an alternative to mouthpiece IPPV (41). In 1987, Bach (42) reported its utility as a means for 24-hour ventilatory support. A number of commercially available continuous positive airway pressure (CPAP) masks became available ·and have been used for nasal IPPV. All were designed to provide a leak-free interface for CPAP users at pressures that are generally less than 15 mm Hg. These masks are held in place by headgear or a strap assembly. They are simple, inexpensive, durable, and readily available but they are not designed for air delivery at the higher pressures required for IPPV rather than CPAP. Even when used for the delivery of CPAP, however, 20 to 30% of patients with obstructive sleep apnea syndrome cannot tolerate them. CPAP masks are inadequate for as many as 50% of IPPV users (19).

A custom acrylic nasal interface (38) (Fig. 27.4) is a molded hard plastic butterfly-shaped shell that covers the nose tip and nostrils and extends over the cheeks. It has a soft inner gasket around the nasal opening. The interface forms a reservoir to deliver air to both nostrils. It is comfortable and durable and provides leak-free air delivery for most

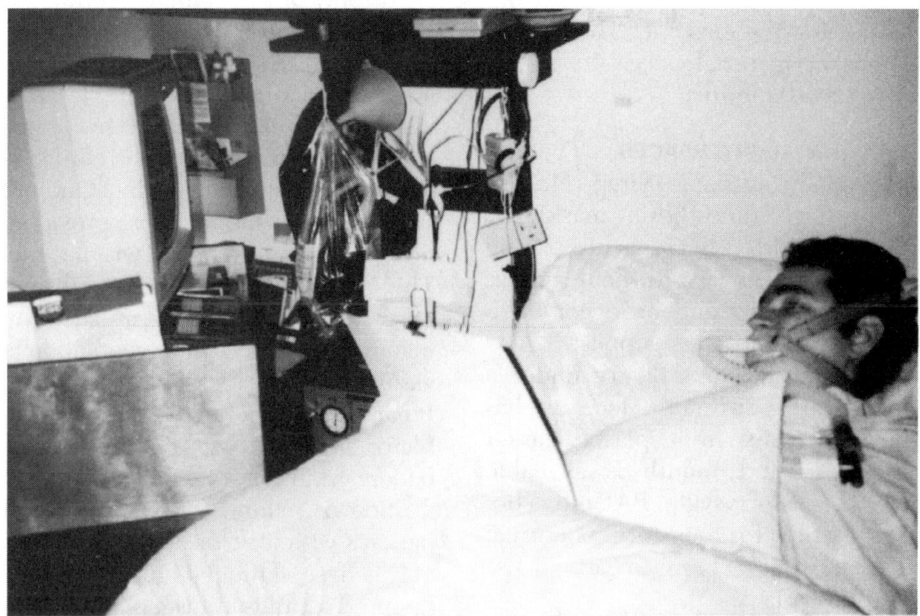

Figure 27.3. Twenty-five-year-old ventilator user with Duchenne muscular dystrophy. Patient has ventilator-free breathing ability of less than 2 minutes, using nocturnal mouthpiece intermittent positive-pressure ventilation with lipseal (Puritan-Bennett Inc., Boulder, CO) retention.

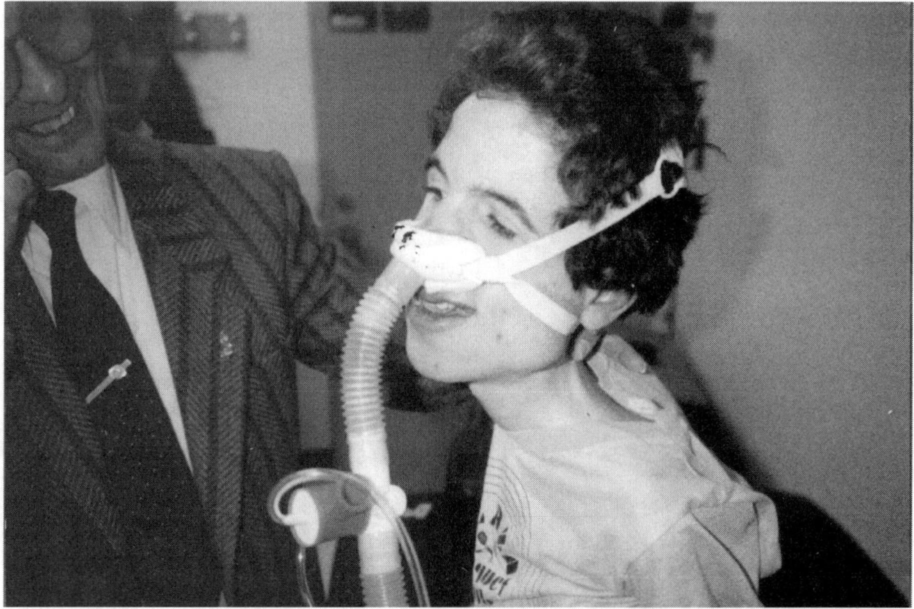

Figure 27.4. Twenty-four-year-old 24 hr/day ventilator user with Duchenne muscular dystrophy using a custom-prepared nasal interface (SEFAM kit, available from Lifecare International Inc., Lafayette, CO) for intermittent positive pressure ventilation.

patients. It must, however, be custom-made from a facial impression prepared with the patient supine for the best fit. The cost is $625, and gasket material needs to be replaced every 4 to 10 months.

IPPV VIA ORAL-NASAL INTERFACES. The use of a commercially available strap-retained oral-nasal interface (anesthesia mask) for IPPV has been reported in the acute setting (43). These interfaces are difficult to fit snugly and comfortably and have not been used for long-term ventilatory support. A new interface that permits air delivery under a transparent shell that covers the face and has a thin, flexible, transparent plastic gasket around the nose and mouth is available (Respironics Inc., Murrysville, PA) and is being used successfully for long-term nocturnal nasal IPPV (personal communication, Dr. William Marino) (Fig. 27.5).

Glossopharyngeal Breathing

Enabling the patient to learn and master GPB and the safety that it provides is one of the most important reasons for avoiding tracheostomy or switching from tracheostomy to noninvasive IPPV and allowing the tracheostomy site to close. GPB is the use of the tongue and pharyngeal muscles to add to a maximal inspiratory effort by projecting boluses of air past the vocal cords. The vocal cords close with each "gulp." One breath consists of six or more gulps, providing normal tidal volumes to patients with little or no VC. The usual GPB rate is 12 breaths per minute for ventilatory support. Many such patients can maintain normal minute ventilation and blood gases indefinitely while awake by GPB alone. It can be a most effective and inexpensive ventilator support backup and can thus free the patient from fear of sudden ventilator disconnection or failure. GPB has permitted many patients with little or no measurable VC hours of time free of their ventilators (34). It can also be used during transfers between different types of noninvasive ventilatory support.

Effective GPB also permits patients to add large volumes to their usual tidal volumes. The deeper insufflations are critical for

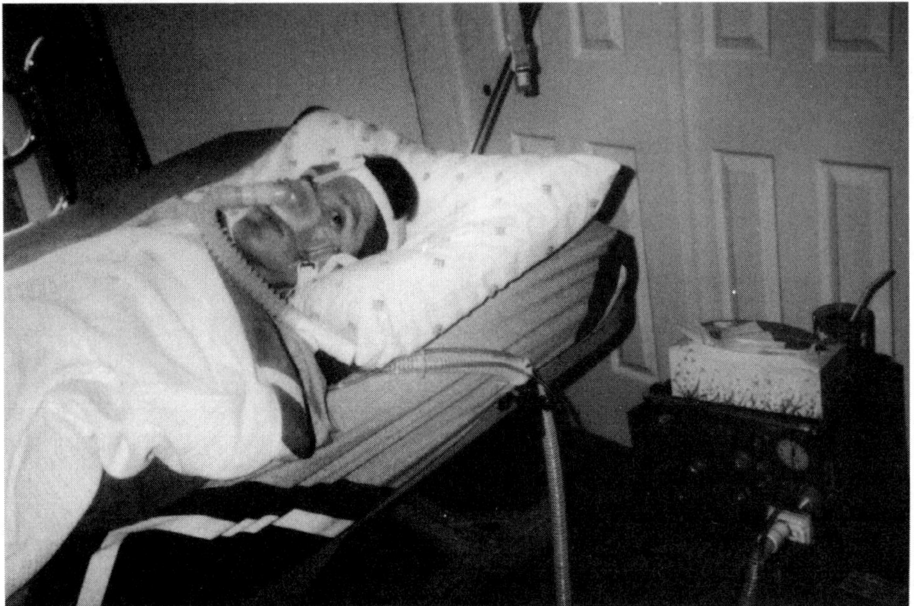

Figure 27.5. Thirty-two-year-old 24 hr/day ventilator user with Duchenne muscular dystrophy using a transparent custom acrylic nasal interface for intermittent positive-pressure ventilation (available from the Physical Medicine and Rehabilitation Department, University of Medicine and Dentistry of New Jersey Medical School)

effective manually assisted coughing (34) and to improve or maintain dynamic pulmonary compliance and prevent microatelectasis. They can also normalize the volume and rhythm of speech and permit the patient to shout. GPB can rarely be used as an alternative for ventilatory support in the tracheostomized patient because of air leakage around the walls of the tube and out the tracheostomy site.

Patients with VCs below 500 mL, functional oropharyngeal muscles, and little ventilator-free breathing ability are the best candidates for learning GPB. It can be introduced at any point in which the tracheostomy cuff is deflated and the tube plugged or removed for patients converting from tracheostomy IPPV to noninvasive ventilatory support. The amount of air (in milliliters) per gulp, the number of gulps per breath, and the number of breaths per minute should be observed to monitor patient progress with the technique. It may also be useful to monitor SaO_2 during GPB training. Training manuals and videos are available (44, 45).

Introduction and Evaluation of Noninvasive Ventilatory Support in the Home

Pulse oximetry biofeedback, assisted coughing, and noninvasive IPPV are critical for maintaining patients free of respiratory complications. There are three key diagnostic parameters that indicate the appropriate interventions. A full battery of pulmonary function studies is rarely necessary, since these patients rarely have chronic intrinsic pulmonary disease. A simple portable spirometer is used to regularly measure the patient's VC. The VC should be evaluated with the patient sitting, supine, side-lying, and with and without wearing a thoracolumbar orthosis when applicable, since the VC can be very different in all of these situations. The supine VC is generally the most important, since it is in this position that the patient should be sleeping and hypoventilation is often worst during sleep. Sleep oximetry should be performed for any

patients with symptoms suggestive of GAH, for patients with rapidly decreasing VCs, and for any patients with supine VCs below 1000 mL or about 30% of predicted normal.

Lung Expansion Techniques

Lung expansion techniques should be used when the VC decreases to 50 to 60% of predicted normal. Chronic lung hypoinflation is associated with alteration in the static mechanical properties of the lung and is characterized by decreased distensibility and static compliance due primarily to diffuse longstanding microatelectasis (46). In the absence of effective deep insufflations, microatelectasis can begin after about 1 hour (47). Although short periods of deep insufflation can briefly increase dynamic pulmonary compliance (48) and may enhance surfactant secretion (49), diffuse microatelectasis and pulmonary fibrosis will not be improved by such treatment if initiated late in the course of the disease. Methods of regular deep insufflation such as GPB, maximal insufflation IPPV or the use of a manual resuscitator, blower (Zephyr, Lifecare Inc., Lafayette, CO), or portable ventilator for the same purpose need to be introduced early with the goal of maintaining the maximum insufflation capacity (the maximum inflatable lung volume) at or close to the predicted normal inspiratory capacity.

Pulse Oximetry Biofeedback and Respiratory Tract Infections

The second key parameter is oxyhemoglobin saturation (SaO_2). Once respiratory chemotaxic receptors begin to reset because of shallow breathing, there is a relentless downhill process of increasing lung restriction and hypoventilation, which are associated with an increased risk of pneumonia and, eventually, cor pulmonale. Appropriate noninvasive IPPV trials need to be introduced. The goal is to maintain SaO_2 greater than 94%, and therefore maintain adequate alveolar ventilation around the clock without supplemental oxygen administration. It is often helpful to set an SaO_2 alarm at 93 or 94% and instruct the patient to maintain SaO_2 greater than these levels during daytime hours. Supplemental oxygen is not administered in the home, because if adequate oxygenation cannot be maintained with the use of respiratory muscle aids, the patient usually has sufficient acute lung pathology to require hospitalization. Oximetry biofeedback cannot be used, and nocturnal noninvasive IPPV is less effective for patients receiving supplemental oxygen.

The patient is instructed to maintain his or her SaO_2 at or above the target level all day either by unassisted breathing or, when tiring, by taking assisted breaths via a mouthpiece (IPPV) from a portable ventilator. The patient sees immediately that by taking slightly deeper breaths his or her SaO_2 will quickly exceed 95%. As more normal alveolar ventilation is maintained, the often present metabolic alkalosis is reversed, chemotaxic response normalizes to blood oxygen and carbon dioxide tensions, and nocturnal ventilatory support by noninvasive IPPV becomes increasingly effective (50).

Most patients with GAH require overnight ventilatory assistance months or years before their condition deteriorates to the point that 24-hour aid is needed. Overnight assistance alone can correct daytime blood gases for a time. The fundamental management goals continue to be maintenance of normal ventilation 24 hours a day, prevention of chest tightness, and effective elimination of airway secretions when present. The resetting of respiratory control centers is further advanced by providing mouthpiece IPPV during sleep using a Bennett lip seal, since with this system alveolar ventilation can be normalized during sleep even without intact chemotaxic drive (51).

Respiratory infections can cause exacerbation of respiratory muscle weakness (52) and the possibility of bronchial mucus plugging. In this setting, the VC and peak cough expiratory flows (PCEFs) often plummet. This may require extension of the daily regimen of assisted ventilation. Frequent "sighs" are necessary to facilitate manually assisted coughing.

Peak Cough Expiratory Flows

The third key parameter is PCEFs. Normal PCEFs reach 6 to 12 L/second depending on sex, height, and age (53). The effectiveness of mucus clearance is largely dependent on the magnitude of the PCEF (53, 54). When assisted PCEFs cannot exceed 3 L/second, elimination of airway secretion is ineffective. PCEFs are measured by peak flow meters (Access Peak Flow Meter, HealthScan, Cedar Grove, N.J.). Unassisted PCEFs are often under 1 L/second for ventilator users with neuromuscular disease. If the VC is less than 1500 mL, a maximum insufflation should precede the abdominal thrusts used in manually assisted coughing (Fig. 27.6).

Mechanical Insufflation-Exsufflation

Manually assisted coughing can usually raise neuromuscular ventilator users' PCEFs to greater than 4 L/second. However, when pulmonary compliance is severely decreased (or when there is irreversible airway obstruction, severe scoliosis, abdominal distention, or other factors that decrease the effectiveness of manually assisted coughing), mechanical insufflation-exsufflation becomes vital (Fig. 27.7). The In-Exsufflator (Emerson Co, Cambridge, MA) can be essential to prevent macroscopic atelectasis and pneumonia.

The In-Exsufflator consists of a two-stage axial compressor that delivers, usually via an anesthesia mask, a deep insufflation followed by a forced exsufflation created by a decrease in pressure of approximately 80 cm H_2O in 0.2 second. The insufflation and exsufflation pressures and timing are independently adjusted for comfort and efficacy, and the exsufflation is usually sustained for 1 to 3 seconds. With the use of mechanically assisted coughing in this manner mucus plugs can be eliminated, SaO_2 returned to normal levels, and VC as much as doubled to approach the levels attained before the respiratory infection or the appearance of mucus plugging. When possible, an abdominal thrust should be used simultaneously with the exsufflation phase of mechanical insufflation-exsufflation. The provision of 24-hour attention by well-trained attendants or family members and the use of assisted coughing as often as every 15 minutes as necessary can permit even patients with little or no VC to be safely managed at home

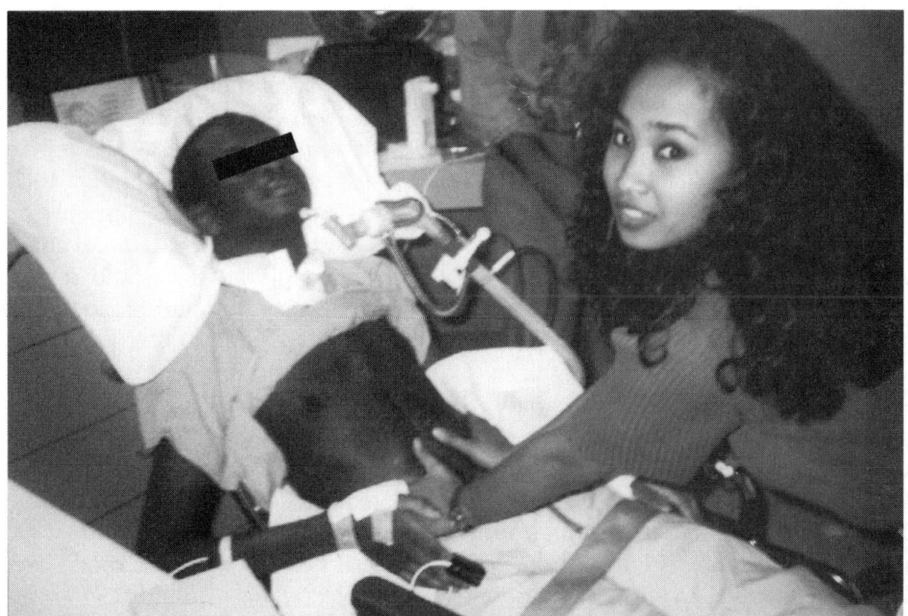

Figure 27.6.   Following deep insufflation from the mouthpiece near this patient's mouth, an abdominal thrust provided as pictured and timed to the patient's glottic opening increases peak cough flows to greater than 5 L/second in this traumatic tetraplegic patient.

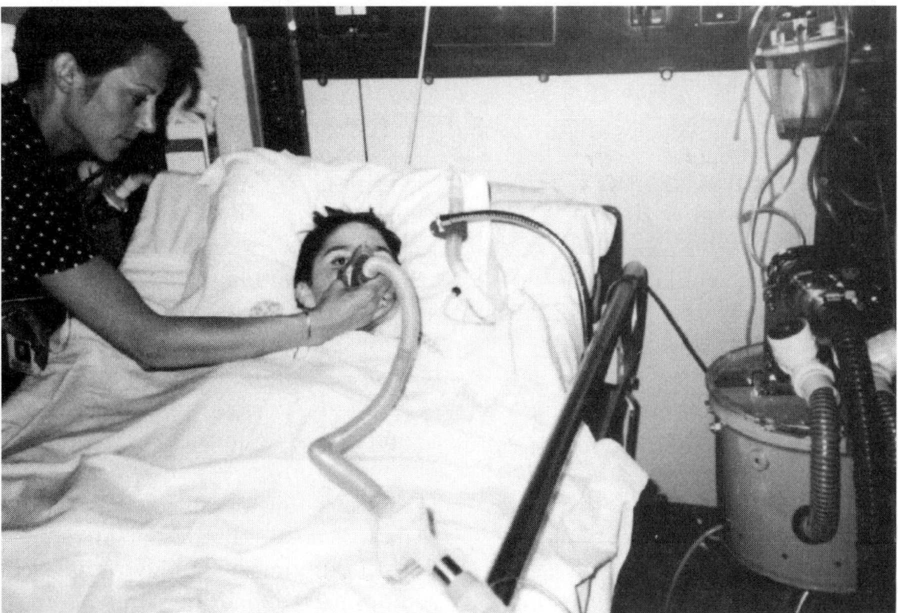

Figure 27.7.   Mechanical insufflation-exsufflation was provided to facilitate elimination of airway secretions for this postsurgery patient with Duchenne muscular dystrophy (pictured on the right: In-Exsufflator, Emerson Company, Cambridge, MA).

when they have upper-respiratory infections. Many long-term ventilator users have become expert at training their attendants how and when to use these measures.

Nocturnal IPPV and Monitoring of Efficacy

Home screening of nocturnal ventilatory function is conveniently performed by continuous SaO_2 monitoring. End-tidal PCO_2 monitoring can also be helpful (5). Oximeters and end-tidal PCO_2 monitors (capnographs) with memory or continuous printout capabilities that can tabulate and summarize the data should be used. When the patient is symptomatic from GAH or when his or her supine VC is less than 50% of normal and during sleep either PCO_2 exceeds 50 mm Hg or the mean SaO_2 is less than 95%, the patient undergoes a trial of nocturnal noninvasive IPPV. The rate of progression of the patient's condition should also be taken into account when considering the timing of the initiation of nocturnal noninvasive IPPV. Overnight SaO_2 monitoring is also done once a year or so to monitor the ongoing efficacy of nocturnal IPPV (19).

Introduction of Noninvasive IPPV in the Home

Noninvasive methods of ventilatory support can be introduced to the patient safely in the home. The simplest methods should be tried first. The indication of one method over another depends on the clinical situation, home environment, and personal choice. For the patients who require 24-hour aid, GPB, mouthpiece IPPV, and the IAPV are the preferred methods for daytime aid. Use of the IAPV frees the mouth for activities of daily living with a mouth stick. Most patients using daytime mouthpiece IPPV also prefer mouthpiece IPPV with the Bennett lip seal for nocturnal support.

When nocturnal support alone is indicated, nasal IPPV should be tried first with CPAP masks. A portable positive-pressure or volume ventilator can be used, but when introducing noninvasive IPPV it is preferable to use a ventilator without a low-pressure alarm. The ventilator should be set at a pressure or volume that decreases the patient's PCO_2 below 40 mm Hg while awake and maintains mean SaO_2 at 94% or greater during sleep. Volumes of 1000 mL or more are commonly used. If there is not adequate improvement in nocturnal blood gases and relief of symptoms, resorting to mouthpiece IPPV with a lip seal is the simplest alternative. A custom-molded oral interface or the use of nasal cotton pledgets may also be considered, as noted earlier (55).

During respiratory infections, sedatives and oxygen administration should be avoided to reduce the progression of respiratory failure and hospitalization. Broad-spectrum antibiotics, adequate humidification, and hydration should be provided as necessary. On-call respiratory therapists of homecare companies can play key roles in providing instruction to patient and family and in maintaining ventilatory equipment (e.g., an In-Exsufflator and an oximeter) in the home.

Tracheostomy Indications

Versatility in the use of noninvasive respiratory aids and effective management of respiratory infections are paramount in averting tracheostomy and hospitalizations and in optimizing quality of life. Tracheostomy is indicated for ventilator users when:

1. Assisted PCEFs cannot exceed 3 L/second and mechanical insufflation-exsufflation is ineffective;
2. There is a history of substance abuse;
3. Patient cooperation is lacking;
4. Intrinsic lung pathology requires oxygen administration in the home to maintain adequate oxygenation;
5. There is a seizure disorder, or
6. Orthopedic conditions interfere with the use of IPPV interfaces, i.e., osteogenesis imperfecta, facial fractures.

Cost

The cost of long-term ventilator use in an institutional setting depends on whether hospital intensive care facilities or "step-down" units are used or whether the patient is managed in lower-cost specialized respiratory care units in nursing or chronic rehabilitation facilities. In a study comparing the total costs of maintaining 10 totally dependent ventilator-supported individuals in the least expensive institutional setting with that of maintaining them in the community with 24-hour personal care attendants, it was calculated that total expenses were half or less in the community setting (56). Other studies have corroborated these findings (26). Government-funded organizations like Concepts of Independent Living Inc. (57) assist motivated, self-directed ventilator users in choosing, training, and directing personal care attendants and in facilitating social and vocational activities (58). Unfortunately, such organizations are limited to only a few states at this time.

Costs can be further reduced by the use of noninvasive techniques of ventilatory support. For example, monthly ventilator rental can cost as much as $900 for a patient maintained at home on tracheostomy IPPV without including the cost of a backup ventilator. Although this was found to be one-fourth to one-tenth as expensive as the equipment costs would have been for the more complex hospital ventilators and accessory equipment during a hospitalization (59), simpler, less expensive alarmless ventilators can be used safely by many patients using noninvasive aids who have mastered GPB. Indeed, many noninvasive ventilatory support setups have been under rental for over 30 years (i.e., from Lifecare Inc., Lafayette, CO) for as little as $60 per month.

Other aspects of the transition from hospital to homecare—including psychological considerations, equipment needs, rehabilitation, manipulation of the home environment, choice of equipment vendor, and mobilization of community resources—are simpler for patients using noninvasive aids than for those with tracheostomies (58). Perhaps the most invaluable source of information is from the personal experiences of patients who have been maintained at home for decades (59).

Activities of Daily Living

Patients should be encouraged to pursue personal goals, and their level of functioning should be maximized (60). Referral to occupational therapists should be made for training in the use of energy-saving devices and techniques, and environmental control systems when appropriate. Physical therapists can train the patient and caregivers in range-of-motion and other appropriate exercises. Speech pathologists specializing in management of dysphagia, dysarthria, and augmentative communication should also be involved in patient care if these problems arise.

Overeating and obesity should be avoided, as should extremes of temperature, humidity, and activities that cause excessive fatigue, since all of these conditions can exacerbate respiratory failure or decrease ventilator-free breathing time. Appropriate flu and bacterial vaccinations should be provided. Crowded areas or exposure to anyone with a cold should be avoided; however, extensive vacations and even transcontinental travel can be done safely, provided that they are well planned. The medical service of the airline should be notified at least 1 week in advance so that a transformer can be placed under the patient's seat to allow ventilator use with airline current. Appropriate electrical adapters and external batteries also need to be provided. Patients with little ventilator-free time who are not proficient in GPB should bring along a manual resuscitator. The public transit system in most major cities will provide for wheelchair-accessible transport from most major airports, provided that they are contacted in advance. Equipment regulations are available in the "Incapacitated Passengers Air Travel Guide," which is available from the International Air Transport Association, Quebec, Canada. Travel agents that specialize in travel for the disabled include Flying Wheels Travel, Inc., Owatonna, MN, and Uniglobe Action Travel Inc., Creve Coeur, MI.

Summary

Ventilatory support for the patient with advanced neuromuscular disease can be provided in the home, often by use of noninvasive methods. This has resulted in significant improvement in quality of life for affected patients and reduces the cost of therapy. Developments in the field will extend homecare applications for a greater number of these patients.

References

1. Rideau Y, Gatin G, Bach J, Gines G. Prolongation of life in Duchenne muscular dystrophy. Acta Neurol 1983;5:118–124.
2. Bach J, O'Brien J, Krotenberg R, Alba A. Management of end stage respiratory failure in patients with Duchenne muscular dystrophy. Muscle Nerve 1987; 10:177–182.
3. Curran FJ, Colbert AP. Ventilator management in Duchenne muscular dystrophy and postpoliomyelitis syndrome: Twelve years' experience. Arch Phys Med Rehabil 1989:70;180–185.
4. Alexander MA, Johnson EW, Petty J, Stauch D. Mechanical ventilation of patients with late stage Duchenne muscular dystrophy: management in the home. Arch Phys Med Rehabil 1979;60:289–292.
5. Bach JR, Alba AS, Bohatiuk G, Saporito L, Lee M. Mouth intermittent positive pressure ventilation in the management of postpolio respiratory insufficiency. Chest 1987;91:859–864.
6. Splaingard ML, Frates RC, Jefferson LS, Rosen CL, Harrison GM. Home negative pressure ventilation: report of 20 years of experience in patients with neuromuscular disease. Arch Phys Med Rehabil 1985;66: 239–242.
7. Splaingard ML, Frates RC, Harrison GM, Carter RE, Jefferson LS. Home positive-pressure ventilation: twenty years' experience. Chest 1984;4:376–382.
8. Leger P, Jennequin J, Gerard M, Robert D. Home positive pressure ventilation via nasal mask for patients with neuromuscular weakness or restrictive lung or chest-wall disease. Respir Care 1989;34:73–79.
9. Bach J, Alba A, Pilkington LA, Lee M. Long-term rehabilitation in advanced stage of childhood onset, rapidly progressive muscular dystrophy. Arch Phys Med Rehabil 1981;62:328–331.
10. Bach JR. A comparison of long-term ventilatory support alternatives from the perspective of the patient and care giver. Chest 1993;104:1702–1706.
11. Braun NMT, Faulkner J, Hughes RL, Roussos C, Sahgal V. When should respiratory muscles be exercised. Chest 1983;84:76–84.
12. Higgins ITT. Epidemiology of bronchitis and emphysema. In: Fishman AP, ed. Pulmonary Diseases and Disorders, 2nd ed. New York: McGraw-Hill, 1988: 1237–1246.
13. Bach JR. Inappropriate weaning and late onset ventilatory failure of individuals with traumatic quadriplegia. Paraplegia 1993;31:430–438.
14. Ishikawa Yuka, Bach JR, Sarma RJ, Tamura T, Ishikawa Yuki, Minami R. Cardiovascular considerations in the management of neuromuscular disease. Semin Neurol 1995;15:93–108.
15. Historical perspective on mechanical ventilation: from simple life support system to ethical dilemma. Am Rev Respir Dis 1989;140:2s-7s.
16. Johanson WG, Pierce AK, Sanford JP, Thomas GD. Nosocomial respiratory infections with gram-negative bacilli: the significance of colonization of the respiratory tract. Ann Intern Med 1972;77:701–706.
17. Johanson WG, Seidenfeld JJ, Gomez P, De Los Santos R, Coalson JJ. Bacteriologic diagnosis of nosocomial pneumonia following prolonged mechanical ventilation. Am Rev Respir Dis 1988; 137:259–264.
18. Craven DE, Kunches LM, Kilinsky V, Lichtenberg DA, Make BJ, McCabe WR. Risk factors for pneumonia and fatality in patients receiving continuous mechanical ventilation. Am Rev Respir Dis 1986;133: 792–796.
19. Bach JR, Alba AS. Management of chronic alveolar hypoventilation by nasal ventilation. Chest 1990;97: 52–57.
20. Niederman MS, Ferranti RD, Ziegler A, Merrill W, Reynolds HY. Respiratory infection complicating long-term tracheostomy: The implication of persistent gram-negative tracheobronchial colonization. Chest 1984;85:39–44.
21. Fishburn MJ, Marino RJ, Ditunno JF Jr. Atelectasis and pneumonia in acute spinal cord injury. Arch Phys Med Rehabil 1990;71:197–200.
22. Pingleton SK. Complications of acute respiratory failure. Am Rev Respir Dis 1988;137:1463–1493.
23. Hedden M, Ersoz C, Safar P. Tracheoesophageal fistulas following prolonged artificial ventilation via cuffed tracheostomy tubes. Anesthesiology 1969;31:281–289.
24. Logemann JA. Evaluation and Treatment of Swallowing Disorders. San Diego, CA: College-Hill Press, 1983:119.
25. Bonanno P. Swallowing dysfunction after tracheostomy. Ann Surg 1971;174:29–33.
26. Bach JR, Intintola P, Alba AS, Holland I. The ventilator-assisted individual: cost analysis of institutionalization versus rehabilitation and in-home management. Chest 1992;101:26–30.
27. Riordan J. Electrophrenic respiration. Resp Ther 1980; Nov/Dec:69–71.
28. Bach JR, O'Connor K. Electrophrenic ventilation: a different perspective. J Am Paraplegia Soc 1991;14:9–17.
29. Weese-Mayer DE, Morrow AS, Brouillette RT, Ilbawi MN, Hunt CE. Diaphragm pacing in infants and children: a life-table analysis of implanted components. Am Rev Respir Dis 1989;139: 974–979.
30. Lee MY, Kirk PM, Yarkony GM. Rehabilitation of quadriplegic patients with phrenic nerve pacers. Arch Phys Med Rehabil 1989;70:549–552.
31. Oakes DD, Wilmot CB, Halverson D, Hamilton RD. Neurogenic respiratory failure: a 5-year experience using implantable phrenic nerve stimulators. Ann Thorac Surg 1980;30:118–122.
32. Kinnear WJM, Talonen P, Shneerson JM. Electrophrenic respiration using quadripolar electrodes. Thorax 1987;42:229.

33. Adamson JP, Lewis L, Stein JD. Application of abdominal pressure for artificial respiration. JAMA 1959;169: 1613–1617.

34. Bach JR, Alba AS, Bodofsky E, Curran FJ, Schultheiss M. Glossopharyngeal breathing and non-invasive aids in the management of post-polio respiratory insufficiency. Birth Defects 1987;23:99–113.

35. Ellis ER, Bye PTP, Bruderer JW, Sullivan CE. Treatment of respiratory failure during sleep in patients with neuromuscular disease, positive-pressure ventilation through a nose mask. Am Rev Respir Dis 1987;135: 148–152.

36. Kerby GR, Mayer LS, Pingleton SK. Nocturnal positive pressure ventilation via nasal mask. Am Rev Respir Dis 1987;135: 738–740.

37. Bach JR, Alba AS, Shin D. Noninvasive airway pressure assisted ventilation in the management of respiratory insufficiency due to poliomyelitis. Am J Phys Med Rehabil 1989;68:264–271.

38. McDermott I, Bach JR, Parker C, Sortor S. Custom-fabricated interfaces for intermittent positive pressure ventilation. Int J Prosthod 1989;2:224–233.

39. Alba A, Solomon M, Trainor FS. Management of respiratory insufficiency in spinal cord lesions. In: Proceedings of the 17th Veteran's Administration Spinal Cord Injury Conference, 1969. Publication 0–436-398 (101). Washington. DC: U.S. Government Printing Office, 1971.

40. Bach JR, Alba AS, Saporito LR. Intermittent positive pressure ventilation via the mouth as an alternative to tracheostomy for 257 ventilator users. Chest 1993;103: 174–182.

41. Delaubier A. Traitement de l'insuffisance respiratoire chronique dans les dystrophies musculaires. In: Memoires de certificat d'etudes superieures de reeducation et readaptation fonctionnelles [Dissertation]. Paris: Université René Descartes, 1984:1–124.

42. Bach JR, Alba A, Mosher R, Delaubier A. Intermittent positive pressure ventilation via nasal access in the management of respiratory insufficiency. Chest 1987;92:168–170.

43. Meduri GU, Conoscenti CC, Menashe P, Nair S. Noninvasive face mask ventilation in patients with acute respiratory failure. Chest 1989;95:865–870.

44. Dail C, Rodgers M, Guess V, Adkins HV. Glossopharyngeal Breathing Manual. Downey, CA: Professional Staff Assoc. of Rancho Los Amigos Hospital, Inc, 1979.

45. Dail CW, Affeldt JE. Glossopharyngeal Breathing (video). Los Angeles: Department of Visual Education, College of Medical Evangelists, 1954.

46. De Troyer A, Deisser P. The effects of intermittent positive pressure breathing on patients with respiratory muscle weakness. Am Rev Respir Dis 1981;124:132–137.

47. Miller WF. Rehabilitation of patients with chronic obstructive lung disease. Med Clin North Am 1967;51: 349–361.

48. Bergofsky EH. Cor pulmonale in the syndrome of alveolar hypoventilation. Prog Cardiovasc Dis 1967;9: 414–437.

49. Slonim NB, Hamilton LH. Respiratory Physiology, 5th ed. St. Louis: CV Mosby, 1987:80–81.

50. Bach JR, Robert D, Leger P, Langevin B. Sleep fragmentation in kyphoscoliotic individuals with alveolar hypoventilation treated by nasal IPPV. Chest 1995; 107:1552–1558.

51. Bach JR, Alba AS. Sleep and nocturnal mouthpiece IPPV efficiency in post-poliomyelitis ventilator users. Chest 1994;106:1705–1710.

52. Mier-Jedrzejowicz A, Brophy C, Green M. Respiratory muscle weakness during upper respiratory tract infections. Am Rev Respir Dis 1988;138:5–7.

53. Leith DE. Cough. In: Brain JD, Proctor D, Reid L, eds. Lung Biology in Health and Disease: Respiratory Defense Mechanisms, Part 2. New York: Marcel Dekker, 1977:545–592.

54. Bach JR. Mechanical insufflation-exsufflation: comparison of peak expiratory flows with manually assisted and unassisted coughing techniques. Chest 1993;104: 1553–1562.

55. Bach JR, Saporito LS. Indications and criteria for decannulation and transition from invasive to noninvasive long-term ventilatory support. Respir Care 1994;39: 515–531.

56. Motwani JK, Herring GM. Home care for ventilator-dependent persons: a cost-effective, humane public policy. Health and Social Work 1988/Winter:20–24.

57. Schnur S, Holland I. Concepts—a unique approach to personal care attendants. Rehabilitation Gazette 1987; 28:10–11.

58. O'Donohue WJ, Giovannoni RM, Goldberg AI, Keens TG, Make BJ, Plummer AL, Prentice WS. Long-term mechanical ventilation: guidelines for management in the home and at alternate community sites. Chest 1986; 90(Suppl):1s-37s.

59. Laurie G, Headley JL, Mudrovic WM, eds. Rehabilitation into Independent Living. St. Louis: Gazette International Networking Institute, 1989;29:1–128.

60. Bach JR. Comprehensive rehabilitation of the severely disabled ventilator-assisted individual. Monaldi Arch Chest Dis 1993;48:331–345.

28

SLEEP DISORDERS AND SLEEP APNEA

Monroe Karetzky

CHAPTER AT A GLANCE: There is a growing recognition of sleep-related breathing disorders and their relationship to excess morbidity. Hypertension and cardiac arrhythmias related to obstructive sleep apnea–induced hypoxemia and surges in sympathetic nerve activity may contribute to premature death. This chapter reviews sleep architecture, normal physiology, and pathophysiological considerations. Diagnostic techniques are covered in detail, especially the technical aspects of monitoring with polysomnography. Home studies are discussed with regard to indications, advantages, and shortcomings, as well as the instrumental criteria to be looked for in available devices. The chapter provides an extensive review of treatment modalities. Great strides have been taken in our understanding of the pathophysiology of sleep disorders and sleep apnea. This has fueled the growth in diagnosis and treatment options.

Introduction

Current concepts of cerebral neurohumoral transmission, blood flow distribution, and regional metabolism do not solve the enigma of defining the physiological role of sleep. It has generally been assumed that sleep serves as a period of restorative physiological processes. These serve to rejuvenate the brain by allowing for protein synthesis, facilitated by a low rate of cellular work and an elevation of cellular "energy charge" (1).

However, the neuroanatomical and biochemical mechanisms involved in the induction of sleep or the maintenance of wakefulness remain to be elucidated (2). Numerous endogenous sleep-promoting substances (somnogens) have been identified, including neurotransmitters, neurohormones such as prostanoids, and neuroimmunogens characterized as cytokines

(3). Current evidence now suggests that sleep, like fever, is also a manifestation of infectious disease and that systems regulating the immune response, sleep, and body temperature are closely interrelated. There is accumulating data to suggest a link between sleep, thermoregulation, and metabolism (4).

The study of sleep abnormalities, particularly as related to disorders of breathing, has as yet received only limited attention in medical training programs. The most important of these abnormalities are the sleep apnea syndromes. Increasing evidence suggests that, if left untreated, sleep apnea leads to multiorgan dysfunction and cardiopulmonary death. This "natural" history is often interrupted by acute events such as fatal accidents resulting from daytime somnolence. Obstructive sleep apnea (OSA) is amenable to treatment and successful palliation, and subsequent cures are available.

Characteristics of Normal Sleep

Architecture and Effects of Aging

Sleep architecture, which is species specific, describes the pattern and distribution of sleep stages. There are two separate sleep stages based on electroencephalographic (EEG) and physiological parameters termed non–rapid eye movement (NREM) and rapid eye movement (REM) sleep. Apneas generally occur in REM sleep with mild OSA but can occur in both phases in severe cases. The minimum stimulus to wake someone, termed the arousal threshold, differs between individuals and varies in the same individual under different circumstances. The arousal threshold increases with deeper NREM (delta) sleep but is variable with REM sleep.

Sleep-related disordered breathing events (DBEs) produce symptoms of excessive daytime sleepiness and impaired cognitive function. Significant morbidity and shorter survival are observed (5).

Physiological Adaptation to Sleep—Nonrespiratory

Cardiovascular

The effects of sleep on cardiac rhythm are variable. There can be ectopy induced during REM and NREM sleep. Cardiac electrical activity can also be disrupted during the transition to wakefulness (6). Circadian changes in left ventricular ejection fraction (LVEF) have been reported and may be related to the decreases in cardiac output previously reported during early-morning awakening (1, 2, 7). It has not been established if this impairment is related to primary vascular resistance or diurnal variations in cardiac contractility.

Thermoregulation and Metabolism

Sleep is closely associated with the regulation of temperature and metabolic rate. The metabolic rate during REM sleep is greater than that during NREM sleep because of the contribution of cerebral metabolism during REM sleep. Cerebral blood flow and cerebral metabolic rate reflect energy utilization for cerebral synaptic activity during sleep (8). The variables associated with NREM sleep indicate that overall cerebral synaptic activity is progressively reduced by 3 to 10% in stage II to approximately 50% during deep sleep. Moreover, there is a superimposed thermoregulatory change with sleep, as determined by the interaction of REM and slow-wave sleep (SWS) (9).

The nocturnal rise of the hypothermic hormone melatonin generates much of the circadian decline in core body temperature. In the elderly there is an aging-associated reduction in the temperature response to melatonin. This is attributable in part to a modification of melatonin receptors (10).

Respiratory Effects of Sleep

Upper Airway

Airway Resistance

Changing from the erect to supine posture causes narrowing of the upper airway in conscious subjects. This is exaggerated during NREM sleep in the elderly (11). The increased resistance to flow in the upper airway during sleep results from a decrease in the inspiratory neuromotor activity of upper-airway dilator muscles (Fig. 28.1) (12). The increase in respiratory drive compensates somewhat and limits the fall in tidal volume (Fig. 28.2) (13). An increase in thoracoabdominal muscle activity also occurs, and there are increased esophageal pressure swings.

Snoring

Snoring and OSA lie on a continuum. Snoring results from narrowing or partial obstruction of the pharyngeal airway and the resultant vibration of upper-airway soft tissues, especially the soft palate. Snoring alone, without apnea, may cause sleep disruption due to arousal. It is associated with alpha intrusions on EEG, and excessive daytime somnolence (EDS). This has been termed the upper-airway resistance syndrome (UARS).

Nonapneic snorers may also be predisposed to morbidity and mortality, as observed in patients with overt OSA (Fig. 28.3) (14, 15).

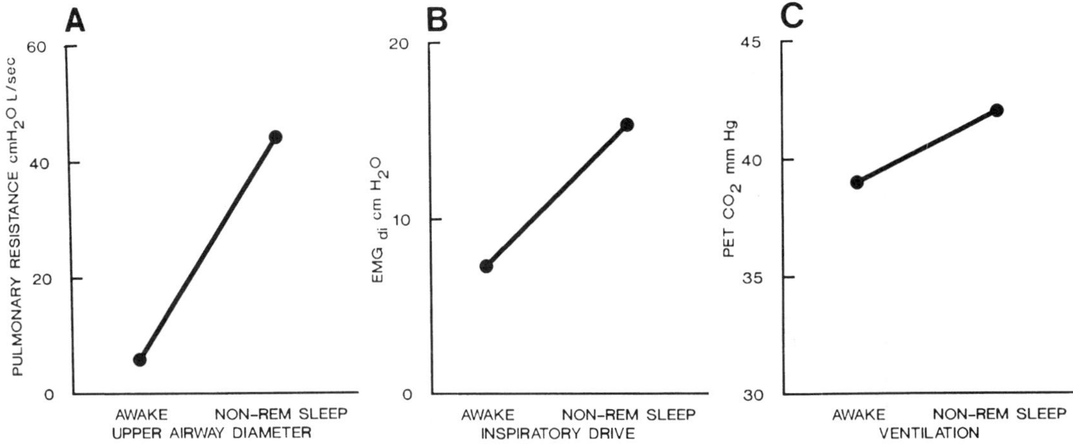

Figure 28.1.   **A,** The diameter of the upper airway diminishes during sleep; this is reflected by an increase in airway resistance. **B,** The perception of airway closure during sleep results in an increase in inspiratory drive as measured by transdiaphragmatic force. **C,** The increased ventilatory effect is not quite great enough to avoid a small rise in Pco_2 despite the decrease in CO_2 production that occurs during sleep.

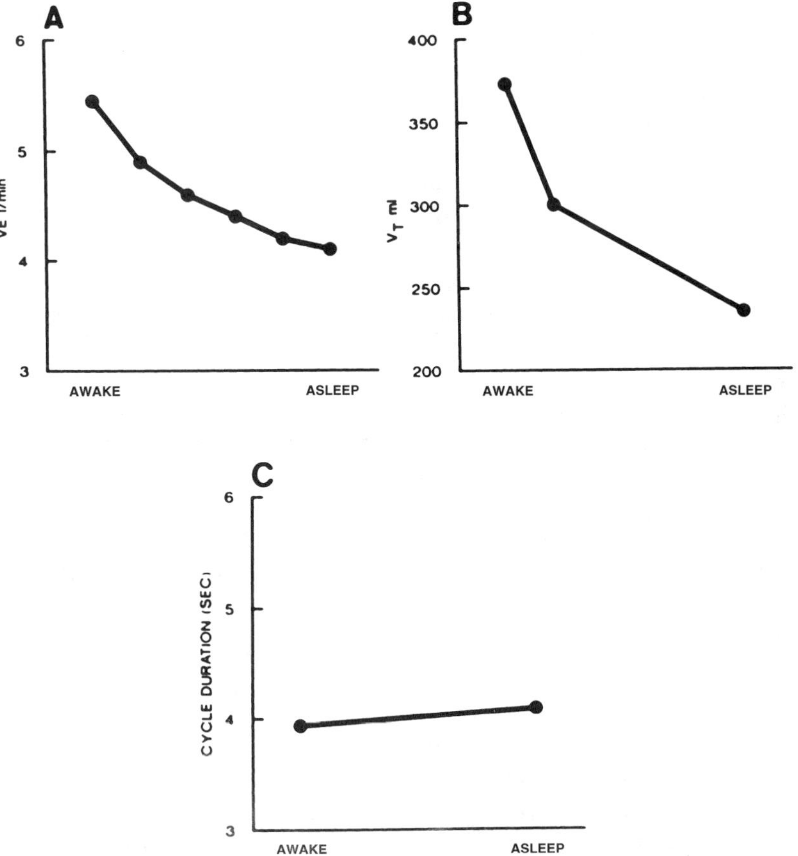

Figure 28.2.   **A,** Ventilation decreased progressively from the awake to the sleep stage (stage 2). **B,** The decrease in ventilation occurring during sleep reflects a decrease in tidal volume. **C,** The respiratory frequency remains relatively unchanged during sleep in comparison to the awake state.

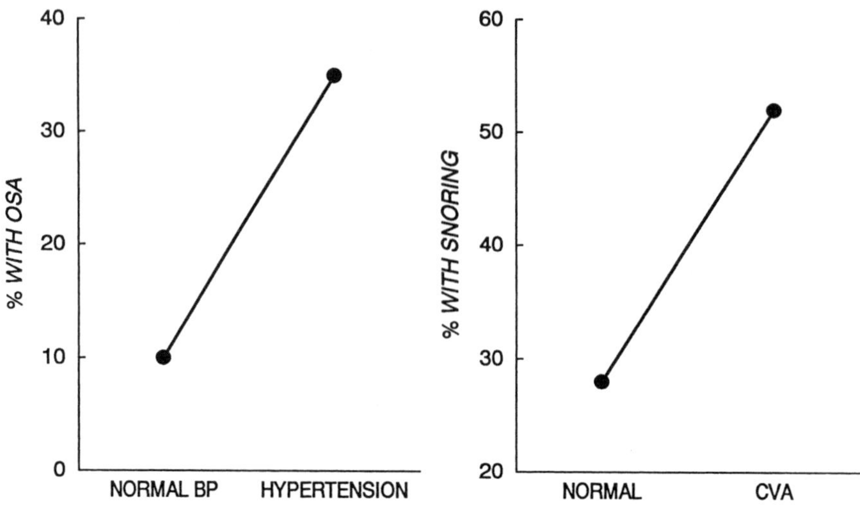

Figure 28.3. **A,** The association of hypertension with an increased incidence of OSA. **B,** The association of stroke with an increased incidence of snoring. (CVA, cerebrovascular accident [stroke]).

Upper-airway resistance is greater in obese snorers than in nonobese controls. However, it has been demonstrated that volume-dependent compliance differences exist between obese snorers with and without associated OSA (Fig. 28.4) (16). These differences have been attributed to greater neuromotor compensation in the nonapneic obese snorers.

Snoring is characteristically loud in sleep apnea and its absence makes OSA unlikely. Nasal resistance has been shown to be an important determinant of snoring frequency, and nasal obstruction predisposes to the development of sleep apnea. Moreover, nasal airflow has a stimulant effect on breathing during sleep that may be a mechanism of the therapeutic benefit of nasal ventilatory assistance techniques.

Ventilation

The central nervous system controls minute ventilation (V_E) by controlling the tidal volume (V_T) and the durations of inspiration (T_I) and expiration (T_E). The central nervous system controller loses several important primary inputs for ventilatory rhythmogenesis and "tone" with the onset of sleep. These include a decreased "wakefulness stimulus" to breathe and its associated nonchemical inputs as well as the alteration of responsiveness to chemosensor and mechanoreceptor afferent stimuli.

An illustration of this effect is observed when O_2 is administered during NREM sleep to hypocapnic subjects. This results in a rapid decline in V_E. In contrast, the effect of O_2 on V_E when subjects are awake is variable (17). Other studies evaluating the mechanisms of arousal from sleep have concluded that increasing ventilatory effort serves as the ultimate stimulus to arousal from sleep. The administration of oxygen prolongs the time course of the increase in inspiratory effort but not the level of effort (threshold) needed to induce arousal. Similarly, an increase in P_{CO_2} shortens the time for arousal from NREM sleep with airway occlusion by increasing the inspiratory effort and the rate of increase in effort (18).

Apnea

Apnea in Children

Children who experience loud snoring, sniffling, or choking during sleep, especially combined with nocturnal enuresis and very restless sleep, may have OSA. In this case, adenotonsillectomy may be beneficial. How-

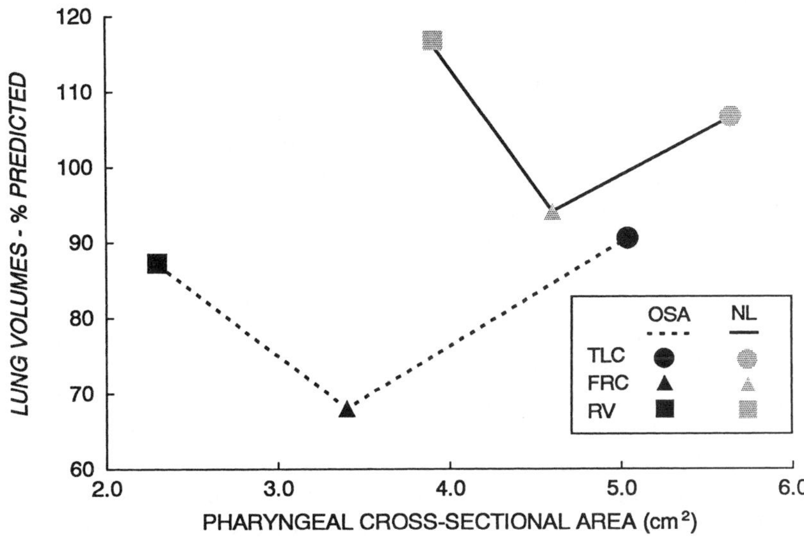

Figure 28.4.   The effects of lung volume (TLC, $\bigcirc$; FRC, Δ; RV, $\square$) on pharyngeal cross-sectional area in obesity, indicating greater inflation dependence in patients ($n = 9$) with OSA (*solid figures*) than in seated obese subjects ($n = 10$) without OSA (*shaded figures*).

ever, surgery should not be performed on the basis of history alone. The diagnosis should be confirmed by polysomnography. Moreover, the criteria for diagnosing OSA in adults do not apply; recently published pediatric normative data should be utilized instead (19).

Central Apnea

This term denotes sleep apnea devoid of apparent respiratory effort. Apneic events have been related to hypocapnia, as the central nervous system controller is exquisitely sensitive to a small reduction in the P_{CO_2}, especially at sleep onset. Individual predisposition to develop central apnea or periodic breathing at sleep onset appears to be linked to an individual's CO_2 "apneic threshold." The greater the activity of the respiratory center with decreased damping of ventilatory fluctuations, the greater the potential for "paradoxical" ventilatory depression by a Pa_{CO_2} below the "apneic threshold."

Obstructive Sleep Apnea

Definition and Epidemiology
DBEs occur along a spectrum of severity. This progresses from the arousal phenomenon,

elicited by the increased respiratory efforts required to overcome the resistive load (UARS), to completely ineffectual efforts with "obstructive" apneas (obstructive sleep apnea syndrome [OSAS]). The findings may be either apneas (of at least 10 seconds' duration) or hypopneas (less than 50% of normal inspiratory flow, decrease of 4% or more in oxyhemoglobin saturation). The consequences of hypopneas are comparable to those of apneas, justifying the use of the combined incidence of apneas and hypopneas into a respiratory disturbance index (RDI). The combination of apneas plus hypopneas per hour—the apnea plus hypopnea index (AHI)—is empirically defined as significant when it is greater than 10. These episodes recur throughout the night, rousing the patient from sleep. The arousals do not imply a return to full consciousness. Many are electroencephalographic in nature (microarousals). So while these episodes effectively interrupt restful sleep (fragmentation), there is frequently no awareness of the disruption on the part of the patient.

It is suspected that these "awakenings" are the result of the mechanoreceptor stimuli, reflected by large negative endoesophageal pressure changes combined with the subsequent arousal response to hypoxia. Both OSA and UARS have similar symptomatology and response to treatment. The sleep apnea syndrome also has a strong familial component, particularly in women, that may be characterized by differences in facial structure and narrower upper airways. In addition to anatomic risk factors and ventilatory control abnormalities, a complex genetic predisposition seems to be involved in some families (20). Furthermore, recent studies suggest that the frequency of OSA in women has been underestimated and in part may be a consequence of the absence of the full range of symptoms characteristic of OSA in men.

Pathophysiology

Patients with OSA have three characteristic abnormalities of the upper airway: increased supraglottic resistance, decreased pharyngeal area, and more compliant walls (21). The latter readily close with negative intraluminal pressure (Fig. 28.5).

Various anatomical abnormalities such as pharyngeal fat, retrognathia, and hypertrophied tonsils decrease the resting length of the pharyngeal muscles, resulting in a lower tension for a given efferent stimulus. Improvements seen with weight loss in OSA obese patients suggests that parapharyngeal fat pads compress the upper airway and collapse its walls. Recently the fat pad volume as measured by MRI was found to correlate with the severity of the OSA.

Other structural and neurological abnormalities also predispose to upper-airway closure by increasing transmural pressure. This is further enhanced by the supine posture and low lung volume, which narrow the retropalatal airway (Fig. 28.4). OSA patients are very heterogeneous with respect to where the site(s) of narrowing and presumed obstruction occurs. Narrowing at the level of the soft palate is common and is usually a severe or "primary" narrowing; however, in most patients two or more sites of narrowing coexist (22).

Clinical Features

Early investigations suggested a causal relationship between OSA and elevations in nocturnal pulmonary arterial pressure (PAP) and systemic arterial pressure (SAP). These may become fixed during waking hours as a result of vascular remodeling. The pulmonary hy-

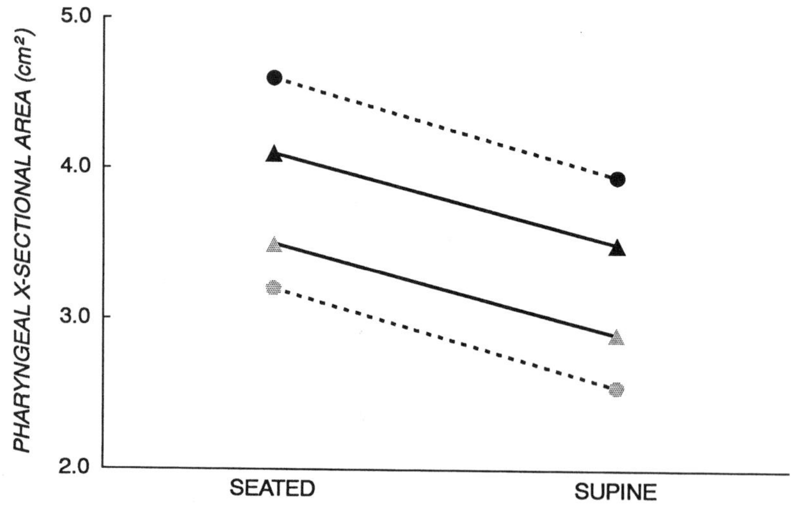

Figure 28.5.   The effects of posture and pressure on pharyngeal cross-sectional area in obesity (all snorers), indicating smaller size and increased compliance (distensibility) of upper airway in patients ($n = 12$) with OSA (○) than in obese subjects ($n = 6$) without OSA (△). (*Shaded figures* = 0 cm H_2O; *solid figures* = 5 cm H_2O).

pertensive peaks, which occur when intrathoracic pressure returns toward postapneic normal values at the nadir of O_2 saturation, are blunted by oxygen administration and are potentiated by hypercapnia.

The time course of changes in SAP during OSA is similar to that of PAP: lowest at the beginning of an apneic event and progressively increasing to a peak "overshoot" postapnea. The latter are attributed to an effect of hypoxia that is potentiated by the arousal reaction, both cortical and subcortical. This pressure response is mediated by sympathoadrenal neurohumoral activation and, as with the rise in PAP, is attenuated by the administration of oxygen. However, hypoxia is clearly not the sole cause of OSA-induced hypertension (23).

Recent studies have indicated that OSA has comorbidity with a variety of other systemic conditions, including pregnancy. It is suggested that OSA might then be responsible for impaired fetal development and episodes of fetal distress. The enlarged uterus might critically load the diaphragm in the predisposed woman on the threshold of developing the syndrome spontaneously.

Similarly, metabolic factors in the patient with end-stage renal disease appear to contribute to the pathophysiology behind the reported increased incidence of OSA in patients with chronic renal failure. The role of hemodialysis is not clear. Peritoneal dialysis may predispose to obstructive events because of respiratory muscle loading. Finally, the apparent frequent coexistence of chronic obstructive pulmonary disease and the sleep apnea syndrome has been suggested to be the critical factor differentiating the "blue bloater" from the "pink puffer."

Diagnostic Techniques

History

Numerous studies have attempted to predict sleep apnea from the presenting clinical features, but have generally been unsuccessful. This is partially due to differences in clinical features between men and women. Patients are also unreliable historians, as illustrated by the discordance between patients' and their bed partners' reports of snoring.

Physical Examination

Central obesity with an increased mean waist-hip ratio correlates with the severity of OSA. For a given degree of upper-body obesity, men have more severe OSA than women (24). Neck fat circumference has also been shown to be a valuable adjunct to screening tests for OSA. Obesity, however, is by no means a prerequisite for having OSA. Recent experience shows that the majority of patients with OSA are less than 130% of ideal body weight.

Diagnostic Examinations

Fiberoptic laryngoscopy may be very useful in the evaluation of OSA. Cephalometrics and computed tomographic (CT) scanning can detail craniomandibular abnormalities and soft-tissue contours of the nasal and oral airway, allowing determination of minimal orifice diameter. Anatomical landmarks of interest in OSA patients include the hyoid bone, which may be abnormally low, and the retropalatal airway, which is often significantly narrowed. Recently, magnetic resonance imaging (MRI) has been used to determine the distribution of fat within the airway and to measure pharyngeal volume as well as soft-tissue water (reflecting upper-airway mucosal edema).

Blood values that should raise suspicion are polycythemia and hypercapnia. Disorders in ventilatory control have been considered to have important implications in OSA. Those with the pickwickian syndrome may have a decreased ventilatory response to CO_2, while patients with eucapnic OSA are characterized by increased respiratory drive, as reflected by both $P_{0.1}$ and V_T/V_I (25).

Spirometry may reveal characteristic abnormalities, such as sawtoothing, caused by vibration of redundant pharyngeal tissue, or flattening of the inspiratory limb of the flow-volume loop. These are sometimes present only in the supine position (Fig. 28.6).

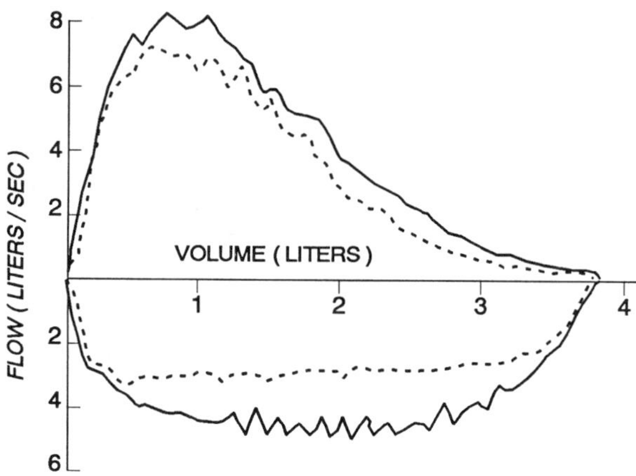

Figure 28.6. Maximal flow-volume curve demonstrating flattening of the inspiratory limb in the upright position. The "sawtooth" pattern appears during inspiration in the supine posture.

Polysomnography

Strategy

A polysomnographic study is indicated in patients with a history of EDS, loud sonorous snoring, and reported respiratory pauses. Multiple parameters can be monitored noninvasively. Sleep staging with a four-lead EEG montage, two-lead electro-oculography (EOG), and submental electromyography (EMG) is routine.

Thoradoabdominal Displacement

Strain gauges, magnetometry, inductance plethysmography, and impedance pneumography are the various technologies used to detect thoracoabdominal movement or displacement. This determines whether respiratory effort is being made. While motion is not observed in central apnea, paradoxical motion of the rib cage and abdomen occurs in patients with OSA as a result of the ineffectual respiratory efforts. The detection of thoracoabdominal discoordination or "paradoxical" inward movement of the rib cage readily assists in characterizing an apnea as obstructive in nature. The abdominal contents behave as an incompressible liquid and act as a hydraulic coupler between the diaphragm and the anterolateral abdominal wall.

Muscle Paresis and Movement

Electromyography (EMG) of the peripheral tibialis should be monitored to allow for the detection of aberrant limb activity. This is done in addition to the submental EMG. Leg movement during sleep is a cause of arousal that increases in prevalence with age. It may be an important cause for fragmented sleep in the elderly. Periodic leg movement (PLM) is associated with various systemic diseases and is related to the restless leg syndrome (RLS).

Oximetry and Arrhythmia Detection

Pulse oximeters allow for noninvasive monitoring of oxygenation. The extent of oxyhemoglobin desaturation is determined by a number of factors, most significantly the duration of the apnea. The basal (control) state of oxygenation is important because preexisting hypoxemia will cause a greater fall in oxygenation during apnea. Lower lung volume at the onset of apnea also produces greater desaturation. For a given duration of apnea, the degree of postapneic desaturation is influenced by apnea type (greater for obstructive than for central apnea) and sleep stage (greater during REM sleep than during non-REM sleep).

Oximeters that record pulse and blood pressure as well as saturation reveal the vagal slowing of heart rate and systemic hypertensive responses to apneic desaturation. The vagal response and sympathetic surge predispose to bradycardia and other conduction abnormalities, so heart rate and rhythm should also be monitored with an ECG precordial lead. OSA-related heart rate changes are so characteristic that they may suggest the diagnosis of the OSA syndrome. The heart rate decreases during apneas and increases abruptly immediately postapnea. This pattern recurs cyclically during sleep. The subsequent arousal stimulus results in inhibition of the vagal suppression of the sinoatrial pacemaker. Similarly, the postapneic tachycardia appears to be the result of interaction of the autonomic nervous system and hypoxia with the arousal reaction, causing increased sympathetic nervous activity and a decrease in parasympathetic tone. However, the overall prevalence of cardiac arrhythmias appears to be surprisingly low in patients without serious coexisting cardiac or pulmonary disease.

Recently, studies that allow for beat-to-beat monitoring of stroke volume have shown that both right (26) and left (27) ventricular stroke volumes decrease abruptly postapnea. Although heart rate increases with recovery, the increase is not sufficient to compensate for the decreases in stroke volume and cardiac output in the early recovery phase (Fig. 28.7) (27). The decrease in flow occurring coincident with the nadir of oxygen saturation

may significantly compromise regional oxygen delivery. This may be related to the clinical ischemic episodes reported to be associated with OSA, cerebral strokes, and acute or chronic syndromes of myocardial ischemia such as infarction or cardiopathy, with manifestations varying from ST-segment depression to heart failure.

Air Movement

Qualitative measurement of airflow is sufficient to determine the duration and frequency of apneas. The movement of air is detected by the increased P_{CO_2} (capnography) or temperature (thermistry) of expired air. The detectors are placed in the oronasal path of the airflow. Evaluation of snoring with a simple acoustic monitor using a microphone and tape recorder can be a useful tool, while more sophisticated spectral analysis allows for characterization of snoring. This establishes the diagnosis of apnea, and the detection of chest movement determines whether it is central or obstructive in character.

Nap Study

While nap studies can provide valuable preliminary and/or screening information, strict criteria for their interpretation must be applied. For example, daytime naps following sleep deprivation should include at least one

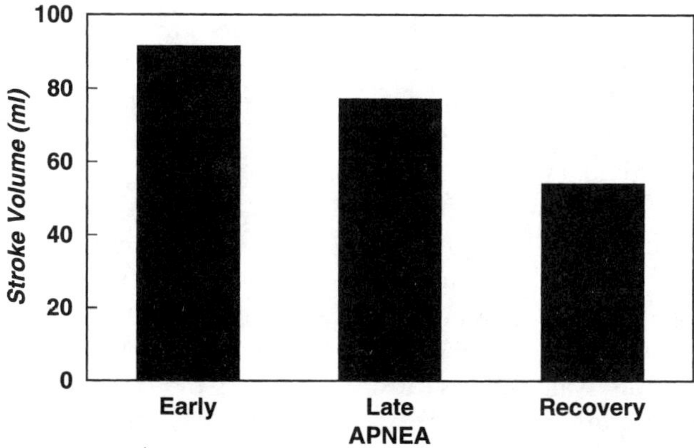

Figure 28.7. Effects of apnea on the cardiac output. There is a progressive decrease with obstruction and an abrupt decrease with restoration of a patent airway and resumption of ventilation. These hemodynamic changes are related to alterations in heart rate during the apnea and to stroke volume postapnea.

REM period with a minimum length of 10 minutes; nap studies should preclude positional apnea by demonstrating multiple sleep positions; and no therapy should be instituted without nocturnal polysomnography. Nap studies in comparison to all-night polysomnography in patients with OSA have a diminished percentage of REM sleep and a lower apnea index. Oxygen desaturation is also less severe during nap studies and is attributable to the decrease in apnea duration. False negatives can occur due to the lack of REM sleep, often the only time apnea is noted in some patients.

Multiple Sleep Latency Test

For patients without EDS, the multiple sleep latency test (MSLT) provides an objective way to quantify sleepiness and to evaluate the results of treatment. It is a measure of the tendency or length of time required to fall asleep. This value is determined by EEG criteria, with a structured series of 4 to 5 naps at fixed 2-hour intervals, usually starting at 9:00 AM. The degree of sleepiness as determined by the mean sleep latency (SL) is strongly influenced by the amount of nocturnal sleep. Therefore, to have a valid MSLT the adequacy of the previous night's sleep must be documented. For this reason the MSLT is usually performed on the day following the all-night polysomnogram. The study utilizes a recording montage solely for sleep staging (EEG, EOG, EMG). Each test is ended 20 minutes after "lights out" or sooner, since the patient is awakened after 15 minutes of sleep. The mean SL in normal subjects is 10 to 15 minutes, while in OSA patients it is generally exceedingly short (less than 5 minutes) and is frequently associated with sleep-onset REM periods (SOREMS), as seen in narcolepsy.

While the MSLT quantifies sleep propensity and detects an abnormal tendency to achieve REM, it has recently been suggested that the ability to stay awake is best measured by the maintenance of wakefulness test (MWT). This tests the patient's ability to remain awake; the results may be discordant with the MSLT, suggesting separate brain mechanisms for sleep and wakefulness that may be differentially affected.

Self-administered questionnaires, such as the Stanford or Epworth Sleepiness Scale (ESS), have also been evaluated as indicators of excessive daytime sleepiness and have been shown to be a valid and inexpensive way of assessing sleepiness in patients. Just as the MSLT is an essential measure of sleepiness and can help detect false-negative polysomnograms, the ESS may clarify the mechanisms underlying the patient with "subjective sleepiness without objective findings" (28).

There is currently no uniform agreement on a specific test for determining unacceptable driving risk. However, the profile of a high-risk driver must be recognized. These individuals should be educated, and the effectiveness of treatment should be judged within 2 months.

Home Study

Overnight monitoring in a sleep laboratory is a labor-intensive, time-consuming procedure. Recent studies have shown that the "first-night" effect encountered with in-laboratory studies does not exist with ambulatory monitoring, allowing patients to sleep in their own beds and in familiar surroundings. The "first-night" effect includes lengthening of sleep onset latency and REM latency and an increase in the percentage of wakefulness and stage 1 sleep. Furthermore, inadequate acclimatization of the patient to the laboratory surroundings not only risks alteration of natural sleep architecture and duration but the frequency and duration of apneic episodes as well. Because of these factors, along with recent studies suggesting a much greater prevalence of OSA, a simpler test that can be performed more quickly, more conveniently, and at less cost has been sought.

Some studies utilize video systems or activity (actograph) rather than EEG monitoring for determination of sleep and wake states. Since patients with OSA invariably exhibit increased motor activity during sleep, activity monitoring has been proposed as an inexpensive and convenient monitoring technique for diagnosis. Motor activity is continuously recorded by a solid-state activity monitor on the wrist, allowing for the calculation of activity indices. However, such actimetry assessment by itself with a sleep log has not been found to be reliable in identifying patients with OSA (29), although this technique has proved to be of value in studying sleep habits in general of large numbers of subjects (30).

In principle, current technology and available instrumentation allow for recording all noninvasive functions under ambulatory conditions with the same accuracy as an examination in the sleep laboratory. These systems have their origins in 24-hour EEG monitoring for seizure activity. The technology was then introduced into sleep medicine and modified with the addition of pneumography. A variety of portable monitoring systems have been developed, and a variety of systems are now available for home study, including such products as Sleep I/T, Poly-G, Snoresat, Eden Trace, Nightwatch, Vitalog, Medilog, and Mesam. The recording variables, which are limited depending on the system used, are grouped under sleep staging (EEG, EOG, EMG), apnea, respiratory effort (impedance or strain gauge), airflow (thermistry or capnography), heart rate (ECG), and oximetry. The montage selected must be valid for the purpose of the study for which it is being used. Theoretically, home recordings also offer the ideal technology for studying the frequency and duration of daytime naps. Microphones for home tape recording of bedroom sounds may also be used for screening and evaluating therapeutic intervention, particularly for snoring.

These currently available systems generally incorporate two or more respiratory recording techniques coupled with solid-state, disc, or tape-based storage technology to allow for ambulatory or home monitoring. However, adequate evaluation of recordings can only be made if the complete course of the original raw data curve is available for playback with high resolution. Therefore, a high-quality, calibrated signal recorded with a sufficiently high sampling rate, as dictated by the highest-occurring signal frequency, is required. Finally, the ambulatory system must be attached to the patient by specially trained technicians. The technician may visit the patient in his or her home to apply the electrodes and other necessary transducers and to calibrate the equipment. Alternatively, the patient attends the sleep laboratory or office during the afternoon or on the way home from work before the night study for this "hookup." The technician either collects the equipment the next morning or the patient returns to the sleep laboratory/office to be disconnected. The advantages are obvious: the ability to have a single technician connect several patients in an afternoon and to have no staffing requirements during night hours.

Ideally, a home study can also be used to evaluate treatment in a patient diagnosed with a sleep disorder, such as for follow-up of patients after initial continuous positive airway pressure (CPAP) therapy or surgery for OSA. The system must be equipped to measure peripheral EMG, if treatment for a movement disorder is to be evaluated, and EEG if narcolepsy is to be evaluated. Muscle interference of EEG patterns may, however, be formidable. Most commonly, apnea monitoring is used to diagnose and assess the severity of OSA by the number, duration, and type of nocturnal disordered breathing events as well as by the degree of desaturation. Systems that do not include EEG recordings determine estimated sleep recording time rather than actual total sleep time for determining the conventional respiratory disturbance indices. While this may be adequate for screening purposes, the lack of sleep-stage monitoring will not allow the detection of the microarousals in the absence of apneas characterizing the UARS.

The advantages—cost and convenience—can be outweighed by the restricted number of channels available for monitoring (8 versus 16). The current generation of home testing devices are capable of overcoming this shortcoming. Recently, home screening for apnea has been shown to demonstrate excellent agreement between an "out-of-laboratory" system and complete polysomnographic monitoring in a sleep laboratory. Current technology has suggested to some a two-stage diagnostic approach: first, an unattended home study followed by a more detailed study in the sleep laboratory, especially for the assessment of treatment intervention such as titration of nasal CPAP (n-CPAP) for patients with OSA.

A substantial benefit of home studies may exist for patients with low probability of a sleep disorder and a "split-night" study in the laboratory for those with high probability of a sleep disorder, specifically OSA. It has been reported that in patients with OSA, the severity of the disordered breathing (respiratory disturbance index [RDI]) during the first half of the night is sufficiently representative of the entire night that the second half of the night can be utilized for the initial therapeutic trial. Thus, rather than having the expense of two nights of study (the initial for diagnosis and the second for evaluating a nonsurgical therapy), the entire evaluation is accomplished in a single night. Recently, n-CPAP titration has been successfully accomplished in attended as well as in unattended home studies (31, 32).

It has been suggested that for unattended home or in-hospital bedside studies, electrophysiological recording is not necessary for accurate diagnosis. A recording of breathing pattern and time in bed with an estimate of sleep time may be sufficient. Furthermore, the more parameters that are monitored, the greater the chance of unattended patients becoming inadvertently detached from or entangled in the electrodes and bands used, thus affecting the quality of recording and sleep and negating the cost advantage. With an established protocol, a less than 5% repeat rate due to technical problems should be experienced. Neurophysiological recording of sleep, however, must be utilized for measuring daytime sleepiness and for detecting the presence of SOREMS. Unanticipated disruptions at home have been found to complicate adherence to the MSLT protocol.

Further attempts to simplify diagnostic strategy and limit the number of patients sent to a sleep laboratory have included using only oximetry for home studies. The results, however, have been conflicting: some studies suggest low sensitivity and false-negative results but high specificity (33), while others suggest low specificity but high sensitivity (34). In ad-

dition, neither expired (P_{ETCO_2}) nor transcutaneous (P_{tcCO_2}) CO_2 monitoring for evaluation and therapy of sleep-disordered breathing has been found to accurately reflect the arterial value (Pa_{CO_2}).

Screening with oximetry alone on an ambulatory basis may result in a high false-negative rate, especially among patients beginning with normal awake oxygenation with their arterial set point atop the plateau of the O_2 dissociation curve. It must be realized that while patients with severe OSA show a consistent number of apneas per hour from night to night, those with mild OSA show a highly variable apnea index. Therefore, a single negative sleep study should be considered insufficient to exclude OSA in patients with clinical characteristics of the syndrome. Such variability might be attributable to alteration of sleep architecture or posture, nasal occlusion, unknown drug (e.g., alcohol) use, or poorly understood chronobiological factors.

Treatment

Weight Loss

Weight loss cures OSA in most obese patients (Fig. 28.8). Resting hypoxemia, hyperventilation, variable extrathoracic upper-airway obstruction, and food-induced thermogenesis all change accordingly once weight loss is achieved. Weight loss results in significant reduction in upper-airway collapsibility and the resolution of abnormalities in the flow-volume curve. This is presumably related to structural as well as functional alterations in the pharynx, such as widening of the pharyngeal aperture with diminished mass loads on pharyngeal structure from lipid deposition. Enhanced neuromuscular activity of upper-airway dilators may also serve to increase pharyngeal cross-sectional area with weight loss.

Posture and Oxygen Therapy

In some patients, maintaining the upright or decubitus posture alone is enough to alleviate mild OSA (Fig. 28.9) (35). However, it is difficult to maintain this position during sleep.

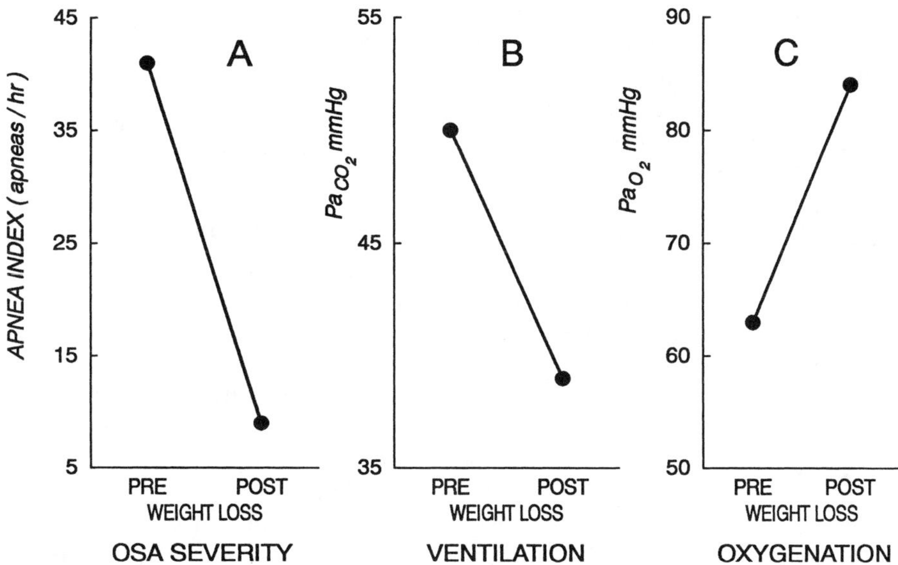

Figure 28.8.   Effect of weight loss (50 lb) achieved by diet in 18 obese patients (165% ideal body weight). **A,** The severity of obstructive sleep apnea decreases. **B,** The resting awake ventilatory status improves. **C,** The resting awake arterial saturation increases, resulting in a smaller fall in oxygenation for any duration of apnea.

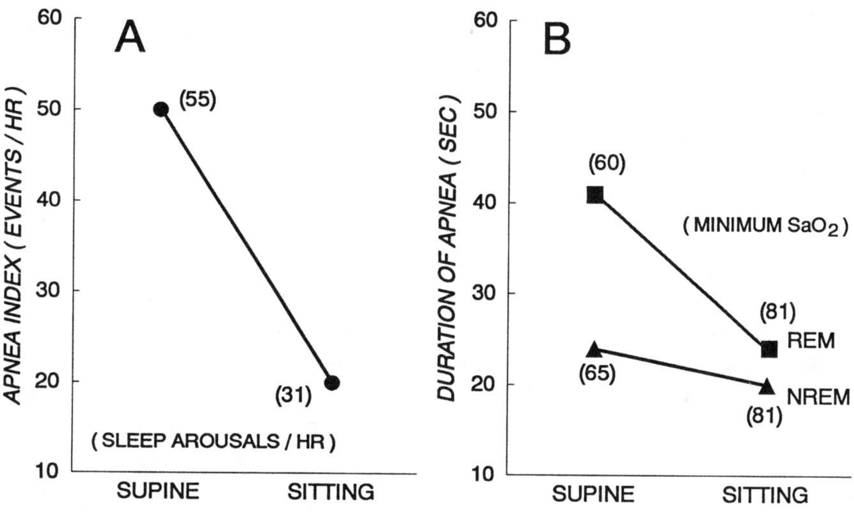

Figure 28.9.   **A,** Effect of changing from the supine to the upright position during sleep on the severity of apnea. The number of arousals also decreases in the sitting position. **B,** The durations of the apneic episodes during both REM and NREM sleep diminish in the upright sleep position. The resulting arterial desaturation decreases.

O_2 therapy has also been reported to ameliorate not only the hypoxemia in central and obstructive sleep apnea but the number of disordered breathing events as well. This mode of therapy is ideally reserved for patients with mild OSA but with a disproportionate degree of resulting hypoxemia due to associated lung disease. Oxygen, administered below the site of upper-airway obstruction by means of a transtracheal catheter, has been found to be more effective than nasal oxygen in reducing the frequency of disordered breathing events in patients with OSA (36). This has been attributed to the development of an increase in mean airway pressure, and an aerodynamic effect similar to that seen with nasal CPAP may be operative.

Drug Therapy

Currently there is no apparent role for drug therapy in the management of OSA. Progesterone is no longer considered an effective mode of therapy, although early reports of success had made it a standard drug regimen in the past. Similarly, hormone replacement therapy in the management of OSA in obese postmenopausal women has not been found to be effective. In contrast, acromegalic patients with sleep apnea improve markedly when treated with octreotide, a somatostatin analog. The drug inhibits growth hormone secretion and may decrease OSA in patients with acromegaly by decreasing upper-airway soft-tissue swelling, thus increasing upper-airway dimensions.

Protriptyline, a tricyclic antidepressant, is another drug that had initially favorable reports of efficacy. As do other drugs in this class, it decreases the amount of REM and is useful primarily for patients with mild REM-associated apnea. Other pharmacological efforts, including administration of theophylline derivatives and L-tryptophan, have not proved useful. Various studies suggesting a pathogenic role for increased endogenous opioid activity led to therapeutic trials of naloxone. The activation of opioid receptors may be related, however, to the need for "load compensation." Therefore, the use of an antagonist may be expected to have mixed results. However, the most effective drug treatment for OSA is avoidance of drugs that depress upper-airway muscle tone. These include alcohol, sedatives, hypnotics, and narcotics. Androgens also enhance OSA, but the mechanism is unknown.

Nasal Continuous Positive Airway Pressure

The use of nasal continuous positive airway pressure (n-CPAP) is often the treatment of choice for patients with OSA. The applied pressure is initially adjusted to alleviate complete obstructive events and then, progressively, hypopneas (desaturation episodes) and finally partial obstructive events reflected by snoring. We use a derived formula to determine a starting point that facilitates titration. The determination of pressure requirements is related primarily to the degree of obesity and the severity of OSA. This mode of noninvasive ventilatory support is now used for other respiratory disorders as well. n-CPAP has also been shown to be an effective therapeutic modality in a variety of forms of "periodic breathing" such as the Cheyne-Stokes pattern of respiration observed in congestive heart failure.

n-CPAP provides an aerodynamic splint for the upper airway, with positive pressure maintaining patency of the pharyngeal lumen. Positive intraluminal pressure directly depresses pharyngeal dilator EMG activity, promoting airway closure. However, the physical forces generated externally enhance distention and overcome the suction pressure. This reverses net transmural collapsing pressure resulting from diaphragmatic and intercostal muscle contraction. n-CPAP also increases functional residual capacity (FRC), which reflexively decreases upper-airway resistance by stimulating airway dilators.

Another proposed mechanism accounting for the efficacy of CPAP postulates the reduction of upper-airway collapsibility by hydrostatically decreasing pharyngeal vascular congestion or interstitial fluid (edema). An additional mode of improvement in airway tone may be the result of reversing the central nervous system depression associated with

OSA and increasing airway dilator activity. These various factors may account for the apparent progressive decrease in the required magnitude of n-CPAP with use.

Patient compliance is a critical factor in successful treatment and is dependent on expert technical teaching and explanation. Patient motivation is generally based on the degree of relief from EDS. Although therapy with n-CPAP is highly effective in the majority of patients with OSA, the combined immediate and long-term failure rate measures 25 to 40%, with no reliable predictors for compliance. It is especially high in nonapneic snorers. Many use the therapy only for limited hours during sleep (37). Effort-sensitive, "intelligent" devices are being developed that may improve compliance.

Drugs that the patient receives, including antihypertensives or other cardiotonics, have to be taken into account. With the alleviation of the OSA, blood pressure can be expected to return to normal and the continued use of antihypertensive medication may result in hypotension. Determination of the CPAP level required in patients who have a significant history of alcohol ingestion is also problematic. Empirically, these patients require higher levels of support. Bilevel positive airway pressure (BiPAP) is derived from CPAP and allows for differential setting of expiratory (EPAP) and inspiratory (IPAP) positive airway pressures to maintain airway patency but the lower expiratory pressure (38). Although most patients with OSA can be titrated with a "split-night" study, many will require alterations in mask fitting, pressure, pressure modality, or the use of endonasal cushions.

Effective therapy results in the immediate relief of sleep fragmentation. The patient often reports "the best night's sleep ever." Tests of cognitive function as well as daytime sleepiness improve immediately. The patient should be monitored closely at home for the first 1 to 4 weeks of treatment. Follow-up sleep studies should be performed after 1 year, which may serve as the most useful role for home studies. Side effects and adverse reactions such as allergies, abrasions, dry nose, and conjunctivitis are commonly reported. They are not correlated with the level of pressure used nor alleviated with the use of a humidifier. Recurrence of symptoms after successful treatment may imply mask leak, weight gain, or alcohol or other drug use.

Nasopharyngeal Tube and Tongue-Retaining and Orthodontic Devices

The nasopharyngeal tube (NPT) was originally introduced in the emergency treatment of upper-airway obstruction. This was generally perceived as an interim step until definitive surgical correction could be achieved (i.e., tonsillectomy or tracheostomy). The procedure involves the insertion of an uncuffed pediatric endotracheal tube through the nares that extends distally to the hypopharynx (Figs. 28.10 and 28.11).

The therapeutic efficacy of dental or tongue-retaining anti-snoring devices in OSA has not been thoroughly evaluated. Preliminary studies have not been encouraging. The tongue-retaining device at best improves rather than cures OSA, and the patient must have a patent nasal airway for it to be effective. Similarly, a variety of orthodontic appliances have been utilized in the treatment of patients with OSA. These devices are designed to advance the mandible and the tissues inserted on it, particularly the genioglossus. Such procedures do not have adequate data to prove long-term efficacy in sleep apnea, though they may be effective in alleviating snoring. Devices that externally dilate the nares are of little benefit.

Surgery

Tracheostomy once held the only therapeutic answer to OSA. Today, surgery is appropriate for the few patients with anatomical abnormalities and those who cannot tolerate n-CPAP. More recently, redundant oropharyngeal mucosa, a long soft palate, a long wide uvula, and retrognathia have also become relative indications for surgical intervention. The goal is to select the patient with airway closure at the level of the palatopharyngeal sphincter (soft palate) and not at the base of the tongue (39).

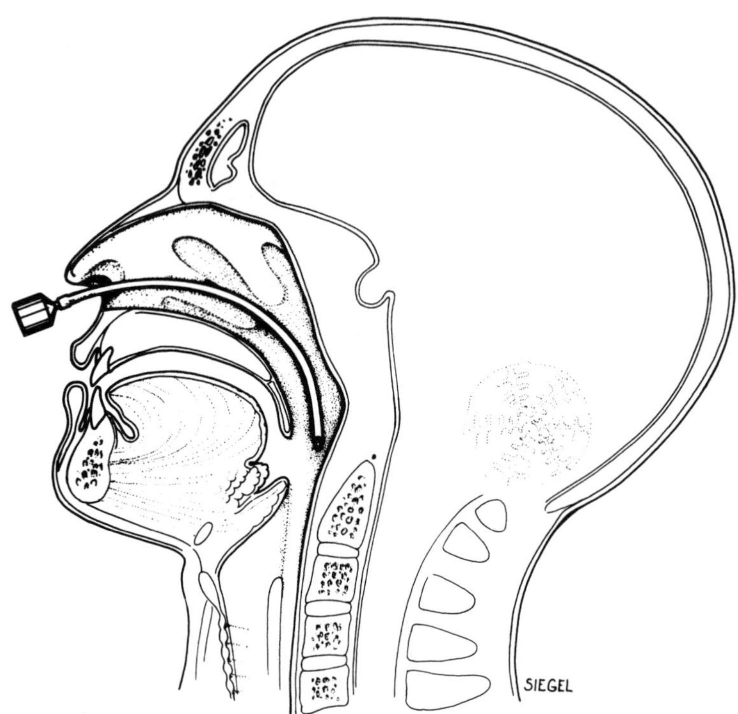

Figure 28.10. Idealized model of nasopharyngeal tube placement above the epiglottis.

Cephalometric examination supplemented by CT scanning can aid in determining the suitable candidate. The procedures currently performed for these anatomical abnormalities are uvulopalatopharyngoplasty (UPPP), anterior sagittal osteotomy of the mandible, hyoid myotomy and suspension, and maxillomandibular and hyoid advancement. The single or combination procedure is selected after consideration of the surgical anatomy and the expertise of the surgeon. Since these are new and innovative surgical techniques, few experienced practitioners exist.

UPPP was initially introduced to treat snoring; however, in OSA the initial overall success rate is less than 50%, and recurrence of apneas frequently occurs after 1 or 2 years. The use of CPAP after UPPP is sometimes found intolerable, as the seal between the soft palate and the tongue is gone. Thus, air blown in through the nose exits the mouth and fails to splint the upper airway. As with tonsillectomy in children, the patients should have

postoperative polysomnography, since OSA may persist even after snoring has been alleviated. Recently, an office-based surgical procedure, laser-assisted uvulopalatoplasty (LAUP), has been promoted as a treatment for snoring. Adequate controlled studies validating the procedure do not exist.

UPPP does not seem to be effective in patients with severe OSA, and compliance with nasal CPAP tends to be lower in patients with mild OSA. Results that have been reported in patients treated either with CPAP or UPPP showed no objective differences in AHI or snoring in the near term (40). After 6 years there was no difference in the long-term survival between the two treatment groups (41).

Finally, the route of respiration (oral versus nasal), which is influenced by palatal position, is known to be a significant factor in OSA. During nasal breathing the oral route is occluded by the tongue adhering to the soft palate as well as by the closed lips. A change

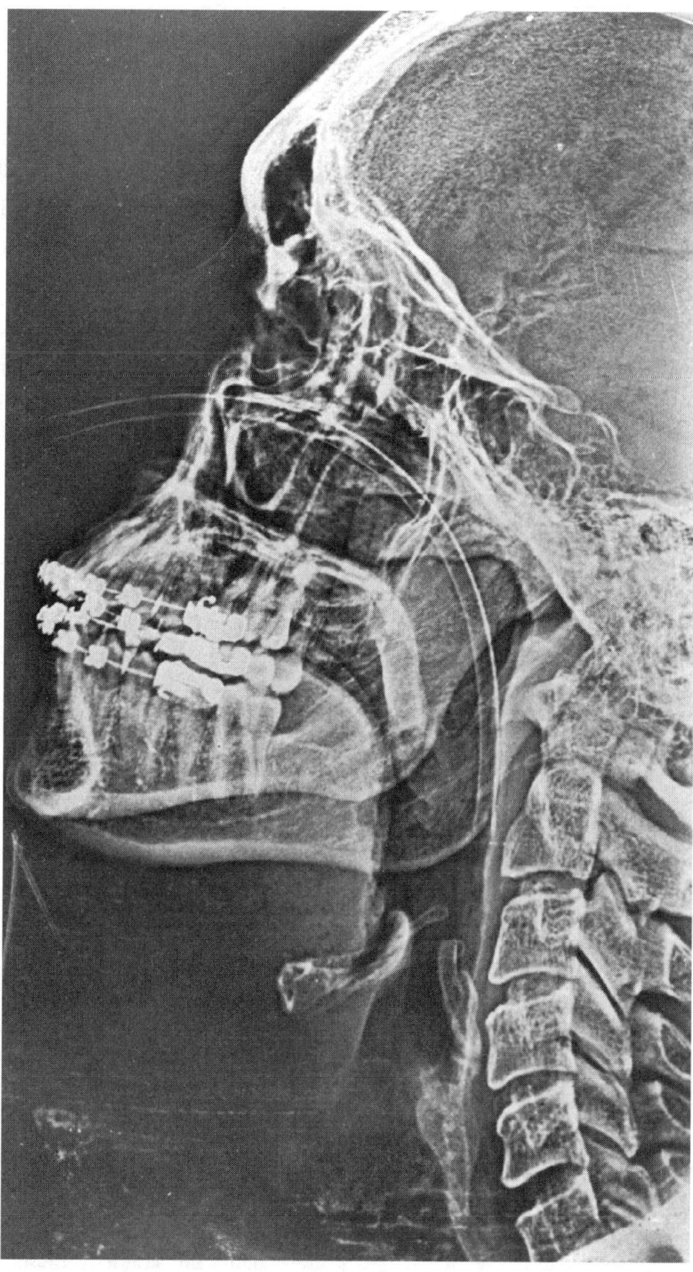

Figure 28.11. Xerograph of tube placement in one subject.

from nasal to oral breathing in response to nasal occlusion is rarely possible during NREM sleep without arousal (42). This is of presumed significance, since nasal occlusion induces OSA in normal subjects and significant nasal pathology has been reported in two-thirds of series of patients with OSA. However, while success has been reported anecdotally for submucosal nasal resection and a variety of other nasal procedures for OSA (correction of septal deviation, polyps, and hypertrophied turbinates), such therapeutic procedures remain poor forms of curative surgery for snoring or OSA.

Prognosis

The natural history of sleep apnea begins with the concept that OSA is a progressive disease that evolves from simple snoring. It is a relatively common condition, but if untreated has major public health implications. Recent reports provide support for the concept of an evolution from mild to more severe sleep pathology. There is ongoing debate over whether the suggested cardiovascular consequences of snoring and untreated sleep apnea are associated with reduced survival (43). Obstructive sleep apnea may present as systemic hypertension, cerebrovascular or coronary artery disease with ischemic symptoms, or heart failure from a dilated cardiomyopathy. Aside from the suggested excess of cardiovascular morbidity, including myocardial infarction and cerebrovascular accidents, OSA results in pulmonary hypertension in about 25% of patients and predisposes to cor pulmonale and right ventricular dysfunction, especially in patients with confounding lung disease.

However, despite a reduction in biochemical markers of sympathetic activity, n-CPAP was not able to demonstrate an overall reduction in blood pressure or left ventricular mass index (44). This suggests other confounding structural and functional mechanisms in the hemodynamic manifestations of OSA that may not readily regress or be reversible with treatment.

The benefits of n-CPAP as expressed by quality-adjusted life years (QALYs) of survival have been shown to be real. The treatment is well tolerated and has a favorable cost-utility ratio (45). However, palliative treatment with nasal CPAP must be continuous. Failure to use it for even a single night can result in the reappearance of pretreatment levels of nocturnal sleep disturbance and daytime hypersomnolence. Moreover, while significant improvements in objective sleepiness and mood have been shown to occur as a result of long-term treatment with nasal CPAP, these studies show no evidence of major improvement in cognitive function (46). This includes persistent memory deficits that are related to the level of nocturnal hypoxemia, suggesting that irreversible anoxic central nervous system damage occurs prior to diagnosis and treatment in severe OSA.

References

1. Adam K, Oswald I. Protein synthesis, bodily renewal and the sleep-wake cycle. Clin Sci 1993;65:561–567.
2. Steriade M. Basic mechanisms of sleep generation. Neurology 1992;42(Suppl 6):9–18.
3. Inoue S, Kreuger JM, eds. Endogenous Sleep Factors. The Hague, Netherlands: VSP Academic Publishing, 1990.
4. Szymusiak R, McGinty D. Brainstem and forebrain regulation of sleep onset and slow-wave sleep. In: Saunders NA, Sullivan CE, eds. Sleep and Breathing. Lung Biology in Health and Disease, vol. 71. New York: Marcel Dekker, 1994:27–45.
5. Ankle-Isreal S, Coy T. Are sleep disturbances equivalent to sleep apnea syndrome? Sleep 1994;7:77–83.
6. Khatri I, Freis ED. Hemodynamic changes during sleep. J Appl Physiol 1967;22:867–873.
7. Veale D, Fagret D, Pepin JL, Bonnet C, Siche JP, Levy P. Circadian changes of left ventricular ejection fraction in normal subjects. Chronobiol Int 1994;11:200–210.
8. Madsen PL, Vorstrup S. Cerebral blood flow and metabolism during sleep. Cerebrovasc Brain Metab Rev 1991;3:281–296.
9. McGinty D, Szymusial R. Neurobiology of sleep. In: Saunders NA, Sullivan CE, eds. Sleep and Breathing. Lung Biology in Health and Disease, vol. 71. New York: Marcel Dekker, 1994;71:1–26.
10. Cagnacci A, Soldani R, Yen SSC. Hypothermic effect of melatonin and nocturnal core body temperature decline are reduced in aged women. J Appl Physiol 1995;78:314–317.
11. Hudgel DW, Devadatta P, Hamilton H. Pattern of breathing and upper airway mechanisms during wakefulness and sleep in healthy elderly humans. J Appl Physiol 1993;74:2198–2204.
12. Warner G, Skatrud JB, Dempsey JA. Effect of hypoxia induced periodic breathing on upper airway obstruction during sleep. J Appl Physiol 1987;62:2201–2211.
13. Colrain IM, Trinder J, Fraser G, Wilson GV. Ventilation during sleep onset. J Appl Physiol 1987;63:2067–2074.
14. Fletcher EC, DeBehnke RD, Lovoi MS, Gorin AB. Undiagnosed sleep apnea in patients with essential hypertension. Ann Intern Med 1985;103:190–195.
15. Partinen M, Palomaki H. Snoring and cerebral infarction. Lancet 1985;2:1325–1326.
16. Hoffstein V, Zamel N, Phillipson EA. Lung volume dependence on pharyngeal cross-sectional area in patients with obstructive sleep apnea. Am Rev Respir Dis 1984;130:175–178.
17. Gleeson K, Sweer LW. Ventilatory pattern after hypoxic stimulation during wakefulness and NREM sleep. J Appl Physiol 1993;75:397–404.

18. Berry RB, Mahutte CK, Light RW. Effect of hypercapnia on the arousal response to airway occlusion during sleep in normal subjects. J Appl Physiol 1993;74: 2269–2275.

19. Marcus CL, Omlin KJ, Basinki DJ, Bailey SL, Rachal AB, Von Pechman WS, Keens TG, Ward SLD. Normal polygraphic values for children and adolescents. Am Rev Respir Dis 1992;146:1235–1239.

20. Pillar G, Lavie P. Assessment of the role of inheritance in sleep apnea syndrome. Am J Respir Crit Care Med 1995;151:688–691.

21. Brown IB, McClean PA, Boucheer R, Zamel N, Hoffstein V. Changes in pharyngeal cross-sectional area with posture and application of continuous positive airway pressure in patients with obstructive sleep apnea. Am Rev Respir Dis 1987;136:628–632.

22. Morrison DL, Launois SH, Isono S, Feroah TR, Whitelaw WA, Remmers JE. Pharyngeal narrowing and closing pressures in patients with obstructive sleep apnea. Am Rev Respir Dis 1993;148:606–611.

23. Okabes S, Hida W, Kikuchi Y, Taguchi O, Ogawa H, Mizusawa A, Miki H, Shirato K. Role of hypoxia on increased blood pressure in patients with obstructive sleep apnea. Thorax 1995;50:28–34.

24. Kissebah AH, Krakower GR. Regional adiposity and morbidity. Physiol Rev 1994;74:761–811.

25. Beniloch E, Cordero P, Morales P, Soler JJ, Macian V. Ventilatory pattern at rest and response to hypercapnic stimulation in patients with obstructive sleep syndrome. Respiration 1995;62:4–9.

26. Bonsignore MR, Maronne O, Romanos S, Pieri D. Time course of right ventricular stroke volume and output in obstructive sleep apneas. Am J Respir Crit Care Med 1994;149:155–159.

27. Garpestad E, Katayama H, Parker JA, Ringler J, Lilly J, Yasuda T, Moore RH, Strauss HW, Weiss JW. Stroke volume and cardiac output decrease at termination of obstructive apneas. J Appl Physiol 1992;73:1743–1748.

28. Johns MW. Sleepiness in different situations measured by the Epworth Sleepiness Scale. Sleep 1994;17: 703–710.

29. Middelkoop HAM, Neven AK, Van Hilten JJ, Ruwhof CW, Kamphuisen HAC. Wrist actigraphic assessment of sleep in 116 community based subjects suspected of obstructive sleep apnea syndrome. Thorax 1995;50:284–289.

30. Reyner A, Horne JA. Gender and age related differences in sleep determined by home recorded sleep logs and actimetry from 400 adults. Sleep 1995;18:127–134.

31. Waldhorn RF, Wood K. Attended home titration of nasal continuous positive airway pressure therapy for obstructive sleep apnea. Chest 1993;104:19–25.

32. Coppola MP, Lawee M. Management of obstructive sleep apnea syndrome in the home: the role of portable sleep apnea recording. Chest 1993;104:19–25.

33. Gyulay S, Olson LG, Hensley MJ, King MT, Allen KM, Saunders NA. A comparison of clinical assessment and home oximetry in the diagnosis of obstructive sleep apnea. Am Rev Respir Dis 1993;147:50–53.

34. Series F, Marc I, Cormier Y, LaForge J. Utility of nocturnal home oximetry for case finding in patients with suspected sleep apnea hypopnea syndrome. Ann Intern Med 1993;119:449–453.

35. McEvoy RD, Sharp DJ, Thornton AT. The effects of posture on obstructive sleep apnea. Am Rev Respir Dis 1986;133:662–666.

36. Farney RJ, Walker JM, Elmer JC, Viscomi VA, Ord RJ. Transtracheal oxygen, nasal CPAP and nasal oxygen in five patients with obstructive sleep apnea. Chest 1992;101:1228–1235.

37. Kribbs NB, Pack AI, Kline LR, Smith PL, Schwartz AR, Schubert NM, Redline S, Henry JN, Getsy JE, Dinges DF. Objective measurements of patterns of nasal CPAP use by patients with obstructive sleep apnea. Am Rev Respir Dis 1993;147:887–895.

38. Reeves-Hoche MK, Hudgel DW, Meck R, Witteman R, Ross A, Zwilich CW. Continuous versus bilevel positive airway pressure for obstructive sleep apnea. Am J Respir Crit Care Med 1995;151:443–449.

39. Launois SH, Feroah TR, Campbell WN, Issa FG, Morrison D, Whitelaw WA, Isono S, Remmers JE. Site of pharyngeal narrowing predicts outcome of surgery for obstructive sleep apnea. Am Rev Respir Dis 1993;147: 182–189.

40. Keenan SP, Burt H, Ryan F, Fleetham JA. Long-term survival of patients with obstructive sleep apnea treated by uvulopalatoplasty or nasal CPAP. Chest 1994;105: 155–159.

41. Miljeteig H, Mateika S, Haight JS, Cole P, Hoffstein V. Subjective and objective assessment of uvulopalatopharyngoplasty for treatment of snoring and obstructive sleep apnea. Am J Respir Crit Care Med 1994;150: 1286–1290.

42. Tangel DJ, Mezzanotte WS, White DP. Influences of NREM sleep on activity of palatoglossus and levator palatini muscles in normal men. J Appl Physiol 1995; 78:689–695.

43. Sforza E, Addati G, Cirignotta F, Lugaresi E. Natural evolution of sleep apnea syndrome: five year longitudinal study. Eur Respir J 1994;7:1765–1770.

44. Hedner J, Darpo B, Ejnell H, Carlson J, Caidahl K. Reduction in sympathic activity after longterm CPAP treatment in sleep apnea: Cardiovascular implications. Eur Respir J 1995;8:222–229.

45. Tousignant P, Cosio MG, Ley RD, Groome PA. Quality adjusted life years added by treatment of obstructive sleep apnea. Sleep 1994;17:52–60.

46. Naegele B, Thouvard V, Pepin JL, Levy P, Bonnet C, Perret JE, Pellat J, Feuerstein C. Deficits of cognitive executive functions in patients with sleep apnea syndrome. Sleep 1995;18:43–52.

Suggested Readings

Chokroverty S, ed. Sleep Disorders Medicine: Basic Science, Technical Considerations and Clinical Aspects. Boston: Butterworth-Heinemann, 1994.

Cooper R, ed. Sleep. London: Chapman and Hall Medical, 1994.

Issa FG, Suratt PM, Remmers JE, eds. Sleep and Respiration. New York: Wiley-Liss, 1990.

Kryger MH, Roth T, Dement WC, eds. Principles and Practice of Sleep Medicine, 2nd ed. Philadelphia: WB Saunders, 1994.

Miles LE, Broughton RJ, eds. Medical Monitoring in the Home and Work Environment, New York: Raven Press, 1990.

Saunders NA, Sullivan CE, eds. Sleep and Breathing. Lung Biology in Health and Disease, vol. 71. New York: Marcel Dekker, 1994:1–959.

29

PERITONEAL DIALYSIS: ALTERNATIVES TO IN-CENTER TREATMENT

Ghias U. Butt and James F. Winchester

CHAPTER AT A GLANCE: Intermittent machine-delivered peritoneal dialysis (PD) is growing rapidly in the United States and the world. It is used specifically for convenience, since most patients use the machine at night. It is also used to enhance the efficacy of peritoneal dialysis in patients who require a larger and more frequent exchange regimen. The three major methods of delivery of dialysate are continuous peritoneal dialysis, nocturnal peritoneal dialysis, and tidal peritoneal dialysis. The three methods differ in concept and delivery cycle.

Introduction

Peritoneal dialysis is an established alternative form of renal replacement therapy. Toward the end of 1992, approximately 80,000 patients were on some form of peritoneal dialysis, representing 16% of the global dialysis population. Of these, 15% were on machine-delivered dialysis (automated peritoneal dialysis [APD]) (1).

Automated peritoneal dialysis, using specially designed delivery machines, consists of four forms of chronic peritoneal dialysis: intermittent peritoneal dialysis (IPD), continuous cycling peritoneal dialysis (CCPD), nocturnal peritoneal dialysis (NPD), and tidal peritoneal dialysis (TPD). At the end of 1992, the number of patients using automated machines of some sort for delivery of peritoneal dialysis was 5650, compared to 326 in 1988 and 816 in 1981.

In general, automated peritoneal dialysis uses a regimen of hourly exchange of peritoneal dialysis fluid over a period of 10 hours or more. It is performed by the patient, with or without the help of a family member, using a specially designed machine. The dialysis regimen consists of an inflow time, a dwell time, and an outflow time. The volume of dialysis fluid used is usually 1 to 3 L per cycle.

Machines and Fluids Used for APD

Increasingly sophisticated machines are being introduced to deliver APD. Older machines made use of gravity to deliver peritoneal dialysis, but newer machines are semiautomated or fully automated and pump driven and do not require the use of gravity. These newer machines have heated cradles, onto which peritoneal dialysis fluid from a larger reservoir (plastic bags of 5 L) is delivered to be heated prior to delivery into the peritoneal cavity (Fig. 29.1). Either the cradle

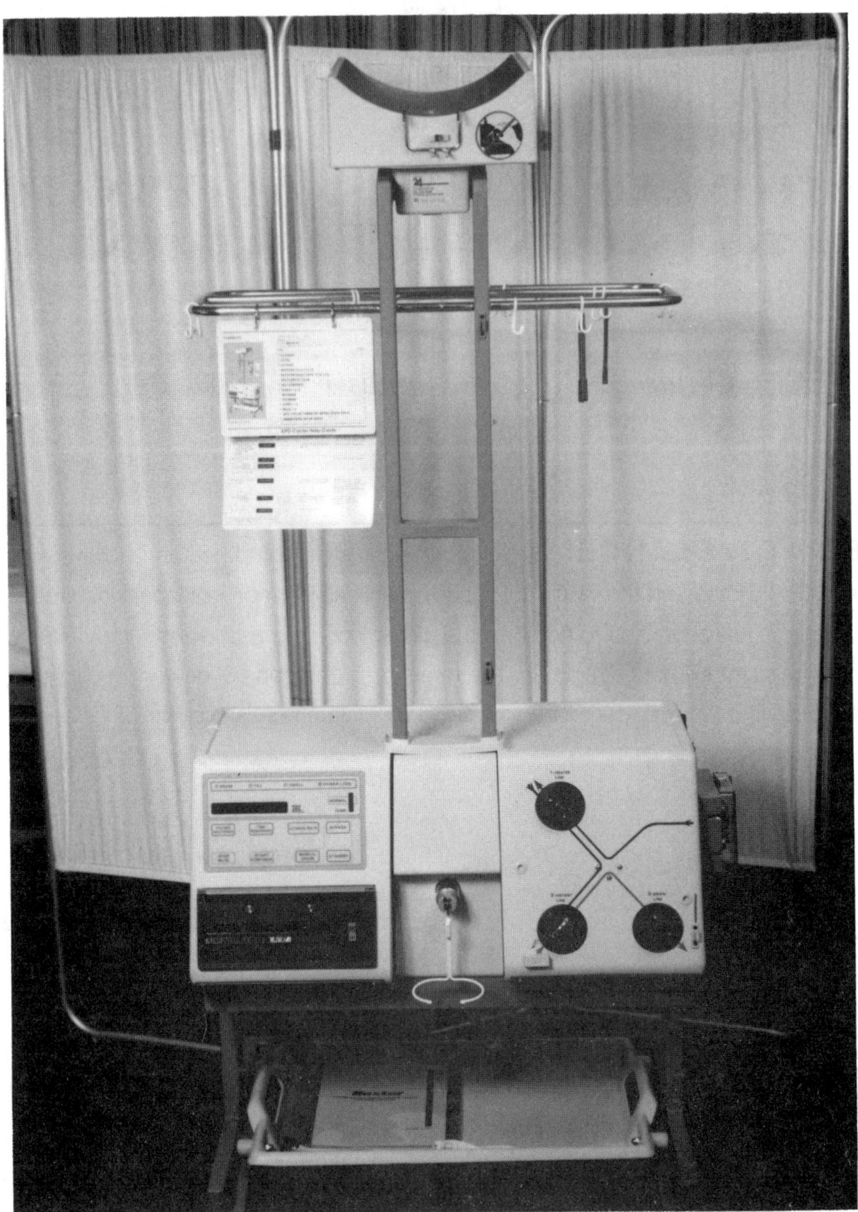

Figure 29.1. A typical peritoneal dialysis cycler (Baxter Pac-X).

functions as a scale, or the pump in the machine measures the actual amount of the peritoneal dialysis fluid being delivered. This information can be stored in the machine's memory for later use to assess and adjust the delivered dose of dialysate.

Peritoneal dialysis fluid used in automated peritoneal dialysis is similar to that used in continuous ambulatory peritoneal dialysis (CAPD). The most commonly used fluid utilizes dextrose as an osmotic agent, but dextran, polyglucose (glucose polymer), glycerol, and amino acids can also be used (2). The concentration of solutes in a typical solution is given in Table 29.1.

In automated peritoneal dialysis, when a short dwell time is used to effect ultrafiltration, hypernatremia may ensue. In this situation,

Table 29.1. Typical Solute Concentrations in Commercial Peritoneal Dialysis Fluids

Constituent	Abbott	Baxter	DelMed	Gambro
		Manufacturer		
Na (mEq/L)	132	132	134	131
K (mEq/L)	0	0	0	0
Cl (mEq/L)	102	96	103.5	94
Mg (mEq/L)	1.5	0.75	0.5	0.5
Ca (mEq/L)	1.75	1.75	1.75	1.75
Lactate (mmol/L)	35	35	40	40
Dextrose (g/dL or %)	a	a	a	a
Osmolality (mOsm/kg)	b	b	b	b
Average pH	5.5	5.2	5.3	5.5
Volumes (Ml)	c	c	c	c

[a]1.5, 2.5, and 4.25% dextrose

[b]350,400, and 480 mOsm/kg corresponding to dextrose concentrations.

[c]250 mL to 3 L, depending on manufacturer.

PD fluid containing lower sodium concentrations should be used (3).

Factors Governing the Efficiency of Peritoneal Dialysis

Two important factors for determining the efficiency of peritoneal dialysis separate automated peritoneal dialysis and CAPD. Solute and osmotic fluid removal differ physiologically because of variations in cycle duration used in APD.

Ultrafiltration

Peritoneal ultrafiltration is governed by the osmotic gradient between dialysate within the abdominal cavity and plasma in peritoneal capillaries and by peritoneal permeability. The osmotic gradient is determined by variation in the concentration of the osmotic agent in the dialysis fluid.

Ultrafiltration is *maximal* at the highest dextrose concentration (4.5%) of the dialysate and is lowest when dextrose has been absorbed through the peritoneal membrane and has reached equilibrium across the peritoneal membrane. Ultrafiltration can thus be maximized by short dwell times (thereby preventing the dextrose concentration in dialysate from falling to a level at which the osmotic gradient is too low to effect ultrafiltration) and by using higher concentrations of dextrose in dialysate.

Maximal ultrafiltration occurs within the first 2 or 3 hours of dwell time. Using 1.5% dextrose dialysate solution, a net ultrafiltration of 1.7 to 2.5 L in 10 hours is easily achieved. Better ultrafiltration will be achieved at higher dextrose concentration or by using shorter, more frequent exchanges (4).

Solute Transport

The diffusive clearance of a solute from the intravascular compartment into the peritoneal cavity depends on the concentration gradient across the peritoneal membrane. This is particularly important for removal of substances such as urea, creatinine, and uric acid. It is also important for the removal, addition, or equilibration of other substances such as potassium, magnesium, and calcium. These substances are (or can be) given separately, in various concentrations as desired. Solute diffusion for low–molecular weight solutes is maximal within the first 3 hours of dwell time, and rapidly falls with little increase in peritoneal diffusibility thereafter. Equilibrium is the state at which transfer of a given solute across the peritoneal membrane is minimal, with a dialysate to plasma ratio approaching 1.

Transport of low–molecular weight solutes can be enhanced by either maintaining the concentration gradient or increasing the splanchnic blood flow. The stagnant fluid film in contact with the peritoneal membrane will limit solute transport; efficient mixing of dialysis fluid (akin to that in hemodialysis) significantly increases the clearance of small solutes. Also, as mentioned earlier, solute diffusion is maximal in the first 3 hours. Therefore, by reducing dwell time, solute transfer can be maximized.

Larger molecules are removed by the process of convection, which depends on peritoneal membrane permeability, ultrafiltration, and time. Automated peritoneal dialysis is inferior to CAPD in the removal of higher–molecular weight solutes, due to shorter dwell times in APD (5).

Intermittent Peritoneal Dialysis

Intermittent peritoneal dialysis (IPD) was introduced in 1923 by Ganter (6). It was the first successful form of renal replacement therapy. IPD was a major contributor to the growth of home dialysis in the 1970s. The major obstacles to its success were the development of adequate chronic peritoneal dialysis access (Tenckhoff catheter) (7) and the supply of sterile dialysate (8). Both were introduced by the dialysis research team under Dr. Scribner in Seattle, Washington. Another necessary development in enabling IPD was the invention of a reverse osmosis proportioning system. This system combined sterile pyrogen-free water with chemical concentrate in the correct proportions to deliver a physiological dialysate to the patient (9).

A further necessity for the maximal utilization of IPD was the development of adequate machinery to control the inflow volume, the length of dialysate dwell, and the outflow times. In addition, such equipment provided safety monitors and alarms to allow the simplified use of the machinery in the home setting (10).

IPD is a viable alternative to hemodialysis in patients with poor or absent vascular accesses. It also provides dialysis without the use of systemic heparinization and is relatively well tolerated in patients with cardiovascular problems. It is easily learned by patients and partners, and training is much more simple than that for hemodialysis. Lastly, because it is intermittent, it allows the patient periods of freedom from dialysis. In general, IPD uses a regimen of hourly exchanges of peritoneal dialysis fluid over a 10-hour period performed by the patient or family member or with an automated machine. The dialysis regimen consists of an inflow time, a dwell time, and an outflow time. The volume of the dialysate fluid is usually 1 to 2 L. Sessions are repeated four times weekly. Weekly clearance rates for solutes are given in Table 29.2.

Contraindications

Contraindications to IPD include abdominal adhesions, recent abdominal surgery, large hernias, and, in most centers, the presence of an ostomy (ileostomy, colostomy). A relative contraindication would be poor vascular status of the lower limbs. Blood flow to the legs may be compromised by high intra-abdominal pressure caused by the presence of fluid in the peritoneal cavity.

Initially, IPD was believed to be comparable to hemodialysis, but studies failed to evaluate the long-term effects of IPD on patient survival. A disconcerting reduction in survival seemed to occur after 2 to 3 years of therapy. This may have resulted from inadequate dialysis due to a fall in glomerular fil-

Table 29.2. Weekly Solute Clearances (liters/week) for Different Peritoneal Dialysis Techniques

Solute	IPD	NPD	TPD	CCPD	CAPD
Urea	60	54	79	56	57
Creatinine	38	37	57	42	44
Middle molecules[a]	17	19	-	34	38

[a]Measured as vitamin B_{12} clearance.

Table 29.3. Complications of Peritoneal Dialysis

Mechanical
   Hernias, abdominal and diaphragmatic,
     peritoneal leaks
   Hemorrhoids, bladder prolapse
   Impaired vascular supply to lower extremities
   Dialysate inflow pain, low back ache
   Catheter malfunction
   Hydrothorax
   Respiratory complications (atelectasis,
     pneumonia, hypoventilation)
   Impaired cardiac return (heart failure)
   Bowel perforation (catheter impingement)
Metabolic
   Hyperglycemia, hyperlipidemia
   Hypernatremia, hyponatremia
   Calcium deficiency, magnesium excess
   Uncorrected acidosis, metabolic acidosis
   Hyperosmolality
   Amyloidosis
   Nephrolithiasis (oxalate)
   Pancreatitis?
Nutritional
   Protein and amino acid losses
   Trace metal deficiencies and excesses
Technology Related
   Peritonitis, exit-site and tunnel infections, and
     pyrogen reactions
   Particulate contamination of peritoneum
   Sclerosing peritonitis? (disinfectants,
     formaldehyde, etc.)
   Eosinophilic peritonitis?
Membrane Related
   Ultrafiltration failure
   Hyperabsorption or hypoabsorption of
     dextrose
   Hemoperitoneum, chyloperitoneum?

tration after the first 18 months. At the end of this period, with reduction in native kidney function, solute clearance becomes inefficient in correcting the uremic state (11).

Boen et al. (12) proposed a minimum total creatinine clearance rate of 4 to 5 mL/min as the standard compatible with adequacy of peritoneal dialysis, along with a middle-molecule clearance rate of 3 mL/min. In an anuric patient, IPD is clearly inadequate for correction of the uremic state.

In some patients, peritoneal transport may be greater than normal and may contribute to total solute clearance. The same may be true in patients with body weight less than 50 kg. IPD should be avoided in patients with endogenous creatinine clearance below 2 mL/min, since adequate biochemical profiles are not achieved with IPD alone (Table 29.3).

Complications

The most significant complications are infection around the catheter exit site and peritonitis (13). Unlike those associated with continuous ambulatory peritoneal dialysis, most studies with IPD have reported more common infections with Gram-negative than with Gram-positive organisms. This is particularly true if IPD was performed in the hospital. Peritonitis can generally be treated with standard antibiotic regimens such as vancomycin (single weekly doses of 1 to 2 g intraperitoneal) or gentamicin (1.5 mg/kg loading dose and 5 mg/L during the cycling periods). If definitive identification of the organism is achieved, a change in antibiotics may be appropriate.

Exit site infections and subcutaneous tunnel infections may also complicate IPD. It has been shown that more resistant infections occur with upward-pointing than with downward-pointing catheters; most catheters are now placed in a downward-directed fashion (14). Placement of catheters is extremely important even within the abdominal cavity, since peritoneal leaks, omental wrapping, and catheter obstruction are other common complications of IPD.

Most catheters are placed with a trocar through direct visualization or through fiber optic catheter placement techniques. The internal cuff of a two-cuff Tenckhoff catheter is anchored within the rectus sheath and rectus muscle (15). The exit site should be 2 cm or more distal to the external cuff.

It cannot be overstated that IPD *is* less efficient than CAPD and CCPD and that careful attention must be paid to the metabolic control achieved with this type of dialysis. Weight increases between dialysis periods, hyponatremia, and hypokalemia have all been reported in IPD patients. The latter may require addition of potassium chloride in varying concentrations to achieve the desired post-treatment level in individual patients. Hyponatremia may be due to reverse osmosis proportioning system failure. In contrast, hypernatremia may be due to rapid removal of water.

Respiratory alkalosis may result from hyperventilation. While metabolic alkalosis is rare, it is seen with rapid cycling and with hyperosmolar solutions (16). Metabolic acidosis usually improves significantly in IPD. However, it can be precipitated by the use of lactate-containing dialysate in the presence of liver failure and the impairment of hepatic lactate metabolism. Trace metal disturbances may occur in peritoneal dialysis, but such complications are rare (17).

Since temperature control may be impaired by heater malfunction, hypothermia or hyperthermia may occur. Excessively heated dialysate can give rise to abdominal pain, paralytic ileus, and metabolic acidosis.

Continuous Cycling Peritoneal Dialysis

CCPD is a regimen with automated delivery of dialysis fluid with a long-dwell peritoneal dialysis time. It is similar to CAPD, with measured inflow volume, dwell times, and outflow times. A diurnal dwell of a volume of peritoneal dialysis fluid occurs to continue solute removal during the day. CCPD is an example of prolonged-dwell peritoneal dialysis with close resemblance to CAPD in its efficiency and clinical results. CCPD provides automated exchanges. This minimizes the duration of dialysis and maintains a steady state and improved efficiency in comparison to CAPD (18). Patient groups that benefit from CCPD are children and patients with severe visual and neuromuscular impairment. These patients generally require the help of a trained partner to perform the procedure. CCPD is also useful for patients with occupational or other time constraints.

Cyclers for CCPD are almost identical to those used for IPD but are adjustable to allow for longer dwell times. Since a smaller total volume for nocturnal delivery is required, dialysis tubing connections are less complex than those for IPD. The usual prescription consists of three to five 2-L exchanges per night over a period of about 10 hours, with a single diurnal exchange lasting 14 hours. The solution delivered is identical to that for CAPD. However, the diurnal cycle usually utilizes a more hypertonic solution than that delivered during the night. This is done to achieve higher solute clearance as well as to maintain ultrafiltration.

Similar to CAPD, CCPD can be terminated by disconnection from the automated cycler without carrying an empty dialysis container attached to the catheter. In this respect, it affords freedom like that achieved with disconnection from CAPD or IPD. Extensive clinical experience with CCPD has demonstrated that the procedure is clinically comparable to CAPD. There is little difference in the biochemical profile or in the incidence of most complications. The technique is also similar to that of CAPD, and patient survival rates are similar. There are some subtle differences in complications. Some studies have reported that peritonitis occurred less frequently with CCPD than with CAPD (19, 20). While the lower incidence of peritonitis could be due to the smaller number of connections required in CCPD, it could also result from different flow patterns of the dialysis fluid after connection, or from flushing of the lines (and contaminating bacteria) before attachment to the cycler. Newer studies suggest the probable role of longer daytime dwell in causing the increased peritoneal macrophage phagocytic activity and opsonic activity of the dialysis fluid effluent (21). The better peritonitis profile in CCPD is not supported by the results published in the national CAPD registry in 1988 (22). Since the diurnal cycle is associated with maximal net ultrafiltration 4 hours after infusion, complications from high intra-abdominal pressure are also seen. This has led some practitioners to prescribe a smaller diurnal cycle volume (1250 to 1500 mL), which results in reduced intra-abdominal volume while maintaining clearance of small and middle molecules (Table 29.2).

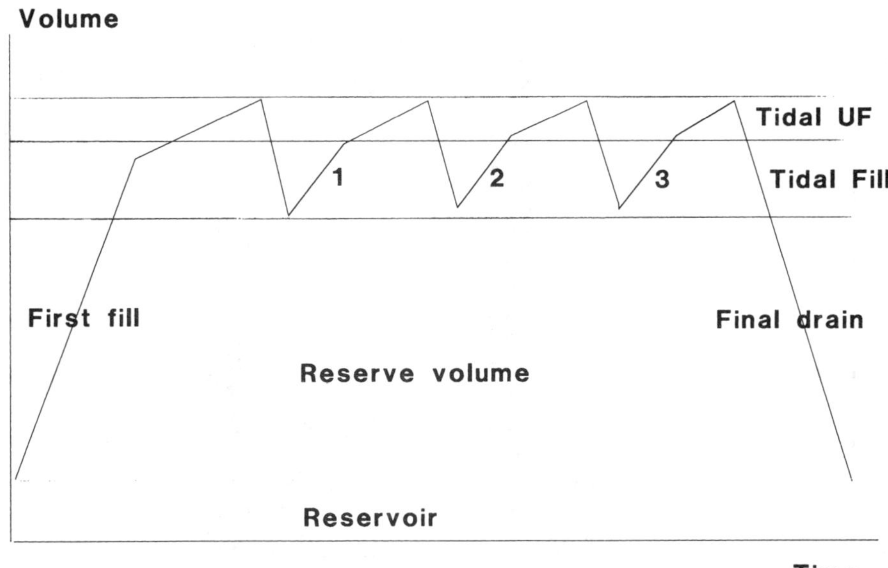

Figure 29.2. The peritoneal dialysis volume schema. Numerals 1, 2, and 3 refer to tidal fill cycles. (Data from Twardowski ZJ. New approaches to intermittent peritoneal dialysis therapies. In: Nolph KD, ed. Peritoneal Dialysis, 3rd ed. Dordrecht, Netherlands: Kluwer Academic Publishers, 1988:169–183.)

Nocturnal Peritoneal Dialysis

Nocturnal peritoneal dialysis (NPD) is essentially identical to intermittent peritoneal dialysis. It basically consists of nocturnally delivered intermittent peritoneal dialysis. However, there is no diurnal dwell of dialysis fluid. Nocturnal peritoneal dialysis is also similar to CCPD, except that the diurnal cycle is omitted. Equilibration testing (as designed by Twardowski and colleagues) to calculate the dialysis prescription is probably necessary before beginning NPD (23). The dialysate to plasma ratio for creatinine at 1, 2, 3, and 4 hours of dwell time is calculated, as is the ratio of dialysate glucose at 2 and 4 hours dwell time to dialysis glucose at 0 dwell time. As seen in Figure 29.2, a low transport rate for creatinine and a higher drain volume would be considered inadequate parameters for nocturnal PD but good for standard or high-dose PD, as outlined in Table 29.4. A variation on NPD uses low-volume,

Table 29.4 Solute Transport Rates and Choice of Peritoneal Dialysis Regimen

Parameter[a]	Value[b]	Comment	PD Prescription
Dextrose D/D_0	0.12–0.26	High	IPD, NPD, CCPD
	0.26–0.38	High average	IPD, NPD, CCPD
	0.38–0.49	Low average	IPD, TPD
	0.49–0.61	Low	TPD, hemodialysis
Creatinine D/P ratio	0.34–0.50	Low	Hemodialysis, TPD
	0.50–0.65	Low average	IPD, TPD
	0.65–0.81	High average	IPD, NPD, CCPD
	0.81–1.03	High	IPD, NPD, CCPD

[a]D/D_0, Ratio of dialysate dextrose at 4-hour equilibration (dwell) to dialysate dextrose at time 0. (High ratio correlates with poor ultrafiltration; low ratio, with high ultrafiltration). D/P ratio, Ratio of creatinine concentration in dialysate to concentration in plasma after 4-hour equilibration. (Low ratio correlates with poor solute clearance; high ratio, with high solute clearance). IPD, NPD, TPD, and CCPD are defined in the text.

[b]Data from Twardowski ZJ. New approaches to intermittent peritoneal dialysis therapies. In: Nolph KD, ed. Peritoneal Dialysis, 3rd ed. Dordrecht, Netherlands: Kluwer Academic Publishers, 1988:169–183.

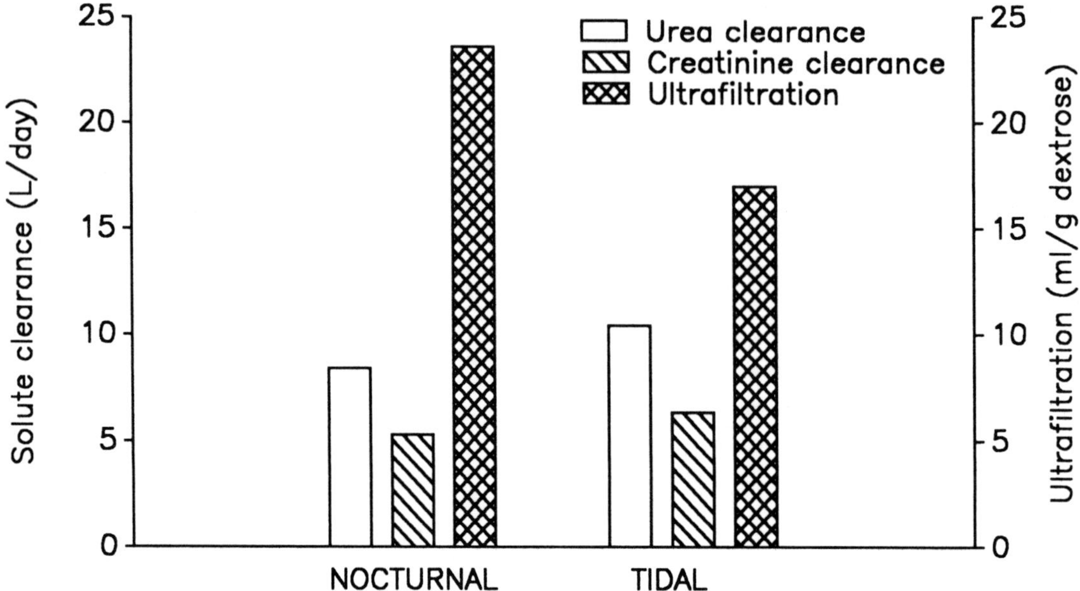

Figure 29.3.   Effect of tidal peritoneal dialysis on solute clearance and dextrose absorption. TPD resulted in significant increases in average urea (8.4 to 10.4 L/day) and creatinine (5.3 to 6.3 L/day) clearances and reduced dextrose absorption over NPD. (Data from Twardowski ZJ. New approaches to intermittent peritoneal dialysis therapies. In: Nolph KD, ed. Peritoneal Dialysis, 3rd ed. Dordrecht, Netherlands: Kluwer Academic Publishers, 1988:169–183.)

high-flow peritoneal dialysis techniques such as the recently introduced tidal peritoneal dialysis (see below).

Tidal Peritoneal Dialysis

Tidal peritoneal dialysis (TPD) is the performance of dialysate delivery and removal of a small volume. Frequent exchanges occur only on the tidal volume, leaving behind a residual volume of fluid in the abdomen. Theoretically, dialysis exchange occurs only on a tidal volume, similar to that of respiration. There is a residual volume and a reserve volume, with exchanges occurring only with the tidal volume (Fig. 29.2). Twardowski and colleagues (24) have examined the role of tidal peritoneal dialysis using a special automated delivery machine that can deliver small volumes between 0.3 and 0.9 L, with dwell times on the order of 1 to 9.9 minutes, to deliver 14 to 26 L over an 8-hour period. In patients with low mean average conventional peritoneal clearances of urea

and creatinine, clearance increased significantly with tidal peritoneal dialysis. Clearance exceeded that achieved with nocturnal peritoneal dialysis, which was slightly increased from that of CAPD (Fig. 29.3). The mean ultrafiltration volume per mass of absorbed glucose was also higher in patients with below-average urea and creatinine clearances (Table 29.5). It is too early to say what the impact of tidal peritoneal dialysis will be in patients with low solute clearances, but the future appears to be dependent on production and cost of the peritoneal dialysis solutions. The delivery of up to 30 L of fluid per 8-hour schedule is extremely costly in present-day terms. Technical problems also surround the delivery machines and the control of ultrafiltration.

Table 29.5 Tidal Peritoneal Dialysis Prescription

Tidal volume 0.3–0.9 L
Residual volume 1.1–2.1 L
Total dialysate volume delivered 23–27 L

Summary

Machine-delivered peritoneal dialysis is a growing therapy for treatment of patients with end-stage renal disease, the most common of which are continuous cycling peritoneal dialysis and intermittent peritoneal dialysis. Solute transport is increased for small molecules with machine-delivered peritoneal dialysis with new techniques called nocturnal peritoneal dialysis and tidal peritoneal dialysis; the latter utilizes a concept similar to that of tidal volumes in respiratory function. It appears that machine-delivered peritoneal dialysis offers several advantages to conventional CAPD and hemodialysis. In the former, there is a reduction of peritonitis, and in the latter, home delivery is easier. Weekly solute clearances with machine-delivered peritoneal dialysis are slightly less for middle molecules and slightly greater for molecules of the size of urea (64 daltons).

References

1. Westman J. Worldwide dialysis update [annual survey]. Deerfield, IL: Baxter Healthcare Inc., 1993.
2. Feriani M, La Grace G, Kriger FL, Winchester JF. CAPD systems and solutions. In: Gokal R, Nolph KD. The Textbook of Peritoneal Dialysis. Dordrecht, Netherlands: Kluwer Academic Publishers, 1994:233–270.
3. Nolph KD, Sorkin ML, Moore H. Autoregulation of sodium and potassium removal during continuous ambulatory peritoneal dialysis. Trans Am Soc Artif Internal Organs 1980;26:334–338.
4. Henderson LW, Leypoldt JK. Ultrafiltration with peritoneal dialysis. In: Nolph KD, ed. Peritoneal Dialysis, 3rd ed. Dordrecht, Netherlands: Kluwer Academic Publishers, 1988:117–132.
5. Popovich RP, Moncreif JW, Pyle WK. Transport kinetics. In: Nolph KD, ed. Peritoneal Dialysis, 3rd ed. Dordrecht, Netherlands: Kluwer Academic Publishers, 1988:96–116.
6. Ganter G. Lieber die Beseitigung Giftiger Dtoffe aus dem Blute durch Dialyse. Muench Med Wochenschr 1923;70–11:1478–1480.
7. Tenckhoff H, Schechter H. A bacteriologically safe peritoneal access device. Trans Am Soc Artif Intern Organs 1968;14:181–186.
8. Boen ST, Molinari AS, Dillard DH, Scribner BH. Periodic peritoneal dialysis in the management of chronic uremia. Trans Am Soc Artif Intern Organs 1962;8:256–262.
9. Tenckhoff H, Meston B, Shilipetar G. A simplified automatic peritoneal dialysis system. Trans Am Soc Artif Intern Organs 1969;15:103–108.
10. Diaz-Buxo JA. Peritoneal dialysis, reverse osmosis machines and cyclers. In: Nissenson AR, Fine RN, eds. Dialysis Therapy. Philadelphia: Hanley and Belfus, 1986:41–47.
11. Diaz-Buxo JA. Intermittent peritoneal dialysis. In: Briggs D, Junor B, Rodger S, Winchester JF, eds. Renal Dialysis. London: Chapman and Hall, 1993.
12. Boen ST, Haagsma-Scouten WAG, Birnie RJ. Long-term peritoneal dialysis and a peritoneal index. Dial Transplant 1978;7:377–379.
13. Vas SI. Peritonitis. In: Nolph KD, ed. Peritoneal Dialysis, 3rd ed. Dordrecht, Netherlands: Kluwer Academic Publishers, 1989:261–288.
14. Khanna R, Twardowski ZJ. Peritoneal dialysis access. In: Nolph KD, ed. Peritoneal Dialysis, 3rd ed. Dordrecht, Netherlands: Kluwer Academic Publishers, 1988:319–342.
15. Helfrich GB, Pechan WB, Alijani MR, Barnard WF, Rakowski TA, Winchester JF. Reduction in catheter complications with lateral catheter placement. Peritoneal Dial Bull 1983;3(Suppl): S2-S4.
16. Winchester JF. Pulmonary function and peritoneal dialysis [Editorial]. Chest 1981;4:267–269.
17. Winchester JF, Rotellar C, Mackow RC, Rakowski TA, Argy WP. Trace metals in CAPD patients. In: La Grace G, Chiaramonte S, Fabris A, Feriani M, Ronco C, eds. Peritoneal Dialysis. Milan: Wichtig Editore, 1988:241–245.
18. Diaz-Buxo JA. Continuous cyclic peritoneal dialysis. In: Nolph KD, ed. Peritoneal Dialysis, 3rd ed. Dordrecht, Netherlands: Kluwer Academic Publishers, 1988:169–183.
19. Diaz-Buxo JA, Walker PJ, Chandler JT, et al. Experience with intermittent and continuous cyclic peritoneal dialysis. Am J Kidney Dis 1984;4:242–248.
20. Price CG, Suki WN. Newer modification of peritoneal dialysis. Am J Nephrol 1981;1:97–104.
21. De Fijter CW, Verburgh HA, Oe LP, et al. Peritoneal defenses in continuous ambulatory versus cyclic peritoneal dialysis. Kidney Int 1992;42:947–950.
22. Lindblad AS, Novak JW, Nolph KD et al. Complications of treatment. In: Final Report of National CAPD Registry of the National Institutes of Health. Washington, DC: U.S. Government Printing Office, 1988:4-1–4-13.
23. Twardowski ZJ, Nolph KD, Khanna R, et al. Peritoneal equilibration test. Peritoneal Dial Bull 1987;7:138–147.
24. Twardowski ZJ, Nolph KD, Khanna R, et al. Tidal peritoneal dialysis. In: Proceedings of the IVth Congress of the International Society of Peritoneal Dialysis (in press).

30

HOME HEMODIALYSIS

Christopher R. Blagg

CHAPTER AT A GLANCE: The use of home-based hemodialysis offers significant quality-of-life improvement for the patient and family. While many patients still opt for in-center treatment, home hemodialysis programs are expanding. The author details the concept, including historical background, patient selection, and specific practical aspects. His extensive personal experience in the field brings special insight to this review.

Introduction

In considering the use of complex medical treatments in the home, hemodialysis (Fig. 30.1) is of particular interest. This was the first high-technology medical procedure to be transferred to the home setting and to be undertaken by the patient with assistance from a family member. While it was initially developed for economic reasons in the early 1960s, it soon became obvious that self-treatment at home also increased the opportunity for independence and rehabilitation for patients with end-stage renal disease (ESRD). For those of us involved in the exciting early days of home hemodialysis, it has been interesting to see how, as other home technologies have developed, each has resulted in rediscovery of the advantages of home treatment and patients' involvement in their own care. Many of the lessons learned from the use of home hemodialysis over the last 30 years have application to other technologies.

Historical Review

The first practical artificial kidney was developed by Willem Kolff in Holland in 1942 (1), and hemodialysis came to be quite widely used for treatment of acute renal failure during the 1950s. Long-term intermittent hemodialysis for ESRD did not become a reality until 1960, when Belding Scribner and colleagues at the University of Washington in Seattle developed the Teflon arteriovenous shunt (2). Once convinced of the success of this treatment, Scribner and James Haviland, then President of the King County Medical Society, obtained funds from the John A. Hartford Foundation to establish the nonprofit Seattle Artificial Kidney Center (now the Northwest Kidney Centers) in 1962 as the world's first free-standing outpatient dialysis unit (3). Before that time, hemodialysis was regarded as a major in-hospital procedure, using cumbersome equipment and needing the presence of at least one physician throughout the treatment. Surgery was required to cannulate an artery and vein prior to

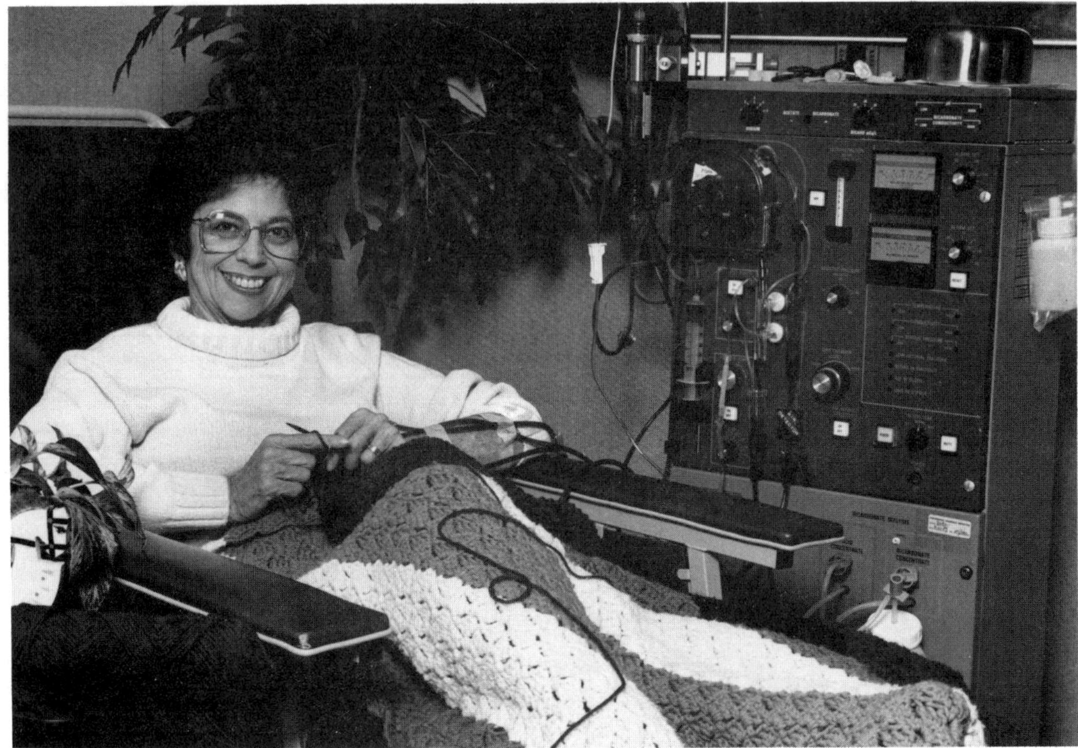

Figure 30.1.   Home hemodialysis.

each dialysis and to remove the cannulas afterwards. The Teflon arteriovenous shunt, by connecting the arterial and venous cannulas between dialyses, made repeated dialysis treatments possible (4). Development of new equipment and modification of the Kiil dialyzer (5) led to a much less fearsome and more routine procedure for hemodialysis of ESRD patients. As a result, when the Seattle Artificial Kidney Center opened, dialysis was supervised by nurses, without the presence of a physician (6).

Throughout the 1960s, Scribner and colleagues at the University of Washington and the Seattle Artificial Kidney Center described most of the medical complications and social, financial, and ethical problems associated with ESRD treatment. It was the financial problems in particular that highlighted the ethical issues and also led to the development of home hemodialysis as a treatment modality.

By the time the Seattle Artificial Kidney Center opened, knowledge about the success of long-term dialysis in Seattle was spreading throughout Washington State and elsewhere. Even so, the cost of this treatment was not yet covered by private insurance or other funding agencies, and demand for treatment already far exceeded available resources. The only support for almost all patients was the use of funds raised from the local public. Consequently, the Seattle Artificial Kidney Center and the King County Medical Society appointed an anonymous Admissions and Policy Committee to screen potential patients for long-term dialysis (7). The committee was chaired by a clergyman, and members representing the community were a banker, a housewife, a lawyer, a state government official, a labor leader, and a surgeon. Patients who met very strict medical criteria were referred to the committee, which decided who would be accepted for treatment and who would not (8). This committee continued in operation until 1971, by which time private insurance and state support had become sufficient to treat all patients referred to the Seattle Artificial Kidney Center.

This approach to patient selection has since proved to be a fertile field for discussions by ethicists, social scientists, and physicians (9), and it has been regarded by some as the origin of bioethics as a separate discipline. At the time, it seemed the most practical response to the unprecedented difficulty (at least in civilian practice) of triage in a population of patients who would inevitably die without treatment and who lacked the resources to pay for the treatment.

One criterion used in selecting patients for dialysis at the Seattle Artificial Kidney Center was an age between 18 and 45 years. Consequently, in 1963, when the 15-year-old daughter of a friend of Albert Babb, Professor of Nuclear Engineering at the University of Washington and one of Scribner's collaborators, developed ESRD, she was not accepted for treatment. Babb and Scribner were already developing an automated system using a central proportioning unit to make dialysate for distribution to several stations in the University of Washington Clinical Research Center (10). The logical next step was to make a smaller version of this—a single-patient dialysate proportioning machine incorporating various monitors for safety during dialysis (11). This, the precursor of all present-day hemodialysis equipment (Fig. 30.2), was first used by this girl in 1964 to treat herself at home, with assistance from her mother (12).

She was not the first patient to be treated by hemodialysis at home. In 1961 in Japan, Dr. Yuki Nosé had treated a patient in the home using a coil dialyzer placed inside a domestic washing machine (13). Scribner himself had visited India in 1963 to train a physician to do hemodialysis at home for a wealthy Madras businessman.

In 1963 and 1964, two other groups were looking at home hemodialysis as a less expensive alternative to outpatient dialysis. In Boston, John Merrill and coworkers began using the twin-coil dialyzer for this purpose, at first having a nurse go to the home to carry out each treatment (14). Concurrently, in London, Stanley Shaldon and colleagues began treating patients by home dialysis, initially using a static tank of dialysate and a

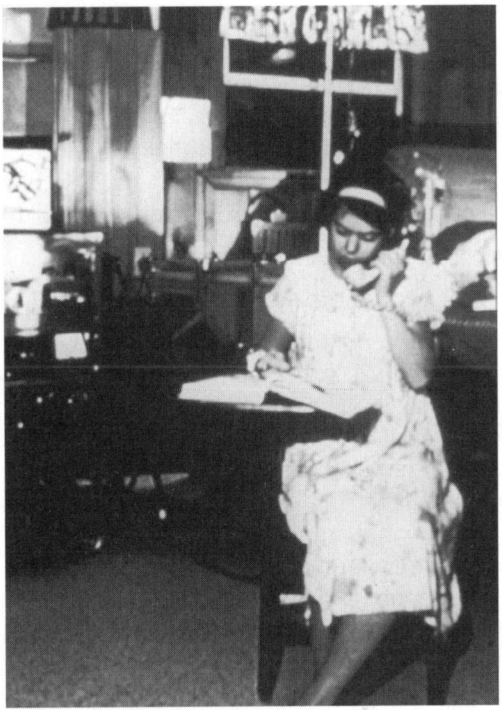

Figure 30.2. The first Seattle home hemodialysis patient using the dialysate proportioning machine developed at the University of Washington, 1964.

modified Kiil dialyzer, and later with a system resembling that used in Seattle (15). It was Shaldon who first began using overnight home hemodialysis. This was possible because the proportioning equipment included fail-safe monitoring, and use of a Scribner shunt and a low-resistance Kiil dialyzer allowed hemodialysis without a blood pump. Treatment was relatively inefficient, requiring some 10 hours of dialysis two or three times weekly, and so it was logical to use overnight dialysis with the patient sleeping at least part of the time.

It soon became apparent that home hemodialysis was as effective as hemodialysis on an outpatient basis, and that it was considerably less expensive because it did not require the presence of nursing staff. Scribner and colleagues in Seattle and Shaldon in London pursued further development of equipment and procedures to simplify dialysis for the patient and to ensure that treatment was as safe as possible. Fail-safe monitoring similar to that developed by Scribner and Shaldon is now a feature of almost all single-patient hemodialysis equipment (16, 17).

By 1967, the Seattle Artificial Kidney Center had exhausted its original grant support from the John A. Hartford Foundation and the U.S. Public Health Service. As a result, it was having serious financial difficulties in supporting even the carefully selected patient population. Consequently, the Center's Board of Trustees decided that all new patients must be treated by home hemodialysis; thereby making funds available to treat the largest possible number of patients. At the same time, patients already receiving outpatient dialysis at the Center were encouraged, cajoled, and persuaded to go on home hemodialysis.

Support for these changes came from Scribner and his colleagues, who had recently developed the University of Washington's Coach House dialysis facility. This center was situated in a motel and consisted of several rooms modified to serve as a freestanding home dialysis training unit. More than 50 patients were trained for home dialysis at this unit during the 1960s, including patients from the Seattle Artificial Kidney Center and from elsewhere in the United States and abroad (18).

Staff from the Coach House helped Seattle Artificial Kidney Center staff develop their own training program, and by 1970 more than 90% of dialysis patients in western Washington were being treated by home hemodialysis. With the aid of an educational consultant, the Center also pioneered use of a videotape-based training program that shortened training time significantly (19).

Early experience with home hemodialysis soon showed the advantages of this to the patient. Besides a reduced risk of hepatitis and other infections, benefits included increased independence, feelings of control and accomplishment, and greater opportunity for rehabilitation compared with patients treated by outpatient hemodialysis. The latter tend to become dependent on the facility and its staff (20) and develop what Seligman has called "learned helplessness" (21). These same benefits have since been recognized in other pa-

tient populations using home technologies. Examples include self-administration of antihemophiliac globulin by hemophiliacs (22), long-term total parenteral nutrition (23), various forms of respiratory support (24), and various cardiovascular devices.

Meanwhile, as these developments with hemodialysis were occurring, long-term peritoneal dialysis for ESRD patients was also being pursued at the University of Washington. Fred Boen and Henry Tenckhoff developed a closed peritoneal dialysate supply system that minimized the risk of peritonitis (25). Tenckhoff also devised the first effective indwelling peritoneal catheter, still used by most peritoneal dialysis patients (26), and equipment using heat sterilization that made home intermittent peritoneal dialysis (IPD) possible (27). He then developed an automated system for on-line preparation of sterile peritoneal dialysate using reverse osmosis and ultraviolet light (28). While this was used successfully by some patients in the Northwest Kidney Center program and elsewhere, it became obvious that home IPD did not provide adequate dialysis once residual renal function was lost (29). As a result, home peritoneal dialysis was not widely used prior to the introduction of continuous ambulatory peritoneal dialysis (CAPD) by Robert Popovich and Jack Moncrief in Austin, Texas, in 1976 (30). Since then, as discussed in Chapter 29, CAPD and modifications such as continuous cyclic peritoneal dialysis (CCPD) (31), have become the most widely used forms of home dialysis in the United States.

Selection of Patients

Various factors have to be considered in selecting patients for home hemodialysis. These include the medical condition of the patient, living circumstances, availability of suitable accommodation, learning ability, and patient and family anxiety. In Seattle we have trained more than 2500 patients to do home hemodialysis over the last 30 years. Our experience has shown that anyone physically capable of doing hemodialysis can be trained to perform this safely at home, provided the patient is motivated and is suitably encouraged by the training staff.

Medical problems, such as severe cardiovascular disease with angina or arrhythmias during dialysis, may be a contraindication to home hemodialysis. Nevertheless, other physical handicaps such as blindness, deafness, or relative immobility in themselves are not necessarily absolute contraindications to home dialysis (32, 33). Apart from serious cardiovascular problems, patient compliance with the treatment regimen is perhaps the most important consideration in the decision to recommend home dialysis.

Another essential element for successful home hemodialysis is blood access that is easy for the patient to use. The arteriovenous fistula, introduced in 1965 by Cimino and colleagues (34), provides a longer-lasting blood access site than the external Teflon shunt but requires use of a blood pump for dialysis. The fistula—or, when the patient's veins preclude fistula construction, a Gore-Tex or other synthetic arteriovenous graft—allows the use of higher blood flows and shorter dialysis time. Currently, home hemodialysis usually takes 3 to 5 hours, three times weekly. The use of disposable dialyzers without reuse also reduces time spent in preparing and ending dialysis. Thus, for many years it has not been necessary or practicable to do home hemodialysis overnight while sleeping. As discussed elsewhere in this chapter, this may be changing.

As far as age is concerned, home hemodialysis can be used for patients of all ages, with the possible exception of infants and very young children, for whom CAPD has proved particularly helpful while waiting for early renal transplantation. Early transplantation also is usually preferred for older children and adolescents, but both home hemodialysis and CAPD can work very well for them. With home hemodialysis in adolescents, it is often better for the patient to be assisted by someone other than a family member in order to break dependency ties.

At the other extreme of age, there is a widespread belief among nephrologists that elderly patients are not good candidates for home hemodialysis. This has not been our experience or that of others (35). In Seattle, half of the home hemodialysis population are aged 60 or more, and there have been many successful patients in their 70s or 80s. Apart from the greater likelihood of medical complications, the most common problem for elderly patients is lack of a suitable family helper. This limitation can be overcome by providing a paid dialysis helper (36).

Another factor to be considered is whether the patient is married and, if not, whether he or she has a relative or other individual who is prepared to assist with home hemodialysis. We discourage single patients from dialyzing at home alone, although this has been done successfully (37). Nevertheless, there is some increased risk under these circumstances, and a paid dialysis helper should be considered.

Suitable accommodation with adequate electricity and water supplies is also essential. This should be assessed early on by the training staff so the patient can be given advice on making the best use of space available for dialysis and for supply storage, and on any necessary electrical or plumbing changes (38, 39).

Ability to learn safe home hemodialysis does not seem to be correlated with intelligence per se, but rather with the patient's motivation. Some years ago we measured the IQ of 100 consecutive patients successfully trained for home hemodialysis and found the average to be 103, ranging from 78 to 147. Obviously, an illiterate patient or one who does not understand English will have more difficulties. However, with illustrations, videotapes, and suitable translation, we have found it possible to train a number of such patients.

While motivation and compliance are important, another important psychological aspect of home dialysis is the degree of anxiety manifested by the patient or the family. Some patients find CAPD preferable because of its simplicity, but for all forms of home dialysis anxiety can usually be relieved by an appropriate approach to patient and family. Whenever possible, they should be introduced to home dialysis before the need to start treatment, and they should also be given an opportunity to meet a successful home hemodialysis patient. It is important not to overlook the stresses home hemodialysis has on family members, whether or not they assist with dialysis (40).

In Seattle, we have developed a separate orientation unit for treatment of new patients. Patients are dialyzed in single rooms and are provided with detailed teaching and information on available social and nutrition services, exercise programs, and medical issues. After learning about their options, patients can the make an informed decision about which modality of treatment to undertake: transplantation, home hemodialysis, some form of home peritoneal dialysis, or outpatient dialysis in the facility (41).

Training

Home hemodialysis training is best begun as soon as possible after the patient starts on dialysis, so independence can be encouraged more easily. Once patients are stable and have suitable blood access, they should be taught to insert their own fistula needles. This is often the biggest psychological hurdle for the patient to overcome. Training should commence as soon as the patient is reasonably competent at inserting his or her access needle.

Whenever possible, training should be done in a separate area, preferably a single room, away from the main dialysis area. Training staff should be chosen for teaching ability as well as knowledge of dialysis, and must be able to take a hands-off approach, allowing patients to learn and make mistakes during training. Training materials should provide information about kidney disease, blood access, diet, medications, the various treatment modalities, the dialysis procedure, and the availability of support services. Written materials, slides, posters, and videotape programs can be specially developed to assist with training (19). Once fistula puncture is learned, home hemodialysis training can be completed by almost all patients in 3 to 6 weeks of thrice-weekly dialysis. Currently at the Northwest Kidney Center, the average number of training hemodialyses is less than nine.

Home hemodialysis may itself contribute to rehabilitation for some patients, as they learn new skills and develop self-confidence in their ability to control their own treatment and eventually their life in general. Every effort should be made during training to show that dialysis is relatively simple and safe if done properly, rather than a dangerous medical procedure. From the earliest dialyses, patients should learn that in the event of a serious problem such as a major blood leak, dialysis can always be stopped by clamping both arterial and venous blood lines, with no greater danger than loss of the blood in the dialyzer.

Patients must be trained to take as much responsibility as possible for their own care to avoid becoming overdependent on a spouse, family member, or paid helper. However, there have been major societal changes since the early days of home hemodialysis in the 1960s. In particular, in many families both partners work outside the home and they and other relatives have less time or inclination to assist with dialysis. Thus, the availability of a paid dialysis helper may be very important and also helps reduce the impact of home dialysis on the family. Use of paid home dialysis helpers, pioneered by the Northwest Kidney Center in the early 1970s, is a cost-effective way to provide home hemodialysis, but always carries the danger of making the patient too dependent. Consequently, successful home dialysis requires careful assessment of patient and family, careful selection of a compatible paid helper if one is required, and ongoing follow-up and support by a social worker. As discussed below, new technological developments may encourage many patients to dialyze themselves in the future, thereby increasing their independence.

During training, patient and family member or paid helper must have their progress assessed at regular intervals to ensure they have acquired the necessary skills and knowledge. They do not need to learn the intricacies of the dialysis procedure or the equipment. Rather, they must learn how to do dialysis safely; what emergency procedures to use when medical or technical problems occur during dialysis; and how, when, and where to call for assistance and advice. This assistance must always be available by telephone at all times.

Specific Requirements

Successful home hemodialysis requires blood access that is easy to use. Most patients can learn to insert their own needles into a well-developed arteriovenous fistula or graft, and, whenever possible, this should be the patient's responsibility. Dialyzer, duration of dialysis, and ultrafiltration rate should be chosen to ensure adequate dialysis while minimizing the likelihood of symptoms occurring during treatment. Hypotensive drugs should always be used with caution in home dialysis patients. Equipment should be chosen for reliability, adequacy of monitoring, ease of use, and ready availability of maintenance and repair services. The patient must have accommodation with suitable sources of water and electricity, and the associated water treatment must be based on analysis of the individual patient's home water supply.

Ongoing Support Services

Home hemodialysis patients require follow-up by a nephrologist, usually in the office, on a monthly basis unless there are problems. They must have a monthly blood sample obtained for analysis, the reports being sent to the nephrologist, the training program, and the patient. The patient must also maintain records of each dialysis, and copies of a monthly log sheet must be sent to the training program and the nephrologist.

Arrangements must be made to deliver dialysis supplies to the patient's home and for equipment maintenance and repair. This can be done through the supplier or manufacturer, or a large dialysis program can provide these services directly.

Besides access to the patient's nephrologist for consultation, a training nurse must be available by telephone at all times to answer questions and provide directions for handling problems. Nutrition advice and social work support, including advice and referral for re-

habilitation services and exercise programs, are also important and should be readily accessible. In addition, the training unit must have a system to ensure patients are updated on changes in technique or supplies as these occur.

Another essential requirement is availability of backup dialysis in a facility when medical or equipment problems prevent dialysis at home. This is also useful to allow occasional relief for the spouse and to give an opportunity for the spouse or paid helper to take a vacation away from the patient. Home dialysis patients themselves are also able to travel and to go on vacation. They may visit elsewhere in the United States after arrangements have been made for outpatient dialysis at a local center. Alternatively, suitably trained patients can take dialysis equipment with them in the form of either the Redy Sorbent–based cartridge system (42) or a simple portable system such as the suitcase kidney (43).

Patient Survival

Individual dialysis programs have reported a mortality rate for home hemodialysis patients that is substantially less than that of patients on center hemodialysis or CAPD (44–47). This has generally been attributed to differences in patient selection, as home hemodialysis patients in general differ in terms of age, race, sex, cause of renal failure, and comorbid conditions. This issue has been readdressed using data from the U.S. Renal Data System Special Study of Case Mix Severity (48). Data were from a nationwide random sample of 4892 ESRD patients who started treatment in 1986 and 1987. An intent-to-treat analysis was used to compare mortality in home hemodialysis patients with that of patients on outpatient hemodialysis. Stratification was based on race, sex, and diabetes as cause of renal failure, using the Cox proportional hazards model, and with adjustment for comorbid conditions present prior to the onset of ESRD. The sample included 3102 patients on center hemodialysis and 70 selected for home hemodialysis.

In general, the home hemodialysis patients were younger; were more likely to be white, male, and nondiabetic; and had fewer comorbid conditions. Mortality risk was adversely affected, particularly by history of stroke, obstructive pulmonary disease, congestive heart failure, peripheral vascular disease, myocardial infarction, smoking, and insulin therapy. A reduction in risk was associated with higher serum albumin levels and with obesity. When adjusted for age, sex, race, and diabetes, the relative risk (RR) of death was 44% lower in home hemodialysis patients when compared with center hemodialysis patients (RR = 0.56; p = 0.02). When additionally adjusted for comorbid conditions, the relative risk increased marginally (RR = 0.58; p = 0.03). Thus, in this sample of patients, adjustment for age, sex, race, diabetes, and comorbid conditions explains only a small part of the strikingly lower risk of death associated with home hemodialysis.

Quality of Life

Two major studies have looked at quality of life of dialysis and transplant patients. The first study examined quality of life and rehabilitation in 859 patients randomly selected from 11 dialysis and transplant centers across the United States (49); the second studied a similar number of patients from dialysis facilities in one geographic area in the Northeast (50). In both studies, quality of life and rehabilitation were best in patients with a successful kidney transplant. Among dialysis patients, even when statistical adjustment was made for medical and other demographic differences between the various patient populations, home hemodialysis patients had a better quality of life and were more often rehabilitated than patients treated by outpatient hemodialysis. Patients on CAPD were intermediate between the two hemodialysis modalities. These studies confirm one of the major advantages of home hemodialysis, and to a lesser extent of CAPD.

Medicare ESRD Program

At the time the Medicare ESRD program began in 1973, home hemodialysis was being used for almost 40% of the 11,000 dialysis patients in the United States. However, the proportion of patients treated with home hemodialysis began to decline once Medicare reimbursement became available. This resulted from several factors.

First, with almost universal coverage by Medicare, the patient population changed rapidly from that of the 1960s (51) and has continued to change. Between 1977 and 1992, the median age of new patients increased from 54 to 63 years, and there was an increase in patients with ESRD due to diabetes from 7.7% to more than 35% of patients starting dialysis (52, 53). The number of black and Native American patients treated also increased rapidly because of the very high incidence of hypertensive renal disease and diabetes in these populations (53). In 1992, blacks, who comprised 12.4% of the U.S. population, accounted for 28.9% of all new ESRD patients (53).

These changes in the patient population have meant that there are now many more dialysis patients who are unsuited for home dialysis on either medical or social grounds. Also, with readily available financial coverage, patients have become much freer to choose their modality of treatment for themselves, and where and by whom this will be performed.

In addition, in 1973 both physician and facility reimbursement from Medicare for outpatient dialysis was much higher than for home dialysis. As a result, there was a rapid increase in the number of dialysis facilities across the country, providing much better access to care, but there was also a financial disincentive to the use of home dialysis. The financial situation also encouraged development of for-profit dialysis facilities, and these now treat more than 55% of dialysis patients in the United States. In the past, for-profit units have been reluctant to encourage selection of home dialysis by their patients (54), and this may be continuing.

Physician bias is also an important factor (55, 56). A survey of selected U.S. nephrologists under the age of 50 showed most would prefer home hemodialysis to kidney transplantation or CAPD for themselves if they developed ESRD (57). There was also a marked disparity between what physicians reported they would prefer as treatment for their patients and their actual practice. In addition, many younger nephrologists do not have personal experience with home hemodialysis, and so are skeptical of its safety and its reported effectiveness and benefits.

Another problem is that the relative complexity of hemodialysis requires a structured 3-to 8-week training program that does not exist in most dialysis facilities. This is in contrast to the 1 to 2 weeks needed for CAPD training. Similarly, in terms of support, home hemodialysis needs a more extensive system to provide supplies and also prompt maintenance and servicing of equipment.

As a consequence of these and other factors, the proportion of ESRD patients treated by home hemodialysis in the United States declined throughout the 1970s, and by 1980 was only 4.6% (52). However, with the introduction of CAPD, home dialysis overall has increased in recent years. Between 1980 and 1992, the percentage of dialysis patients on some form of home dialysis increased from 6.2 to 16.8%. In this same time period, the number of patients on CAPD and other peritoneal therapies increased from 1.6 to 15.5%, while patients on home hemodialysis declined from 4.6 to 1.3% (52, 53). Thus, until recently, the increased use of home dialysis has been solely due to the increase in the use of peritoneal dialysis.

By virtue of being a form of home dialysis, CAPD has many of the same advantages for the patient as home hemodialysis, and is also less expensive to perform than outpatient hemodialysis. Unfortunately, fewer than 40% of patients who start CAPD or CCPD are still on this treatment after 2 years (53), because dialysis becomes inadequate in many patients when residual renal function is lost (58) and because of problems with peritonitis (59). Unfortunately, most patients who experience CAPD

failure are not subsequently trained for home hemodialysis, and so these patients lose the advantages associated with home treatment.

Despite these issues, in Washington State 25.1% of all dialysis patients are still treated by home dialysis, and 45.4% of these are on home hemodialysis (60). In the Northwest Kidney Center's program, 15.4% of more than 800 dialysis patients are on home hemodialysis and 11.3% on peritoneal dialysis. Thus, home hemodialysis can still be very successful where a dialysis program is committed to this as an option for patients.

One major change in the Seattle program since the early years is that in many cases home hemodialysis is now being done with a paid dialysis helper rather than a family member or close friend. This has proved extremely useful (36). Because of the success of this approach in Seattle, some years ago the Health Care Financing Administration (HCFA) funded three multicenter studies of home hemodialysis using "paid aides." These studies showed that the number of patients choosing home dialysis could be increased significantly by making funding available to pay a dialysis aide or a family member, and this was particularly effective in hemodialysis programs associated with nonprofit dialysis facilities (61).

Although the studies showed significant variation in cost among individual programs, the cost of an aide averaged 17% of total home hemodialysis costs. The average cost per home hemodialysis with an aide was $119 per treatment; this was 77% of the cost of outpatient hemodialysis at the same facility and 82% of the cost at 23 "control" facilities. Thus, it was possible to fund payment of an aide or family member to help with home hemodialysis without the total cost per dialysis exceeding that of outpatient hemodialysis. Despite this evidence, Congress introduced "composite rate" reimbursement in 1983, which pays the same for each dialysis, whether done in a center or in the home, and specifically excludes payment for a home dialysis aide as a Medicare-allowable charge. As a result, a home dialysis program using paid aides under the composite rate has to pay for these from its "profits."

Several years ago, Congress asked the HCFA to undertake another demonstration of the use of staff-assisted home hemodialysis, this time for patients who had severe medical problems and a life expectancy of no more than 6 months. The study was undertaken despite concerns expressed by those experienced with home hemodialysis that such patients are not the population that can benefit and are generally better treated in a facility. So few patients met the criteria for inclusion that the study has been abandoned.

In contrast to some other home treatments such as parenteral nutrition and home respiratory therapy (62), home hemodialysis has not generally been regarded as a major revenue generator. However, several years ago a for-profit supplier used an alternative method of Medicare reimbursement for home hemodialysis and used paid aides to provide treatment to more 1700 patients. This was possible because the company was charging some $250 per dialysis, twice the usual reimbursement for dialysis, and so was able to cover the costs of the aide while maintaining a large profit margin. The HCFA regarded this payment as grossly excessive, and so Congress passed legislation in 1989 capping reimbursement for home dialysis at the more usual rate. Following this, the supplier involved closed down this operation. Apart from this, home hemodialysis has generally not been attractive to for-profit companies.

The last year has seen something of a revival of interest in home hemodialysis in the United States, in part because of several recent reports. At the 1994 American Society of Nephrology meeting, the late Robert Uldall reported on six patients treated by nightly home hemodialysis (63). Patients dialyzed for 8 hours during sleep, at least six nights a week, using a Silastic jugular vein catheter for blood access and modified Fresenius dialysis equipment. Special precautions were taken to prevent accidental blood line separation. Monitoring of dialysis functions was carried out remotely via modem. Dialyzer and blood lines were reused in situ to minimize expense and patient effort. Dialysate flow was 100 mL/min, blood flow was 300 mL/min, and

with a 0.4 m² polysulfone dialyzer there was greater than 90% equilibration of urea between plasma and dialysate effluent.

With this regimen, patients' serum urea and creatinine levels were close to normal throughout the week, and cumulative weekly urea kinetic modeling (KT/V) was 6.2 compared with 4.5 with very adequate conventional hemodialysis. Patients were able to stop phosphate binders, increase dietary phosphate intake, and stop taking ACE inhibitors and calcium channel blockers, treating their hypertension with β blockers only, or in some cases without drugs. Patients slept soundly and had greatly increased energy and stamina, and all their days were free for work and other activities.

At a session on daily home hemodialysis at the 1995 Annual Conference on Peritoneal Dialysis and at the 1995 Annual Meeting of the American Society for Artificial Internal Organs (ASAIO), in addition to a further report by Uldall, Rod Kenley of AKSYS described work on development of equipment designed specifically for home hemodialysis (64). This highly automated equipment should allow many patients to do home hemodialysis without a helper, and may be available for testing within 1 to 2 years. If this device fulfills its potential, it will help make home hemodialysis readily available again.

Finally, the last several years have seen increasing concern with hepatitis C infection in dialysis and transplant patients. This is the most frequent cause of liver disease in ESRD patients and occurs in some 20 to 30% of dialysis patients (65). While the potential risk is low and the routes of transmission in dialysis units are uncertain, hepatitis C is potentially serious because it is a frequent cause of cirrhosis and liver failure. One way to reduce the risks of this and other infections is the use of home hemodialysis (66).

In light of these developments and the reports of the better survival, quality of life, and opportunity for rehabilitation with home hemodialysis, this seems a most appropriate time to reexamine the question of how to make home hemodialysis available on a wider scale through existing dialysis facilities and at a more economic cost. Because a successful home hemodialysis training and support program may be difficult to establish in smaller dialysis units, the best way to provide this would be to regionalize home hemodialysis programs in the same way that kidney transplantation and other tertiary services are regionalized. Under this approach, patients from a given region could be referred for home hemodialysis training to a central training program. After completion of training, they would return to the medical care of their nephrologist. Support services could be provided by the regional dialysis training center. Any backup dialyses required would be provided by the patient's original dialysis facility.

Summary

Home hemodialysis, a healthcare technology that has been available for more than 30 years, is still used by only a minority of ESRD patients in the United States. Nevertheless, experienced physicians and programs believe this provides major benefits to patients in terms of survival, quality of life, and opportunity for rehabilitation. CAPD and other forms of home peritoneal dialysis have some of the same advantages, although probably not to the same degree. New technologies under development will increase the attractiveness of home hemodialysis to both patients and facilities. While this treatment clearly works, as with many of the other technologies now used in the home, its future depends to a large extent on reimbursement, both the amount and the methodology for setting the rate. What is clear is that home hemodialysis, properly organized and supported, is a treatment with several advantages to patients that can be provided at a lower cost than the same treatment in a dialysis facility. With the pressures on health care costs now and in the future, there will be increasing need for technological treatments to be moved to the home. Now is the time to reexamine all home therapies to ensure that they are provided in the optimum way and in a cost-effective manner.

References

1. Kolff WJ. First clinical experience with the artificial kidney. Ann Intern Med 1965;62:608–619.
2. Quinton W, Dillard D, Scribner BH. Cannulation of blood vessels for prolonged hemodialysis. Trans Am Soc Artif Intern Organs 1960;6:104–113.
3. Haviland JW. Experiences in establishing a community artificial kidney center. Trans Am Clin Climatol Assoc 1965;77:125–129.
4. Scribner BH, Buri R, Caner JEZ, Hegstrom R, Burnell JM. The treatment of chronic uremia by means of intermittent hemodialysis: a preliminary report. Trans Am Soc Artif Intern Organs 1960;6:114–122.
5. Pendras JP, Cole JJ, Tu WH, Scribner BH. Improved technique of continuous flow hemodialysis. Trans Am Soc Artif Intern Organs 1961;7:27–36.
6. Murray JS, Tu WH, Albers JB, Burnell JM, Scribner BH. A community hemodialysis center for the treatment of chronic uremia. Trans Am Soc Artif Intern Organs 1962;8:315–319.
7. Alexander S. They decide who lives, who dies: medical miracle and a moral burden of a small committee. Life Magazine, November 9, 1962:102–125.
8. Darrah JB. The committee. Trans Am Soc Artif Intern Organs 1987;33:791–793.
9. Fox RC, Swazey JP. The Courage To Fail: A Social View of Organ Transplants and Dialysis, 2nd ed. Chicago: University of Chicago, 1974.
10. Grimsrud L, Cole JJ, Lehman GA, Babb AL, Scribner BH. A central system for the continuous preparation and distribution of hemodialysis fluid. Trans Am Soc Artif Intern Organs 1964;10:107–109.
11. Babb AL. Design and construction of a portable, single patient, dialysate proportioning machine at the University of Washington 1964–65. ASAIO J 1995;41:1–10.
12. Curtis FK, Cole JJ, Fellows BJ, Tyler LL, Scribner BH. Hemodialysis in the home. Trans Am Soc Artif Intern Organs 1965;11:7–10.
13. Nosé Y. Discussion. Trans Am Soc Artif Intern Organs 1965;11:15.
14. Merrill JP, Schupak E, Cameron E, Hampers CL. Hemodialysis in the home. JAMA 1964;190:468–470.
15. Baillod RA, Comty C, Ilahi M, Konotey-Ahulu FID, Sevitt L, Shaldon S. Overnight hemodialysis in the home. Proc Eur Dial Transplant Assoc 1965;2:99–103.
16. Grimsrud L, Cole JJ, Eschbach JW, Babb AL, Scribner BH. Safety aspects of hemodialysis. Trans Am Soc Artif Intern Organs 1967;13:1–4.
17. Eschbach JW Jr, Wilson WE Jr, Peoples RW, Wakefield AW, Babb AL, Scribner BH. Unattended overnight home hemodialysis. Trans Am Soc Artif Intern Organs 1966;12:346–356.
18. Blagg CR, Hickman RO, Eschbach JW, Scribner BH. Home hemodialysis: six years' experience. N Engl J Med 1970;283:1126–1131.
19. Stinson JW, Clark MF, Sawyer TK, Blagg CR. Home hemodialysis training in three weeks. Trans Am Soc Artif Intern Organs 1972;18:66–69.

20. Blagg CR, Cole JJ, Irvine G, Marr T, Pollard TL. How much should dialysis cost? Proceedings, Workshop on Dialysis and Transplantation, Transactions ASAIO, Washington, DC: Georgetown University Press, 1972: 54–60.

21. Seligman MAP. Depression and learned helplessness. In: Friedman RJ, Katz MN, eds. The Psychology of Depression. Contemporary Theory and Research. Washington, DC: VH Winston and Sons, 1974:83–125.

22. Oremland EK. Work dynamics in family care of hemophiliac children. Soc Sci Med 1988;26:467–475.

23. Howard L. Home nutritional support: the patient point of view. Nutr Clin Pract 1989;4:49–50.

24. Pierson DJ, George RB. Mechanical ventilation in the home: possibilities and prerequisites. Respir Care 1986;31:266–270.

25. Boen ST, Mulinari AS, Dillard DH, Scribner BH. Periodic peritoneal dialysis in the management of chronic uremia. Trans Am Soc Artif Organs 1962;8: 256–262.

26. Tenckhoff H, Shilipetar G, vanPaasschen WJ, Swanson E. A home peritoneal dialysate delivery system. Trans Am Soc Artif Intern Organs 1969;15:103–107.

27. Tenckhoff H, Schechter H. A bacteriologically safe peritoneal access device. Trans Am Soc Artif Intern Organs 1968;14:181–186.

28. Tenckhoff H, Meston B, Shilipetar G. A simplified automatic peritoneal dialysis system. Trans Am Soc Artif Intern Organs 1972;18:436–439.

29. Ahmad S, Gallagher N, Shen F. Intermittent peritoneal dialysis: status reassessed. Trans Am Soc Artif Intern Organs 1979;25:86–89.

30. Popovich RP, Moncrief JW, Dechard JB, Bomar JB, Pyle WK. The definition of a novel portable/wearable equilibrium peritoneal dialysis technique [Abstract]. Trans Am Soc Artif Intern Organs 1976;5:65.

31. Diaz-Buxo JA. Continuous cyclic peritoneal dialysis. In: Nolph KD, ed. Peritoneal Dialysis, 3rd ed. Dordrecht, Netherlands: Kluwer Academic Publishers, 1989: 169–173.

32. Roberts CM. Home dialysis in the haemophiliac paraplegic patient. Proc Eur Dial Transplant Nurses Assoc 1979;7:62–66.

33. Roberts CM, Davis B, Pavitt L, et al. Home dialysis training in a blind patient and a deaf patient. Proc Eur Dial Transplant Nurses Assoc 1973;1:41.

34. Brescia MJ, Cimino JE, Appel K, et al. Chronic hemodialysis using venipuncture and a surgically created arteriovenous fistula. N Engl J Med 1966;275: 1089–1092.

35. McDonald M, McPhee PD, Walker RJ: Successful self-care home dialysis in the elderly: a single center's experience. Perit Dial Int 1995;15:33–36.

36. Clark MF. Experience with paid dialysis helpers. J Am Assoc Nephrol Nurses and Technicians 1977;4(Suppl): 39–44.

37. Baillod RA, Moorhead JF. Review of ten years' home dialysis. Proc Eur Dial Transplant Assoc 1974;11:68–75.

38. Baillod RA. Home dialysis. In: Drukker W, Parsons FM, Maher JF, eds. Replacement of Renal Function by Dialysis, 2nd ed. Boston: Martinus Nijhoff, 1983: 493–513.

39. Sawyer TK, Blagg CR. Home preparation and installation for home dialysis. In: Nissenson AR, Fine RN, eds. Dialysis Therapy, 2nd ed. Philadelphia: Hanley & Belfus, 1993:52–54.

40. Brunier GM, McKeever PT. The impact of home dialysis on the family: literature review. ANNA J 1993;20: 653–659.

41. Eschbach JW, Seymour M, Potts A, Clark M, Blagg CR. A hemodialysis orientation unit. Nephron 1983;33: 106–110.

42. Shapiro WB: REDY sorbent hemodialysis system. In: Nissenson AR, Fine RN, eds. Dialysis Therapy, 2nd ed. Philadelphia: Hanley & Belfus, 1993:146–149.

43. Friedman EA, Blagg CR, Sullivan JF, Briefel GR, Galonsky RS, Delano BG, Hutchisson JT. Collaborative field trial of suitcase travel dialyzer (STD) [Abstract]. Trans Am Soc Artif Intern Organs 1977;6:24.

44. Vollmer WM, Wahl P, Blagg CR. Survival with dialysis and transplantation in patients with end-stage renal disease. N Engl J Med 1983;308:1553–1558.

45. Burton PR, Walls J. Selection-adjusted comparison of life-expectancy of patients on continuous ambulatory peritoneal dialysis, hemodialysis, and renal transplantation. Lancet 1987;1:1115–1119.

46. Mailloux LU, Belluci AG, Napolitano B, Mossey T, et al. Survival estimates for 683 patients starting dialysis from 1970 through 1989: identification of risk factors for survival. Clin Nephrol 1994;42:127–135.

47. Grant AC, Rodger RS, Howie CA, Junor BJ, Briggs JD, MacDougall AI. Dialysis at home in the West of Scotland: a comparison of hemodialysis and continuous ambulatory peritoneal dialysis in age- and sex-matched controls. Perit Dial Int 1992:365–368.

48. Woods, JD, Stannard D, Blagg CR, Held PJ, Port FK. Comparison of mortality with home hemodialysis and center hemodialysis: a national study (in press).

49. Evans RW, Manninen DL, Garrison LP, Hart G, Blagg CR, Gutman RA, Hull AR, Lowrie EG. The quality of life of patients with end-stage renal disease. N Engl J Med 1985;312:553–559.

50. Bremer BA, McCauley CR, Rona RM, Johnson JP. Quality of life in end-stage renal disease: a reexamination. Am J Kidney Dis 1989;13:200–209.

51. Evans RW, Blagg CR, Bryan FA. Implications for health care policy: a social and demographic profile of hemodialysis patients in the United States. JAMA 1981; 245:487–491.

52. U.S. Renal Data System, 1989 Annual Data Report. Bethesda, MD: National Institutes of Health, National Institute of Diabetes and Digestive and Kidney Diseases, August 1989.

53. U.S. Renal Data System, USRDS 1995 Annual Data Report. Bethesda, MD: National Institutes of Health, National Institute of Diabetes and Digestive and Kidney Diseases, April 1995.

54. Rettig RA. Implementing the End-stage Renal Disease Program of Medicare. Santa Monica, CA: Rand, 1980.

55. Friedman EA. Physician bias in uremia therapy. Kidney Int 1985;28(Suppl 17):S38–S40.

56. Mattern WD, McGaghie WC, Rigby RJ, Nissenson AR, Dunham CB, Khayrallah MA. Selection of ESRD treatment: an international study. Am J Kidney Dis 1989;13:457–464.

57. Dunham C, Mattern WD, McGaghie WC. Preferences of nephrologists among end-stage renal disease treatment options. Am J Nephrol 1985;5:470–475.

58. Harty J, Gokal R. Does CAPD provide adequate dialysis? Nephrol Dial Transplant 1995;10:1115–1117.

59. Maiorca R, Cancarini GC, Brunori G, Camerini C, Manili L. Morbidity and mortality of CAPD and hemodialysis. Kidney Int 1993;43(Suppl 40):S4–S15.

60. Annual Report, 1994 Northwest Renal Network. Seattle, WA: Northwest Renal Network, 1995.

61. Orkand Corporation. Evaluation of the home dialysis aide demonstration. Contract HCFA 500–79-0054. Silver Spring, MD: The Orkand Corporation, 1982.

62. Lutz S. Home care's growth hinges on winning over the physicians. Modern Health Care 1989;19:20–30.
63. Uldall R, Francouer R, Ouwendyk M, Wallace L, Langos V, Ecclestone A, Vas S. Simplified nocturnal home hemodialysis (SNHHD). A new approach to renal replacement therapy [Abstract]. J Am Soc Nephrol 1994;5:428.
64. Kenley R. Tearing down the barriers to hyper-frequent home hemodialysis and achieving the highest value dialytic therapy through holistic product design. Adv Ren Replace Ther (in press).
65. Davis CL, Gretch DR, Carithers RL. Hepatitis C virus in renal disease. Curr Opin Nephrol Hypertens 1994;3:164–173.
66. Pascual J, Tereul JL, Liano F, Ortuno J. Home hemodialysis protects against hepatitis C virus transmission [Letter]. Nephron 1993;64:314.

INDEX